81195X

HEALTH SCIENCE

THIRD EDITION

HEALTH SCIENCE

THIRD EDITION

Kenneth L. Jones
Louis W. Shainberg
Curtis O. Byer

MT. SAN ANTONIO COLLEGE

HARPER & ROW, PUBLISHERS
New York   Evanston   San Francisco   London

Grateful acknowledgment is made to the following individuals and organizations for their kind permission to use the photographs that appear at the opening of each chapter.

Chapter 1: Bruce Roberts, Rapho Guillumette; Chapter 2: Joel Gordon; Chapter 3: New York Public Library Picture Collection; Chapter 4: Bob Combs; Chapter 5: Henry Monroe, DPI; Chapter 6: Bob Combs; Chapter 7: Paolo Koch, Rapho Guillumette; Chapter 8: Lynn McLaren, Rapho Guillumette; Chapter 9: Carnegie Mellon University; Chapter 10: Bob Combs; Chapter 11: Bob Combs; Chapter 12: Alice Kandell, Rapho Guillumette; Chapter 13: Sigrid Owen, DPI; Chapter 14: New York Public Library Picture Collection; Chapter 15: Joel Gordon; Chapter 16: Beckwith Studios; Chapter 17: American Cancer Society; Chapter 18: Beckwith Studios; Chapter 19: Lew Merrim, Monkmeyer; Chapter 20: Joel Gordon; Chapter 21: Wide World; Chapter 22: Ray Ellis, Rapho Guillumette.

Sponsoring Editor: Alvin A. Abbott
Project Editor: Robert Ginsberg
Designer: Rita Naughton
Production Supervisor: Stefania J. Taflinska

HEALTH SCIENCE, Third Edition

Library of Congress Cataloging in Publication Data
Jones, Kenneth Lamar, 1931–
  Health science.

  Bibliography: p.
  1. Hygiene. I. Shainberg, Louis W., joint author.
II. Byer, Curtis O., joint author. III. Title.
[DNLM: 1. Medicine–Popular works. WB120 J77h 1974]
RA776.J692 1974   613   73-8372
ISBN 0–06–043427–9

Contents

Preface

The trend in health education, as in all branches of science, is toward more relevant knowledge. We feel that the first edition of *Health Science* was one of the texts that helped generate a scientific, yet practical, approach to health education. It is an academic subject, imparting knowledge that will be useful to an individual preparing to be an informed and conscientious adult.

Health is an applied science that draws upon many fields, disciplines, and areas. It is an ever-changing body of knowledge, which must be kept up to date or ahead of the needs of the population. The material must be presented in such a manner that one is able to understand it and explain the basic principles to his children whenever they need it.

The chief purpose of this text has not changed since the first edition, but much of the information has changed. The young person in a college health education course either is a new parent or may be one soon. He is interested in learning the scientific basis of health practices. *Health Science* is intended to be a scientific guide for the individual and his growing family. It is a textbook for the student and a reference book for the family.

Complete outlines of all chapters are given as Summaries, for use as study tools and quick reference. Important words have their pronunciations, derivations, and meanings given in the Glossaries. The Appendixes are useful informational tools and contain reference materials for both student and instructor.

This text is the product of a one-semester health-education course at Mt. San Antonio College. We constantly experiment, rework, and readapt the course, trying to produce as complete, informative, and interesting a program as is feasible.

We have updated every chapter in this third edition of *Health Science* and have made some major revisions, such as those in the chapters on emotional health, on drugs, and on marriage. We thank the many instructors and students whose suggestions have guided us.

We are grateful to the many people who helped make this book possible. We wish to express special gratitude and appreciation to Robert E. Carrel, M.D., Neurologist and Pediatrician, for his review and comments on Chapters 2 and 3; to Robert W. Earle, Ph.D., Senior Lecturer, Department of Medical Pharmacology and Therapeutics, University of California at Irvine, for his ideas on the continuum of drugs; to Karl Menninger, Director, Menninger Foundation, Topeka, Kansas, for permission to use his concepts throughout Chapter 2; to Paul A. Thornton, Ph.D., Chairman, Department of Clinical Nutrition, Albert B. Chandler Medical Center, University of Kentucky, for his reviews and comments on Chapters 7 and 8; to Bob W., member of Alcoholics Anonymous, for his perceptive contributions to the sections on the abuse of alcohol; to Donovan W. Byer, M.D., Obstetrician and Gynecologist, for his suggestions and comments on Chapter 11; to Nelson Miller, Certified Marriage Counsellor, American Institute of Family Relations, for his review and counsel on Chapter 12; to Robert M. Klein, D.D.S., for his suggestions on Chapter 7; to Garret Hardin, Ph.D., Professor of Biological Sciences, University of California at Santa Barbara, for providing us with his personal ideas on the critical issue of abortion and ethics in contemporary society; to Gary Romig, the artist who prepared the original drafts of the line illustrations for this book; to Morey R. Fields, Ph.D., for his fine comments and excellent review of the entire manuscript; and to George A. Middendorf, Executive Editor, College Department, Harper & Row, Publishers, for his guidance, friendship, and constant encouragement.

KENNETH L. JONES
LOUIS W. SHAINBERG
CURTIS O. BYER

HEALTH SCIENCE

THIRD EDITION

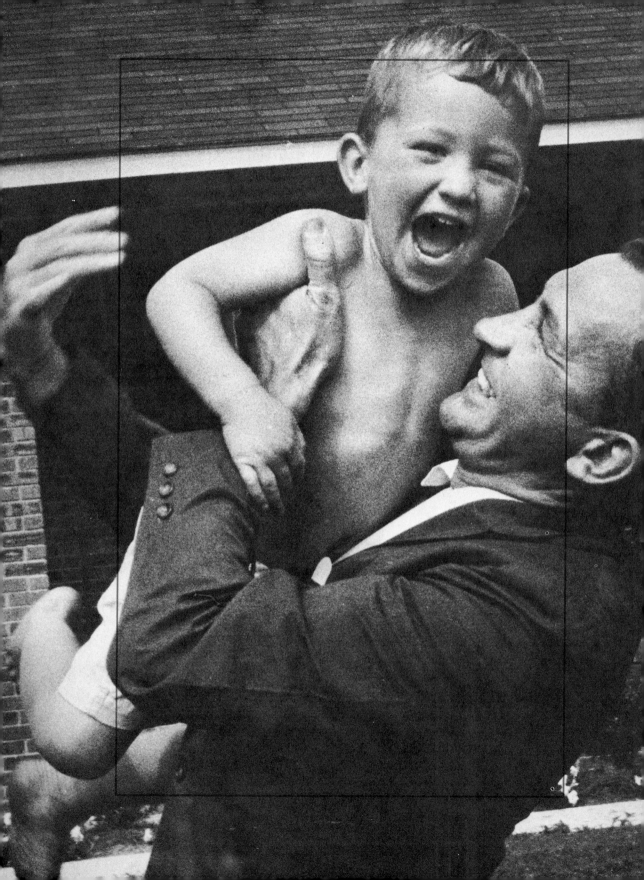

A lifetime of health

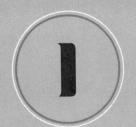

We are now witnessing the most rapid scientific and technological development in the history of Man—a development that could lead to a greater fulfillment of human aspirations than Man has ever known. To achieve it, however, Man must apply his newly gained skills with care, he must avoid whenever possible the creation of new problems, and he must find satisfactory solutions of those problems that have already appeared.

At no time in history has Man's future held such uncertainty as it does today. Modern technical and medical advancements have proven to be a mixed blessing. Technology and education have, on the one hand, raised standards of living and freed millions from degrading menial jobs; on the other they have created social upheaval, the threat of nuclear annihilation, and a physical environment so poisoned that continued survival is being seriously questioned by prominent authorities. Medical science has been able to overcome many of the traditional causes of illness and early death, but that has resulted in a world population growth rate that threatens with massive famine and populations so dense that living can become a burden instead of a pleasure. All these developments relate directly to our physical and emotional health and so are an important part of our study of health science.

1

MEANINGS OF HEALTH

Health has many meanings and definitions. To the man on the street it usually means freedom from disease. To him who has lost health it means the loss of his most priceless possession: he may have every material possession, but without health he has nothing. To the psychologist health is principally the normal functioning of the mind; to the physician it is principally the normal functioning of the body. To the quack it is a fee, payable in advance.

The problems faced by Man today require that health be defined in very broad terms. Health cannot be defined as merely the absence of disease or as a purely personal condition. The World Health Organization's constitution defines health as "a state of complete physical, mental, and social well-being and not merely the absence of disease or infirmity." The health of the individual and of society are mutually dependent. Individual health cannot reach its fullest development within an ailing society, nor can a society composed of physically or emotionally ill individuals be truly healthy. The health of the individual contributes to the health of society; the health of society helps build the health of the individual.

Another definition of health is "the ability to function effectively within man's environment." Health is seen as the consequence and the evidence of a successful adaptation to the conditions of physical and emotional existence and disease as a failure in adaptation. Since the environment is constantly changing, this definition of health implies an ongoing, continuous process of adaptation. When one's ability to adapt to a changing environment fails, then his health is affected. Such failure could result from an individual loss of adaptive ability (physical or emotional) or from an environment that changes beyond the inherent limits of a person's adaptive potential.

FACTORS INFLUENCING HEALTH

Mental outlook on life

Mental health is recognized today as an essential and inseparable part of one's total health. Poor mental health is at least as handicapping in life as is poor physical health. Not only do emotional problems severely limit the pleasure one derives from living, but also they frequently result in physical illness. The abuse of alcohol or other drugs is today properly regarded as an emotional health problem.

Intelligent use of foods

Today's methods of growing, processing, and shipping foods make possible good nutrition for people of even modest income; yet there are those in all income brackets who show signs of poor nutrition. Commonly observed today is the symptom of overnutrition, excessive weight. Nutritional deficiencies also are common, especially among families of low income or poor education and among those who rely upon nutritional fads.

Living with others

Individual, national, and world welfare depend strongly upon people's understanding each other socially, because social stresses can becloud the lives of millions. A high level of emotional health is essential for pleasant relationships with neighbors, productive relationships with coworkers, and peaceful relationships among members of different ethnic and social groups. As the world population increases, international tensions increase. The quest for world peace requires finding solutions to many problems that relate to physical and emotional health.

Sexual adjustment

Adequate sexual adjustment is important for individual happiness and fulfillment. Each of us needs to achieve a sense of sexual adequacy and to define the most appropriate context for the satisfaction of our sexual needs. For many people, this context is still marriage in its traditional form. But success in marriage depends on individual readiness and the careful selection of marriage partners. The prevention of unwanted births and the limitation of total family size is important for the happiness and welfare of both parents and children.

Disease prevention

Among the most traditional of factors promoting health is the prevention of disease. Methods for the prevention of most communicable diseases are now available. Some of them are public health concerns, such as the control of mosquitoes and the assurance of safe foods and drinking water, but much disease prevention remains the responsibility of the individual as, for example, the procuring of immunizations and the prevention of venereal diseases. The prevention of the chronic degenerative diseases, now still largely in the research stages, will, when understood, probably rest mainly upon the efforts of the individual.

Choosing best health services

The individual is responsible for selecting the best health services from those available in the community. Individuals must choose their medical practitioner carefully, checking his training, skill, and ethical standards. Quacks still flourish in many cities. Even among legitimate practitioners a wide range in skills exists. The choice of hospitals often determines the quality of care received. Many of the nation's hospitals do not meet the minimal standards for accreditation. The choice of a poor practitioner often restricts the patient to a poor hospital, which compounds the situation. The quality of care received often depends upon the ability to pay, which, for the average family, depends upon the type of health insurance it carries: health insurance policies vary greatly in coverage and value received, and many people unsuspectingly select very poor health insurance plans.

Protecting the environment

Man's continued survival on earth depends upon his maintaining an environment favorable to his welfare. Fortunately, in recent years there has been an increasing awareness of the relationship between Man and his environment. One of the most critical problems is the pollution of that environment. Man can afford no further pollution of his air, soil, and water; it is not only esthetically unpleasant but also a definite health hazard.

Greater attention must also be given the significant problem of world population dynamics. There must be worldwide recognition of the fact that we live on a finite earth with finite resources and that even with the most efficient application of those resources there is a limit to the number of people the earth can support.

Today's college student has at hand the possibility of a lifetime of health and happiness for himself and his family. The remaining chapters of this book will acquaint the reader with the means of attaining such a life.

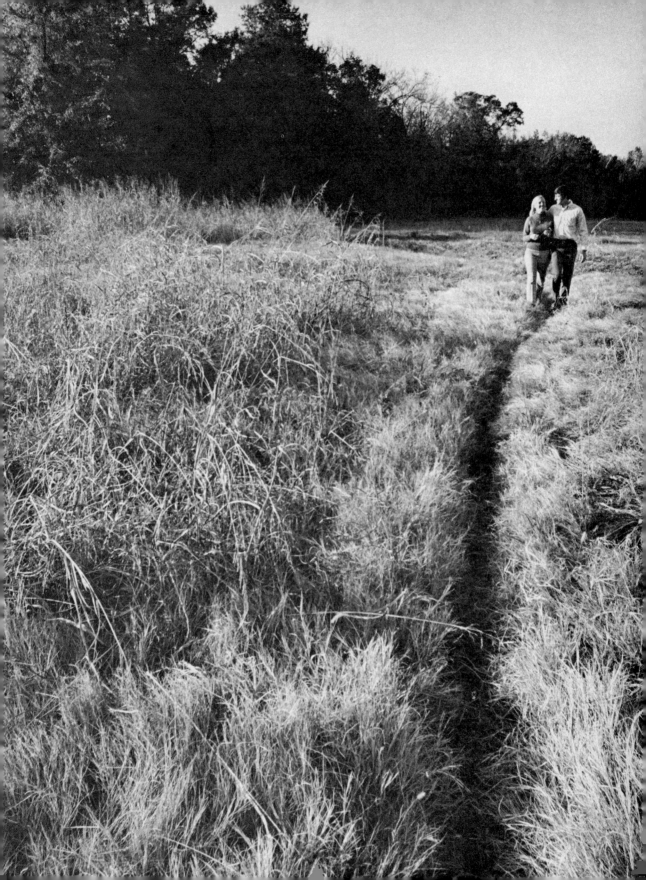

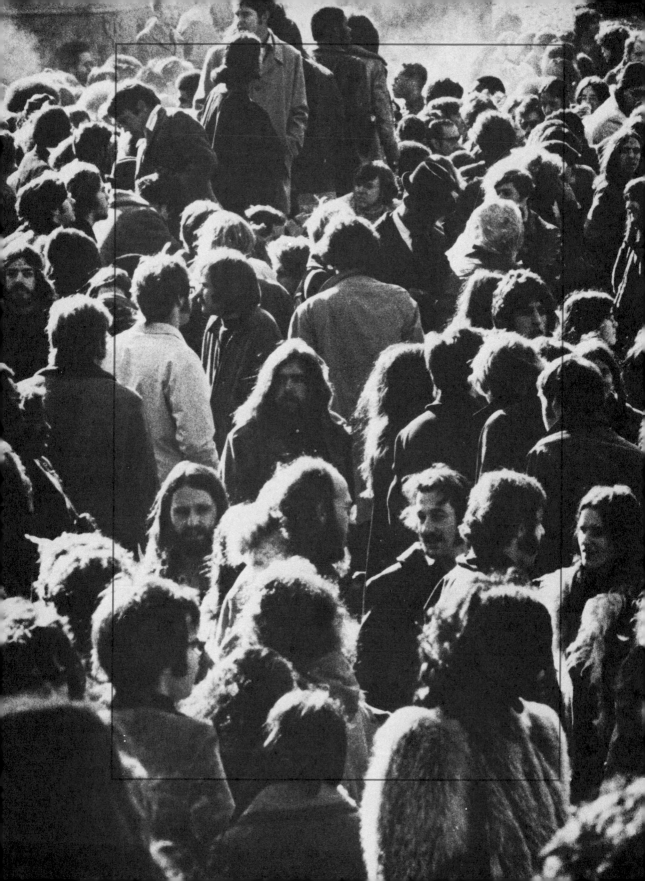

Emotional health

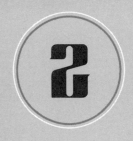

Emotional health differs from other areas of health in that often we are dealing with opinions and not facts. Some day, we hope, the formula for maintaining emotional health will be as definitely established as the formula for maintaining a balanced diet. In the meantime we must to some extent content ourselves with educated guesses. Because of this lack of finality, we must also be prepared to receive different answers from equally competent authorities for a given emotional problem.

THE STRUCTURE OF PERSONALITY

Personality may be defined as the total reaction of a person to his environment. Many things influence personality. A child is conceived with a definite genetic makeup, and the personality he will eventually develop depends upon this original endowment and all of the environmental factors to which he is exposed. His personality will also include the ways in which he interprets his environment and how he learns to deal with the conflicts between his basic inner needs and the obstacles he meets that frustrate his attempts to fulfill those needs.

Thus we find four forces that influence the personality: genetic makeup, environment, interpretation of the environment, and learned ways of dealing with conflicts. The first two forces are mainly beyond our power to control:

7

we have no control over our genetic makeup and only a limited one over our environment. Nevertheless, it is through our *interpretation* of *environment* and our learning to deal with frustration that our personalities can be developed and improved. Personality should be viewed as *dynamic*, changing throughout life in response to continuing environmental changes.

Freudian concept of personality

The pioneer psychoanalyst Sigmund Freud (1856–1939) conceived of two basic *levels* of thinking and feeling, the conscious and the unconscious. According to his scheme, the conscious mind is the surface, or "skin," which is observable. It covers the great bulk of the mind, the unconscious, which is not directly observable.

Freud divided the personality into the *id*, the *ego*, and the *superego*, which roughly describe *processes* of the conscious and unconscious levels of thinking and feeling.

The id processes   At the time of birth the child brings with him a bundle of inborn tendencies necessary for survival. These represent the unconscious strivings of the human organism to live and enjoy life, his id. Since they work for the individual's biological survival, they are aggressive and selfish. They operate for his pleasure and gratification. The id does not distinguish between good and evil or between what is realistic and what is not. It operates under the pleasure principle ("whatever brings pleasure is good"), so the child must be educated to control its processes. Maturing of the individual and pressure from society both tame the aggressive id.

The ego processes   The ego processes largely spring from the conscious self. It is through the ego that we are aware of reality. The ego processes act as regulators, controlling and balancing the needs of the id with the demands of society and of the superego, or "conscience." The ego maintains contact with the outside world by means of the individual's perceptual and motor apparatuses; the conscious self responds on the basis of what it hears, sees, feels, tastes, and smells. Since the individual at birth lacks training with respect to such responses, the processes of the ego develop gradually and gain strength as the individual grows older and responds to the pressures of society.

Instinctive, aggressive impulses that arise in the id must be accepted or rejected for expression by the ego. The ego processes may be thought of as the rational thinking that results from experiences of trial and error. Therefore there is constant communication between the id and the ego. If an impulse is unwelcome in terms of the ego's experience with reality, the ego places barriers against the impulse's entering consciousness, striving to restrict its action to what is *possible*. The ego may be described as a controlling agency that recognizes, receives, stores, discriminates, and acts by restraining, releasing, modifying, and directing impulses. Thus the ego processes may be considered the guardian of the vital balance of the person.

The superego processes   The superego represents the judgment processes with respect to right and wrong, good and evil. The superego advises and "threatens" the ego. The very young child has little concept of what is right and wrong, but as the codes and values of his parents and society are impressed upon him, he gradually develops his superego.

The word *conscience* is sometimes used to describe the superego, but actually the conscience is only the conscious *portion* of the superego. A more important element of the superego is unconscious, and it produces conflicts that are unconscious. Any violation of the judgment of the superego produces guilt, at either the conscious or unconscious level of the mind. Because guilt causes an extremely uncomfortable feeling, a person may go to great lengths, either consciously or unconsciously, to avoid it. Whenever possible, a person simply avoids behavior that would produce guilt, but when he doesn't, he may use certain ego-defense mechanisms to escape guilt, such as blaming his behavior on someone else.

It is possible for a person with a weakly developed superego to live according to the pleasure principle, without regard for the rights and privileges of others, yet suffer little or no guilt. On the other hand, it is also possible for a person with a strongly developed superego to be so rigid and severe in life that he enjoys almost no pleasure, regardless of the situation. The most healthy superego is one that produces behavior within the limits imposed by society yet allows guilt-free pleasure within those limits.

Basic human needs

Since human behavior is largely directed toward the fulfillment of basic needs, and since emotional illness is often a response to the frustration of those needs, it seems useful at this point briefly to examine the basic needs of Man. Although we might expect them to be clearly understood by now, there is still disagreement on the subject. Perhaps the needs of all of us are not exactly the same, and some authorities may have generalized their own needs as being true of everyone. We present the basic needs listed by the late A. H. Maslow in his classic book *Motivation and Personality*.

Physiological needs   The most basic of human needs are the physical drives, such as hunger, thirst, sleep, and sexual expression. Unsatisfied physical needs may be strong enough to push all other needs into the background. Not only may the immediate interest in the higher needs be lost, but the entire outlook on life may be modified. For example, a starving man may think that, if only he were guaranteed plenty to eat for the rest of his life, he would never want anything more, and a young person with the strong sexual drive characteristic of youth may direct his behavior toward obtaining sexual satisfaction with little regard for the present or future fulfillment of his higher needs.

Security   The need for a feeling of security or safety is nearly as basic as the physiological needs. It is most easily observed in the fright reactions of infants and children, because adults in our society have generally been taught to hide or inhibit such reactions. However, they do so often regardless of the cost, for when they feel their security threatened, they may not react openly but, rather, with masked anxiety and physical changes, such as a faster heartbeat.

The need for security is great in children, and parents must make every effort to provide them with it. The relationship between the parents is especially important to a child; parental quarrels may be quite upsetting to a youngster. The child also gains security from a certain amount of routine in the daily schedule of the family. It is also important that parents be consistent in the degree of rigidity or permissiveness with which they govern their children. A child feels more secure when he knows what his parents expect of him and how they will react to his behavior.

Love and belonging Most of us feel a strong need for love and acceptance. Yet many of us find it difficult to establish close interpersonal relationships. Several barriers may stand in the way of honest and meaningful relationships. Our society has a strangely inhibited and cautious attitude toward love and affection and especially toward their possible expression in sexuality. This attitude has made it difficult for some persons to establish close relationships, including those in which sex would play no role. Of course, love and sex are not synonymous. There may be strong love relationships in which sex is not involved, just as there may be sexual relations in which love is not a factor.

It is of the utmost importance that parents be responsive to the love needs of their children. The child who feels unloved and rejected by his parents may experience great difficulty at home and at school and may bear lifelong emotional scars. The child who has felt parental rejection may in adult life be reluctant to attempt close personal relationships for fear of further rejection, so that he may never be able to give and receive love adequately. The person who has "loved and lost" may similarly fear further rejection; however, to a reasonably secure person the fulfilling of love needs is worth the risk involved.

Esteem Every normal person has a need for self-esteem, which means a feeling of personal value or worth, of success, achievement, self-respect, and confidence in facing the world. In addition, most people have a need for respect or esteem from other people, as seen in their striving for status, dominance, attention, and appreciation.

The need for esteem generally requires finding some area of constructive activity in which to excel. Its satisfaction leads to feelings of self-confidence, value, strength, adequacy, and usefulness, and its frustration may produce feelings of inadequacy, inferiority, dependency, weakness, and despair. A vicious circle may be set up, in which a person lacks the self-confidence to attempt the very activity in which his success could build his feelings of self-esteem. Something must be done to break his cycle of helplessness and begin the building of self-respect.

It seems that as a person's self-respect is strengthened, his need for esteem from others is diminished. A constant seeking of praise suggests insecurity. However, it is important to recognize that everyone has a need of recognition from others, and sincere praise is one of the foundations of good interpersonal relationships.

Self-actualization   The need for self-actualization is the need to achieve self-fulfillment, to reach one's full potential, to do what one is capable of doing. If an artist is to be at peace with himself, he must paint; a poet must write; a musician must make music. Maslow says, "What a man can be, he must be." This statement means that, to feel fulfilled, an individual not only must do the kind of thing he is able to do but also must do it as well as he is capable of doing it.

Characteristics of good emotional health

It is difficult to set up an exact standard by which an individual's level of emotional normality may be judged. Certainly, no line neatly divides the emotionally healthy from the emotionally ill, and there are many degrees of emotional health. The characteristics described below are all signs of good emotional health. The temporary lack of one or more of them does not necessarily indicate emotional illness, since few, if any, of us show all these traits at all times, but a consistent failure to display any one of them might be symptomatic of emotional illness.

Ability to deal constructively with reality   The emotionally healthy person faces reality, whether it is pleasant or not. He does not generally attempt to escape from it by retreating into mental fantasies or excessively using alcohol or other drugs. Nor does he take the opposite path—becoming preoccupied with his own problems and spending much time worrying or brooding. When a problem arises, he attempts to correct it, if the solution seems within his ability, or else he realistically accepts the situation as being beyond his power to change.

Ability to adapt to change   We all show a natural tendency to resist change, since security is found in familiar things and situations. But the world constantly changes, and the emotionally healthy person is able to change with it. He welcomes new experiences and new ideas and does not live in fear of the future.

Reasonable balance of independence and dependence   A person in good emotional health functions independently, thinks for himself, and makes plans that he can follow through. He also demonstrates a reasonable reliance upon the judgment and experience of others, and when important decisions are to be made, he seeks advice from qualified persons. He accepts fair criticism of his faults and errors without regarding it as a threat to his personal security.

Moderation in negative emotions   The emotionally healthy person does not allow negative emotions such as anger, hatred, jealousy, or guilt to overpower his rational control over his own actions. He can take life's irritations and disappointments in his stride, minimizing the unpleasant aspects.

Ability to make long-range choices   The mature person is willing to sacrifice some immediate pleasures for the sake of long-range goals. He values pleasure, but he plans his life to yield the greatest net satisfaction over the long run. His plans involve choices of career, management of finances, and matters concerning marriage and children. He looks beyond the immediate situation to the future.

Ability to love and understand others   The mature person does not have a large number of childish needs that are striving for expression. He has the ability to initiate expressions of affection for other people. Such an ability extends beyond his mate and children. He can accept people of racial, religious, and cultural backgrounds different from his own. He can afford such feelings, because they reflect a sense of inner security.

Ability to work productively   It is widely agreed among authorities that one of the prime indicators of emotional health is the ability to work effectively and productively. In school it is often found that the student who is having academic difficulty is suffering from emotional conflicts. Similarly, the chronically unemployed adult is often suffering from emotional problems that inhibit him from actively looking for a job, that work against him in job interviews, or that lower his productivity to the point where he repeatedly loses jobs. The emotional problems of a housewife may be reflected in her inability to do her housework or in the fact that routine household chores consume all of her available energy.

DEALING WITH STRESS

Stress-producing situations are a part of life. Everyone develops ways of coping with them, and their purpose is to avoid a conscious feeling of anxiety. Anxiety-preventing devices have been called by different authorities "defenses against anxiety," "ego-defense mechanisms," or just "defense mechanisms."

Defense mechanisms are not abnormal; everyone makes use of them. They are recognized by most authorities as necessary and valuable in dealing with the stress situations we all face throughout life. It is doubtful whether anyone could successfully go through life without making use of them.

Defense mechanisms in themselves are neither desirable nor undesirable. The value of a particular mechanism usually depends on the context and on the extent to which it is used. Used in moderation and in the proper situation a mechanism may be of great value, but used to excess or in inappropriate situations it may be quite undesirable. The more important defense mechanisms are described below.

Avoidance   One of the simplest and most common methods of defense against anxiety is to avoid the situations that would produce it. Everyone uses this defense to some degree. For example, a person with a fear of flying travels by surface, and a person who feels uneasy speaking in front of groups doesn't make speeches. Neither is abnormal or even particularly unusual behavior. But avoidance can become so intense as to indicate emotional illness, as when a person is so generally fearful that he refuses to leave his home for *any* reason. Thus it may be seen that a defense mechanism may be either normal and harmless or seriously disabling, depending on its intensity.

Denial   In using denial, a person protects his ego from a stressful situation by refusing to recognize it. Denial usually is an unconscious process, or at least largely so; one usually is not consciously aware that he is denying anything. Like avoidance, denial can be either a helpful or harmful defense, depending on the situation in which it is used and the extent to which it is used. For example, we must admit that the world is a dangerous place, every day each of us facing the possibility of being cut down by fatal disease, war, murder, an automobile accident, fire, flood, tornado, lightning, or a building's collapse, to name but a few of life's hazards. Of course, the probabilities on a given day are extremely remote, and if one continually thought about all the dangers he faced, he would be in a constant state of anxiety. Thus, in some respects denial makes it possible to ignore remote dangers and live a normal life, but it is harmful if it results in failure to take precautions against the more immediate dangers. For example, some fail to take physical examinations because they deny the possibility of illness, and others fail to use automobile seat belts because they deny the possibility of an accident. When any clear or present danger is denied, denial is an obvious misuse of the defense mechanism.

Repression   Repression is a process of forgetting purposefully. A person unconsciously tries to forget those events in his past or present that cause him pain or discomfort—a kind of emotional block. He tries to keep them from being expressed; in other words, he feels one way and tries to act another. His feelings are not to be denied, however, and will find expression one way or another. They may express themselves as dreams, amnesia, slips of the tongue, or absentmindedness. Since repressed feelings can create anxiety and guilt, many psychologists believe it is better for a person's emotional health that he find reasonable ways of expressing them.

Rationalization   In attempting to find excuses for failures and shortcomings a person may resort to rationalization, a kind of mental deception that allows him to feel blameless. For example, the student excuses his poor performance on an examination by feeling that it was an unfair test or that he was unprepared for it (although he may have studied thoroughly). This mechanism helps to ease the letdown of failure.

Although the use of rationalization at times helps one to feel more comfortable and may even be justified, the overuse of this kind of thinking encourages an individual to put off solving problems. It is better to admit one's shortcomings and then either to accept them or to work out a plan for correcting them.

Projection   Projection is the denying of one's own weakness by placing the blame for a situation on another person or persons. For example, an executive fires a subordinate for a mistake he himself has made and for which he is responsible. Some people, having certain weaknesses, are very adept at seeing the same weaknesses in other people and are quick to condemn them in place of themselves. Children show projection by running to their parents and tattling on a brother or sister who has done something they themselves have done. We tend to project those feelings that bother us most. If we despise someone, we may not find it difficult to think that he despises us, so that we easily "justify" becoming mean or sarcastic.

Substitution   Everyone has his strengths and weaknesses. To satisfy emotional needs one may substitute the satisfactions he gains from some activities for the disappointments he experiences in others. A person particularly adept in some athletic activity, for example, may substitute the pleasure he gets from it for the disappointment he feels in his chosen profession. Everyone practices some substitution, but it is important not to choose substitutes for disappointments one has the ability to overcome. It is equally important not to choose substitutes that can harm oneself or others, such as excessive use of alcohol or other drugs.

Regression   Regression is the reversion to childlike and immature behavior when one is faced with difficult situations. It represents a retreat from the present frustrations to the fancied security of some time in the past. A person displays regression when he reacts to a situation as he reacted in childhood: going into a tantrum when he cannot have his way, not playing unless he is captain, or throwing his bat away if an unfavorable call is made against him in a baseball game. Although such behavior may not gain him the treatment he wants, he temporarily feels more comfortable.

Identification   Identification is a kind of hero worship, a person identifying himself with people or institutions that represent ideal qualities. The process can be very helpful to developing children who identify themselves with persons or groups representing high goals and ideals. College students frequently seek to be identified with individuals or groups that can bring them attention and prestige. Identification is desirable when the ideal represents high standards, and on the whole it can be one of the most satisfying mental mechanisms, but overidentification or overreliance upon one's family, school, or other group may hinder personal development and even detract from good mental health.

Fantasy and daydreaming   Daydreaming can be helpful if not overdone. The fantasy a child creates is an important part of his development. Adults use it in constructive imagination, as shown by the artist. We can escape from the pressures of reality through the pleasures of fantasy. It is possible to relax by entering the world of illusion found in fiction, drama, and poetry. The mechanism becomes harmful, however, when it is overused, to such a point that one no longer distinguishes reality; then it is a serious disturbance of emotional health.

EMOTIONAL DYSORGANIZATION

It has been indicated how the ego tries to regulate events that tend to disturb a person's adjustment inside himself and with society. The ego tries to level off the disturbances as best it can. Sometimes, however, an individual is in situations that disturb him deeply. He experiences frustrations or alarm; the primitive, aggressive impulses of the id, over which the ego has maintained control, are aroused and threaten that control. From the other side, the super-ego's ideal may be so high as to be impossible to attain, so that the ego, which tries to regulate the self with regard to the *possible*, may give way. The inability of the ego processes to maintain normal control constitutes what is commonly called emotional, or mental, illness (the two terms are synonymous).

   Instead of using the traditional concept of mental illness, complete with definitive labels and diagnoses, the authors of this text follow the lead of Dr. Karl Menninger, a founder of the Menninger Clinic, a psychiatric hospital in Topeka, Kansas. His is a simple yet broad approach, which regards emotional illness as a continuum that ranges from relative emotional normality to emotional collapse or death. Dr. Menninger has coined the word *dysorganization* to describe the increasingly painful or disturbing experiences the ego goes through in trying to maintain successful control over the id. The prefix *dys-* means "painful"; thus this word refers to the pain or disturbance the person experiences in trying to maintain an organized emotional balance. The word *disorganization* means the state of being disarranged; in dysorganization the organization is only impaired and neither lost nor destroyed.

   Starting with a relatively normal adjustment, Menninger takes increasing degrees of emotional dysorganization as representing increasing degrees of mental illness. As the pressure from anxiety becomes greater, one's whole self becomes more and more threatened. At the extreme one may even die, since the whole system, both emotional and physical, may collapse under the unbearable strain of dysorganization.

   For purposes of explanation Menninger distinguishes five "levels" of emotional dysorganization, ranging from mild to severe on a continuum (some emotional states fall between levels); see Fig. 2.1.

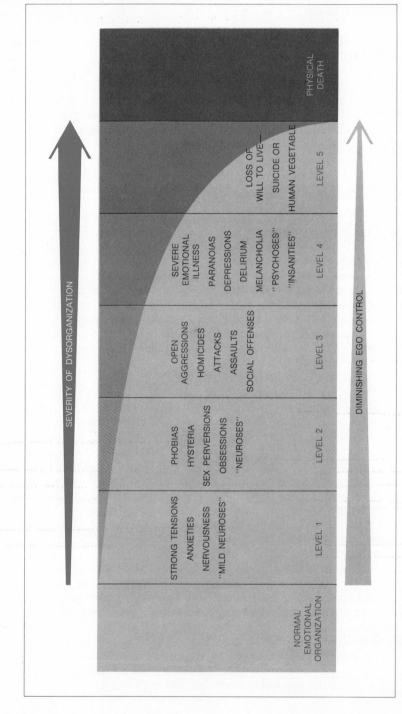

Figure 2.1 Levels of emotional dysorganization. A continuum of progressively more severe emotional illness.

First level of dysorganization

The person with the beginnings of emotional dysorganization experiences a somewhat more than normal amount of tension and shows it through "nervousness." The ego is aware of an increase in aggressive impulses coming from the id—fear, anger, frustration. Although the person may not recognize these events as a threat to the ego, he knows that he is using more than his usual willpower to master his internal reactions. He may respond by determining not to notice these rising tensions or may even try to convince himself that everything is all right. Normally he is able to manage them by using one or more of the defense mechanisms previously described. But, just as a person who is physically ill may be conscious of his breathing or the beating of his heart (activities we normally take for granted), the emotionally disturbed person becomes aware of emotional disturbances and is made uneasy by them. He may exert conscious effort to control them, minor as they are.

At the same time the ego processes become increasingly alert, *hyperalert*, to events. A hyperalert person may hear mysterious noises in the night or detect the slightest irregularity in the appearance of something. Some alertness is normal, but in the first level of dysorganization alertness becomes exaggerated. The person looks for possible dangers—sounds are exaggerated, lights are more intense, and his entire perception is keener. He unconsciously refuses to relax at night during sleep. He may show increased touchiness, tearfulness, irritability, nervous laughter, moodiness, or depression. He may appear overactive by displaying restlessness—walking the floor, biting his fingernails, or driving aimlessly about in his car. He may worry or think obsessively about something, anxiously reflecting on it time and again. He may daydream excessively, impairing realistic thinking and effective action, or be overzealous in identifying with some cause. He may experience certain psychosomatic ailments—itching skin, twitching eyes, diarrhea, upset stomach, or pain. The symptoms are both uncomfortable and expensive in terms of medical treatment, yet they serve to protect a person's ego and thus save him.

The degree of disturbance we have just described is sometimes labeled *mild neurosis* or, by some authorities, *mild hypochondriasis*. The presence of one or several of the symptoms surely would not be positive proof of illness, yet the presence of several symptoms over a period of days or weeks might well indicate some inability to cope satisfactorily with life situations.

Usually the emergency device disappears the moment the stress that originally caused it disappears. Many persons showing such simple dysorganization over a period of time eventually recover, although some remain as chronic cases and some become worse. If the symptoms continue for too long a period of time, they are physically wearing. A headache can be endured for a few hours, but one that lasts for days or weeks can lead to more severe dysorganization. If a person already undergoing some stresses encounters new ones, deeper dysorganization may result. If the ego is unable to control behavior with the mild devices discussed here, the ego processes are led to increased activity. Something else must be done, other ego-saving devices must be called upon, and they lead to the second level of dysorganization.

Second level of dysorganization

The emotional changes that occur at the second level are still moderate, yet they may cause definite detachment of the person from his environment. He becomes a little more unrealistic. Although his actions may or may not appear changed in the eyes of others, he further shuts off the real world. The isolation means less contact with the normal flow of stimulation and information. The ego processes become more impaired. At this stage the person is aware that his emotional state is neither comfortable nor pleasant. He may feel a sense of failure, uselessness, or disappointment with himself or others; he experiences less joy in productive work. Others begin to appear to him deliberately provocative or indifferent. He keeps doing things he does not want to do and saying things he does not want to say. Saint Paul made a related comment when he wrote, "The good which I would, I do not; but the evil which I would not, that I practice." In almost every case of second-level impairment are hidden drives toward *aggressiveness.* The individual is, however, still functioning in society and handles his own unconscious aggressive impulses by any of various means. Some are emergency devices, lasting only a short time; some are chronic, playing a permanent role in the personality. Certain syndromes (groups of symptoms characterizing a disease) are described in the following paragraphs.

Withdrawal A person may unconsciously sever contact with the outside world temporarily. He can do so by means of fainting, total lapse of memory, selective blindness, selective deafness, selective amnesia, or *phobias.* Phobias are the attaching of strong negative feelings to objects or situations, such as thunderstorms, cars, high places, snakes, cats, or public speaking. Sometimes persons with phobias express their anger and fear by embracing, rather than withdrawing from, that which they fear. They may become pathologically daring, for example, by playing "chicken" (a game in which cars approach each other head on at high speed, the first driver to swerve being defeated). This extreme boldness can be typical of the second level of dysorganization.

Physical affliction Some persons feel such intense hostility toward another, a group, or a situation that they cannot get it out of their systems merely by swatting flies or playing a hard game of tennis. Instead, they take it out on themselves. Usually the self-punisher operates quietly. He expresses aggressions unconsciously in accidental injury, peptic ulcers, hypertension, or obesity. Although physically painful, such expressions probably provide him with salvation because he actually feels jeopardized.

Some go through vivid fantasies accompanied by real pain or *psychosomatic illnesses.* Some women even demonstrate pseudocyesis, a false pregnancy characterized by an interruption of menstruation, enlargement of the abdomen, and increased pigmenting of the nipples. Menninger cites the following psychosomatic case history:

A psychiatrist in Columbus, Georgia, last week detailed the amazing case history of a woman who spent seventeen of her twenty-eight years in a *psychosomatic marathon.* Her ailments included hives, headaches, hacking cough, constant sore throat, nausea, earaches, muscular soreness, and numbness in her right leg. The patient was never without some of these symptoms. She had paid 602 visits to 22 physicians and one chiropractor and was hospitalized five times. She received 33 different kinds of medication, 600 tests, and 1,500 injections. Nothing helped. Finally, the last physician advised her that she was "emotionally ill" and needed psychiatric help. After 32 consultations spread over eight months, her symptoms had all but disappeared, and she was dismissed. The patient's total bill: some $2,700 for medical care, $500 for psychiatry.[1]

Physiological reactions are in all instances considered to be accompanied by psychological reactions, and vice versa.

Compensating acts   Certain acts may be used in place of the carrying out of aggressive impulses, and they may so well mask the impulse as to be almost symbolic.

· RITUALS   All of us use some rituals or ceremonies every day. They may bring us pleasure, but sometimes they are accompanied by discomfort and inconvenience. They may be calisthenics, dietary fads, daily enemas, abdominal massage, or even certain religious practices. These are symptoms of a problem when they become ends in themselves and no longer serve another purpose, but merely carrying them out affords some release.

· COMPULSIONS   Acts that seem quite unreasonable and unnecessary to a rational person but are irresistible to the person doing them are compulsions. Two examples are eating more food than one needs and hoarding above and beyond the amount required for a secure and comfortable future. Everyone indulges in some such behavior at times, but carried to excess it may indicate advancing emotional dysorganization.

· OBSESSIONAL THINKING   In spite of having the appearance of thoughtful consideration in preparation for action, obsessional thinking actually takes the place of action. As such thinking becomes more intense, effective actions and productivity diminish. Obsessional thinking may be another device for handling increasing emotional problems.

· SEXUAL PERVERSION   Sexual perversion and compulsive sexual behavior, like other psychiatric symptoms, represent emotional compromises. Among the various forms of perversion are *fetishism* (deriving erotic satisfaction from objects instead of people), *pedophilia* (the seduction of children), *exhibitionism* (exposing one's sexual organs to the gaze of others), *sadism* and *masochism* (inflicting pain and cruelty upon another person or having such pain inflicted), and *voyeurism* (looking at others' sexual activities). Psychiatrists believe that behind these acts lies hate, so that the perversions represent a type of cover-up for deeper aggressions. The person must get his sexual gratification at any cost, so he engages in actions that are condemned by our society and that may be very destructive to him.

Personality deformities   In some cases defensive devices become a permanent part of the personality. Society's tolerance of the individual depends

---

[1] K. Menninger et al., *The Vital Balance: The Life Process in Mental Health and Illness*, New York, Viking, 1964, pp. 187–188.

on his social standing, power, and wealth. Whether a person is considered sick or not depends on society's opinion of him. If he is wealthy, he may be considered eccentric; if he is poor, he may be rejected or even judged criminal. Not knowing causes, people find it easy to assign motives.

Of the various personality deformities, such as the infantile (beautiful but useless) and the narcissistic (excessively vain and selfish) only the dependency-prone is considered here.

In the light of the millions of Americans who are dependent upon alcohol and other drugs, this category represents the largest single psychiatric affliction in the United States. In spite of the fact that dependency is painful and can disable a person, there is a general misunderstanding about this illness or disease. It is too often considered simply a vice that the victim has voluntarily chosen. In reality it often represents a "chemically induced escape from reality," which may be innocent in its beginnings but later become a successful substitute for the things from which the victim wishes to escape. Thus it represents, like the other processes, a degree of ego failure.

Traditionally the second level of dysorganization is called by such familiar names as *neurosis, psychoneurosis,* and *hysteria.* Dr. Menninger strongly suggests that these old names are wrong and obsolete in that ailments of this second level are not the result of inflammation of the nerves, excess sexual activity, or exhaustion of the mind. The devices used on the second level represent an attempt to control and reduce a state of tension. They may avert more serious consequences. If they tide one over the emergency, they may disappear and anxiety be *reduced.* If they are not sufficient, however, stress and tension may *increase* and the threat to the person continue. Such a person may move on to the third level of dysorganization.

Third level of dysorganization (open aggression)

In the third level of dysorganization the uncontrolled aggressive impulse is expressed directly on the environment. The ego rationalizes itself into believing the expression is actually a way of self-defense. Are not all wars fought, in the eyes of either side, for self-preservation? Individuals use the same reasoning. The aggressive person usually does not try to give logical reasons for his behavior, either to himself or to others; he may not even know why he carried out an act of vengeance or perpetrated an assault.

Society today no longer considers open aggression demonstrative of manliness or necessary for survival. Capital punishment, for instance, is interpreted by many as a kind of corporate aggressive expression that is socially undesirable and, furthermore, ineffective as a deterrent to crime. Others believe that, if it is to be a deterrent to potential criminals, it should be conducted openly, for all to see, rather than in its usual setting of almost complete secrecy.

The muggings, clubbings, and shootings displayed each day on television represent a kind of reverting to the past, when such aggression was more acceptable. This type of expression is highly satisfying to the weak individual. Thus, as our society becomes more and more civilized, not only should the reasons for personal violence become fewer, but also physically aggressive people should be less tolerated. Cases of open aggression today often give strong evidence of ego failure. The sick person who commits an aggressive act is showing that all or nearly all control has been lost. In general he may be described as follows.

He no longer conceals his aggressive impulse.
He shows disregard for laws and social customs and little heeds his conscience.

His judgment, consciousness, and perception may be impaired during the aggressive act.
After the aggressive act is over, his emotional tension is relieved.

In the following paragraphs are described some syndromes characterizing the third level of dysorganization.

Chronic, repeated aggressions   Some people are rebels in search of never-found causes; they do not know what they are against but, whatever it is, they are against it. Their behavior is self-damaging, and they do not seem to learn from experience. A typical example is the boy who seems to make all the wrong turns throughout school life, however long that may last, for, although seemingly a promising student, he goes from bad to worse. Once out of school he cannot hold down a job, because he is always breaking some trust or responsibility.

The characteristics of "antisocial" behavior are similar at all ages, differing only in the nature of the work and play activities. Antisocial persons are more lacking in common sense, more unrealistic, more detached from a sense of the past, more lacking in a reasonable vision of the future, and slower in seeking help, than are persons on the second level.

Occasional violence   Some persons display spectacular, once-in-a-lifetime, or very infrequent outbursts of violence. These may, nevertheless, be severe enough to lead to corrective measures of some type. Senseless beatings, suicide, and murder are examples.

A murder may be bizarre and senseless, and the murderer usually is just as puzzled as anyone about why it all happened. Even though such acts are often violent, the murderer has been successful in putting off something he fears more—his own destruction. The murder is a substitution used by him to preserve his own life, which he prizes more highly than that of his victim. At the moment the murder was the only solution the crippled ego of the murderer could find.

Thus, in summary, the expression of open, direct aggression, except in certain socially acceptable forms, is evidence of acute or chronic ego failure. The acts are often explosive and destructive. Open aggression represents a weaker ego situation than that of the second level of dysorganization: there is more detachment from reality and more injury to the victim, to the environment, and to the perpetrator. Yet open aggression is thought to represent an attempt to avoid an even greater ego failure.

Fourth level of dysorganization

Formerly we dismissed the preceding three levels of dysorganization as eccentricity, perversion, or viciousness; thus persons acting on those levels were not often under the care of a physician. Such illness does not generally happen suddenly but usually develops over a span of years. If the condition worsens, it may lead to the fourth level of dysorganization, sometimes called *psychosis* (known in the past as *lunacy* or *insanity*). It may have any of various causes. Certain forms develop gradually from increasing stress, but there is evidence that other forms have a biochemical or hereditary basis. Regardless of causes, the effects may appear similar.

In the fourth level pretense of control is no longer effectively maintained. Aggressive impulses break into consciousness and into action so easily that the ego processes appear to have disintegrated. The person loses contact with the world of reality and the sense of loyalty he felt toward it. To him the world appears distorted, and he responds with emotions that are inappropriate, exaggerated, and unpredictable. Effective productivity in the home or on the job is gone. Sometimes the patient appears scarcely human. However odd, senseless, or fantastic he may appear, a therapist nevertheless can see some pattern in the patient's talk which matches his past experience.

Certain syndromes are typical of the fourth level. Although the names assigned to these disorders may be helpful in treatment, in legal decisions, and for general communication, it should not be thought that they are well-defined disorders; we consider them, rather, only forms of a further dysorganization of the personality.

Melancholia, depression   The patient has feelings of sadness, guilt, despondency, and hopelessness, with convictions of inadequacy, incompetence, unworthiness, or wickedness. Physical reactions may be retarded. Delusions, with feelings of guilt, defection, unworthiness, and self-abasement, along with fantasies of imaginary offenses and punishments, are common.

Mania, delirium, furor, frenzy   The patient demonstrates erratic and disorganized excitement or excessive talking, acting, elation, and excitement. His actions are self-injuring, bizarre, exhibitionistic, or annoying. A characteristic feature is the great and continuing overflow of poorly controlled energy.

Chronic delirium, chronic deterioration, or autism   The patient is overly absorbed with himself, or silly, or he has bizarre delusions with irrelevant and incoherent speech and apparent indifference to social mores or standards. He is inert or mute, has hallucinations, or displays occasional sudden, impulsive outbursts of speech or actions.

Paranoia   The patient is preoccupied with persecution and shows defensiveness, resentment, and suspiciousness. Still, he may appear dignified and sensible at times.

Dementia, delirium   The patient appears confused, delirious, bewildered; he may suffer from amnesia or hallucinations. These symptoms are also connected with severe injury, intoxication, or brain inflammation.

Once again, according to the concept used in this text, these disorders are not separate diseases but varieties of one disease. In other words, this is one illness with various expressions. The symptoms are reversible, except in cases of brain injury. Persons with such advanced cases may recover when favorable situations once again surround them. Then the evidence of extreme crisis and dysorganization may well be left behind. When circumstances are not favorable, patients rarely die but, instead, continue to live in a world of chronic, long-term maladjustment. Some modern psychiatrists believe this condition is the result of neglect or ignorance on the part of society.

Fifth level of dysorganization

The fifth level represents the greatest extreme to which the ego processes may be pushed. The ego completely disintegrates and rejects life itself; the will to live is gone. All that is left is a determination to end life or to settle for minimal existence.

The extremely ill person either commits suicide or becomes a human "vegetable," refusing to eat, drink, or make any contact with other persons. Force-feeding may be necessary to prevent his starving.

The earnest suicide attempts of fifth-level persons are quite different from the half-hearted ones displayed at the first three levels. The exhibitionistic suicide consciously or unconsciously is hoping and planning for a last-minute rescue, as when he takes sleeping pills and then immediately calls for help. Such an effort should be interpreted as a desperate cry for help. Whoever indulges in it should have professional therapy, since it has often been found that such persons make repeated suicide attempts, and another time might well succeed.

SUICIDE

Suicide is the tenth leading cause of death in the United States today. The "official" annual suicide rate is about 12 per 100,000 persons, and more than 24,000 deaths per year are recorded as suicides. The actual suicide rate probably is nearly double the official rate, because many suicides are disguised as accidents or natural deaths for the purpose of avoiding a loss of insurance money or the stigmatization of the survivors.

No group or class of people is free from suicide. Every person is a potential suicide, and almost everyone at some time during his life considers suicide. However, the probability of suicide relates to certain characteristics.

The most significant pattern in the incidence of suicide is its increase with advancing age: suicide is rare under fourteen years of age, but its rate rises sharply in adolescence, sharply again in early adulthood, again in middle age, and finally in old age.

Several factors are commonly associated with suicides of college students, the most frequent of which is academic failure. Failure brings not only the disappointment and disapproval of parents but also the shattering of self-confidence and self-esteem. The next most frequent factor is the end of a love affair. When romance ends, there is more than just disappointment: there is the overwhelming feeling of being rejected and abandoned, the complete loss of self-esteem. College suicides often are the reserved, introverted, or shy students who, lacking social contacts, tend to internalize their problems. Despite the alarming college suicide rate, many colleges offer little or no on-campus therapy for emotional problems.

The suicide rate rises again in middle age. The male realizes that his career or financial goals have not been attained and are in fact now unattainable. The middle-aged woman feels "finished" as a woman at menopause, or no longer useful and needed after her children's departure from home.

The suicide rate reaches its peak among the elderly, who today suffer from a host of emotionally crippling influences. Many older people feel useless, lonely, bored, and frustrated. In addition, they may suffer great financial insecurity, physical pain, or terminal illness.

Women "attempt" suicide more often than men, but a greater percentage of successful suicides are carried out by men. In recent years the suicide rate for females has risen sharply, while the rate for males has remained fairly constant. This has been attributed to various causes, such as an increasing dissatisfaction with the traditional woman's role of "wife and mother," and increasing career opportunities for women. The chance to succeed in a particular career field is also the chance to fail in it. Increasing social and sexual expectations among women may also be involved. It seems that women may now be commiting suicide for reasons that were formerly more characteristic of men.

In general, suicide is less frequent among the married than among the single, divorced, and widowed, except for married people under twenty-four years of age, among whom the rate is quite high.

Social isolation is a common factor in those who resort to suicide. The more intimately one is involved with others, the less likely he is to consider suicide. Unfortunately, the severe depression that commonly precedes suicide is likely to lead to social alienation and isolation, further increasing the chance of suicide. Suicide may be considered the final outcome of a progressive failure of adaptation, with the isolation and alienation from the usual network of human relationships that support us all and give meaning to our lives.

With today's high incidence of suicide any one of us might at any time be in a position to help dissuade someone from the act. The crucial element that makes its prevention possible is *ambivalence*. Most suicidal people are not fully intent on dying; though their wish to die may be extremely strong, there is almost always an underlying wish to live. But the suicidal person does not wish to live as he is living, for that is seen as being the same as, or even worse than, death. To prevent a suicide, you must grasp the delicate thread that remains of the person's will to live. The first step is to establish communication. As an opening line, the National Save-A-Life League suggests asking, "Are you thinking of killing yourself?" This may seem brutally direct, but in crisis intervention the communication must be open and direct to be effective. You must remain calm and convey attitudes of helpfulness, hopefulness, and genuine concern, building upon the suicidal person's ambivalence about dying and convincing him that he really does want to live.

Everyone has some strengths. The severely depressed person often loses sight of his own strengths or his ability to use them. In talking to a suicidal person you should keep emphasizing his strengths so as to decrease his feelings of helplessness and hopelessness.

Remember that the role of the layman in the suicide crisis is much the same as in any first-aid situation. It is to preserve life until professional help can be reached—it is not to "play doctor." Telephone or walk-in crisis intervention services may be valuable during the crisis. As soon as the immediate threat of suicide seems to have abated, the person should be encouraged to seek competent professional help. *Suicide impulses recur;* it is dangerous to assume there will be no further ones.

THE PROBLEM OF EMOTIONAL ILLNESS

The problem of emotional illness may be considered from several points of view. In addition to the incidence of emotional illness and the number of patients in hospitals we must consider the personnel providing mental care, the facilities available for providing this care, and the methods of therapy being used.

Prevalence of emotional illness

The incidence of emotional illness will depend somewhat upon how "emotional illness" is defined. According to the concept used in this text, even the early stages of emotional dysorganization, beginning with symptoms of anxiety and nervousness (which may not impair a person), constitute emotional illness. Thus everyone might be considered emotionally ill at some time in his life. In the opinion of Dr. Menninger, everyone *is* emotionally ill at some time. Anxiety and stress are widespread. It is estimated that perhaps as many as 10 percent of the United States population are now suffering from some form of *serious* emotional illness or will be at some time in their lives.

There are ways of measuring the prevalence of emotional illness. More than half of the hospital beds in the country are occupied by mental patients. Each year more than one million persons receive treatment in our mental hospitals and in the psychiatric wards of general hospitals.

Since 1900 the rate of hospitalization for emotional illness has more than doubled. This is not evidence of an increased prevalence in emotional illness; it may be the result of a growing awareness of the problems of mental health, a higher percentage of people living in urban areas, the gradual aging of the population, and a significant increase in mental health facilities. Although the rate of hospitalization for emotional illness in this country is one of the highest in the world, there is not necessarily a higher percentage in the United States than elsewhere. This country has the most facilities for the care of such illness and has made greater attempts to understand it than have many other countries. In some countries relatively little is done.

Fortunately, the number of resident patients in mental hospitals has been decreasing since 1955, despite an increase in the general population. Although the number of new admissions to mental hospitals has been increasing, the net number of releases has been increasing faster, according to the Mental Health Statistics of the U.S. Department of Health, Education, and Welfare. These developments are due to the new drugs used in therapy. Over all, it does not appear that the rate of mental illness is increasing in this country.

Methods of treatment

Much progress has been made in the treatment of emotional illness. Today the patient who receives prompt treatment with modern methods stands an excellent chance of complete recovery. The more common forms of treatment may be divided into several major categories.

Individual psychotherapy Psychotherapy most commonly involves a dialogue between the patient and a specially qualified person, usually a psychiatrist, psychoanalyst, psychiatric social worker, or clinical psychologist. The therapy should result in the patient's having a better understanding of himself and of the ways to handle his affairs. The patient should learn to replace ineffective or undesirable coping devices with more appropriate ones. Psychotherapy is administered in outpatient clinics, offices, hospitals, and schools. Persons with minor problems may need only a few sessions, but those with more serious impairments may require months or years of continued treatment.

Group therapy The general category of group therapy includes a wide variety of forms of psychotherapy in which there is interaction among several patients and one or more therapists. In recent years there has been a growing appreciation of the value of group therapy.

Besides the obvious advantage of lower cost to the patient, there is the more important advantage of greater effectiveness for many types of problem, than individual psychotherapy can offer. Group therapy is largely based on the same theoretical principles as individual psychotherapy, but it has additional dimensions, which often enhance its usefulness.

For example, personality disorders may be difficult to treat individually if the patient does not feel that he has a problem but believes that the problem is within his environment (most of us tend to blame our problems on others). In group therapy the attitudes and behavior of the patient can be directly observed, and his distorted views can be challenged by other members of the group and by the therapist.

Often the passive, dependent person does better in group therapy because individual therapy offers him simply another opportunity for dependency (upon the therapist) and little motivation for dealing with his basic problem. In a group the attention of the therapist must be shared with others, and for this reason the frustration of dependency desires becomes obvious to the patient in his increased anxiety, and he thus becomes motivated toward effective psychotherapeutic work. A major portion of the role of the therapist is to provide a certain amount of anxiety and frustration by not meeting every demand and wish of every group member.

The presence of other patients helps draw the patient out of himself and promotes partial identification with other people. The patient tends to identify with those traits, styles, and attitudes of the other patients which are more attractive or effective than his own; the patients use each other as positive role models. They also use each other as negative role models. Often through observing someone else the patient sees a caricature of his own behavior, and it becomes apparent to him why his methods of relating to people are ineffective or antagonistic.

Group therapy provides a "safe" environment for experimentation with new modes of social behavior. Within the protection of the group each patient has the opportunity of testing ways of relating to others and of discovering how others respond without risking the repercussions possible in other settings.

Group members often report that for the first time in their lives they have found a feeling of acceptance and belonging. They can be very antagonistic toward each other and still feel that each is very much a part of the group. The group provides a setting in which a façade of strength, compatibility, accomplishment, or passive accommodation is not necessary to prevent rejection. Group acceptance helps the individual develop a sense of importance, status, and self-esteem, which he can often extend to the world at large.

Finally, the observations and criticisms of peers are often given much greater acceptance than those of a therapist. A therapist, after all, represents an extremely authoritarian figure, and many patients identify him with past authority figures, such as parents and teachers, and reject what he says accordingly. What a therapist says often has a much greater effect when it is seconded by group members or, even better, when he is in the position of seconding interpretations by members of the group.

Drug therapy The discovery of the *ataractic* drugs (those that free one from confusion), also known as the *major tranquilizers,* has been an outstanding pharmaceutical development in recent years. They have become primary means of treatment in mental hospitals; in fact, their use has stopped the increase in the number of hospitalized patients. They suppress emotional disturbance and make the patient more docile, cooperative, and accessible for psychotherapy. They have been the most effective with the very severely disturbed. Milder drugs, known as *minor tranquilizers,* have been widely used to reduce mild forms of anxiety. Although the milder drugs, such as Librium, have fewer undesirable side effects than do the major ones, they are more habituating. Another of these, meprobamate, marketed under the trade names Equanil and Miltown, has the distinct advantages of usually not interfering with clarity of consciousness and not causing drowsiness, as do the major tranquilizers. Other drugs stimulate depressed patients; they are called *antidepressants*. Combinations of these agents are used with some patients. The *sedative* drugs, such as phenobarbital, are used for combatting anxiety, overactivity, and insomnia. Although tranquilizers have cut down on the widespread use of sedative drugs, they have not eliminated them.

Soma therapy

Electroconvulsive therapy Owing to the discovery of the ataractic and antidepressive drugs, the use of electroconvulsive therapy (ECT) has greatly declined. It is of value for certain types of severe depression as well as for patients who do not respond well to drugs.

Other forms of physical therapy used in the past are hydrotherapy, massage, and insulin shock therapy. These modalities are very rarely used today. However, insulin shock therapy may be helpful for certain patients who do not respond well to other forms of treatment.

Psychosurgery Psychosurgery is used today only when all else fails, and even then with reluctance. A number of techniques have been tried, but the most frequently used is the *lobotomy*, in which nerve tracts between the frontal lobes and the thalamus of the brain are severed. At best it is used for patients whose condition is very poor and for whom any improvement is better than none.

Professional workers and the emotionally ill

Most hospitalized patients today are treated by a specially trained group of people rather than by an individual. The group is known as the psychiatric team. In addition to physicians and nurses it may include social workers, psychologists, occupational therapists, physical therapists, and others concerned with specialized aspects of the patient's rehabilitation.

Psychiatrist The psychiatrist is a physician who has been qualified by the American Board of Psychiatry and Neurology. As the leader of the psychiatric team he is responsible for diagnosing the case, prescribing treatment, administering psychotherapy, and supervising and directing the work of other members of the team. He delegates much of the total program to others of the team.

Psychoanalyst A psychoanalyst is a psychiatrist who has had additional specialized training in psychoanalytic methodology and has fulfilled the requirements for membership in a psychoanalytic association.

Clinical psychologist The clinical psychologist does not go through medical school but, instead, does graduate study in psychology. He usually holds the degree of doctor of philosophy (Ph.D.) or master of arts (M.A.) in psychology. He gives psychological tests, makes diagnoses, and engages in psychotherapy. He does not administer drugs or shock therapy, since those may be employed only by medically trained persons. In mental hospitals he often works in association with a psychiatrist.

Psychiatric social worker   The psychiatric social worker usually has taken two years of graduate study, holds a master's degree in social work, and has had training in psychology. He makes contact with relatives, friends, employers, and others associated with the patient. He assists in making any changes in the patient's environment that seem necessary for the patient's recovery.

Psychiatric registered nurse   The psychiatric nurse is a registered nurse who has had special training and experience with the emotionally ill. She may supervise a hospital ward and administer treatments under the direction of a psychiatrist.

Mental health aide or assistant   The aide or assistant, referred to as a *psychiatric technician* in several states, is charged with the actual physical care and custody of the hospitalized patient. The aide or technician is a highschool graduate who has received on-the-job training. A few colleges are now establishing training programs for psychiatric technicians. Aides are important because of the great amount of time they spend with the patient and the personal influence they may have over him. A good relationship between aide and patient can greatly aid the recovery process.

Treatment facilities

Outpatient clinics   Many patients with minor or moderately severe emotional illness can be successfully treated today while they continue to live at home. Psychotherapy sessions and mild drugs usually play an important part in such treatment. The professional worker administering this care can be in private practice (supported entirely by patient fees) or in a community clinic (supported partly or entirely by government agencies or charity). Often community clinics have a sliding scale of fees, determined by the ability of the patient to pay.

Outpatient clinics are also quite important in providing care for the patient who has had short-term hospitalization during the acute stage of his illness and is completing his recovery at home. Such follow-up treatment can greatly reduce the chances of his need to return to the hospital.

Psychiatric sections of general hospitals   There is a growing trend in general hospitals to build or reserve certain sections specially for the treatment of emotional illness. These facilities provide the severely disturbed patient with psychiatric treatment in a hospital setting without requiring him to travel far from home. They also help reduce the social stigma of emotional illness by treating it in the same context as any other disorder.

State mental hospitals   In the past emotional illness often required prolonged hospitalization because no effective methods of treatment were available. Some patients received only custodial care: they were given humane shelter but no specific treatment. Since hospitalization was so prolonged, the responsibility for its cost usually was assumed by the state government. The main purpose of the hospitals for the mentally ill (then called *asylums*) was to confine patients where they could not bother anyone.

Most states are now applying the newer approaches to the treatment of emotional illness, with results often comparable to those obtained in private hospitals. It has been shown that if a state is willing to spend enough money to provide intensive care for newly admitted, acutely ill patients, then money will be saved in the long run. Given intensive care, many patients leave the hospital in a short time; without such care the same patients might require hospitalization at state expense for years and perhaps even for life. The states that recognize this principle have been able to reduce the population of their mental hospitals despite rising general populations.

Private mental hospitals In recent years increasing numbers of privately owned hospitals for the exclusive treatment of people with mental and emotional problems have opened. Some treat all kinds of mental problems, while others are restricted to certain kinds, such as adolescents, elderly persons, and alcoholics.

Comprehensive community mental-health centers Unfortunately, there is still an enormous gap between what should be done and what actually is being done for the emotionally ill. In many communities facilities are non-existent. Where available, they are often priced beyond the reach of all but the most fortunate. Treatment for emotional illness is often specifically excluded from payment by health-insurance policies.

To stimulate the development of comprehensive community mental-health centers, the federal government has made available financial aid to centers that meet certain standards of qualification. The centers offer complete inpatient and outpatient services and emergency services available at all times. The number of such centers remains limited, and they are particularly scarce outside the major metropolitan areas. While it may be impossible for a small community to build and maintain a center, it is often feasible for several neighboring communities to do so cooperatively.

Preventing emotional illness

Much more can be done by both individuals and communities to foster emotional health.

Each individual should make a conscious effort to lead a well-balanced life, attempting to understand both himself and others. As a parent he can provide his children with loving care and consistent discipline. As a citizen in the community he can give matters of mental health his active support.

The members of a community who come into close contact with people—for example, teachers, social workers, lawyers, public-health workers, and housewives—should learn to detect emotional stress in themselves and others. Upon early detection the individual should be referred to a community clinic or local physician. Mass tests of students in schools may detect certain cases of emotional illness before they become apparent. Such prevention requires cooperation between voluntary and public agencies on all levels.

SUMMARY

I. The structure of personality
   A. The total reaction of a person to his environment
   B. Changes throughout life
   C. Freudian concept of personality
      1. The id processes.
      2. The ego processes.
      3. The superego processes.
   D. Basic human needs (after Maslow)
      1. Physiological needs.
      2. Security.
      3. Love and belonging.
      4. Esteem.
      5. Self-actualization.
   E. Characteristics of good emotional health
      1. Ability to deal constructively with reality.
      2. Ability to adapt to change.
      3. Reasonable balance of independence and dependence.
      4. Moderation in negative emotions.
      5. Ability to make long-range choices.
      6. Ability to love and understand others.
      7. Ability to work productively.
II. Dealing with stress
   A. Defense mechanisms used to avoid anxiety
   B. The mechanisms include
      1. Avoidance.
      2. Denial.
      3. Repression.
      4. Rationalization.
      5. Projection.
      6. Substitution.
      7. Regression.
      8. Identification.
      9. Fantasy and daydreaming.
III. Emotional dysorganization
   A. Concept of Dr. Karl Menninger.
   B. Commonly called emotional or mental illness.
   C. Results from difficulty in maintaining control of id by ego.
   D. Has levels representing increasing degrees of emotional illness.
      1. First level, commonly called "nervousness."
      2. Second level, sometimes called "neurosis."
      3. Third level, open aggression (the escape of destructive id impulses).
      4. Fourth level, loss of contact with reality, sometimes called "psychosis."
      5. Fifth level, loss of will to live.

IV. Suicide
   A. Tenth leading cause of death in the United States today.
   B. Rate increases with age.
   C. Social isolation a common factor in suicide.
   D. To prevent, grasp suicidal person's remaining thread of will to live.
   E. Suicide impulses recur.
V. The problem of emotional illness
   A. Prevalence of emotional illness; everyone "emotionally ill" at some time
   B. Methods of treatment
     1. Individual psychotherapy—conversation between patient and therapist.
     2. Group therapy:
       a. psychotherapy involving a group of patients and one or more therapists.
       b. many varieties.
       c. sometimes more effective than individual psychotherapy.
     3. Drug therapy—many mood-modifying drugs used.
     4. Electroconvulsive therapy—for the severely depressed or those not responding to drugs.
     5. Psychosurgery—rarely used; nerve tracts in brain severed.
   C. Professional workers and the emotionally ill
     1. Psychiatrist.
     2. Psychoanalyst.
     3. Clinical psychologist.
     4. Psychiatric social worker.
     5. Mental-health aide (psychiatric technician).
   D. Treatment facilities
     1. Outpatient clinics.
     2. Psychiatric sections of general hospitals.
     3. State mental hospitals.
     4. Private mental hospitals.
     5. Comprehensive community mental-health centers.

Glossary

If you cannot find the word you wish in this glossary, check the index for text and glossary references.

aggression (ə gresh'ən) (L. *ad-*, to; *gradi*, to step). A forceful, attacking action, either physical, verbal, or symbolic; it may be realistic and self-protective or unrealistic and unprovoked; it may be directed outward to other things or directed inward to oneself.

amnesia (am nē'zhə) (G. *amnesia*, forgetfulness). A loss of memory due to brain injury, disease, shock, or repression.

ataractic drugs (at ə rak'tik) (G. *a*, not; *taraktos*, disturbed). A group of drugs used to decrease anxiety; essentially the same as tranquilizers.

autism (aw'tizm) (G. *autos*, self; *ismos*, state of). A form of thinking which gratifies unfulfilled desires without regard to reality; a form of fantasy thinking.

avoidance (ə voi'dans). In psychology, refers to the avoidance of anxiety-producing situations.

compulsion (kəm pul'shən) (L. *compellere, compulsum,* to drive, to compel). An insistent, irresistible urge to perform an act which is contrary to a person's ordinary conscious wishes or standards.

continuum (kən tin'yoo əm) (L. *continuus,* continuous). A series in which the discrete parts are united by a common character.

delirium (di lēr'ē əm) (L. *de-,* from; *lira,* furrow or track, thus, "off the track"). A temporary mental state characterized by confusion, disorientation, and illusions.

dementia (di men'shə, di men'shē ə) (L. *de-,* from; *mens,* mind). An old term denoting madness or insanity; now used to denote organic loss of intellectual functioning.

depression (di presh'ən) (L. *de-,* down; *premere,* to press). In psychology a morbid sadness, dejection, or melancholy.

dysorganization (dis or gə ni zā'shən) (G. *dys,* difficult or painful; *organon,* instrument for work). A state of impaired and inefficient emotional organization resulting from a person's inability to cope with internal conflicts and external reality.

ego processes (ē'gō pros'es əz) (L. *ego,* I; *pro-,* forward; *cedere,* to go). According to Freudian theory, one of three major divisions of the psychic apparatus, which consciously acts as mediator for the impulses of the id, the prohibitions of the superego, and the demands of reality.

fetish (fet'ish) (L. *facticius,* artificial). A material object—natural (such as a foot or other part of the body) or artificial (such as an article of clothing)—which is symbolically endowed with special meaning; sometimes necessary for the completion of the sexual act.

hallucination (hə loo si nā'shən) (L. *hallucinatio,* to wander mentally). A false perception of sounds, sights, etc., that are not actually present; may occur in any of the senses.

hyperalert (hī'pər ə lurt') (G. *hyper,* above; It. *all' er ta,* on the lookout). Abnormally and excessively watchful of activities around oneself.

hypochondriasis (hī'pō kən drī'ə sis) (G. *hypo,* under; *chondros,* cartilage). Persistent overconcern with the state of one's health, accompanied by various body pains without evidence of disease; it is so called because the area of the abdomen called the hypochondrium was once thought to be the seat of the disorder.

identification (ī den ti fi kā' shən) (L. *identicus,* identity). An ego defense by which a person identifies himself with persons or institutions which represent ideal qualities to him.

id processes (id pros'es əz) (L. *id,* it; *pro-,* forward; *cedere,* to go). According to Freudian theory, one of the three main divisions of the psychic apparatus; the id harbors the unconscious instinctive desires and strivings of the person.

impulse (im'puls) (L. *in,* on; *pellere,* to drive). A psychic striving to act; usually referring to an instinctive urge.

instinct (in'stingkt) (L. *in,* on; *stinguere,* to prick). An inborn drive which includes self-preservation, sexuality, aggression, and certain social patterns.

lobotomy (lə bot'ə mē) (G. *lobos,* lobe; *temnein,* to cut). Incision, or cutting, into a lobe of the brain, severing certain fibers connecting that lobe to the rest of the brain.

mania (mā'nē ə) (G. *mania,* madness). A mental disorder characterized by a preoccupation with some desire, idea, or activity; a morbid compulsion.

masochism (mas'ə kizm) (named after Sacher-Masoch, 1835–1895). Sexual perversion in which one finds pleasure in receiving physical or psychological pain.

melancholia (mel ən kō'lē ə) (G. *melas,* black; *chole,* bile; *-ia,* condition). Severe depression with inhibition of mental and bodily activity.

narcissism (nahr' si sizm) (from Narcissus, a character in Greek mythology who fell in love with his own image reflected in the water). Self-love rather than love of another person.

neurosis (noo rō'sis) (G. *neuron*, nerve; *-osis*, a process). A psychic disorder due to unresolved unconscious conflicts; sometimes considered a major category of emotional illness. Also called *psychoneurosis*.

obsession (əb sesh'ən) (L. *obsessio*, obsession). A persistent, unwanted idea or impulse that cannot be eliminated by logic or reasoning.

paranoia (par ə noi' ə) (G. *paranoia*, madness). A tendency toward excessive or irrational suspiciousness and distrust of others; delusions of persecution.

pedophilia (pē'də fil'ē ə, ped'ə fil'ē ə) (G. *pais, paidios*, child; *philein*, to love). A morbid interest in children, often expressed in sexual behavior.

personality (per sə nal' i tē) (L. *persona*, mask or person). The total reaction of a person to his environment.

phobia (fō'bē ə) (G. *phobos*, fear). A persistent, unrealistic fear of an external object or situation.

projection (pro jek' shən) (L. *proicere*, to throw). The attribution of one's own thoughts, feelings, or actions to others.

pseudocyesis (soo'dō sī ē'sis) (G. *pseudes*, false; *kyesis*, pregnancy). A false pregnancy.

psyche (sī'kē) (G. *psyche*, soul). The mind; the mental life, including both conscious and unconscious processes.

psychiatrist (sī kī'ə trist). A physician trained in psychiatry.

psychiatry (sī kī'ə trē) (*psych-*; *iatreia*, healing). That branch of medicine which deals with disorders of the mind.

psychoanalysis (sī'kō ə nal'i sis) (G. *psyche*, soul; *ana-*, backward; *lysis*, dissolution). A psychological theory of human development and behavior that dreams, emotions, and behavior can be traced to the repressed instinctual drives of the id and the defenses of the ego against them.

psychologist, clinical (sī kol'ə jist, klin'i kal) (G. *psycho-*; *logos*, reason; *klinikos*, pertaining to a bed). A psychologist with a graduate degree (usually a Ph.D.) who specializes in research, diagnosis, and psychotherapy in the field of emotional disorders.

psychosis (sī'kō'sis) (G. *psych-*; *-osis*, a process). A major mental disorder of organic or emotional (functional) origin in which there is a departure from normal thinking, feeling, and acting; commonly characterized by loss of contact with reality, lessened control over impulses, and distortion of perception.

psychosomatic (sī'kō sə mat'ik) (G. *psycho-*; *soma*, body). Pertaining to the interaction of the mind and the body.

psychosurgery (sī'kō sur'jə rē) (G. *psycho-*; L. *chirurgia*, from G. *cheir*, hand; *ergon*, work). Brain surgery for the treatment of psychiatric disorders by removal or interruption of certain nerve pathways.

psychotherapy (sī'kō ther'ə pē). (G. *psycho-*; *therapeia*, to nurse). Any type of treatment based primarily upon verbal or nonverbal communication with the patient, in contrast to other forms of treatment, such as the use of drugs.

rationalization (rash ən əl i zā'shən) (L. *rationalis*, reason). The process of justifying by reasoning one's acts as an ego defense.

regression (rē gresh'ən) (L. *regressus*, to go back). Reversion to childlike and immature behavior in response to stress situations.

repression (rē presh' ən) (L. *repressus*, to reprimand). The process of selectively restricting to the unconscious mind those thoughts, feelings, or memories that would cause anxiety. An ego defense mechanism.

sadism (sā'dizm) (named after Marquis de Sade, 1740–1814). Sexual perversion in which pleasure is derived from inflicting physical or psychological pain on others.

schizophrenia (skit'sə frē'nē ə, skiz'ə fren'e a) (G. *schizein*, to split; *phren*, mind). A severe emotional disorder often characterized by a retreat from reality accompanied by delusions, hallucinations, regression, and emotional disharmony. Once called *dementia praecox*.

self-actualization. Reaching one's full potential.

soma (sō'mə) (G. *soma*, body). The body as distinguished from the mind.

substitution (sub sti tu' shən) (L. *substituere*, to put in place of). An ego defense mechanism in which the satisfaction of one emotional need substitutes for the satisfaction of another.

superego processes (soo'pər ē'gō pros'es əz) (L. *super*, above; *ego*, I; *pro-*, forward; *cedere*, to go). According to the Freudian theory, one of the three main divisions of the psychic apparatus, associated with ethics, standards, and self-criticism; these standards help form the "conscience."

syndrome (sin'drōm) (G. *syndrome*, concurrence). A group of symptoms which occur together and whose occurrence indicates a recognizable illness.

unconscious (un kon'shəs) (AS. *un-*, not; L. *conscius*, aware). In psychological theory, that part of the mind which is only rarely subject to awareness; it includes data which were never conscious or were once conscious but have been repressed.

voyeurism (vwah yur'iz əm, voi yur'iz əm) (Fr. *voir*, to see; G. *ismos*, the act). A compulsive, often sexually motivated, interest in watching or looking at the genitals and/or sexual behavior of others; roughly the same as being "a peeping Tom."

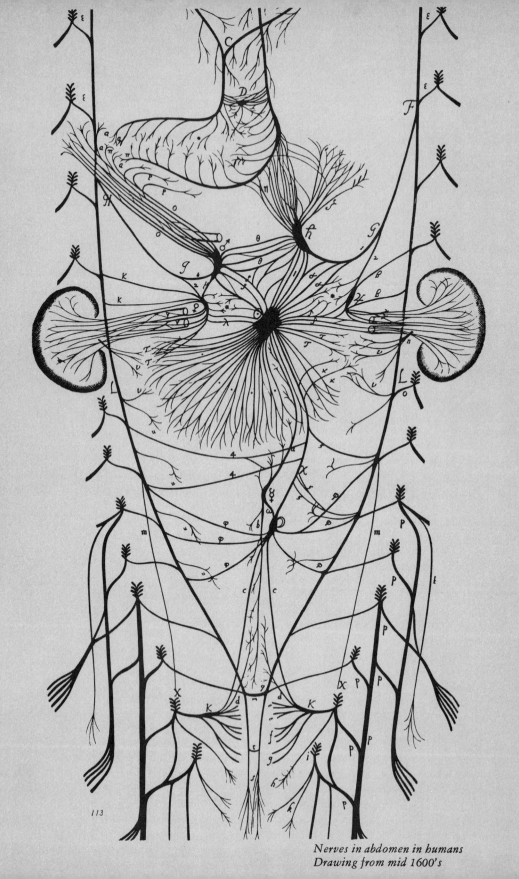

113

Nerves in abdomen in humans
Drawing from mid 1600's

Structure and disorders of the nervous system

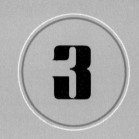

In Chapter 2 we examined emotional conflict. The various levels of emotional dysfunction discussed there usually have no definite organic basis—they are not the result of organic brain damage. Such psychological disorders are spoken of as *functional* disorders because no actual tissue impairment can be found: the brain merely is not functioning properly.

In this chapter we shall examine the nervous system from a more biological standpoint, considering the *organic* disorders: those in which there is definite damage to the structures of the nervous system or impairment of its bio-chemical functioning. Such problems are also called *neurological* disorders. Organic damage to the nervous system can impair mental and emotional function so that the symptoms produced are much like those of the emotional disorders discussed in Chapter 2. Even highly qualified psychiatrists and neurologists sometimes have difficulty in determining if the symptoms a patient exhibits are the result of psychological or neurological causes. Once again we see that mind and body act as a unit and that the health of each is dependent on the other.

STRUCTURE OF THE NERVOUS SYSTEM

As dynamic living organisms, humans are continuously carrying on physical activities—transforming food into energy, metabolizing stored food into available energy, maintaining respiration, balancing themselves against gravity, or recoiling from pain. All these activities are under the continuous control and coordination of the nervous system. The more than 12 billion nerve cells, or *neurons*, which make up the human nervous system are organized into brain, spinal cord, nerve tracts, and sense organs. The work of this system has been appropriately compared to that done by an electronic computer—but far more efficient and concise than any man-made computer yet developed.

The nervous system basically is *nervous tissue*, consisting of neurons (see below), which are simply cells that receive and transmit impulses, and supporting cells. Generally speaking, neurons constitute the sensory apparatus, which *receives* stimuli; the nerves and central nervous system, which *transmit* impulses; and the *effectors*, which convert impulses into action.

The nervous system is divided into *central* and *peripheral* portions. The central nervous system consists of the *brain* and the *spinal cord*. The peripheral nervous system consists of *cranial nerves* that carry impulses to and from the brain and *spinal nerves* that carry impulses to and from the spinal cord. Those of the peripheral nerves that control specific internal functions are called the *autonomic nervous system*.

Certain highly developed and important structures are called the *sense organs*. They receive messages or sensations from outside or from within a person. Some of them, such as the eye, ear, nose, and tongue, receive stimuli special to themselves; others, such as the skin, are more generalized. In this chapter two special sense organs, the *eye* and the *ear*, will be described.

The neuron

The basic functional unit of the nervous system is the neuron, or nerve cell. Neurons are the most specialized cells of the body. Like other cells, the neuron has a *nucleus* located within its *cell body* (Fig. 3.1); if the nucleus is destroyed, the cell dies and is never restored. The neuron has *fibers* extending from the cell body; those which carry impulses toward the cell body are called *dendrites*; those which carry impulses away from the cell body are called *axons*. The axon of one neuron may lead to the dendrite or cell body of the next. The junction of two neurons is called a *synapse*, which contains a space, across which impulses are carried from one neuron to the next by chemicals known as *neurotransmitters*.

A bundle of *nerve fibers* is a *nerve*; one nerve may contain thousands of fibers. Since the cell bodies of nerve fibers are located mainly in or near the central nervous system, the nerve fibers may be several feet long, running, for example, all the way from the spinal cord to the toes. Damage to nerve fibers disrupts sensation and control in some part of the body. However, within the peripheral nervous system damaged fibers may gradually regenerate, as long as the cell body has not been destroyed.

The central nervous system

The brain consists of three major divisions: the *cerebrum*, the *cerebellum*, and the *brain stem*; see Figs. 3.2 and 3.3.

The largest part of the brain is the cerebrum, which is divided into two *cerebral hemispheres*, a right and a left, connected by tracts of nerve fibers. The surface, or *cortex*, of each hemisphere is composed of the so-called *gray matter*, made up of millions of neurons. The cortex is divided into four lobes, the *frontal, parietal, temporal,* and *occipital* (Fig. 3.2). Neurologists have been able to locate areas of the cortex that are responsible for certain body functions, such as vision control, speech, hearing, and motor activity. Internally the cerebral hemispheres are made up largely of *white matter*. The white matter at the base of each hemisphere surrounds a few islands of gray matter called *basal ganglia*, which are groups of nerve cells that regulate

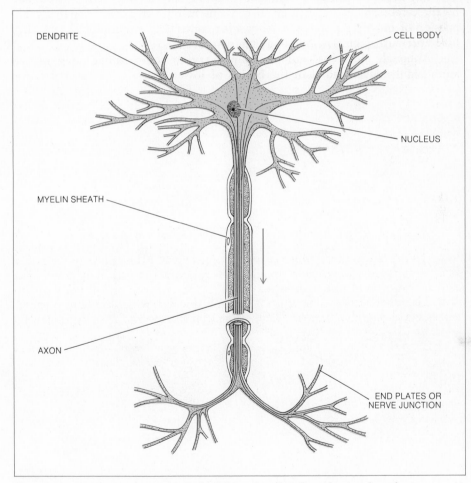

Figure 3.1   Typical neuron. Arrow indicates the direction of nerve impulses in the cell.

motor impulses arising in the cortex and being transmitted to various parts of the body. Inside the hemispheres are several cavities filled with *cerebro-spinal fluid* (Fig. 3.3). The functions of the cerebrum include control of the voluntary muscles, the interpreting of impulses from the sensory organs, and the control of learned behavior. The cerebrum serves as the center for all intellectual and rational activities.

The cerebellum, located below the hind portion of the cerebrum, has the functions of coordinating motor impulses between the cerebrum and other parts of the body and helping to maintain body balance and muscle tone. The surfaces of the cerebrum and cerebellum are wrinkled and folded into ridges; the folds make for a large surface area without increasing the brain's total size.

The brain stem may be thought of as the core of the brain, surrounded by the cerebrum and cerebellum. It contains many nerve tracts for the transmission of impulses and nerve centers for controlling respiration, heart beat, blood pressure, digestion, and body temperature.

Although individual human brains vary to some extent, they are all more highly developed than the brains of lower animals. In particular, the

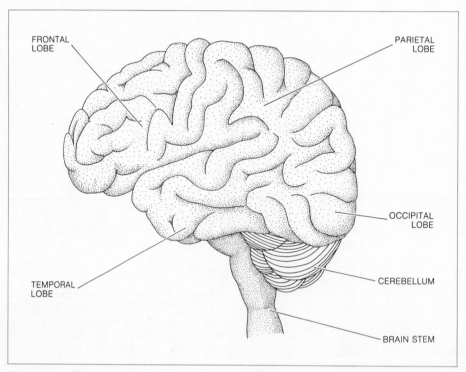

Figure 3.2   The divisions of the brain and the lobes of the cerebral hemisphere (left view).

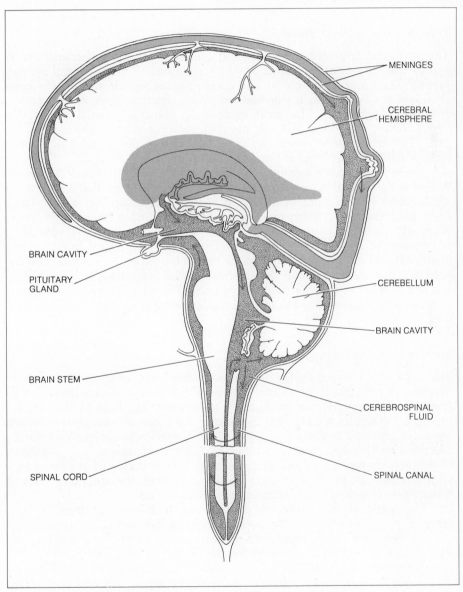

Figure 3.3   Midsection of the brain and the spinal cord. Arrows indicate the direction of circulation of the cerebrospinal fluid.

human cerebrum shows the highest level of development of any living thing; it is responsible for man's ability to learn and to reason.

The spinal cord occupies the *spinal canal* inside the *vertebral column* (Fig. 3.3). It serves as a main line connecting the brain and the spinal nerves. In cross section it is seen to be made up of a large center section of gray matter and an outer sheath of white matter.

The peripheral nervous system

The peripheral nervous system (Fig. 3.4) consists of 12 pairs of cranial nerves and 31 pairs of spinal nerves, all of which are attached to the central nervous system (brain and spinal cord). The cranial nerves, which arise in the brain stem, are involved in such functions as vision, hearing, speech, eye motion, and facial expression. The most extensively branched cranial nerves, the vagus nerves, pass down through the neck to serve most of the internal organs. The spinal nerves, emerging along the sides of the spinal cord, control most of the body functions of the neck and below.

An impulse from a sense organ travels over a neural pathway, or circuit. A simple example of a neural pathway is the *reflex arc;* see Fig. 3.5. A reflex arc involves two or more neurons and at least one organ: (1) a *receptor,* a specialized ending of a sensory nerve fiber associated with a special sense organ, (2) a *sensory neuron,* which carries the impulse to the spinal cord, (3) a *motor neuron,* which carries the impulse from the spinal cord to an effector organ, (4) *end plates* at the endings of the motor nerve, and (5) an *effector,* such as a muscle or a gland, that carries out the response. Physicians often use this reaction to test the condition of certain nerve tracts; for instance, by tapping the knee area they can test the nerves between the knee and the spinal cord.

The autonomic nervous system

The autonomic nervous system is not an anatomic entity, since it consists of neurons of both the central and peripheral systems, but is named for its *function:* the regulation of involuntary body activities, those of the internal organs for example; see Fig. 3.4. Its counterpart is the somatic system, which regulates activities under voluntary control; the somatic system will not be described in this text. Such activities as heart beat, respiration, digestion, blood-pressure regulation, and sexual arousal are controlled by the autonomic system. Although not under direct conscious control, the autonomic system is extremely responsive to the emotional state at any time.

Two parts of the autonomic system act in direct opposition to each other: the *sympathetic* and the *parasympathetic* divisions. The sympathetic division responds to emotions such as fear, anger, worry, and anxiety, and its function is, in general, to prepare the body for emergency action. The parasympathetic division responds to a state of emotional well-being, and its function is, in general, to restore and conserve energy. Some of the actions of the two divisions are compared in Table 3.1. Although sympathetic stimulation is valuable during emergency situations, its prolonged action may be

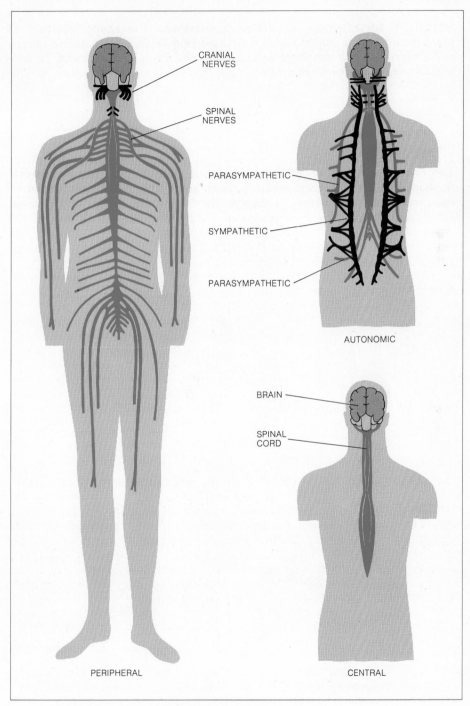

Figure 3.4   Divisions of the nervous system.

responsible for a variety of destructive processes. The emotional states of many people cause almost constant stimulation of the sympathetic nerves, contributing to such problems as ulcers, heart disease, and problems in male and female sexual response.

THE EYE

Structure of the eye

The eye is a complex organ about an inch in diameter and nearly spherical in shape; see Fig. 3.6. Its essential features are a lens mechanism formed by the curved transparent front of the eye, the *cornea*, and a *crystalline lens* inside. Together they focus an image on the light-sensitive back wall of the

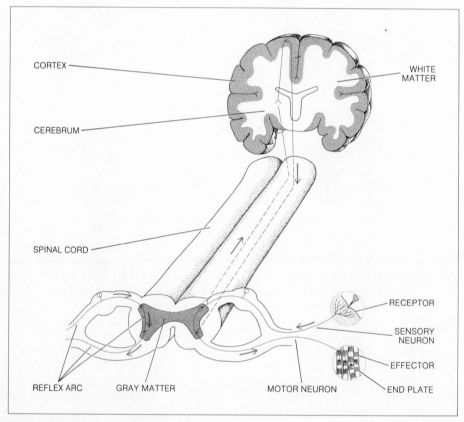

Figure 3.5   The nerve pathways. Nerve impulses pass from a receptor cell, along a sensory neuron, through a reflex arc, to the brain and return along a motor neuron to a muscle.

Table 3.1 *Functions of the sympathetic and parasympathetic divisions of the autonomic nervous system*

organ affected	sympathetic action	parasympathetic action
Heartbeat	Increases rate	Decreases rate
Iris of eye	Dilates pupil	Contracts pupil
Digestive system	Inhibits secretion of digestive juices except stomach acid	Stimulates secretion of digestive juices
Sweat glands	Causes "cold sweat"	Regulates normal functioning
Sex organs	Inhibits sexual arousal	Stimulates sexual arousal
Blood vessels	Diverts blood from internal organs to skeletal muscles	Stimulates flow of blood to internal organs

eye, the *retina*. The cavity between the cornea and the lens contains a watery fluid, the *aqueous humor;* the cavity between the lens and the retina contains a jellylike material called *vitreous humor.*

The wall of the eyeball is made up of three layers of tissue. The outermost layer, the *sclera*, is a strong, fibrous tissue; it is commonly spoken of as "the white of the eye." Its anterior portion is the cornea.

The middle layer, the *choroid*, is composed almost entirely of blood vessels, which supply the retina (the innermost layer). As the choroid extends forward and nears the lens, it becomes a structure known as the *ciliary body*. This body is composed of some muscle, which surrounds and contracts the lens, and some epithelium, which produces the aqueous humor. The ciliary body extends farther forward, over the front edges of the lens, and becomes the *iris*. The iris is pigmented with *melanin*, giving color to the eye. It consists of blood vessels and smooth muscles; the latter are responsible for dilating and constricting the *pupil*, the round opening in the center of the iris. The pupil, which appears black, acts as an adjustable light diaphragm.

The innermost layer of the eye, the *retina*, is the light-sensitive part of the eye. It is composed of a layer of pigmented cells and three layers of neurons. The pigmented cells are attached to the choroid layer, and over them (touching the vitreous humor) are the neurons, called photoreceptors. There are two types of photoreceptor, *rods* and *cones*, so named because of their shape. The rods perceive black and white and the cones perceive both black and white and colors (red, green, etc.). An area of the retina directly behind the lens, the *fovea*, contains only cones; this area is the most active during daylight vision. The rods are most active in the adaptation of the eye to darkness.

Impulses from the photoreceptors are transmitted out the *optic nerve*, which leads away from the eye to the brain. Since there are no photoreceptors at the point where the optic nerve joins the eye, there is a so-called *blind spot* there.

Nature has provided the eye with various structures to protect it from injury or infection. The eye is set in a bony socket that surrounds it. At the anterior end of the socket the eye is protected by eyelids, which are fringed with protective hairs, the eyelashes. Lining the eyelid and covering the exposed surface of the eyeball is a delicate membrane, the *conjunctiva*, which is kept moist by secretions of the *tear glands* (*lacrimal glands*). The tear fluid given off by these glands not only washes away foreign particles but also kills bacteria. Normally just enough tear fluid is secreted to keep a thin film of moisture over the exposed portion of the eye; when excess fluid is given off, it ordinarily drains into lacrimal ducts, which discharge into the nasal cavity.

Disorders of the eye

The good health of the eyes is of incalculable importance. Accordingly, any structural defects, injuries, or diseases which affect the usefulness of the eyes should be given proper medical care. Some of the conditions that may affect the eye and reduce its usefulness follow.

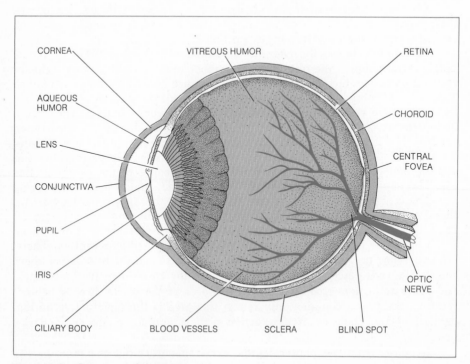

Figure 3.6   Structure of the eye.

Refractive defects In refractive defects images are focused improperly on the retina; see Fig. 3.7. The most common of such defects are myopia (nearsightedness), hyperopia (farsightedness), presbyopia (decreased accommodation as a result of aging), and astigmatism (defective curvature of the cornea).

· MYOPIA One defect of development is an eyeball that is too long, so that usually images are being focused in front of the retina, instead of on it, as in normal vision. Objects that are far away appear blurred; those nearby are clear. This condition is corrected by the use of concave lenses ground thick at the edges and thin at the center, which throws the point of focus back so that it strikes the retina correctly.

· HYPEROPIA When the eyeball is too short or the lens of the cornea is flattened, images come to focus behind the retina. As a result the eye cannot

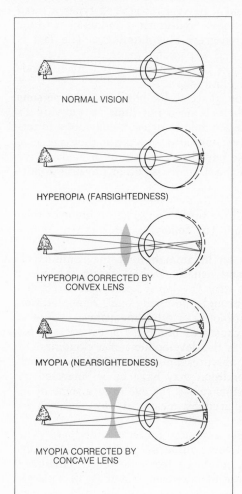

NORMAL VISION

HYPEROPIA (FARSIGHTEDNESS)

HYPEROPIA CORRECTED BY
CONVEX LENS

MYOPIA (NEARSIGHTEDNESS)

MYOPIA CORRECTED BY
CONCAVE LENS

Figure 3.7 Normal and defective focusing. In the normal eye light focuses exactly on the retina, in the farsighted, or hyperopic, eye it focuses behind the retina unless corrected by a convex lens, and in the nearsighted, or myopic, eye it focuses in front of the retina unless corrected by a concave lens.

focus properly on nearby objects. The ciliary muscles may be able to compensate by thickening the lens, but the compensation can be a source of eyestrain. A convex lens that is thin at the edges and thick in the center corrects this condition. The eyes of a person wearing convex lenses may appear larger than their actual size.

· PRESBYOPIA   A loss of the elasticity of the lens causes distant objects to be clearly seen but close objects to be blurred. This condition develops as a person grows older. It too can be corrected with prescribed lenses.

· ASTIGMATISM   When the cornea or the lens has an irregularity in its curvature, its surface does not refract light uniformly. Vision then is blurred or distorted to some degree, and the eyes are strained. Astigmatism can be corrected with lenses ground to compensate for the distortion.

Color blindness   Color blindness is a hereditary, sex-linked condition, appearing in about 5 to 9 percent of all men. Several recognized types are red blindness, green blindness, blue blindness, red-green blindness, red-blue blindness, green-blue blindness, and red-green-blue blindness. The last is achromatic, or total, color blindness, and a person having this type sees objects as black, gray, or white. The most common type is red-green blindness, and the least common is total color blindness.

Since there is no way to prevent or correct color blindness, the persons who inherit it must learn to cope with it. It need not limit an individual's functioning, for most color-blind people are able to detect some subtle differences between the shades they perceive normally and those they perceive abnormally, and some color-blind people have been successful in fields where color detection is important, as in medicine. Usually no other physical abnormality is connected with the condition.

Diseases and inflammations   Despite all the protection given to the eyes they are susceptible to irritation and infection. The following infections are some of the most common:

· CONJUNCTIVITIS   Conjunctivitis is an inflammation of the conjunctiva. The blood vessels become engorged and usually visible, giving the eye a bloodshot appearance. Newborn babies may develop it because of infections they have picked up in their passage through the birth canal. The condition can be controlled by treatment with antibiotics or other medicines.

· CATARACT   One of the common causes of blindness is cataract. It occurs principally among older people. It is the development of a cloudiness or opacity of the lens. When a cataract obscures light transmission so much that it seriously impairs vision, the condition may have to be corrected by the surgical removal of the entire lens; this causes the eye to lose some of its refractive power, but that may be replaced by means of powerful convex lenses.

· GLAUCOMA   Glaucoma is the most common cause of blindness. The condition is characterized by an excessive *intraocular pressure*. Aqueous humor in the normal eye is constantly produced from the blood, circulated through the eye, and reabsorbed into the bloodstream, but if its drainage is reduced and it cannot escape from the eye rapidly enough, the fluid pressure inside the eye begins to rise. As the pressure rises, the contents of the eye compress backwards against the retina and, in particular, against the optic nerve. Then the cells of the optic nerve atrophy and are destroyed, causing permanent blindness.

Some symptoms of glaucoma are headaches, loss of peripheral vision, need of frequent changes of glasses (particularly among older people), and the seeing of halos around lights. Some forms of the disease progress very rapidly, others slowly. Early diagnosis is essential. The malady can often be effectively treated through surgery or the administration of drugs.

Some public clinics conduct tests for excessive intraocular pressure. Testing is done painlessly with an instrument called a *tonometer*, which is placed over the surface of the eye. Everyone over the age of 30 should have this test performed by an ophthalmologist. After the age of 40 he should have the test every two years at least; it is a part of every complete eye examination given by an ophthalmologist to people of this age.

Care of the eyes

We have seen how complicated the eye is and some of the disorders to which it is subjected. Because the eye is so essential, it should be given the best of professional care. Various professional services are available. A physician who specializes in treating diseases, defects of the eye and injuries to it is an *ophthalmologist*. He is a physician who is trained to examine the eyes and prescribe lenses, to prescribe medication, to give treatment, and to perform eye surgery. An *optometrist* is trained to examine the eyes for refractive errors and to prescribe appropriate lenses. He is not a physician and so is neither trained nor permitted to perform eye surgery or to prescribe drugs for the eye. An *optician* is trained to grind lenses and mount them in frames to conform to the face of the patient.

Contact lenses Lenses that are placed directly on the front of the eyeball under the eyelid have been used for a long time by those in the performing arts and in contact sports. Recent improvements in their construction have increased their popularity. Today they are made of lightweight plastic and are unbreakable. They are small and virtually invisible to other people.

Certain types of visual defect can be corrected satisfactorily with contact lenses; others cannot. They are more comfortable to some people than others. Although they may be desirable for appearance, they have drawbacks: they must be placed in the eye and taken out, they are easily lost, the length of time a person may wear them varies with the sensitivity of his eye to them, some people find them too irritating to wear at all, and their cost is considerably greater than that of most regular lenses.

Contact lenses should be purchased only upon the recommendation of a qualified eye specialist. He will be able to do an exact fitting and afterwards carefully observe the eye for its sensitivity to the lens. Since he writes a prescription for an optician to fill, he does not profit from the sale.

Sunglasses Sunglasses should be worn under conditions of bright sunlight or glare to protect the eye against harmful ultraviolet and excessive visible light. Although they come in many styles and shapes, most may be considered safe for wear. Sunglasses purchased without prescription should be checked first for optical flaws that may create eyestrain. The prices of sunglasses vary widely; it is wise to pay a little more for a pair that will give the eye the greatest comfort. A person who wears prescription lenses should either have sunglasses ground to his prescription or wear the type that clips onto his normal glasses. Many sunglasses interfere with color perception. It is not advisable to wear them indoors or on a cloudy day. They never should be worn for nighttime driving or for looking directly at the sun.

Eye exercises   Although much has been said in the past concerning the value of eye exercises, they may be of no value unless the patient has a muscular imbalance. They are of no value in restoring diseased eyes or in changing the proportions of the eyeball. If such exercises are needed, they should be prescribed by an eye specialist.

Eye irritants and injuries   The eye is vulnerable to foreign objects and injury. Stray objects that get into the eye, such as dirt, should always be carefully removed. Debris that becomes embedded in the eye should be removed only by a physician.

Many women today use various cosmetic products to enhance the appearance of the eye, and some of them can cause irritation to the edge of the conjunctiva at the edge of the eyelid, as well as irritate the skin. Hairsprays that get into the eye can irritate the eyeball. The use of anything that causes irritation to the eye should be discontinued.

Eyedrops or eyewashes meant to clear the appearance of the white of the eye, reduce soreness, or clear the eye of dust should be used only upon the recommendation of a physician, since the eye is sensitive and may be damaged by them.

Eye injury frequently is caused by flying objects or sharp instruments and toys. Anyone working near a grinding wheel or other type of high-speed machine or with caustic or explosive chemicals should wear protective goggles made of safety glass. Children should be advised concerning the correct handling of scissors and sharp-edged toys.

Proper lighting   Improper lighting while a person is reading or watching television, although not a cause of blindness, may create eye fatigue. One's reading light should be bright enough, evenly distributed, and without glare, and television viewing is properly done in a partially lighted room.

THE EAR

Structure of the ear

The ear is a combination sense organ, related both to hearing and to equilibrium. Structurally it may be divided into three parts: the *external ear*, which includes the outer projection and a canal, the *middle ear*, which is an air space containing three small bones, and the *internal ear*, the most important part, which contains the sensory receptors for hearing and equilibrium; see Fig. 3.8.

The external ear is composed of the *auricle* ("ear") and the *external auditory canal*. Both pick up sound and direct it toward an opening in the skull. At the end of the auditory canal is the *tympanic membrane* (eardrum), which is a physical barrier between the external auditory canal and the middle-ear cavity. It is a taut, thin membrane that vibrates in response to intercepted sounds.

The middle ear contains three small bones (*ossicles*) for the transmission of sound to the internal ear. The three small bones within this cavity—the *malleus*, the *incus*, and the *stapes* (Latin for "hammer," "anvil," and "stirrup," and sometimes called by the English names)—are united by joints so as to form a lever system that greatly amplifies vibrations picked up from the tympanic membrane and transfers them to another membrane, the *oval window* of the internal ear. Air comes into the middle-ear cavity through the *eustachian tube*, which connects the lower part of the middle-ear cavity with the *pharynx* and has the function of keeping the air pressure on the inside of the eardrum equal to that on the outside. When the air pressure

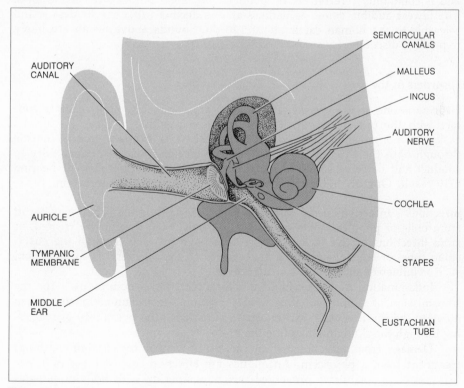

Figure 3.8   Structure of the ear.

changes rapidly, as when one goes through a tunnel or up in an airplane, one may yawn or swallow, which equalizes the pressure in the middle ear by way of the eustachian tube. The mucous membrane that lines the passage from the pharynx, through the eustachian tube, and into the middle-ear cavity is susceptible to infections, particularly in children. At the back of the cavity is an opening into the *mastoid air cells,* spaces inside a portion of the temporal bone of the skull.

The internal ear is the area of sensory reception for hearing and equilibrium. It contains the *cochlea* for hearing and the *semicircular canals* and several other structures for the sense of balance and position. The cochlea is a coiled duct filled with fluid; one portion of it, the *organ of Corti,* has more than 15,000 hair cells (*cilia*) that receive sound. As the fluid within the cochlea is set in motion, it stimulates the hair cells, which transmit impulses to the *auditory nerve* which, in turn, sends them on to the cerebrum.

The cochlea responds to certain properties and qualities of sound. *Pitch* refers to the level (in the musical scale) at which a sound is placed. It depends upon the frequency of the sound waves—that is, the number of waves per second. Generally, young persons can detect sounds with frequencies as low as 30 cycles per second and as high as 20,000 cycles per second; the range is usually reduced with age. *Intensity* is the power of sound waves and is commonly referred to as loudness. Loudness is measured in decibels. The lowest audible sound is defined as one decibel (db); the loudest sound tolerable to the human ear is about 120 db. Sounds above 80 db are likely to produce discomfort.

Disorders of the ear

Hearing is one of the special senses necessary for maintaining accurate contact with the outside world. The ear is very sensitive and can be injured easily. Although embedded within the skull, it is exposed to the outside through both the external ear canal and the eustachian tube. If its ability to conduct and perceive sound is impaired, partial or complete loss of hearing may result. One of the major causes of impaired hearing is infection.

Infections   Infections occur rather easily in the middle ear. They may result from boils or pimples in the outer ear that have been improperly treated, or from infections of the throat or nose that have traveled through the eustachian tube, or from the bacteria and viruses of some general body infection, such as influenza, measles, and scarlet fever.

Inflammation in the middle ear may affect the structures used for the transmission of sound and thus reduce hearing. An inflammation may then move to the mastoid cells, causing *mastoiditis,* with the possibility of spreading through the skull and infecting the brain.

Damage from infections often can be prevented by obtaining prompt treatment from a physician. Antibiotics are effective against most of them. Infections are sometimes prevented by not tampering with boils or pimples in the outer ear, by keeping the ear free from wax, by keeping objects out of the ear canal, and by being careful not to blow the nose so hard that infectious material might be forced up the eustachian tube into the middle ear.

Deafness Anything that interferes with the transmission of sound waves or their interpretation may be responsible for the loss of hearing. There are two basic types of hearing loss: conductive and perceptive. *Conductive deafness* is the result of interference with the passage of sound through the outer and middle ear. The loss is greatest in the lower and middle range of the hearing scale. It may be caused by obstruction of the external ear canal, destruction or damage of the eardrum, inflammation of the middle ear, resulting in swelling and abscesses, or *otosclerosis*, which immobilizes the stapes of the middle ear. Anyone aware of persistent "fullness" in the ears, buzzing or ringing sounds, or dullness in hearing should see an *otologist*, a physician who specializes in ear disorders.

Perceptive deafness is caused by damage to the sensory cells of the cochlea or of the auditory nerve. Loss of hearing with this type of deafness is greatest at the higher range of the hearing scale. It may be the result of infections (mumps, scarlet fever, or measles), injuries, such as blows on the head, or excessive dosages of certain drugs, such as aspirin, quinine, and some of the antibiotics.

Professional workers currently are expressing great alarm over prolonged exposure to loud noises, or "noise pollution." Noises are getting louder. Common examples of noise makers are garbage-disposal units (80 db), vacuum cleaners and city garbage trucks (85 db), food blenders (93 db), farm tractors (98 db), typical discotheques, or rock bands (114 db), and a jet plane taking off (150 db). The exposure to loud and persistent noises very probably causes irreversible hearing loss. High-decibel sounds destroy the hair cells of the inner ear, causing perceptive deafness. It is believed such noises also relate to indigestion, high blood pressure, and emotional troubles, and other nervous disorders. The prevention of such effects includes noise control, construction soundproofing, and the use of earplugs or ear protectors.

Aids to hearing Many people have profited from the development of new medical and surgical techniques for the restoration of hearing. For others restoration is not possible. For some the greatest help in hearing has been the hearing aids. At one time hearing aids were clumsy, obvious, and unpredictable in their operation. Those available today are compact, efficient in operation, and inconspicuous; some are built into the earpieces of eyeglasses.

NEUROLOGICAL DISORDERS

The neurological disorders are many. Some have a single known cause; others have various causes, or the cause may be unknown. The disorders may occur during embryonic development or be the result of accident, faulty metabolism, disease, or something else. A few of the most commonly known neurological disorders are discussed below; they are arranged by cause.

Developmental

During the time of embryonic development a malformation occasionally occurs. It may be due to faulty inheritance or to some sort of developmental accident.

Down's syndrome (mongolism) An unfortunate inherited brain malformation occurring in approximately 0.2 percent of Caucasian live births results in Down's syndrome. The victims are characterized by physical abnormalities of the face, eyelids, tongue, and hands and by a general physical and mental retardation. Mongolism is so called because of the similarity in a fold of the eyelid between the victims and members of the Mongoloid race.

The incidence of mongolism is related to the age of the mother. As the age of the mother advances, the chances of her bearing an affected child are increased considerably; the age of the father seems to have no bearing on the disease. The number of pregnancies the mother may have had preceding the birth of an affected child is not considered a cause of the condition. A mongoloid parent can give birth to a normal child, but when a mongoloid mother is mated to a normal partner, the chances are 50 percent that their children will be mongoloid.

Mongolism occurs in two forms. In one there is an extra chromosome, giving a total chromosome count of 47 instead of the ordinary 46; in the other a part of a chromosome breaks off and reattaches to another chromosome. In either case the imbalance of genetic material can lead to maldevelopment of the child.

Hydrocephalus Cerebrospinal fluid is a clear liquid that is derived from the blood supply that closely surrounds the brain. It flows into the brain cavities (*ventricles*) and circulates through them. It then passes down and around the spinal cord, back up and around the outside of the brain, and is finally absorbed by the veins of the meninges inside the skull (Fig. 3.3).

Hydrocephalus, meaning "water in the head," is an excess of cerebrospinal fluid within the brain. It may be due to excessive fluid's being produced, to obstructed passage inside the brain, or to a too slow reabsorption around the brain. It may also be due to infection or tumors. Whatever the cause, the result is that the brain is compressed against the skull, the head enlarges, and a child may be mentally retarded if untreated.

Success in preventing mental retardation depends upon the extent of damage and the exact tissues affected. The condition may be treated surgically by removal of the obstruction or by tubes (shunts) passed into the brain, which drain off excess fluid into certain blood vessels. Drugs may be given to reduce the fluid formation. Many children born with this condition are now being successfully treated.

Traumatic

Traumatic disorders are caused by wounds or injury, such as injuries to infants during the process of being born, automobile accidents, falls, assaults, and bullet wounds. Accidents of all kinds are the leading cause of death up through the age of 34. Accidental injury to the brain and spinal cord are important factors leading to death and disability.

Head injuries In minor head injury a patient may suffer only momentary loss of consciousness and no brain damage (*concussion*). In moderate injury there may be longer periods of unconsciousness, some actual brain damage, and small hemorrhages of blood vessels around the brain, resulting in clotting and pressure on the brain. Severe injury may lead to prolonged unconsciousness and even to laceration of the brain.

The complications are many and varied; they may be shock, convulsions, motor disabilities, respiratory difficulties, bleeding around the meninges, or infection. Severe cases may culminate in death.

Spinal injuries Spinal injuries are usually the result of accident. Spinal injuries commonly also involve injury to the vertebral column, which may result in paralysis of the body parts below the area of damage. Additional complications may be shock, respiratory failure, pneumonia, and secondary infections.

Metabolic

In some instances disrupted chemical and physical processes in the body—metabolic disorders—can lead to mental defects or nervous disorders. Only one metabolic disorder is discussed below.

Phenylketonuria (PKU) is a hereditary disease which, if untreated, usually brings on mental retardation during the first several years of life. It is found in either sex, and it is transmitted by a recessive gene. About one in every 10,000 babies is a victim.

Although children with this disease appear normal at birth, they lack a certain liver enzyme needed to convert phenylalanine, an amino acid, into tyrosine, another amino acid; see Fig. 3.9. Because of the absence of the enzyme phenylalanine accumulates in the body in 20 to 40 times the normal amount. This excessive amount interferes with the movement of other important amino acids into the brain, causing incomplete brain development that is permanent and irreversible.

Owing to the fact that brain development goes on for several years after birth, the early detection of PKU is vital. Between the ages of 4 and 24 months affected children show a progressive decline in mentality. Of the untreated patients most have an IQ of less than 50.

Melanin, the pigment responsible for hair and skin color, usually is less evident among PKU children than among normal children, the victims often having blue eyes, blond hair, and fair skin. The victims may not be toilet trained or may not have learned to feed themselves until 8 or 10 years of age, if then. About 1 percent of the patients in institutions for the mentally retarded are PKU victims.

Various tests can detect PKU before any permanent brain damage occurs. Most states require that all newborn infants be tested for PKU. One test is usually given before the baby is released from the hospital, but since PKU cannot always be detected that early, a second test should be performed at about 3 months of age.

PKU treatment must begin early. The older the victim before treatment is begun, the greater the amount of damage; treatment begun after the age of 2 is usually futile. The treatment consists of restricting the patient's dietary intake of phenylalanine. The diet needs to be adjusted as the child matures, but it is not yet known how long such a course needs to be continued.

Degenerative

Some disorders are the result of tissue deterioration. Tissues and organs that were once active lose their ability to function. Examples of neurological degeneration include the following conditions.

Multiple sclerosis   Multiple sclerosis is a progressive disease resulting in the loss and destruction of the fatty myelin sheaths (see Fig. 3.1) that sur-

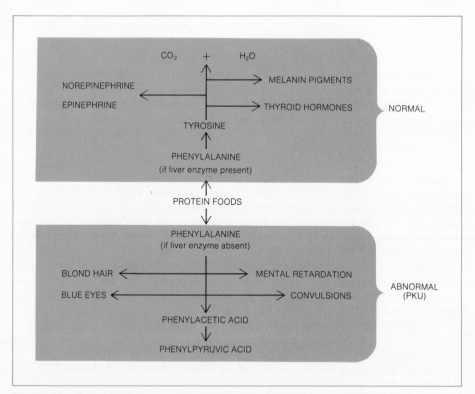

Figure 3.9   The chemical events in the disease phenylketonuria (PKU): the normal protein metabolism and the abnormal protein metabolism characteristic of PKU.

round and insulate nerve cells. Scar tissue forms in the damaged areas, causing the nerve tracts to be "short-circuited," distorted, and eventually blocked. This demyelinization occurs in scattered areas of the brain and spinal cord. Once scar tissue is laid down, the nerve cells can never be restored to normal functioning, and sometimes they die. Thus the communication system of the body is permanently damaged. Messages from the brain to the muscles are either distorted or blocked, and bodily movements the individual wants to make are hampered or prevented. The location and extent of the nerve damage are unpredictable.

This disease is characterized by symptoms such as paralysis and numbness of different parts of the body, loss of coordination, tremor of the hands, double vision, dragging of the feet, impairment of the speech, and loss of bladder and bowel control; any of these symptoms can be significant. The disease usually strikes people between the ages of 20 and 40 years, and it may appear at irregular intervals. It may progress gradually or rapidly. It is of equal incidence among both sexes. Although in some cases the disease is fatal, the life expectancy of most patients is approximately that of the rest of the population. Possible causes of the disease are suspected but still unproved. At the present time there is no known cure. However, many victims of multiple sclerosis are able to adjust to the impairment and live useful lives. The Multiple Sclerosis Society and the United States Public Health Service's National Institute of Neurological Diseases and Blindness are pursuing research on this disease.

Parkinson's disease Also known as "shaking palsy," Parkinson's disease is an abnormal functioning of the basal ganglia of the cerebrum. When the functions of the basal ganglia are interfered with, the motor areas of the brain release nerve impulses more easily than they normally would, causing rapid, involuntary contractions of the muscles. The muscles usually affected are those controlling the head, the hands, and the fingers. As a result the head and hands shake gently when the body is at rest. Along with this shaking, other muscles of the body become abnormally immobile, causing the facial expression to become unchanging and masklike, the walking to become stiff, and the arms to remain motionless when the person is walking. Because of the rigidity of his body muscles the victim hates to move. He slumps, and his speech becomes inarticulate. As the disease progresses, muscles all over the body become affected, and movements of any kind become labored.

Recent studies have led to a new theory concerning this disorder. It is now believed that a balance exists within the nervous system between two parallel motor control pathways. The activity of one pathway is regulated by body-produced amines; the other is regulated with acetylcholine and cholinesterase. Parkinsonism occurs when there is an imbalance caused by a reduction in activity in the amine pathway. Symptoms may be alleviated either by *reducing* activity in the acetylcholine system (through drugs or surgery) or by *increasing* the activity of the parallel amine pathway. Concerning the latter there has recently been much interest in treatment with large doses of the amine, L-Dopa. Surgery may involve the use of alcohol or pinpoint freezing (with liquid nitrogen at $-50°$ C); neurosurgeons locate and deaden certain ganglia. In some cases such an operation is successful in reducing or stopping tremor and lessening muscular rigidity. Treatment merely relieves symptoms; it does not prolong life.

Although the disease is occasionally found among young people, most of the 500,000 victims in this country are older people. The relative mortality risk is less in men than in women. There is no correlation between the rate of progression and the age of onset, severe infection, positive family history, or other neurological disease.

Huntington's chorea Huntington's chorea is also called *hereditary chorea.* The word *chorea* comes from a Greek word meaning "dancing," and the victims display a dancelike movement; the disease is named after an American physician. It is characterized by involuntary jerking movements of body and limbs. The malady consists of a progressive degeneration of the nervous system and leads to gradual physical and mental impairment and the eventual death of the individual. It generally appears in adults; on an average it begins in adults between the ages of 30 and 45. It has, however, appeared in victims as young as 1 year and as old as 60 years.

Although the disease consists of damage to the basal ganglia of the brain somewhat like that found in Parkinson's disease, the damage results in a more spasmodic and extensive involuntary muscular movement.

The disease is inherited and is transmitted from parent to child through a single dominant gene; consequently, children of affected parents have a 50 percent chance of inheriting it. Since the age of onset is variable, the ailment has been known to develop in children before it has shown up in their parents. However, in such cases one of the parents will be expected to show the disease if he or she lives long enough.

It is essential that parents who know of hereditary defects in their lineage tell their children about them. Failure to pass on such information can result in situations similar to the following account. A man developed Huntington's chorea after he had raised his own family of children; only then was it pointed out to him that his mother had died from the same condition. This information given to him earlier could have helped him decide to refrain from having children and so avert possible suffering in the next generation.

Tumorous

Tumors may arise in any of the tissues of the nervous system. They may be either benign or malignant (see Chapter 17); a malignant tumor is one that is capable of *metastasizing* (spreading from one place to another). A tumor originating in any structure adjacent to the central nervous system is of vital importance to health; even a benign tumor may have drastic effects.

When tumors occur within the vertebral column, they affect the spinal cord. Although similar in nature to cranial tumors, they occur much less frequently. When malignancies do occur here, they metastasize to the bones of the vertebrae more commonly than the cranial tumors metastasize to the skull. The treatment for intravertebral tumors is surgical, since they tend to compress the spinal cord against the inside of the vertebral canal.

Some tumors grow in the cells of the structures within the cranium—the meninges, blood vessels, nerve cells, or cranial glands (pituitary or pineal). The effects and symptoms of intracranial tumors vary, depending upon the exact location and condition of the tumor. The development of signs may be gradual or rapid. The parts of the body normally controlled by the affected part of the brain also will be affected and impaired. If treatment is not successful, the tumors are fatal.

Certain kinds of brain tumor respond to radiation, others must be removed surgically, and others need a combination of treatments.

Infectious

Some nervous disorders occur as the result of infection. Such are poliomyelitis, neuritis, abscess, meningitis, and encephalitis. The last two will be discussed here as examples of infectious causes of neurological disorders.

Meningitis   Meningitis is an infection of the meninges caused by the presence of specific organisms. The meninges or linings (Fig. 3.3) become inflamed, the cerebrospinal fluid becomes cloudy, owing to the presence of more white blood cells, brain tissues become congested, and some nerve cells degenerate. The patient may suffer from fever, headache, pain and stiffness of the neck and, sometimes, convulsions. The treatment depends on the organism responsible. Drugs are used, along with blood transfusions and drainage of cerebrospinal fluid.

Since meningitis usually occurs after a primary infection (one first affecting some other body part), effective treatment of other body infections and good nutrition are important in its prevention.

Encephalitis   Encephalitis is an inflammation of the brain, usually caused by a virus. It may be either the result of a primary infection or a complication of a viral disease such as measles, chickenpox, or mumps. The victim may show headache, fever and lethargy, progressing into stupor and coma. Although recovery is usual, there is permanent damage in some cases. Because of this danger it is most important that immunizations against diseases such as measles be given to all people, particularly to children.

Multiple or of unknown causes

Some neurological disorders have a single known cause, some have a number of causes, and others have causes yet unknown. Following are several examples of the latter two types.

Cerebral palsy   Cerebral palsy denotes the symptoms arising from damage to the central nervous system, usually occurring before or during birth but sometimes as long as three years after birth. The damage may be the result of one of a number of things: trauma or head injury during or following birth, premature birth, prenatal anoxia (oxygen deficiency), congenital malformations, malnutrition, encephalitis, meningitis, German measles in the mother during the first six months of pregnancy, or Rh incompatibility between mother and fetus.

The symptoms of cerebral palsy range from mild muscular incoordination to severe spasm or violent convulsions; no two patients have identical symptoms. The most common symptom is an awkward, irregular walk. The patient may lack muscular control, balance, or both. From 25 to 50 percent of cerebral palsy victims have seizures, more than 60 percent are mentally retarded, and 10 to 30 percent have hearing difficulties. The United Cerebral Palsy Association estimates that there are more than 600,000 victims of cerebral palsy in the United States and that 1 in every 170 newborns has cerebral palsy.

The damage does not necessarily have a bearing upon a patient's intelligence, but he is in need of understanding and special education to fit him for tasks in which he can be useful.

Epilepsy   Epilepsy is a symptom of certain forms of neurological impairment. Although it has been known to occur in all animals with brains, it is most common among humans. Ancient physicians thought that a person suffering from epilepsy had been seized, in an attack, by the devil or by an evil spirit; hence the name, which means "seizure" in Greek. The attacks, also called "fits" and "blackouts," involve a disturbance or impairment of consciousness. Often they result in *convulsions*, which are uncontrolled muscular spasms.

The causes of epilepsy are far from known. It is now believed that epileptic seizures may be inherited, represent a chemical imbalance, be acquired from a brain injury, or result from tumors. Most commonly, seizures start during childhood or adolescence.

Convulsion occurs as the result of a disorderly discharge of brain-cell impulses: during the period of seizure the muscles of the patient undergo involuntary contractions, or spasms. Convulsions may be mild and may not result in loss of consciousness, or they may be severe and leave the patient unconscious.

Convulsions, however, are not unique to epileptics. They can be induced in any individual. It was early observed that patients with emotional conflicts who had experienced convulsions obtained some relief from their emotional conflicts. It was thought, therefore, that if convulsions could be artificially induced, some patients with emotional illnesses could be benefited. Thus *electroshock* (*electroconvulsive therapy*), insulin, and Metrazol have been used to induce convulsions in some types of emotionally disturbed individuals. Shock therapy, rarely used today, has been largely replaced by various psychiatric drugs.

Although more than 30 types of epilepsy have been described, the disorder is usually defined in one of the following categories.

Grand mal shows the most severe effects. The victim usually screams because of the constriction of his chest as the air is forced out through his throat. He falls, all the voluntary muscles of the body stiffen, and jerking actions follow. Finally the spasm subsides. When a person is having a grand mal attack, it is important to keep him from hurting himself. A firm, but not hard, object should be placed between his teeth to keep him from biting his tongue. The clothing around his neck should be loosened. Persons subject to grand mal attacks should be encouraged to lie down when they feel an attack coming on. Some of the drugs useful in reducing the frequency of attacks are Dilantin, Mesantoin, phenobarbital, and the bromides.

Petit mal is a minor seizure that differs from the major seizures in that its victim has only blackouts. Though not falling, he becomes suddenly unaware of his surroundings. The attack may last only a few seconds. The victim may go for years without knowing he is having any seizures.

Psychomotor epilepsy is an attack of illusions and disorganized movements, short periods of amnesia, abnormal rage, sudden anxiety, discomfort, fear, incoherent speech, or hallucinations.

Unfortunately, there is still much misunderstanding and stigma surrounding epilepsy. In spite of the fact that known epileptics have contributed significantly to science, government, and the arts (Julius Caesar, Van Gogh, and Handel, for example) some states still prohibit a known epileptic from marriage, from attending public school, or from certain community programs for youngsters. Some states prohibit an epileptic from obtaining a driver's license, even when it can be established medically that his seizures are under medical control.

Far from being rare, epilepsy has been estimated to occur in about 1 percent of the United States' population. There appears to be little relationship between the incidence of epilepsy and intelligence, occupation, economic and social level, age, or sex.

Electroencephalography (EEG) has been of great help in diagnosing epilepsy. All living tissue of the body has some electrical activity, and variations in the electrical activity of brain cells can be picked up from the scalp with electrodes. When amplified and recorded on paper, these fluctuations appear as a wavy line. Neurologists now can recognize a normal wave and certain abnormal ones; see Fig. 3.10. Thus the waves are classified according to their frequency and amplitude and can be used to detect epileptic conditions as well as other brain disorders.

Electroencephalography is not a perfect diagnostic tool, however, since normal individuals give abnormal EEGs in 5 to 10 percent of cases tested, and abnormal persons may give normal EEGs.

Headache   Headaches constitute one of the most common yet most baffling of physical problems. The precise causes of only a few types are known. Where a headache is felt will not necessarily indicate the actual location of the disorder. The disorder may be located inside the cranium (_intracranial_) or outside the cranium (_extracranial_), as discussed below.

Since the brain itself is almost totally insensitive to pain, headaches generally arise outside the brain. Disorders of the blood vessels around the brain or of the membranes (meninges) lining the surface of the brain can lead to headache. The pain may be localized or general. For example, in-

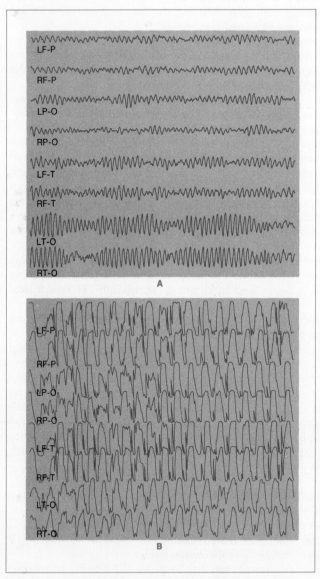

Figure 3.10 Electroencephalographic records: (A) normal tracings; (B) tracings of a patient with petit mal epilepsy.

flammation of all the meninges can cause a severe headache over the entire head. This may be due to meningitis, brain surgery, a brain tumor, or a drop in the pressure of the cerebrospinal fluid around the brain. Other causes are high blood pressure, alcoholic binges, or injections of histamine.

Migraine headache is a special type of headache brought on by temporary disturbances in the arteries supplying the inside of the head. It is believed to be caused by prolonged emotion or tension. It often begins with preliminary sensations such as nausea or partial loss of vision. The vascular disturbance results in a reduced blood supply to the head, followed by dilation of the vessels and intense pulsations for 24 to 48 hours. Certain drugs administered when symptoms begin tend to restore normal blood flow and prevent the intense pains of migraine.

Extracranial causes of headache are various. Spasms in the muscles of the head, scalp, or neck brought on by emotional tension can cause a headache in those areas. Infection or irritation in parts of the nasal structures can cause a headache behind the eyes, above the nose, or in the face. Headaches can originate with the eyes, being brought on by excessive strain on the muscles which focus the eyes, from imbalance in eye muscles, or from exposure of the eyes to excessive irradiation from the sun or an arc light.

Headache constitutes a vast economic problem. Chronic headaches are responsible for approximately as much economic loss as that from the common cold: millions of dollars annually in lost work time. They lead to the spending of $300 million annually in the United States for popular, nonprescription "headache remedies."

SUMMARY

   I. Structure of the nervous system
      A. Neuron
         1. Most specialized kind of body cell
         2. Consists of:
            a. cell body containing nucleus.
            b. fibers leading to and from the cell body, called dendrites and axons, respectively.
      B. Central nervous system
         1. Brain:
            a. cerebrum.
            b. cerebellum.
            c. brain stem.
         2. Spinal cord
      C. Peripheral nervous system
         1. Cranial nerves.
         2. Spinal nerves.
      D. Autonomic nervous system—responsible for control of body functions that are generally self-regulating
         1. Extends from nerve centers down the brain stem and spinal cord.
         2. Consists of two divisions, which act in contrast to each other: sympathetic nerves and parasympathetic nerves.

II. The eye
  A. Structure of the eye
    1. Essentially includes:
      a. lens mechanism formed by the curved, transparent cornea and an internal crystalline lens that focuses an image on the back wall (retina) of the eye.
      b. two internal cavities—one between the cornea and the lens (anterior chamber) filled with a watery fluid (aqueous humor), and one between the lens and the retina (posterior chamber) filled with a jellylike material (vitreous humor).
      c. Wall consists of three layers of tissue—sclera (outermost layer), choroid (middle layer), and retina (innermost layer) consisting of light-sensitive receptor cells called rods and cones.
      d. optic nerve—bundle of neurons leading from retina to brain.
      e. eye protected from injury and infection by the conjunctiva, a delicate membrane lining the eyelid and covering the exposed eyeball surface, which is kept moist by secretions from the tear (lacrimal) glands.
  B. Disorders of the eye
    1. Refractive defects—improper focusing of images on the retina:
      a. myopia—nearsightedness.
      b. hyperopia—farsightedness.
      c. presbyopia.
      d. astigmatism.
    2. Color blindness—hereditary, sex-linked condition.
    3. Diseases and inflammation, which include the following most common types:
      a. conjunctivitis.
      b. cataract.
      c. glaucoma.
  C. Care of the eye
    1. May include the professional services of an:
      a. ophthalmologist.
      b. optometrist.
      c. optician.
    2. Contact lenses—placed directly on the front of the eyeball.
    3. Sunglasses—reduce eyestrain caused by excessive light glare.
    4. Eye exercises are of value only in cases of eye-muscle imbalance.
    5. Eye irritants and injuries may be prevented by protecting the eye from flying objects or sharp instruments.
    6. Proper lighting is necessary to prevent eye fatigue.
III. The ear
  A. Structure of the ear
    1. Sensory organs both for *hearing* and *equilibrium.*
    2. Three structural parts
      a. external ear—auricle, external auditory canal, and tympanic membrane (eardrum).
      b. middle ear:
        (1) consists of three small bones (ossicles)—malleus (hammer), incus (anvil), and stapes (stirrup).
        (2) is adjacent to eustachian tube and mastoid air cells (spaces back of the middle-ear cavity).

      (3) cochlea.

      (4) semicircular canals.

  B. Disorders of the ear most often involve the middle-ear cavity, some the inner ear.

    1. Infections—occur most easily in the middle ear.

    2. Deafness—caused by anything interfering with the transmission of sound waves or their interpretation in the ear.

    3. Aids in hearing—include surgical restoration and the use of some type of hearing aid.

IV. Neurological disorders

  A. Developmental—malformations occurring prior to birth, due to faulty inheritance or a developmental accident.

  B. Traumatic—arise as the result of injury during birth or by accidental means.

  C. Metabolic—result of disrupted chemical and physical processes.

  D. Degenerative—result in deterioration of the tissues and organs of the nervous system.

  E. Tumorous

    1. May arise in any of the tissues of the nervous system, but often in the spinal cord.

    2. May be either benign or malignant, but in either case may cause drastic effects, depending upon the location.

  F. Infectious—result in a number of disorders.

  G. Multiple or of unknown causes—responsible for some of the more baffling neurological disorders.

Glossary

If you cannot find the word you wish in this glossary, check the index for text and glossary references.

acetylcholine (as′e til ko′len). A chemical liberated at the synapse of certain nerve cells and responsible for transmission of the nerve impulse.

amine (am′in). An organic compound containing nitrogen and playing a role in transmission of the nerve impulse.

aqueous humor (ā′kwē əs hyoo′mər)(L. *aqua*, water; *humor*, fluid). The fluid filling the anterior chamber in front of the lens.

astigmatism (ə stig′mə tizm) (G. *a-*, without; *stigma*, point). A structural defect of the cornea or lens that prevents light rays from meeting at a single point, thus forming indistinct images.

auricle (aw′ri kəl) (L. *auricula*, a little ear). The part of the external ear not contained within the head.

autonomic nervous system (aw tə nom′ik) (G. *autos*, self; *nomos*, law). The division of the nervous system that controls the glands and the smooth and cardiac muscles.

axon (ak′son) (G. *axon*, axis). That portion of a neuron fiber which carries the impulse away from the cell body.

basal ganglia (bā′səl gang′glē′ə) (G. *basis*, base; *ganglion*, knot). A group of nerve centers located within the cerebrum, below the cortex, which serve as a center for the transmission of nerve impulses.

blind spot. The small area, insensitive to light, in the retina of the eye where the optic nerve enters.

brain (brān) (AS. *braegen,* brain). The mass of gray and white nerve tissue in the cranium; it includes the cerebrum, cerebellum, and brain stem.

brain stem (brān stem). All of the brain except the cerebrum and cerebellum; it includes the cranial nerve nuclei and sensory and motor tracts.

cataract (kat'ə rakt) (G. *kata-,* down; *rhegnynai,* to break). A disease in which the crystalline lens becomes opaque, causing partial or total blindness.

central nervous system. That division of the nervous system which includes the brain and spinal cord.

cerebellum (ser'ə bel'əm) (L. dim. of *cerebrum,* the brain). The division of the brain behind and below the cerebrum; it is the coordinating center for muscular movements.

cerebral hemisphere (ser'ə brəl hem'i sfēr) (L. *cerebrum,* the brain; G. *hemi,* half; *sphaira,* sphere). One lateral half, or side, of the cerebrum.

cerebral palsy (ser'ə brəl pawl'zē). Paralysis due to a lesion of the brain, usually suffered at birth.

cerebrospinal fluid (ser'ə brō spīn' əl, sə rē'brō spīn'əl) (L. *cerebrum,* the brain; *spina,* a thorn; *fluidus,* fluid). Fluid that occupies spaces in the brain and circulates through the brain, down the spinal canal, and up again.

cerebrum (ser'ə brəm, sə rē'brəm) (L. *cerebrum,* the brain). The main portion of the brain occupying the upper part of the cranium.

cholinesterase (ko'lin es'ter as). An enzyme at the synapse of nerve cells which is necessary for the destruction of acteylcholine.

choroid (kor'oid) (G. *chorion,* leather; *eidos,* form). The dark, vascular layer of the eye between the sclera and retina.

chromatic (krō mat'ik) (G. *chroma,* color). Pertaining to color.

ciliary body (sil'ē er ē) (L. *cilium,* eyelid). A structure of the eye which regulates the convexity of crystalline lens.

cochlea (kok'lē ə) (G. *kochlias,* snail). A spiral-shaped part of the internal ear which receives sound waves and produces nerve impulses for the auditory nerve.

concussion (kən kush'ən) (L. *concussio,* from *con-,* together; *quatere,* to shake). A brain impairment resulting from a violent blow or jar.

cone (kōn) (G. *konos,* cone). The sensitive cell end of the retina that perceives chromatic color.

conjunctiva (kon jungk tī'və) (L. *con,* with; *jungere,* to join). The mucous membrane lining the inner surface of the eyelid and the front part of the eyeball.

conjunctivitis (kən jungk'tə vī'tis). An inflammation of the conjunctiva.

cornea (kor'nē ə) (L. *corneus,* horny). The transparent part of the outer layer of the eyeball, covering the iris and pupil.

cortex (kor'teks) (L. *cortex,* bark of a tree). The outer layer of the brain, consisting of gray matter.

cranial nerves (krā'nē əl) (G. *kranion,* skull). Any peripheral nerve connected with the brain; arranged in twelve pairs.

cranium (krā'nē əm). The skull, especially that part containing the brain.

crystalline lens (kris'tə lin) (G. *krystallos,* ice; L. *lens,* "lentil"). The transparent lens of the eye, located behind the pupil; serves to focus light on the retina.

decibel (des'ə bel) (L. *deci,* tenth; *bel,* unit of sound). A unit of hearing. One decibel is the least intensity of sound at which any given note can be heard. Abbreviated *db.*

dendrite (den'drīt) (G. *dendron,* tree). The branched portion of a nerve cell which carries impulses toward the cell body.

Down's syndrome: see *mongolism.*

effectors (i fek'tər(z)) (L. *ex-*, out; *facere*, to do). A nerve end organ; it serves to distribute impulses that activate a muscle or gland.

electroconvulsive (or **electroshock**) **therapy** (i lek'trō kən vul'siv, ilek'trə shok) (G. *elektron*, amber; L. *con-*, together; *vellere*, to pull). The treatment of emotionally disturbed patients by inducing convulsions; this is done by passing an electric current through the brain.

electroencephalography (i lek'trō en sef'ə log'rafē) (G. *elektron*, amber; *encephalos*, the brain; *graphein*, to write). The recording of electric currents developed in the brain.

encephalitis (en sef'ə līt'is) (G. *encephalos*, the brain; *-itis*, inflammation). Inflammation of the brain.

end plate A disclike expansion at the ending of a motor nerve in a muscle.

epilepsy (ep'i lep'sē) (G. *epilepsia*, seizure). A disease characterized by convulsions and sometimes spells of unconsciousness.

eustachian tube (yoo-stā'shən) (after Bartolommeo Eustachio, an Italian anatomist, 1520–1574). A tube connecting the middle ear and the pharynx.

external auditory canal (ek stur'nəl aw'di tor'ē kə nal') (L. *externus*, outside; *audire*, to hear; *canalis*, a channel). The narrow passage of the external ear leading from the auricle to the tympanum. Also called the *external auditory meatus.*

external ear (ek stur'nəl ēr). The part of the ear that includes the auricle, the auditory canal, and the tympanic membrane (eardrum).

extracranial (ek'strə krā'nē əl) (L. *extr-*, outward; G. *kranion*, skull). Pertaining to something outside the cranium, or skull.

fovea (fō'vē ə) (L. *fovea*, a pit). The area of the retina directly back of the lens; it contains only cones.

frontal lobe (frun'təl lōb) (L. *frontalis*, forehead; G. *lobos*, lobe). One of the four main divisions of the brain, lying directly behind the forehead.

gene, dominant (jēn, dom'i nənt) (G. *gennan*, to produce). The gene, of a pair of genes, that produces an effect in a person, regardless of the nature of the other gene.

gene, recessive (ri ses'iv) (L. *re-*, back; *cedere*, to yield). One of a pair of genes that together produce an effect in a person only when they are inherited from both parents.

glaucoma (glaw kō'mə, glou kō'mə) (G. *glaukos*, gleaming). A disease marked by intense pressure inside the eye, resulting in a hardening of the eyeball and eventual blindness.

grand mal (grahn mahl) (Fr. *grand*, strong, great; L. *malum*, ill). The most severe form of epilepsy, in which there are convulsions preceded by periods of unconsciousness.

gray matter (grā mat'ər). Grayish nerve tissue of the brain and spinal cord, made up of nerve cells and nerve fibers.

Huntington's chorea (hunt'ing tənz kə rē'ə) (G. *choreia*, dance). A convulsive nervous disease characterized by involuntary and jerking movements and progressive dementia. Also called *hereditary chorea.*

hydrocephalus (hī'drō sef'ə ləs) (G. *hydro*, water; *kephale*, head). A condition characterized by an abnormal amount of fluid in the cranium, causing an enlargement of the head, atrophy of the brain, and convulsions.

hyperopia (hī'pə rō'pē ə) (G. *hyper*, above; *ops*, eye). A vision defect in which distant objects are seen more clearly than near ones; *farsightedness.*

incus (ing'kəs) (L. *incus*, anvil). The middle of three ossicles of the middle ear. Also called the *anvil.*

intensity (in ten′ sə ti) (L. *intensus*, intense). The energy or power of sound waves; it is proportional to the amplitude of the waves.

internal ear. The part of the ear that includes the cochlea and semicircular canals. Also called the *inner ear.*

intracranial (in trə krā′nē əl) (L. *intra-*, within; G. *kranion*, skull). Situated within the cranium.

intraocular (in trə ok′yə lər) (L. *intra-*, within; *oculus*, eye). Situated within the eye.

intravertebral (in trə vur′tə brəl) (L. *intra-*, within; *vertebra*, vertebra). Within the vertebrae, or spine.

iris (ī′ris) (G. *iris*, rainbow). The round, pigmented diaphragm surrounding the pupil of the eye.

lacrimal gland (lak′ri məl) (L. *lacrima*, tears; *glans*, acorn). A gland, located above the eye, that produces tears.

malleus (mal′ē əs) (L. *malleus*, a hammer). The outermost of the three ossicles of the middle ear. Also called the *hammer.*

mastoid air cells (mas′toid) (G. *mastos*, breast; *eidos*, form). Spaces inside a part of the temporal bone behind the ear.

mastoiditis (mas toi dī′tis). Inflammation of the mastoid.

melanin (mel′ə nin) (G. *melas*, black). A dark pigment found in the skin, hair, iris, and other parts.

meninges (me nin′jēz) (G. *meninx*, a membrane). The three membranes covering the brain and spinal cord.

meningitis (men in jī′tis). An inflammation of the membranes covering the spinal cord or brain.

metabolic (met ə bol′ik) (G. *meta*, beyond; *ballein*, to throw). Pertaining to the sum total of physical and chemical changes occurring in the body and the transformations by which energy is made available to the body.

metastasis (mə tas′tə sis) (G. *meta*, beyond, over; *stasis*, stand). The spread of disease from one part of the body to another not directly connected with it.

middle ear. The cavity that is interior to the tympanic membrane, includes the ossicles, and connects with the mastoid air cells and eustachian tube.

migraine headache (mī′grān) (G. *hemi*, half; *kranion*, skull). A type of periodically recurring headache, often confined to one side of the head.

mongolism (mon′gə lizm). A kind of congenital mental deficiency, accompanied by facial characteristics resembling those of Mongols. Also called *Down's syndrome.*

motor neuron (mō′tər nyoor′on) (L. *movere*, to move; G. *neuron*, nerve). A neuron carrying impulses from the brain or spinal cord to a muscle or gland.

multiple sclerosis (skla rō′sis) (L. *multiplex*, many folded; G. *sklerosis*, a hardening). A disease in which there is hardening in various portions of the nervous system.

myelin sheath (mī′ə lin) (G. *myelos*, marrow). The sheath of fatlike material around certain nerve fibers.

myopia (mī ō′pē ə) (G. *myein*, to shut; *ops*, eye). A visual defect in which near objects are seen more clearly than distant ones; *nearsightedness.*

nerve (nurv) (G. *neuron*, nerve). A cordlike bundle of nerve fibers surrounded by a protective sheath; carries impulses from one part of the body to another.

nerve fiber. An extension of the cell body of a neuron covered with one or more sheaths.

neurologist (nyoo rol′ə jist) (G. *neuron*, nerve; *logos*, word; *-istes*, one skilled in). An expert in the branch of medicine dealing with the nervous system, both normal and in disease.

neuron (nyoor'on) (G. *neuron,* nerve). A nerve cell, including its cell body and processes or fibers.

nucleus (nyoo'klē əs) (L. *nux,* a nut). A spherical body in most plant and animal cells necessary to growth and reproduction.

occipital lobe (ok sip'i-təl lōb) (L. *occiput,* back of head; G. *lobos,* lobe). The hindmost lobe of the cerebral cortex.

oculist (ok'yə list) (L. *oculus,* eye; G. *istes,* one skilled in). A physician specializing in the treatment of diseases of the eye. An *ophthalmologist.*

ophthalmologist (of thal mol'ə jist) (G. *ophthalmos,* the eye; *logos,* word; *-istes,* one skilled in). A specialist in the branch of medicine dealing with the structure, functions, and diseases of the eye. The old term was *oculist.*

optic nerve (op'tik nurv) (G. *optikos,* pertaining to the eye; *neuron,* nerve). The nerve that arises from the retina of the eye and connects it to the cerebrum.

optician (op tish'ən). A person who makes or sells eyeglasses.

optometrist (op tom'ə trist) (G. *opto-,* vision; *metron,* measure). An expert in the profession of testing the vision and fitting glasses to correct eye defects.

organ of Corti. The terminal portion of the cochlea, containing many auditory cells.

ossicles (os'i kəl[z]) (L. *ossiculum,* little bone). Any small bones. The *auditory ossicles* are the three tiny bones in the middle-ear cavity, the *malleus, incus,* and *stapes.*

otologist (ō tol'ə jist) (G. *otos,* ear). A physician specializing in the branch of medicine dealing with the ear and its diseases.

otosclerosis (ō'tə sklə rō'sis) (G. *otos,* ear; *sklerosis,* hardening). A condition characterized by chronic, progressive deafness. Caused by the formation of spongy bone around the oval window and stapes.

parasympathetic (par'ə sim pəthet'ik) (G. *para,* beyond; *syn,* with; *pathos,* suffering). A division of the autonomic nervous system in which fibers arise from the midbrain, medulla, or the sacral region of the spinal cord.

parietal lobe (pə rī'ə təl lōb) (L. *paries,* a wall; G. *lobos,* lobe). A lobe of the cerebral cortex located centrally between the frontal and occipital lobes and above the temporal lobe.

Parkinson's disease (pahr'kin sənz) (James Parkinson, English physician, 1755–1824). A chronic disease of the nervous system characterized by a fine, slowly spreading tremor, muscular weakness, and rigidity. Also called *shaking palsy.*

peripheral nervous system (pə rif'ə rəl) (G. *peri,* around; *pherein,* to bear). That division of the nervous system which includes the cranial and spinal nerves and their branches.

petit mal (pə tē' mahl) (Fr. *petit,* little; L. *malum,* ill). A minor form of epilepsy in which there may be a brief blackout of consciousness, and which may even go unnoticed by the victim or others.

pharynx (far'ingks) (G. *pharynx*). The pouchlike structure between the mouth and nasal passages and esophagus; the throat.

phenylalanine (fen'il al'ə nēn, fēn'il al'ə nēn). An amino acid found in protein foods.

phenylketonuria (fen'il kēt'ə nyoor'ē ə, fēn'il ket'ə nyoor'e ə). A congenital faulty metabolism of phenylalanine, resulting in the appearance of phenylpyruvic acid in the urine; if untreated, phenylketonuria usually brings on mental retardation. Sometimes called *PKU.*

pitch (pich). The quality of sound that enables one to classify it in a scale from high to low. It depends on the frequency of vibration.

presbyopia (prez"bē ō'pē ə) (G. *presbys,* old; *ops,* eye; *-ia,* a disease). A visual defect caused by the loss of ability to adjust the eye to varying distances; due to hardening of the crystalline lens.

psychomotor epilepsy (sī″kō mō′tər) (G. *psyche*, soul; L. *motor*, mover; G. *epilepsia*, seizure). A form of epilepsy characterized by purposeful motor and/or psychic activity which is irrelevant to the time and place. The patient is amnesic afterwards.

pupil (pyoo′pəl) (L. *pupilla*, girl). The opening at the center of the iris of the eye for the transmission of light.

receptor (ri sep′tər) (L. *recipere*, a receiver). A sense organ; a nerve ending specialized for the reception of stimuli.

reflex action (rē′fleks) (L. *reflexus*, bend back). A reflected action or movement; an action induced by the stimulation of a receptor and carried on without the intervention of the will.

refractive defect (ri frak′tiv) (L. *refringere*, to break apart; *agere*, to do). A defect in the ability of the eye to refract, or bend, light rays entering it, so that a distinct image on the retina is not formed.

retina (ret′ə nə) (L. *rete*, a net). The innermost layer of the eye, which is stimulated by light.

rod (rod) (AS. *rodd*, club). The sensitive element of the retina that perceives dark and light and generates visual impulses.

sclera (sklē′rə) (G. *skleros*, hard). The outer, tough, white layer of the eyeball, except the area of the cornea.

seizure (sē′zhər) (ME. *seizen*, to take possession of). An attack of epilepsy.

semicircular canal (sem′i sur′kyə lər kə nal′). (L. *semis*, half; *circularis*, a ring; *canalis*, a channel). Any of the three looped tubular structures of the inner ear that serve to maintain balance in the person.

sense organ (sens or′gən) (L. *sensus*; G. *organon*, an instrument). An organ that receives a stimulus and transforms it into a sensation.

sensory neuron (sen′sə rē nyoor′on) (L. *sensus*, sense; G. *neuron*, nerve). A neuron carrying impulses from the sense organs to the spinal cord and cerebral cortex.

spinal canal (spīn′əl kə nal′) (L. *spina*, a thorn; *canalis*, a channel). The passage surrounded by the vertebrae, which contains the spinal cord.

spinal cord (spīn′əl kord). That part of the central nervous system which is lodged in the spinal canal.

spinal nerve (spīn′əl nurv). Any peripheral nerve arising from the spinal cord and passing out through the vertebrae; arranged in thirty-one pairs.

stapes (stā′pēz) (L. *stapes*, stirrup). The innermost of the three ossicles of the middle ear. Also called the *stirrup*.

sympathetic nerve (sim pə thet′ik) (G. *syn*, with; *pathos*, suffering). A division of the autonomic nervous system in which fibers arise from the thoracic and lumbar regions of the spinal cord.

symptom (simp′təm) (G. *syn-*, together; *piptein*, to fall). Any functional evidence of a disease or of a patient's condition; a change in a person's condition which indicates a physical or mental change.

synapse (sin′aps) (G. *synapsis*, a connection). The region of contact between adjacent neurons, the junction where an impulse is transmitted from one neuron to another.

temporal lobe (tem′pər əl lōb) (L. *tempora*, the temples; G. *lobos*, lobe). A lobe of the cerebral cortex located laterally and below the frontal and occipital lobes.

tonometer (tō nom′i tər) (G. *tonos*, tension; *metron*, measure). An instrument used for measuring intraocular pressure.

trauma (trou′mə, traw′mə) (G. *trauma*, wound). A wound or injury.

tympanic membrane (tim pan′ik mem′brān) (L. *tympanum*, drum; *membrana*, membrane). The eardrum.

tyrosine (tī′rə sēn, tir′ə sin). An amino essential to the diet.

vertebral column (vur′tə brəl) (L. *vertebra*). The spinal column; bony column of vertebrae.

vitreous humor (vit′rē əs hyoo′mər) (L. *vitreus*, glassy; *humor*, fluid). The semi-fluid, transparent substance which lies between the lens and the retina of the eye.

white matter (hwīt mat′ər). White nervous tissue, composed mostly of myelinated nerve fibers; the conducting portion of the brain and spinal cord.

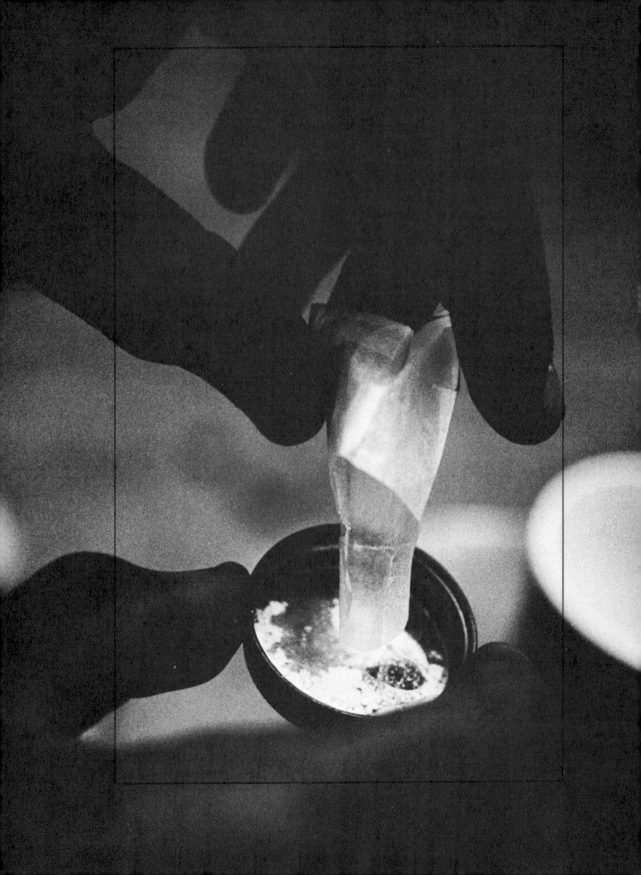

Use and abuse of drugs

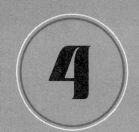

Society is experiencing dramatic changes in drug-abuse patterns. Historically, struggling segments of society have misused the depressant drugs, such as alcohol, barbiturates, and heroin, as escape mechanisms. But many of today's young people are abusing drugs of all kinds "just for kicks." They may be from the struggling or the affluent segments of society. They want not only the feelings of relief, euphoria, or being "stoned" that are produced by the depressant drugs, but also the "new experiences" or "highs" which, they feel, they are unable to obtain without the use of drugs. Many of them mix their drugs, a very dangerous habit.

Another significant change is the spread of drug abuse into age groups both younger and older than that in which most drug abuse was previously concentrated. Yet another is the added social element: the taking of drugs, except for alcohol, was once almost exclusively a solitary activity, but now drug use is often a social function, not unlike social drinking.

The following information is by no means complete, nor does it ensure an understanding of the rapidly changing drug scene, yet we feel that Chapters 4 and 5 contain the information needed for an individual to make meaningful decisions concerning drugs. Alcohol (see Chapter 5) is treated in its proper perspective—as a drug.

The principles and factual bases of drug abuse given herein reflect the authors' view of drug dependence: that it is a sign of deeper emotional and psychological problems in an individual, expressed through the abnormal social behavior characteristic of such an individual.

USE OF DRUGS

In the past twenty-five years scores of new drugs have been introduced to the general public. They have revolutionized the practice of medicine, in many ways bypassing natural law and overcoming death. But, like all revolutions, this one carries with it the risk of excesses—abuse.

Because of the development of the so-called "wonder drugs" many people have built up unrealistic expectations of what drugs can do for them. In fact, the people of the United States are, in general, "drug users." In their zealous search for miraculous cures, they often decide for themselves what drugs and what quantities of drugs are needed, instead of leaving this difficult and delicate decision of drug treatment where it belongs, in the hands of trained physicians and dentists. The authors of this book feel that some understanding of how drugs act and of what can be expected of them may help put the myth of "miracle drugs" into its proper perspective.

How drugs affect the body

The drugs used in our country are so numerous that it would be almost hopeless to attempt to study them without the aid of some system of grouping. Drugs may be classified in various ways: for example, according to their source, according to their chemical composition, according to their actions and effects, and according to their medical use. None of these classifications is entirely satisfactory, but probably the most useful for our purposes is that based on their actions and effects.

How drugs work   A drug may act on the surface of cells, within cells, or in the extracellular fluids of the body. In most cases the action is within a cell.

Drugs enter a cell in the same manner that normal body chemicals do, and usually because some part of their chemical structure is similar to that of normal chemicals. When similar to normal body chemicals, a drug enters a cell and participates in a few steps of the normal sequence of a cellular process. In this manner drugs may interfere with, alter, or replace chemicals of normal cellular life processes (hopefully for the betterment of the individual). Some of these actions seem relatively simple and easy to understand, some are exceedingly complex, and many are at present unknown.

Some drugs act to block a normal manufacturing process, a storage process, a releasing process, or a transport system. Other drugs exert their effects by altering cell-membrane function, either by reducing the membrane's permeability or increasing its permeability to specific substances. This often helps to carry drugs from the cell surface into its interior. Such obstructions or altering of normal biochemical sequences may lead to a piling up of usually insignificant products, which often produces stimulating effects. Some drugs chemically combine with the cell lipids (fats) and so cause a decreased oxygen concentration in the cell, which results in depressed cellular activity.

Major actions and effects of drugs   The present knowledge of the chemical structure of drugs enables scientists to predict what a drug will do and what the results will be. Drugs act on many parts of the body and in a number of different ways. Many act only at the site of application, which is usually on the skin or mucous membranes of the body; their action is said to be *local*. When a drug is absorbed into and distributed through the body, its action is said to be *systemic*. Drugs are most often absorbed and distributed by the blood stream. Systemic action may affect the whole body or it may be restricted to "target" organs within the body.

Terms that are used to describe the major actions and effects of drugs with systemic action are explained in the following paragraphs.

Stimulation is the action of a drug resulting in an increased activity of the cells. For example, caffeine is called a stimulant because it increases the activity of cells in the central nervous system. However, prolonged over-stimulation of cells often results in depression.

Depression is the action of a drug resulting in a decreased power of the cell to function. For example, narcotics depress the ability of the respiratory center to send out nerve impulses to the respiratory muscles, thereby reducing respiration.

Selective action is the ability of a drug to produce a greater effect on some tissue or organ than on others. For example, certain posterior-pituitary hormones have a highly selective action on the functioning of tubular cells of the kidney.

Therapeutic action is the action of a drug on diseased tissues or in a sick individual.

Side effect (*side action*) is any effect or action of a drug other than the one for which it is administered. This effect is not necessarily harmful. Morphine is often given to relieve pain, not for its ability to constrict the pupil of the eye; the constriction is a side effect.

Untoward effect (*untoward action*) is a side effect regarded as harmful to the individual. The action of morphine that results in nausea, vomiting, constipation, and addiction is undesirable and harmful; these are untoward effects.

Cumulative action is the action or effect that may be produced when drugs are excreted or destroyed more slowly than they are absorbed, so that they accumulate in the body. A sufficiently high concentration may be toxic.

Synergism, potentiation, and additive effects are ways in which drugs may work together. Some drugs that may have the same general effect when taken separately produce a much greater effect than the simple sum of the two when taken together. Such drugs are said to be *synergistic*. For example, a combination of barbiturates and alcohol produces an effect much greater than would the two drugs taken separately.

When two or more drugs are given together and their effects represent the action of one plus the action of the other (or others), their effects are said to be *additive*. For example, half a dose of one drug plus half a dose of a similarly acting drug may produce the additive effect of a full dose of either.

When two drugs are given together and one intensifies the action of the other, the one is said to *potentiate* the other. For example, when epinephrine is given with the local anesthetic procaine, it intensifies the effect of the procaine because it produces constriction of the blood vessels and holds the procaine in the area where its action is desired.

Antagonistic drugs are drugs that have opposite effects in the body; one drug is *antagonistic* if it produces temporary effects opposite to those of another drug. This antagonistic action is valuable in treating toxic overdoses or poisonings. Such is the action of some tranquilizers on relieving the effects of LSD.

Idiosyncrasy is any abnormal response of a person to a drug. Not only do different individuals have different reactions to a particular drug, but one individual may react differently at various times to the same drug. This is one of the major reasons why individuals should not prescribe drugs for themselves, use drugs that have been prescribed to treat previous conditions, or use drugs that have been prescribed for others.

Hypersensitivity is an allergic response to a drug. This means that at some time the individual was "sensitized" to a substance, and thereafter any small dose of the drug can produce an allergic reaction, which may vary from slight to severe.

Drug interactions When two drugs are taken together or within a few hours of each other they may interact, altering the expected action of either drug. These interactions occur between prescription drugs, between over-the-counter-drugs, and at times between drugs and foods. Because of the possibility of drug interactions your physician should always know the names of *all* drugs, both prescription and over-the-counter, that you are using at one time.

Drug dosages A dose of a drug is defined as the amount of drug which is given or taken at one time. The degree of response depends upon the effectiveness of the drug; see Fig. 4.1. The doses taken by an individual become an extremely important part of any study of drug abuse. A number of terms are used to describe the amount of a drug in a dose. *Minimal dose* is the smallest amount of a drug that will produce a therapeutic effect (amount needed to treat or heal). *Maximal dose* is the largest amount of a drug that will produce a desired therapeutic effect without any accompanying symptoms of toxicity. *Toxic dose* is the amount of a drug that produces untoward effects or symptoms of poisoning. *Abusive dose* is the amount needed to produce the side effects and actions desired by an individual abusing a drug; this is usually a toxic amount. *Lethal dose* is the amount of a drug that will cause death.

How drugs are administered

Drugs can be administered in a number of ways, and a physician makes the decision as to how to administer drugs on the basis of the effect he wishes to achieve. Figure 4.2 shows the routes of administration of drugs.

Most drugs are distributed throughout the body and delivered to the tissues by the bloodstream. Drugs can enter the bloodstream by being taken *orally* (by mouth) and then being absorbed from the digestive tract into the bloodstream. In general, when a choice of methods is possible, physicians prefer *oral administration*, because drugs taken orally assure a more gradual and sustained effect on the body, are less painful, less likely to produce adverse reactions, are safer than those administered by other methods, and a patient can take them at home by himself.

When a physician prescribes medicines to be taken orally, he usually specifies the time at which they should be taken. If he wants rapid action, he instructs the patient to take the drug before meals, so that the digestion of food will not interfere with the absorption of the drugs into the bloodstream. If the medicines might irritate the stomach or the doctor wants a more sustained action, he instructs the individual to take the drug after meals. Drugs that produce sleep or a sedative effect are, of course, taken at bedtime.

Drugs may be *inhaled* into the lungs and enter the bloodstream there. Inhalation of drugs may be used in the treatment of certain lung disorders or in the administration of an anesthetic.

Certain drugs must be administered by *injection* under the skin, into a muscle, or into a vein. Some medicines cannot be absorbed into the bloodstream through the digestive tract, some are irritating to it or to the lungs,

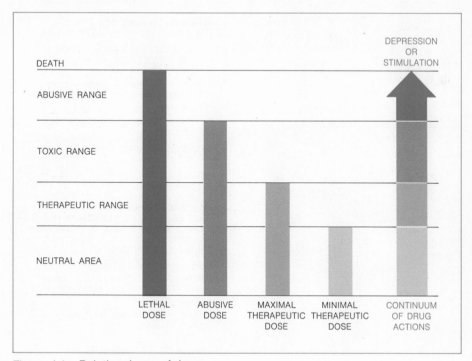

Figure 4.1   Relative doses of drugs.

and some drugs are destroyed by the gastric acid of the stomach. An injection also is used when a particularly large dose is to be given or when rapid action is desirable.

In addition to dosage the physician's directions indicate both when and for what length of time a medicine should be taken. These directions are intended to safeguard the patient from needlessly treating himself after his

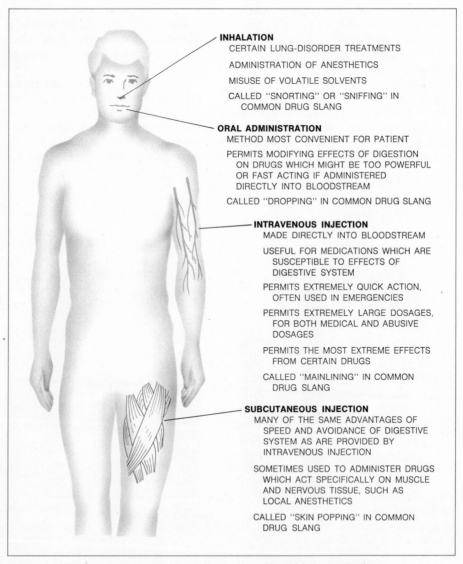

INHALATION
CERTAIN LUNG-DISORDER TREATMENTS

ADMINISTRATION OF ANESTHETICS

MISUSE OF VOLATILE SOLVENTS

CALLED "SNORTING" OR "SNIFFING" IN
COMMON DRUG SLANG

ORAL ADMINISTRATION
METHOD MOST CONVENIENT FOR PATIENT

PERMITS MODIFYING EFFECTS OF DIGESTION
ON DRUGS WHICH MIGHT BE TOO POWERFUL
OR FAST ACTING IF ADMINISTERED
DIRECTLY INTO BLOODSTREAM

CALLED "DROPPING" IN COMMON DRUG SLANG

INTRAVENOUS INJECTION
MADE DIRECTLY INTO BLOODSTREAM

USEFUL FOR MEDICATIONS WHICH ARE
SUSCEPTIBLE TO EFFECTS OF
DIGESTIVE SYSTEM

PERMITS EXTREMELY QUICK ACTION,
OFTEN USED IN EMERGENCIES

PERMITS EXTREMELY LARGE DOSAGES,
FOR BOTH MEDICAL AND ABUSIVE
DOSAGES

PERMITS THE MOST EXTREME EFFECTS
FROM CERTAIN DRUGS

CALLED "MAINLINING" IN COMMON
DRUG SLANG

SUBCUTANEOUS INJECTION
MANY OF THE SAME ADVANTAGES OF
SPEED AND AVOIDANCE OF DIGESTIVE
SYSTEM AS ARE PROVIDED BY
INTRAVENOUS INJECTION

SOMETIMES USED TO ADMINISTER DRUGS
WHICH ACT SPECIFICALLY ON MUSCLE
AND NERVOUS TISSUE, SUCH AS
LOCAL ANESTHETICS

CALLED "SKIN POPPING" IN COMMON
DRUG SLANG

Figure 4.2   The various ways drugs may be introduced into the body.

illness has been brought under control or from prematurely stopping a drug because he thinks he is well.

Treatment of diseases and conditions

A person seeking relief from an illness may understandably respond with impatience and resentment toward a doctor who does not seem to be doing anything to cure him. He may feel that his visit is a waste of time unless he walks out of the doctor's office with a prescription in his hand. However, in many cases the prescribing of drugs is exactly what should *not* be done. A physician should not prescribe until he knows what he is treating, and the process of making a diagnosis may take time. If drugs are prescribed too quickly, they may temporarily relieve the symptoms and mislead both patient and doctor into thinking the illness has been cured, or they may interfere with the diagnostic procedures being used by the physician. Sometimes the physician does not prescribe drugs because he knows the disorder will correct itself without treatment or because another form of treatment would be more effective. In some cases he does nothing other than provide reassurance.

The benefits to be derived from drugs prescribed by a physician and taken in accordance with his instructions far outweigh the possible risks involved in their use. Since the chemistry of the body is subtle and variable, only a physician should have the responsibility of prescribing and directing the use of drugs in the treatment of illnesses.

A person can help himself and assist his doctor by taking drugs only in the amounts and at the times prescribed, by reporting to his doctor any adverse reaction he has to a drug, by being as skeptical as his physician is about new drugs until they have been thoroughly tested, by not treating his own illnesses on the basis of what he reads, sees on television, or hears from the neighbors, and by not taking drugs that have been prescribed for others.

Definitions of drug abuse

To the general public a drug is a "medicine" or a substance used in the treatment of a disease. However, a more complete or scientific definition of a drug is *any substance, other than food, which alters the body or its functions*. The public is familiar with many drugs and their uses—for example, the antibiotics used in the treatment of bacterial infections and narcotics used in relieving pain.

Equally well known is that the actions and effects of all drugs are not alike. Some are rather mild in effect and relatively harmless; others are severe in effect and can be extremely dangerous if not taken exactly as prescribed by a physician. Some drugs, such as LSD, are considered so dangerous that laws have been passed to prohibit their use except in research projects. Other drugs, such as marijuana, have no valid medical use and are sufficiently dangerous when misused to be legally prohibited. No drug is considered safe for the public to use without a prescription, if its effects are a potential hazard to the person using it.

Forms of drug dependence

With the repeated consumption of any mood-modifying or behavior-changing drug a person will develop a *drug dependence*. The intensity of this dependence varies with the individual, with the motivation behind the abuse, and the physical (biochemical) properties of the drug. Drug dependence and continued abuse produce both physical and psychological effects detrimental to the individual and to society.

Researchers in the field of drugs have traditionally attempted to distinguish forms of drug dependence according to the nature of the drug used. In the past drugs have been classified as *addicting, habituating,* or *habit-forming.* These terms may be useful in describing the effects of certain drugs, but when one considers the individual, it is the drug dependence itself, whatever form it takes, that is significant. Habituation and addiction have been redefined in the hope that they may serve the needs, not only of science and medicine, but also of law and society.

The definitions of habituation and addiction most often quoted today are those of the Expert Committee on Addiction-Producing Drugs of the World Health Organization; these are given in Table 4.1.

Habituation The physical properties of a habituating drug must be considered. Habituating drugs do not produce physical dependence or specific withdrawal symptoms (abstinence syndrome) when a person suddenly stops using them. Habituating drugs may or may not produce a tendency to increase the dosage (tolerance) for the desired euphoric, mood-modifying, or behavior-changing effects. Persons abusing habituating drugs are called "drug users" or

Table 4.1 *Definitions of addiction and habituation according to the Expert Committee on Addiction-Producing Drugs of the World Health Organization*

drug addiction	drug habituation
Drug addiction is a state of periodic or chronic intoxication produced by the repeated consumption of a drug (natural or synthetic).	Drug habituation is a condition resulting from the repeated consumption of a drug.
Characteristics:	Characteristics:
1. An overpowering desire or need (compulsion) to continue taking the drug and to obtain it by any means.	1. A desire (but not a compulsion) to continue taking the drug for the sense of improved well-being or effect it produces.
2. A tendency to increase the dose (reaction to tolerance).	2. Little or no tendency to increase the dose (tolerance).
3. A psychic (psychological) and generally a physical dependence on the effects of the drug.	3. Some degree of psychic dependence on the effect of the drug, but absence of physical dependence and hence of abstinence syndrome.
4. Abstinence syndrome of a specific type.	4. Detrimental effects, if any, primarily on the individual.
5. A detrimental effect on the individual and on society.	

"users" in the medical profession. For definitions of some of these terms, see below.

Addiction   Besides psychological dependence, some drugs evoke biochemical and physiological adaptations in the user known as *tolerance* and *physical dependence.*

Tolerance is a fundamental survival mechanism within the body: it permits body cells to be exposed continuously to toxic substances and toxic doses without evoking dangerous (or deadly) responses. Drug tolerance is such a phenomenon. As cells become accustomed to successive doses of a drug, similar amounts of the drug have less and less effect. Thus a person must increase his doses to procure a desired response in himself.

With repeated administration of increasing doses of certain drugs the brain (central nervous system) and other organs are exposed to concentrations of the drug that often bring about a *physical dependence* within the body cells—that is, the drug must be present for the cells to continue functioning in a way similar to the way they functioned before the drug was first introduced into the body. This physical dependence is revealed when sudden withdrawal of the drug brings about an illness, an *abstinence syndrome*, as the cells of the body try to return to normal. The symptoms of withdrawal from certain solvents, opiates, and opium derivatives include irritability, depression, extreme nervousness, pain in the abdomen, and nausea, all of which may be mild or severe; this is called the *narcotic-solvent abstinence syndrome.* The sudden withdrawal from alcohol of a person physically addicted may cause delirium tremens and, from barbiturates, convulsions, delirium tremens, and frequently death; this is called the *alcohol-barbiturate abstinence syndrome.*

The terms *addict* and *user* can be ambiguous. We usually say "addict" to describe someone who is dependent upon the addicting drugs such as opium and its derivatives, synthetic narcotics, barbiturates, alcohol, and solvents. We say "user" for one who is habituated to cocaine, amphetamines, marijuana, LSD, or other hallucinogenic drugs.

Habit-forming drugs   The term "habit-forming" has grown up with the legitimate medical use of drugs and the control of drug manufacture. A drug with the potential of becoming either habituating or addicting on continued use is described as habit-forming. Drug manufacturers are required to so label any drug having this potential.

Abuse of drugs that modify mood and behavior

The use of drugs in medical practice is accepted as legitimate, but the use for purposes other than those intended in medicine is abuse. Abuse is usually associated with drug dosages (abusive doses) many times in excess of those in legitimate medical practice. *When a drug is self-administered in toxic dosages and damages an individual, a society, or both, the drug is being abused.*

As mentioned earlier, in all cases of repeated abuse of a drug or substances containing drugs an individual develops a dependency either upon the effects of the drug or the social patterns associated with its abuse. Some drugs, such as nicotine in tobacco and caffeine in coffee and tea produce dependence in the user but are *socially acceptable* because they do not produce other effects, such as euphoria (an artificial, exaggerated sense of pleasure and well-being) or drastic mood-modifying effects. Alcohol usually produces such effects to some degree when taken in moderate amounts, but its use is still socially accepted. Drugs that consistently produce effects such as these to a marked degree also have the ability to change the general behavior of an individual.

Drugs considered "dangerous" and "unacceptable to society," when used for other than legitimate medical purposes, create problems within society by causing personality changes, euphoria, or abnormal social behavior. Such drugs include narcotics, solvents, hypnotics, sedatives, tranquilizers, alcohol, cannabinols, hallucinogens, cocaine, and amphetamines. They may be called "mood modifiers," "psychotropic drugs," or "psychotoxic drugs." These terms point out the effects of a drug and are not a type of classification. Mood-modifying drugs, no matter how they are classified (as stimulant, depressant, or hallucinogenic), are always associated with an abnormal personality. Whether this personality distortion is the cause or the result of the drug abuse is not known. The abnormal social behavior and modification of moods in such individuals is more of a problem to society than is the drug abuse itself, which is mainly the individual's problem.

In all cases of repeated drug abuse the person who misuses such drugs voluntarily chooses to do so. Once started, his abuse will lead to drug dependence and may well lead to drug habituation or drug addiction according to the physical properties (such as tolerance) of the drug being abused. On the other hand, the person who does not find a pleasurable experience in drug abuse or who is subject to strong social pressures when first experimenting with a drug does not usually continue to abuse drugs—that is, his personality does not lack, or seek, what the drug has to offer, and he therefore tends to reject it.

PHYSICAL ASPECTS OF DRUG ABUSE

Today much of the research into the abuse of drugs is concerned with biochemical actions. Researchers are attempting to establish the chemical characteristics of drugs that are responsible for the mood-, personality-, behavior-modifying, or mind-changing (psychotropic) actions of specific drugs. They are also trying to establish the immediate and long-range damage to the body. In this section we examine the drugs that affect the nervous system and have a potential for being abused by producing personality changes, euphoria, or abnormal social behavior.

Drug-induced effects on the nervous system

The actions of drugs upon the nervous system are what cause the personality changes, euphoria, or abnormal social behavior associated with drug abuse.

Such terms describe the outward signs arising from drug-induced changes on the nervous system and form the usual drug classification used when one is talking about drug abuse. The overall actions and effects of these drugs are mainly those of either a *stimulant* or *depressant*, acting directly upon the nervous system to increase or decrease the activity of nerve centers and their conducting pathways.

A nervous-system stimulant is defined as a drug that temporarily increases body function or nerve activity. At times stimulant drugs produce dramatic effects, but their medical usefulness is limited because of the complexity of their reactions and the nature of their untoward effects. Furthermore, repeated administration or excessive doses may produce convulsive seizures alternating with periods of depression ranging from exhaustion to coma.

Depressants have the ability to temporarily decrease a body function or nerve activity. Drug-induced depression of the nervous system is frequently characterized by lack of interest in surroundings, inability to focus attention on a subject, and lack of motivation to move or talk. The pulse and respiration become slower than usual and, as the depression deepens, sensory perceptions diminish progressively. Psychic and motor activities decrease; reflexes become sluggish and finally disappear. If a stronger depressant drug is used, or if larger (abusive) doses are consumed, the depression progresses to drowsiness, stupor, unconsciousness, sleep, coma, respiratory failure, and death.

Drugs that act on the nervous system do not act on all parts of it (see Chapter 3) with the same degree of intensity. Also, the specific response of an individual to a specific drug depends to a large extent on the personality of the individual and a number of social factors, as well as the nature of the drug itself.

Spectrum and continuum of drug action

The degrees of depression and stimulation of drugs affecting the nervous system are not discrete. As shown in Fig. 4.3, the spectrum of drug actions can be set into a continuum of effects and actions on the central nervous system. The construction of this continuum is an attempt to present them in an orderly and understandable manner. It was devised by Robert W. Earle, Ph.D., Senior Lecturer, Department of Medical Pharmacology and Therapeutics, University of California, Irvine, California. The continuum extends from an overstimulation of the nervous system to death, at the one extreme, to a severe depression of the nervous system resulting in death at the other extreme. The central or neutral area of this continuum is the degree of stimulation and depression usually encountered in everyday living. The drug groups are placed on the continuum according to the actions or effects they produce when normal therapeutic (minimal) doses are consumed by an individual. The action of a drug used for this classification or grouping is called its *major action*. Drugs in different groups may have similar untoward effects even when their major actions differ. For example, narcotics are used to relieve pain (major action), but they may also cause a person to be drowsy or sleepy

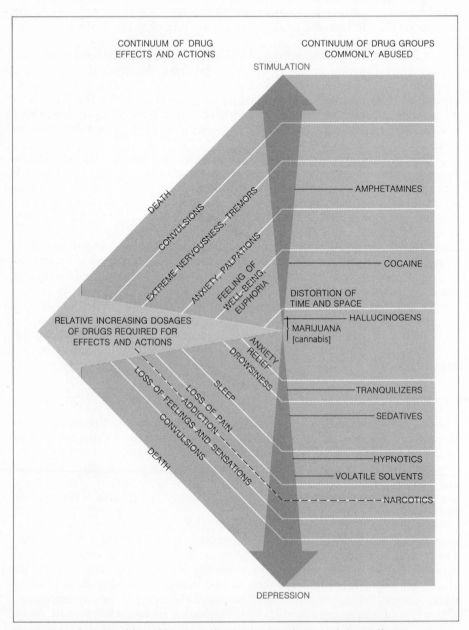

Figure 4.3   Relationships of increased doses to continuum of drug effects. As doses of drugs are increased, the effects progress along a continuum of effects until a lethal dose, producing death, is taken.

(side action). Barbiturates are used for their ability to produce sleep (major action), but they do not have the ability to relieve pain and cannot be used as a narcotic. Thus the sleep-producing effects of these two depressants, narcotics and barbiturates, overlap on the continuum; see Fig. 4.4. All drugs that affect the nervous system have similar properties. Along the chart from the neutral area specific points show where the area of one group of drugs, in terms of an action, overlaps the area of a more powerful group. The weakest groups end nearest the center; the most powerful, at the two extremes.

If doses are increased from minimal, to maximal, to toxic, to abusive, to lethal, any drug group is able to cover the complete range of effects of stimulation on the one hand or depression on the other. Overstimulation or extreme depression produces the effects the drug abuser is seeking. Consequently, the doses taken by abusers are far in excess of those normally used in medical practice. A complete range of effects, produced by increased dosages, also is presented in Fig. 4.3.

Drugs may be arranged on such a continuum because the effects a person is seeking, when abusing drugs, are extremely similar. For example, any of these drugs will produce hallucinations at some dosage. This is why individuals, while preferring one drug over another, will abuse any drug within these groups if it becomes available. As the specific actions of a drug become more familiar and less spectacular, the individual may experiment with new ways to use the drug. He may progress from taking the drug orally to injecting it under the skin or into a muscle ("skin popping") to injecting it directly into a vein ("mainlining"). Or he may seek stronger and stronger drugs to produce more vivid effects, quicker actions, or longer-lasting experiences. Very few drug abusers are satisfied with experiences from just one drug. Most often they will move toward the extremes of the continuum. If the first drug abused was from a group near the center of the continuum, and it did not produce the "high" he wanted, he would either increase the dosage or experiment with stronger drugs up or down the continuum. Such individuals seldom experiment with less potent drugs after this.

The more commonly abused drugs, such as marijuana and the barbiturates, are close to the center of the chart when used in minimal dosages. The strong preference for these drugs lies in the abilities of an individual to control the amount and consequently the relative effect of the drug. In a highly emotional state a user is able to increase the dosage or consume more of the drug to reach a more intense effect. If he is less emotionally distressed at the time of abuse, he often is content with a reduced consumption and effect. This ability to control drugs is offset when addiction levels (Fig. 4.3) are reached with depressant drugs. At addiction levels the dose must be increased regularly to keep the body from entering withdrawal. This increasing dose is needed to keep the person at his normal or neutral level, regardless of his emotional state. Thus he has built himself into a constantly changing artificial continuum of effects. The minimal dose must be used daily to maintain a neutral level, and then additional abusive dosages are needed to reach the levels of effects to satisfy his emotional states.

When abusing stimulant drugs, which do not have the addictive properties of depressant drugs, an individual may not progress from a relatively

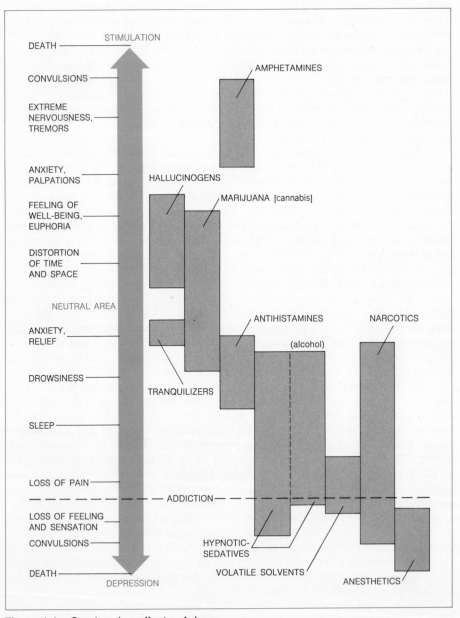

Figure 4.4   Overlapping effects of drugs.

mild drug such as marijuana, because he is better able to control the effects by controlling the amounts consumed. However, some who start on weaker drugs do progress to stronger ones because of the slight differences in the quality or intensity of effect.

The drugs within each group differ slightly in their effects. This is why different drugs are used for different therapeutic uses. The differing effects are regulated by the areas or routes of action within the nervous system. All either stimulate or depress the functions of the cells, tissues, or organs. For instance, caffeine stimulates the function of nerve cells, and barbiturates depress it. Because of the complexity of the body organization a drug action is often complex. The complexity at times makes it extremely difficult to place a group of drugs on a progressive continuum chart. This is more of a problem with the stimulant drugs than with the depressant drugs. Also, at times the complexity of actions leads to apparent paradoxes. For example, if alcohol is a depressor of nerve function, why do people seem stimulated by a small amount of alcohol? The answer is that the brain contains a group of cells whose function is inhibition—cells that normally keep us from acting irresponsibly on every passing impulse. These inhibitory cells are more sensitive to alcohol and similar drugs (such as barbiturates and solvents) than are the other brain cells. As the alcohol concentration in the blood begins to rise, the inhibitory cells are depressed and cease to function properly, so that many impulses that would otherwise be suppressed are acted upon. Therefore, moderate amounts of alcohol, a depressant drug, can cause excitation by depressing an inhibitory function.

The following is the general classification or groupings of the commonly abused drugs based on the continuum of actions associated with their use. The classes to be discussed are narcotics, volatile solvents, hypnotic-sedatives, tranquilizers, marijuana, hallucinogens, and amphetamines. The position and relative depression or stimulation abilities of each group can be obtained by referring to Fig. 4.3.

MOST COMMONLY ABUSED DRUGS

The indiscriminate or excessive use of drugs of various kinds and for various purposes is a matter of grave concern to the public, the medical world, and the private citizen. This section deals with a number of drugs in some detail, under the headings Narcotics, Volatile Solvents, Hypnotic-sedatives, Antihistamines, Tranquilizers, Cannabinol, Hallucinogenics, Cocaine, and Amphetamines. The classification is based on the continuum of actions associated with their use.

Narcotics

The most widely abused drugs throughout the world are the so-called narcotics. The noun *narcotic* comes from a Greek word meaning "to benumb" and is defined here (see the Glossary) as "having the power to produce sleep or drowsiness and to relieve pain." The word in recent years has been used in at least three senses: (1) a central-nervous-system depressant producing a marked reduction in pain, (2) an addicting drug, and (3) any drug that comes under the restriction of the federal narcotics law, the Harrison Narcotics Act.

In this section we describe, for convenience, only the opiates and certain synthetic narcotics as the more well-known "narcotics."

Effects of narcotics   The narcotics are chiefly used for their ability to produce a marked insensibility to pain without producing excessive drowsiness, muscular weakness, confusion, or loss of consciousness, such as happens with anesthetics. Narcotics cannot be used in place of an anesthetic, because in doses large enough to produce a loss of sensation they depress the respiratory center in the brain to a degree that can result in death.

All narcotics have features in common, differing mainly in the degree to which the actions or effects are produced. The general action on the nervous system is one of depression. (Narcotics are also paradoxical in that they produce nausea and vomiting by stimulation of areas in the brain.) Their major depressant actions include *analgesia* (relief of pain) and *sedation* (freeing the mind of anxiety and calming the emotions). These depressant actions lead to the principal use of narcotics in medicine—which is to produce marked analgesia without excessive drowsiness, muscular weakness, confusion, or loss of consciousness.

When abusive doses (see Fig. 4.1) of a narcotic are used, during depression of the nervous system there is an elevation of mood, *euphoria* (an exaggerated sense of well-being and contentment), relief from fear and apprehension, and feelings of peace and tranquility. This intense euphoric, contented state is usually considered the main reason for the abuse of narcotics. After a short period of time this state passes, and the individual becomes apathetic, with a slowing of both mental and physical activities, terminating in sleep.

Recognition of the narcotics user   Abuse of these drugs produces all of the classic symptoms of drug addiction (see Table 4.1), and a *compulsive user* is clearly within the classification of an addict. Recognition of narcotics users, especially when they are regularly obtaining a daily dosage, is extremely difficult. Users will not reveal their condition, and experience makes them very adept at disguising it.

Abusive doses of narcotics, before much tolerance has developed, produce constriction of the pupils of the eyes, as shown in Fig. 4.5. The pupils, constricted to a pinpoint condition, do not react to light—that is, the pupil will not constrict in strong light (even when flashed directly into the eyes) or dilate in weak light (such as when a bright light is quickly pulled away). This condition of the eyes is termed "frozen." After tolerance to a narcotic has developed to some degree, pupillary constriction may not be so pronounced, but the reduced ability to react to light remains the same. When addicted individuals have been without a dose of narcotics for a period of time (from 4 to 6 hours or overnight), they begin to enter withdrawal, in which the pupils of the eyes become dilated but maintain the sluggish reaction to light.

Long-term addicts tend to be pale and emaciated and to suffer from severe constipation. Their appetites are poor, and they show little or no interest in sex. While under the influence of a narcotic, after the initial "flash" of euphoria, they are not particularly dangerous. However, they suffer periods of extreme discomfort if their injections are not taken three or four times daily just to keep from going into withdrawals. Thus, if deprived of their regular and necessary supply of narcotics, they must steal to obtain money for drugs. A heroin addiction can cost up to $75 or more a day. New York City has found that a large proportion of its crime can be traced to heroin

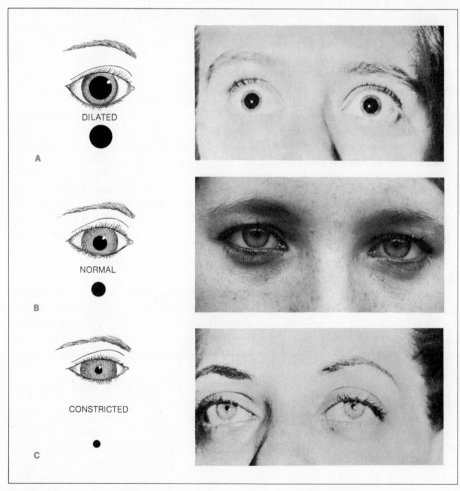

Figure 4.5   Pupil reactions: (A) dilated pupil reaction to a stimulant drug; (B) normal pupil reaction in light of average intensity; (C) contracted pupil reaction to a depressant drug.

addicts. The offenses consist mainly of burglary, shoplifting, prostitution, and other petty offenses related to the addict's need for money.

Administration of narcotics Someone abusing narcotics usually will administer them to himself by injection (Fig. 4.2). Early in the use of narcotics he may "skin pop," that is, inject them under the skin or into a muscle. A "skin pop" gives too slow an action for the confirmed addict, so he resorts to taking intravenous injections, which give the desired effect immediately. This type of injection is known as a "mainline" or "fix."

Because of fear, haste, and a general disregard for themselves, narcotics users, and drug users in general, are not careful about sterilizing their equipment. As a result, infections and diseases such as syphilis and hepatitis can be passed on to other people using the same injecting equipment as an infected individual.

Drugs classified as narcotics The drugs treated below are the more well known of the central-nervous-system depressants that are addictive and of express social concern today.

· OPIUM The drug opium is the dried juice obtained from the Oriental poppy, *Papaver somniferum;* see Fig. 4.6. The fragile red, white, or purple flowering plant grows best in hot, dry climates or in areas with seasonal rainfalls, such as are found in India, Turkey, Egypt, southern Asia, Mexico, and certain parts of Russia and China.

Opium has a bitter taste and a heavy, sweet odor. When it is being smoked, the odor is similar to that of wet, smoldering eucalyptus wood. Opium is generally smoked in a pipe or eaten. American drug users seldom use opium in its raw state, but they do use its derivatives.

· MORPHINE Morphine is the chief derivative of opium. It is produced by the chemical refinement of opium. It may be pure white, light brown, or off-white in color. It may be in the form of a cube, capsule, tablet, powder, or solution. On the illegal market morphine that comes in a gelatin capsule is known as a "cap." The powder folded into a paper square is known as a "paper" or "package."

Unlike heroin, very little morphine is sold by dealers. When morphine is unlawfully possessed, it usually has been stolen from a physician or pharmacist or obtained by means of forgery on a prescription form stolen from a physician.

Some morphine users "skin pop." Again, this type of "shot" gives too slow an action for the confirmed user, who resorts to "mainlining."

· HEROIN Heroin is produced from morphine. In the pure state it is a grayish-brown powder. Because of its great strength the dealer is able to dilute it many times with milk sugar (lactose) and still deliver a potent drug to the user. Consequently, heroin is "cut" in this manner and loses its grayish-brown color, becoming white or off-white, greatly resembling morphine. The legally seized heroin in the United States often is only 4, 3, or even 1 percent or less in purity. Heroin is odorless and has a distinctly bitter flavor.

The wholesale peddler sells heroin by the kilogram or in one-ounce or smaller plastic bags. The retailers or dealers handle it in "bags" or "papers" (folded squares) and in clear or red capsules.

If the heroin is of high quality, such as that sold outside the United States, drug users may introduce it into their bodies through the membranes of the nose by "sniffing" or "snorting" or through the lungs by mixing the heroin with tobacco or marijuana and smoking it (Fig. 4.2). These two routes of administration do not produce tolerance as quickly as when the heroin is injected. In the United States a beginner may "snort" but, because of the poor quality of the heroin, he is soon forced to inject it, to obtain the "kick" he is looking for. Usually addicts begin by injecting it into the fleshy parts of the arm or body, but their rapidly mounting tolerance necessitates injection directly into the veins for the desired euphoric effects. At this point the addict is referred to as a "mainliner."

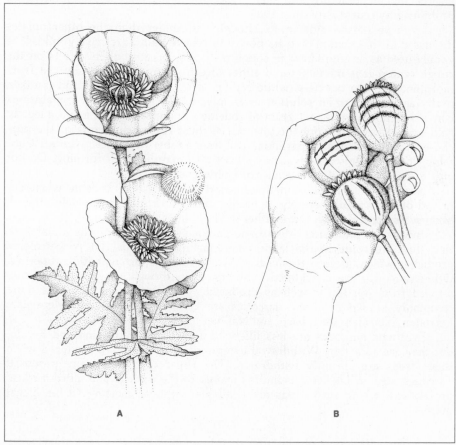

A   B

Figure 4.6   Oriental opium poppy, *Papaver somniferum:* (A) the flower; (B) the capsules, or pods, of the poppy flower, cut to release the opium juice.

A standard hypodermic needle attached to a syringe or common medicine dropper may be used. When a needle is not available, the drug may be forced into the body by opening a blood vessel with a pin or razor blade and administering the heroin directly with the medicine dropper. The equipment needed to inject heroin is termed an "outfit." With constant injection the blood vessels break down, and scars form over the veins, causing the addict to seek new areas for injection, until the entire lengths of the arms are marked by needle punctures. Prolonged addiction results in the necessity to inject between the fingers, in the legs and the neck, above the hairline, inside the mouth or anywhere else on the body.

The danger of addiction to heroin is great because the body's tolerance to the drug builds so rapidly. The addict requires increasingly larger doses within a short time in order to secure the euphoric effects. Addicts prefer heroin to morphine and take morphine only when they cannot obtain heroin.

Legally, heroin is considered extremely dangerous, and, because of its effects, the manufacture and sale of heroin in the United States has been prohibited by federal law since 1922.

· CODEINE (METHYLMORPHINE) Codeine is milder than the other opiates discussed in this section, and its power to relieve pain is relatively mild. It is widely used as an ingredient in cough medicines because of its effects on the cough center. It is manufactured either directly from opium or derived from morphine. It is an odorless, white crystal or crystalline powder and is taken orally as a tablet or in solution or is injected. In many states preparations containing not more than 1 grain of codeine per ounce of fluid may be legally sold over the counter, but the pharmacist must record the name of the purchaser. In some states preparations will bear a label with these words, "Contains Codeine (Opium derivation). WARNING—may be habit-forming. Do not give to children except upon advice of a physician."

Narcotics users will sometimes resort to the use of codeine when deprived of their regular supply of heroin. But the drug is not widely abused, because its euphoric effects are rather mild.

· SYNTHETIC NARCOTICS Synthetic narcotics differ from the opiates in that they are made in the laboratory, starting with coal tar or petroleum products, which, before chemical conversion, have no narcotic properties. Other narcotics are considered synthetic even though they are chemically dervied from opiates as well as produced synthetically. Some of the more commonly known synthetic narcotics are Demerol, methadone, Mepergan, Percodan, Nucodan, Percobarb, and Nalline.

Synthetic narcotics are less likely to addict than morphine and heroin, but they are addictive. Withdrawal symptoms in the user are produced when these drugs are abruptly withdrawn. The abuse of synthetically produced narcotics, such as Demerol, is limited mainly to the medical and allied medical professions, where such drugs are available without resorting to the illegal market.

Volatile solvents

Some volatile (easily vaporized) chemicals, when inhaled, produce a state of intoxication that is characterized by drowsiness, dizziness, a slurring of speech, the loss of consciousness, and often hallucinations. These chemicals are usually the solvents (chemicals capable of dissolving something) contained in lighter fluid, paint thinner, cleaning fluid, gasoline, and model-airplane glue.

Several dangerous solvents are used in the manufacture of "airplane glue" and other cements. The most common are isoamyl acetate and ethyl acetate. Other dangerous solvents used are benzine, toluene (synonym: toluol), and carbon tetrachloride. Prolonged inhalation of any of these solvents may cause death. The labels on many of the fluids containing solvents have the warning "Use only in a well-ventilated, open area." The hydrocarbons in gasoline—such as butane, hexane, and pentane—also cause solvent intoxication when inhaled. Probably the most commonly abused are the airplane cements containing the solvent toluene.

Solvents have a depressant action on the central nervous system similar to barbiturates and narcotics. They are placed between the hypnotic-sedative drugs and the narcotics on the continuum of drugs (Fig. 4.4).

The toxic effects of solvents have been carefully observed. They include irritation (producing cellular death) of the mucous membranes, skin, and the respiratory tract; cellular injury to the heart, liver, and kidneys; and bone-marrow depression, which results in anemia (reduction in red blood cells), leukopenia (reduction in white blood cells), and thrombocytopenia (reduction in platelets in the blood). There have also been reports of brain-tissue deterioration, acute liver damage, and kidney failures; many deaths have occurred after repeated daily use of solvents.

In the beginning stage of solvent sniffing a few whiffs of the vapors will produce a "jag." But, since tolerance to the solvents develops very rapidly, the habitual user must inhale the contents of many tubes of glue in order to experience the desired effects. By this time, many authorities feel, he has acquired an addiction to the solvents.

The effect is one of pleasantness, cheerfulness, euphoria, and excitement, closely simulating the early stages of alcohol intoxication. The abuser acts drunk, exhibits disorientation, and has slurred speech. This period of drunkenness continues for half or three-quarters of an hour after inhalation. Then he may become drowsy, lapse into a stupor, or become unconscious. He may remain unconscious for as long as an hour or more.

An addicted glue-sniffer often has a characteristic unpleasant odor to his breath and excessive salivation. His salivary secretions result from the solvent vapors' irritation of the mucous membranes of his nose and mouth. This irritation requires him to make frequent expectorations. He also suffers from insomnia, nausea, and weight loss.

The strong drug dependence, the psychotoxic effects (during administration), the strong tolerance developed, and the necessity to increase the dose characterize the solvents in abusive dosages as addicting drugs.

Hypnotic-sedative drugs

The hypnotic-sedative drugs are classified together because of their ability to depress the central nervous system into a condition resembling normal sleep. Drugs in this group are mainly general nervous-system depressants and are characterized by their broad range of suppression of brain functions. All these drugs resemble each other in this action in spite of their chemical differences.

The only difference between a hypnotic action and a sedative action is the degree of depression. The hypnotic action is a stronger depression of the nervous system. When a drug of this group is given in a moderate or a maximal therapeutic dose, producing sleep soon after administration, it is known as a *hypnotic*. When it is given in less or minimal doses, even several times a day, to reduce excitement, it is called a *sedative*. With increasing dosages, all drugs in this group tend to produce a continuum of effects from tranquilization and sedation (the allaying of excitement or quieting) to the loss of psychomotor and intellectual efficiency, to artificial sleep, and then to coma and death. When abused (in toxic dosages), these agents greatly reduce anxiety and produce a mild euphoria as a relief for people who tend to live in an uncomfortable, painful, or hyperaroused state.

Bromides The bromides exert a sedative effect on the nervous system. They were once widely utilized in medicine and by the general public. But with the development of much more effective sedatives (the barbiturates) and with the growing recognition of the dangers of chronic bromide intoxication and of the cumulative action of the drugs, the modern physician finds few uses for them. They are still important to a drug study, however, because of the problems of bromide intoxication and poisoning.

The administration of *sodium bromide* or other bromide salts produces sedation, drowsiness, and sleep. Chronic administration of a bromide tends to produce mental depression, confusion, and lethargy. Many persons with bromide intoxication may be suspected of suffering from emotional disorders; in fact, some have been admitted to mental hospitals when the toxic nature of the symptoms was not recognized. In bromide intoxication various skin lesions, intestinal disturbances, and destruction of the membranes of the eyes and respiratory passages are common.

Bromides, although capable of inducing physical dependence, are rarely abused, because they produce no euphoria. They are highly dangerous because of their extreme toxicity.

Alcohol and alcohol derivatives For thousands of years the only sleep-producing drugs that were available were alcohol, opium, and belladonna (a highly toxic drug extracted from *Atropa belladonna,* "deadly nightshade," a plant found in Europe and Asia).

The oldest hypnotic-sedatives used in modern medicine are alcohol and its major derivatives. The first drug derived from alcohol was *chloral hydrate,* used as a sleep-inducing drug since 1869. The next important hypnotic was another kind of alcohol derivative called *paraldehyde,* introduced into medicine in 1882.

Alcohol, when consumed in abusive amounts, is truly addictive, and the sudden withdrawal of alcohol from an addicted person produces serious disturbances. These may vary from a craving for alcohol, anxiety, and tremors to full-blown delirium tremens. Although some psychiatrists believe that delirium tremens is a form of acute toxic psychosis, many experts in the field of alcoholism or alcohol addiction regard it as an "alcohol-barbiturate withdrawal syndrome."

The abuse of alcohol is a problem of such magnitude that a complete chapter of this book is devoted to it.

Chloral hydrate and paraldehyde are effective sleep-inducing drugs. However, the medical use of both has decreased considerably, largely because the barbiturates are much more convenient to administer. Both chloral hydrate and paraldehyde have such disagreeable tastes and odors that they must be taken in special solutions to disguise these unpleasant properties.

Chloral hydrate is usually taken orally. Because it produces rapid and refreshing sleep, it has been used as "knock-out drops." The lethal dose of this drug is highly variable among individuals; thus it is extremely dangerous to administer. Its effects are greatly increased when there is the simultaneous use of alcohol (synergistic action), a condition which has been responsible for many accidental overdoses and deaths.

Paraldehyde is a liquid with a highly disagreeable odor. Oral administration, usually over shaved ice or in some cold drink, induces rapid sleep in most persons. Paraldehyde is seldom used as an ordinary sleeping drug because of its taste and the disagreeable odor, which is noticeable to others for many hours after ingestion. It is given to hospitalized patients in the management of delirium tremens, withdrawal illness, and convulsions.

Abuse of these two alcohol derivatives is very uncommon because of their unpleasant tastes and odors.

Barbiturates   The drugs most widely used for their sleep-producing abilities are the barbiturates. They were first produced in 1864 by combining urea (an animal waste product) with malonic acid (derived from an acid in apples). The compound obtained, a new synthetic, was named "barbituric acid." Since then chemists have produced a great variety of derivatives of barbituric acid. More than twenty-five hundred compounds have been synthesized. The first derivatives used as hypnotic-sedatives were barbital (Veronal) and phenobarbital (sold under the trade name Luminal). About two dozen barbiturate drugs, with various *latencies* (period of time between administration and effect) and *lengths of action* (period of time that drug is effective), have been produced and put on the market. On the illegal market barbiturate drugs are known as "goof-balls," "downers," and "sleeping pills" or by their colors, especially "reds."

The barbiturates are the most versatile of all central-nervous-system depressants. They can produce the whole range of depressant effects, from mild tranquilization and sedation to deep anesthesia—and death. They depress a wide variety of physiological functions in the body: for example, the activity of nerve and muscle cells, cell division, and oxygen consumption by a number of different tissues. This depression reverses after inactivation or removal of the drug. The drug is removed from the body mainly by the kidneys. It is also inactivated by an alteration in the liver. In chronic users or addicts the liver becomes quite active and is able to inactivate (detoxify) larger and larger dosages faster and faster, which is one form of tolerance, requiring increasing dosages.

The organ most sensitive to barbiturates is the brain, which is the chief site of their action. In low and moderate doses it appears that the barbiturates interfere with oxygen consumption and the mechanisms by which energy is derived, stored, and utilized within the cells of the brain. These cells also become tolerant of barbiturates in time, requiring further dosage increases. This depression of brain cell function, results in a general depression of the function of most, if not all, areas of the nervous system. Such depression of cellular activity accounts for the dosage continuum producing suppression of thinking, doing, and feeling abilities of the person taking barbiturates—leading toward sleep, anesthesia, coma, and death.

Depression of areas of the brain is the action enabling certain of the barbiturates—phenobarbital, memphobarbital, and methabarbital—to prevent epileptic seizures.

At higher dosages the nervous-system depression lets barbiturates act as anesthetics. Not only does the individual become unconscious, but his spinal reflexes are depressed so that the muscles are relaxed and manageable for surgery.

However, at extremely high (toxic, abusive) dosages, in the chronic abuser (whose liver is active and able to detoxify these substances quickly), barbiturates produce a state of hyperactivity and excitement before the general suppression of the nervous system sets in. This is an action of barbiturates *antagonistic* to its other actions. The activity seems to be in response to a depression of the brain's inhibitory systems. This inhibition-relieving action of barbiturates is responsible for a number of side actions associated with barbiturates: euphoria, excitement, and release of anxiety. It also is what produces the "truth serum" recovery of memories, the antisocial, mood-modification, and behavioral changes of the "barbiturate" addict, and the occasional excited, sleepness night spent by those who night after night use sleeping pills to go to sleep. The tolerance of the cells of the brain and spinal cord to the effects of barbiturates develops very quickly. This requires the chronic user (or addict, by this time), who is seeking excitement and euphoria, to increase the dose, often to a lethal dose without even suspecting the danger of the massive amounts of the drug he is using.

The barbiturates seem to be the second most popular suicide poison in the United States (carbon monoxide from auto exhaust is first). These pills account for one fifth of all cases of drug poisoning, and most of these are considered suicide attempts. Actually some of the deaths, though self-inflicted, are not suicides but accidents. Many may be overdoses by users. Accidental deaths may occur after a person has taken a moderate (prescribed) dose to go to sleep, but then, in a drowsy, half-asleep, and confused condition due to the effects of the dose, takes another dose, a lethal one. Physicians constantly warn barbiturate-using patients not to keep their bottles of tablets near the bed, where they may stretch out a hand to take more pills while in a confused or even comatose state of mind. The toxic and lethal effects of barbiturates are unpredictable. For some individuals a comparatively moderate or small dose may cause the effects of abuse and be dangerous. With such persons a lethal dose could also be relatively small.

Barbiturates are usually taken orally (barbiturate abusers use the term "dropped"). However, habitual users and addicts have been known to dissolve the compounds and inject them hypodermically. Sometimes they are "dropped" with alcohol and sometimes with Benzedrine or Dexedrine (amphetamines), which are nervous-system stimulants, to overcome the depressing effects of the barbiturates and to increase their antagonistic actions. This use of a stimulant drug to antagonize the depressant drug is dangerous, but the practice, widely used by young people, of combining two depressants, barbiturates and alcohol, is even more dangerous and often results in death. Such a combination interferes with the body's normal disposal of both alcohol and barbiturates through the liver, causing a toxic or lethal level of each to be reached very quickly. Besides, the two drugs working together have a synergistic effect—that is, the total depressant effect is far greater than the sum of their individual effects. Consequently, the consumption of even small amounts of barbiturates and alcohol in combination can be dangerous and may result in death.

A person under the influence of barbiturates acts like someone who has had enough alcohol to show signs of intoxication. How much of the drug is necessary to produce the degree of intoxication observed depends mostly on how tolerant to the drug the person is. Addicts keep taking more and more, and in time they reach amounts that would kill anybody who had not grown tolerant to the drug gradually. Whenever a person acts as if he has had a little or a great deal to drink, but there is no odor of alcohol about him, it is possible that he has been abusing barbiturates. Sometimes when barbiturates and alcohol are taken together, they produce what looks like an ordinary "drunk"—but the "drunk" takes much longer to sober up. The person who gets intoxicated on barbiturates follows the same course as the person who takes a drink of alcohol and keeps on until he passes out. However, barbiturates are more dangerous than alcohol because they are not vomited, and all of the drug that is taken will be absorbed unless the stomach is pumped.

A small abusive dose (the equivalent of a large therapeutic dose) makes an individual feel relaxed, sociable, and good-humored, but he loses alertness and is very slow to react. After taking more, he becomes sluggish, gloomy, antisocial, maybe quarrelsome. His speech becomes "thick," he staggers about for a while, and then he gradually slumps into a deep sleep or, if he has had a large amount of the drug, may suddenly collapse in a coma. He may die in the coma, unless he receives medical attention promptly. Even when there is no apparent sign of life from a person in a coma, a doctor may be able to revive him.

Those who become addicted to barbiturates must have them to prevent going into withdrawal. Without the drug they have seizures which resemble epileptic convulsions. Sudden withdrawal of an addict from large abusive doses of barbiturates without medical attention often results in death.

Nonbarbiturate hypnotic-sedatives   There are drugs that, while not chemically related to the barbiturates, produce reactions very similar to them. Some are being abused more and more as they become available. They are very strong and dangerous depressants, and on the continuum of drug actions their effects overlap with those of the anesthetics. *Glutethimide* (Doriden or "Ciba") is an example of this group. Others are *methaqualone* (Quaalude) and *phencyclidine* (Sernyl), which is called "PCP," "hog," "angel dust," and "the peace pill." There are many others that fall within this group.

Antihistamines

Histamine is a material that occurs naturally and is found in most cells of the body. It has very marked actions in very small concentrations. These actions are often harmful.

It produces a direct stimulation of certain smooth muscles and is a powerful vasodilator in the capillary beds. Upon release of histamine in a person a noticeable dilation of the arterioles and capillaries is seen. This produces a flushing of the skin, a rise in skin temperature, and a fall in blood pressure. There is also vasodilation in the meningeal blood vessels, which is accompanied by an increase in intracranial pressure. The increased pressure often produces headache. *Antihistamines* act by preventing the actions of histamine. They are quite selective in their abilities to block histaminic actions.

Antihistamines find their greatest uses in the relief of such allergic responses as bronchial spasm in asthma, wheals (smooth, elevated, red or pale areas on the skin—a skin reaction to an allergy), and itching of the skin.

One peculiar action of some antihistamines is their ability to relieve or abolish the symptoms of motion sickness. A number of the compounds sold for this purpose are moderate to large dosages of antihistamines, such as dimenhydrinate (Dramamine), which is a chemically changed compound of diphenhydramine (Benadryl).

The antihistamines have been placed on our continuum of drug actions and included in this discussion because of some of their side reactions. Many of the antihistamines produce drowsiness, which can progress into sedation and sleep when used in increasing doses. When this property was first noted, it was considered a minor side effect which, although undesirable, could be tolerated by most individuals. However, today many drug manufacturers have utilized this side effect of drowsiness in the major active ingredients of most over-the-counter "tension relievers" such as Cope and sleep-producing pills such as Sleep-eze. This is because most antihistamines and their compounds can be purchased without a prescription.

There is an increasing use of these compounds, and it should be noted that in some states, such as California, it is a misdemeanor to drive an automobile under the influence of an antihistaminic drug because of the drowsiness it produces. A driver under the influence of such a drug, who is in an auto accident in which there is bodily harm to someone, may be charged with a felony.

Tranquilizers

The tranquilizing drugs are able to relieve or prevent uncomfortable emotional feelings; they relieve tension and apprehension and promote a state of calm and relaxation. As shown in Fig. 4.4, there are overlapping areas of effects with other drug groups. Many tranquilizers have sedative and hypnotic effects like those of the barbiturates, and the barbiturates in turn have some tranquilizing effects. Even the narcotic drugs have tranquilizing actions. The tranquilizers are considerably less addicting than the narcotics, but addiction will occur if large enough dosages are used over a period of time.

The dramatic effects of tranquilizers on the general public and in the treatment of violent, overactive, psychotic individuals have in some instances led to exaggerated expectations regarding their role in the treatment of the mentally ill. Major tranquilizers do not cure mental illness, but they do reverse many of the symptoms of psychosis and make the management of the mentally ill, while they are taking the drug, easier. They also produce a more desirable state of mind for psychotherapy (see Chapter 2).

The major tranquilizers The major tranquilizers are not tranquilizers in the sense that they make a person feel more "tranquil." They are actually powerful *antipsychotic agents,* and their actions are completely different from the actions of minor tranquilizers. They are very effective when used by a psychotic individual, but their effects on normal individuals are varied, usually ranging from deep sleep to a feeling of deep depression. They have had a great impact on psychiatry. These are dangerous drugs; their use is not recommended except when a person has been or is in danger of developing a severe mental disturbance (psychosis). The use of a major tranquilizer for "nervousness," even in the low doses advertised by some drug firms, is dangerous and not justified.

The minor tranquilizers Minor tranquilizers are probably the most widely used *and abused* of the psychotropic drugs. They are used to combat anxiety and tension and all their attendant symptoms, including fast heart rate, tension headaches, gastrointestinal disturbances, restlessness, insomnia, irritability, and oversensitivity—whether *real* or *imagined.*

A large variety of these agents is on the market. Three of the most frequently used minor tranquilizers are *meprobamate* (Miltown and Equanil), *diphenylmethanes* (Phobex, Suavitil, and Atarax), and *chlordiazepoxide* (Librium and Librax).

The minor tranquilizers have replaced some of the barbiturates, though they are more expensive and less effective. The replacement probably is due to advertising by drug firms and physicians' bad experiences with the suicide and addiction of barbiturate users. There have been reports, though, of addiction to meprobamate and of associated suicides; thus many of these drugs are not as harmless as their advertising image suggests.

None of the minor tranquilizers is commonly used illegally, chiefly because they do not produce any euphoric effect. Addiction to them, however, can come from increased doses over a long period of time; therefore, the progressive increase in self-administration of tranquilizers is a very real danger and is a compulsive drug abuse. When large amounts have been taken for long periods of time, a sudden withdrawal may result in muscular twitching, convulsions, and other withdrawal symptoms. The doses recommended by a physician may be maintained for extremely long periods of time without adverse effects.

Cannabinol drug family (marijuana)

The cannabinol drug family has been well known since ancient times. The drugs are produced from the many varieties of *Cannabis sativa* grown throughout the world; see Fig. 4.7. The leaves and flowering tops of the female plant secrete an amber-colored resin containing the chemical cannabine (also called cannabinol, or tetrahydrocannabinol), which is believed to be the active substance causing the mood modifications and behavior changes in the user. *Cannabis* is probably known by more names throughout the world than any other plant. Some of the names for it (and for substances derived from it) are Indian hemp, Canadian hemp, Indian hay, loco (crazy) weed, weed, grass, pot, marijuana (or marihuana), 13, maryjane, kif, hashish, hash, bhang, charas, ganja, THC.

This drug family, more than any other, cannot be accurately discussed without specifying dose levels. The amount and the "potency," of the tetra-hydrocannabinol extracted from a plant vary widely throughout the world

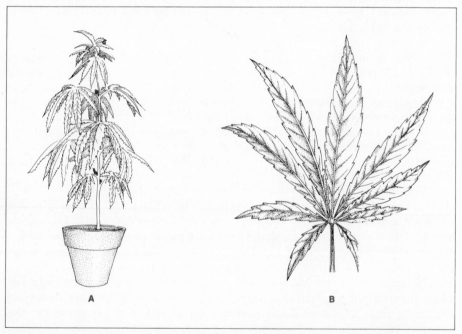

Figure 4.7   Marijuana plant, *Cannabis sativa:* (A) a young potted plant, which grows to a height of 3 to 16 feet; (B) compound leaves of five to eleven leaflets, or lobes (always an uneven number), extending 2 to 6 inches from the center diagonally to the edges, the two outer lobes always very small compared with the others.

according to the genetics of the variety of the plant being used, how the drug is prepared, which parts of the plant are used, and how the drug is stored until it is consumed.

Marijuana, used mostly in the United States, is probably the weakest preparation of the plant used in the world. The most potent preparation is *charas* (used mainly in India), which is the unadulterated tetrahydrocannabinol resin obtained from the female plant or its dried flowers. The term *hashish*, when used correctly, indicates a powdered and sifted form of charas; hashish and a "hash oil" are being sold in the United States.

A synthetic form of tetrahydrocannabinol, THC, has been synthetically produced. It has been used in scientific studies and has been found to be less potent than the naturally occurring form. There have been reports that this material is available on the street, but that seems very unlikely, because of its extremely high cost; if it is so, however, the material probably is not pure and, especially in the liquid state, may be an unknown broad mixture of chemicals—which may be very dangerous.

In great strength, such as is found in hashish or charas, the drug has effects similar to those of hallucinogenic drugs. That is why, for the last few years, it has been classified as a hallucinogen and will continue to be classified as such by many persons. Owing to recent research and reports on the effects of cannabis (such as the *Marihuana and Health* report to Congress from the Secretary of Health, Education and Welfare, 1971) the authors of this book feel it should be given a classification distinct from all other drugs.

Cannabinol has a wide range of action. In high doses it is similar to the hallucinogens (stimulants), and in low doses it is similar to the sedatives, alcohol, and the narcotics (all depressants); for this reason marijuana is in the neutral area on the continuum of drug actions, overlapping both the stimulant and the depressant areas.

The effects of even large doses of cannabinol are milder and more easily controlled than those of LSD or mescaline. The differing "trips" or "highs" of the two classes of drugs are readily distinguishable by users; users of cannabinol, even taking large doses, lack the major anxiety, panic, and stress reactions suffered by hallucinogen users. Cannabinol at any dose level does not show the increased body temperature, increased blood pressure, or pupil reactions of the hallucinogens. Cannabinol use ends in sedation and sleep, whereas wakefulness is characteristic throughout the use of hallucinogenic drugs.

In low strength, such as in marijuana, the effects of cannabis are very similar to those of alcohol; both produce an early excitement and later a sedated phase, which appears faster in the marijuana user. There are some differences, too. The marijuana "high" is completely different from alcoholic intoxication. The appetite and consumption of food are increased by marijuana and decreased by alcohol. Lastly, the "margin of safety in drug abuse" is far greater with cannabis than with alcohol. Large doses of alcohol act as a general anesthetic, producing a continuous depression of the central nervous system; large doses of cannabis, on the other hand, tend to repress and then to backtrack toward the stimulating side of the continuum of drug actions. This down-and-then-up reaction to marijuana, as the individual consumes more, is the reason his behavior can become impulsive and his mood reactions highly variable, unpredictable—and dangerous.

In the United States the most commonly used cannabinol is marijuana, the dried leaves and flowering tops of the female plant. Cigarettes (called "joints") are made by rolling the weed in double, brown, straw papers with the ends tucked in to prevent loss of the prickly, loosely packed weed. The marijuana cigarettes cannot be confused with tobacco cigarettes: marijuana is green rather than brown, the "joint" burns hotter than cigarettes made of tobacco, the burning tip is brighter, and the lighted tip goes out easily unless an effort is made to keep it lit. Burning marijuana has the smell of burning hay, leaves, or weeds; no one can smoke marijuana without easily distinguishing it from tobacco.

Shortly after inhaling marijuana, the user may have a feeling of inner joy (euphoria) that is out of proportion to his actual situation; this is described by users as a "high." If someone smoking marijuana is alone, he may be quiet and dreamy or just sit and watch the passing parade of colored illusions that may occur. In a group he may be talkative and happy and can be easily misled regarding his abilities and intellectual capabilities. His sense of touch and perception are changed, and his ideas about time, space, and speed are distorted. The user's coordination is altered, although he and also others may fail to recognize either this alteration or the impairment of his intellectual capacities. All of his behavioral modifications depend upon his environment, personal feelings, and the amount of marijuana smoked. If he is in a negative mood or in unpleasant surroundings, he may become anxious and apprehensive. If he continues smoking in this environment he may become easily irritated. With increased use at this point he becomes stimulated, confused, disoriented, and afraid. His behavior can become impulsive and his mood reactions highly variable and unpredictable. With increasing doses at this point he may then experience hallucinations and other reactions associated with the more potent hallucinogens.

The total effects of a marijuana experience last from three to five hours, after which the user feels slightly drowsy or sleepy and very hungry.

The compulsive, chronic use of cannabinol does occur. Often individuals recognize the beginning of a *compulsive use pattern* and preoccupation with marijuana by experiencing vague feelings that something is wrong and that they are functioning at a reduced level of efficiency; in this respect the compulsive alcohol and cannabinol users resemble each other. Individuals feel a loss of desire to work, to compete, to face challenges. Interests and major concerns become centered around marijuana. They may drop out of school or work. The reduced efficiency has been termed the "amotivational syndrome"; it produces a life style similar to that of the "skid row" alcoholic.

Controlled research has begun to expand our knowledge of cannabis. Since the National Institute of Mental Health embarked on a cannabis research program in the early 1970s, a supply of standardized natural and synthetic tetrahydrocannabinol has been developed. As time passes, additional information will become available and provide a more complete picture of the implication of cannabis use at various dose levels and in differing patterns.

Hallucinogenic drugs

A drug that creates vivid distortions in the senses without greatly disturbing the user's consciousness is called a hallucinogenic drug. In the popular literature a number of other terms have been used to describe these drugs and their effects, such as *psychedelic* ("mind manifesting") and *pseudohallucinogenic* ("producing false hallucinations"). The terms *psychotomimetic* ("psychosis mimicking") and *psychotogenic* ("psychosis producing") have been used in reference to some hallucinogens because many individuals under the influence of these drugs exhibit behavior that resembles the disturbances seen in the psychotic or severely mentally ill. Some of the drugs seem capable of temporarily producing psychotic behavior in a normal person. It has been necessary to hospitalize some users to prevent them from doing harm to themselves or others during their temporary psychoses.

During recent years psychiatry has had an increasing interest in hallucinogenic drugs. Some researchers have taken these drugs to produce in themselves what they have termed "a model psychosis" to increase their understanding of the severely ill psychiatric patient. Other researchers have tried using the drugs as psychedelics—that is, as expanders of mental potentials. They have tried to use the drugs in this manner in the treatment of a variety of conditions, such as alcoholism, personality problems, and frigidity, to expand the patient's ability to realize thoughts and actions and to visualize shortcomings and problems. The results have been contradictory and have not fulfilled the expectations or intentions of the investigators.

A large number of individuals have acquired the drugs illegally and have taken them without medical supervision in cultlike group experiences, in small groups (two or three individuals), or alone. Frequently a persistent psychotic reaction or a prolonged delirious reaction (called a "bring down," "downer," "bummer," "bad trip") has followed. Psychiatrists have been increasingly needed to help those suffering from these extreme reactions. Thus, for protection of the individual and for its own protection, society has become involved in legislative action against the abuse of any hallucinogenic compounds.

The hallucinogenic drugs are placed only slightly above the neutral area on the continuum of drug effects, because in what would be considered therapeutic or minimal doses all members of the group produce rather mild stimulation of the individual. Within the hallucinogenic group different classes of drugs produce a wide continuum of stimulation and hallucinogenic effects. Many of these drugs produce extreme reactions in almost incomprehensibly small doses; LSD is an example.

There are two major chemical classes of hallucinogenic drugs: the phenethylamines and the indole alkaloids. Tolerance to both groups develops very quickly, and cross-tolerance within the groups also develops.

Phenethylamine drug family (mescaline)   The most significant drug abused in this group is *mescaline* (trimethoxyphenylethylamine), named after the Mescalero Apache Indians of the southwestern United States, who developed the cult of peyotism. Mescaline occurs in peyote, a small, spineless cactus that grows naturally in northeastern Mexico and the watershed of the Rio Grande river. Peyote is carrot-shaped; only the topmost part extends above the ground; see Fig. 4.8. This portion is cut off and, though it may be eaten fresh, it is usually dried to form the peyote or "mescal" buttons. It may also be boiled and the broth drunk.

Mescaline is of interest because it is chemically related to epinephrine, a natural substance in the body. The chemical association seems to be responsible for the effects mescaline produces on the autonomic nervous system prior to the onset of psychic reactions. Soon after one takes mescaline, any psychic experience is preceded by one to three hours of flushing, vomiting (which greatly limits the abuse of this drug by young people), cramps, sweating, increased pulse rate, elevated blood pressure, muscle twitching, and other autonomic phenomena. These effects are followed by four to twelve hours, or several days in some cases, of visual hallucinations (in all ranges of color and fantastic geometric patterns), vast feelings of depersonalization, and great distortions in the sensing of time and space relationships.

Mescaline usually is ingested in the form of a soluble crystalline powder or as a capsule. It must be used in high doses to produce the extreme hallucinogenic effects usually sought. These doses are psychologically dangerous to many individuals, producing psychotic reactions without any prior warning.

Of the other drugs in this group (anhalonine, TMA, MDA, MMDA, etc.) only one, DOM (or "STP," as it is known on the street), has been used to any extent. DOM is an extremely dangerous drug, and during one ten-day period in San Francisco it caused ten "bad trips," one chronic psychosis, and one death.

Indole alkaloids A number of separate drugs comprise this group: DMAT, tryptamines, Harmala family, bufotenin, morning-glory seeds, psilocybin, LSD, and others. Many are found in plants and some in animals. Compounds like the indole alkaloids and that have hallucinogenic potentialities have been synthesized in the laboratory or produced by rearranging the chemical structure of the naturally occurring substances. This rearrangement and synthesis may have almost limitless possibilities which, in the future, could deluge humanity with extremely potent and highly selective drugs affecting the nervous system in yet unknown ways.

DMT, dimethyltryptamine, is found, together with *bufotenin* (which was originally isolated from the skin of toads), in the Caribbean cahobe bean, which is chewed by certain Indians in South America to produce religious illusions and visions. It is also found in the seeds of the domestic morning glory plant, which are abused in the United States for their hallucinogenic effect. *Psilocybin* is the active ingredient of the ritually employed hallucinogenic mushroom *Psilocybe mexicana* of Central Mexico. Another drug, *harmaline*, is isolated from shrubs and used by South American Indians to produce hallucinatory states. A similar compound, *ibogaine*, is used by African natives to remain motionless for as long as two days while stalking game. Hallucinogenic compounds are universal in their distribution around the world and have been known for many years.

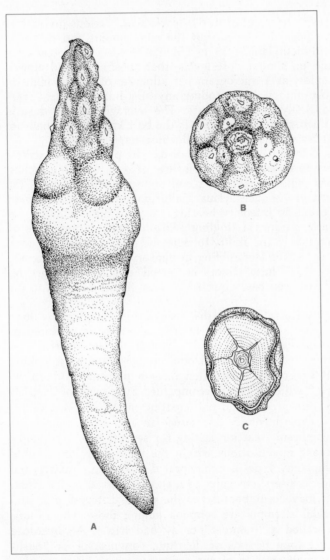

Figure 4.8   Peyote cactus plant, *Lophophora williamsii:*
(A) complete plant; (B) top view of the cut and rounded
top of a plant, called a peyote or mescal "button"; (C)
bottom view of the "button."

Probably the most potent indole alkaloids are the *ergot alkaloids*. These were first isolated from a fungus found on rye and some other grasses; see Fig. 4.9. It is believed that the alkaloids in the fungus were probably responsible for the convulsions, mental confusion, and gangrenous changes in the lower limbs associated with periodic outbreaks, in the Middle Ages, of St. Anthony's Fire, which was probably produced by eating foods containing infected rye.

All ergot alkaloids can be changed into *lysergic acid*. Various derivatives of this compound have been developed, but the most potent and the most famous is *d*-lysergic acid diethylamide-25, or LSD-25. It is such a potent drug (800 times more potent, on similar dose levels, than mescaline) and abused in such small doses (as low as 1 microgram per kilogram of body weight in humans) that it is almost impossible to produce anything but an extreme reaction when one takes illegally prepared doses. The average abusive dose is between 100 and 250 micrograms. Since LSD is the best known, we shall use it as the example in discussing this group of hallucinogens.

LSD is a tasteless, colorless, and odorless drug. The physical side effects and complications seem to be physical discomfort: nausea, vomiting, aches, and pains. It dilates the pupils, raises the blood pressure, and increases the strength of the reflexes. It produces visual hallucinations in all ranges of color. The actions of the drug intensify hearing, increase the sensitivity for feeling texture, and may produce a tingling sensation and a numbness of the hands and feet. Increases in the ability to taste and smell are not frequent. Subjects often report crossover (scrambling at sensory synapses) of sensation; for example, they may "hear" colors or "smell" music. There are reports that individuals have been badly burned because flames felt cool to the touch.

After the initial physical effects of the drug, users experience a high degree of subjective euphoria and a sense of mental clarity or comprehension, although objectively they appear to an observer to be confused, uncoordinated, hallucinating, and disoriented. Upon recovery from a profoundly moving and significant experience they often have a personal (subjective) feeling of being "reborn," which may be accompanied by a sense of deep affection for others who were present and participating in the experience.

LSD was first used experimentally to produce an artificial psychosis resembling an acute schizophrenic reaction lasting for several hours, a "model psychosis." The temporary modifications within the nervous system caused by the drug may produce any type of behavioral disturbance. Anxiety and panic may occur during the users' struggles to maintain control of the situation, and fear reactions may occur because of the users' distorted time and space perceptions. Suicidal attempts are common among those who experience panic or anxiety (called a "bummer" or a "bad trip"). An overdose (toxic dose) may produce long periods of delirium, convulsions, or "flashbacks" in which the dramatic effects of the drug reoccur at intervals of a year or more. These prolonged reactions to any hallucinogen (mescaline, LSD, etc.) seem to be caused by a combination of the drug's effects and the emotional disorders already present in the users, prior to their abuse of drugs.

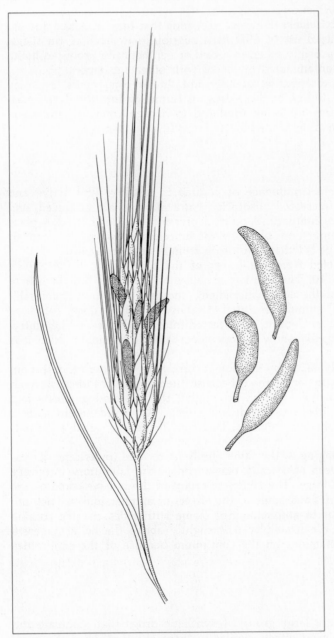

Figure 4.9   The ergot fungus *Claviceps purpurea* shown as it occurs on the head (spike) of a rye plant. The drug LSD (lysergic acid diethylamide) is derived from this fungus.

However, no one has been able to predict who is likely to have such an extreme reaction nor when.

Because of the extremely disturbed reactions that have occurred and are occurring with the illegal use of LSD, it is possible that much of the illegal supplies of LSD and possibly other extracted or synthetically produced hallucinogens are either contaminated or mixed with other substances. Since the legal production and distribution of LSD and similar compounds is closely controlled, very little, if any, of these drugs is funneling into the illegal market. The illegal supplies are being produced in foreign countries and basement laboratories here in the United States.

Cocaine

The individual under the influence of cocaine is talkative and active and feels euphoric. With increased absorption hallucinations are produced, and the individual becomes confused. A quick depression ("letdown") takes place after the period of stimulation, plunging the individual into stupor, sleep, or coma and, if the dosage is lethal, into death from respiratory failure.

Cocaine is extracted from the leaves of the coca shrub, *Erythroxylon coca*, shown in Fig. 4.10. The plant is a native of Peru and Bolivia, where the leaves (containing the active ingredient, cocaine) have been habitually chewed for their mild stimulation (at that relatively benign dose) for more than four hundred years. Cocaine is processed into an odorless, white, fluffy, fine crystalline powder, like snow in appearance; on the criminal market it is commonly referred to as "snow."

Cocaine is usually taken by sniffing it, rarely by hypodermic injection. Sniffing is the most popular method, because the drug is absorbed through the membranes of the nose slowly, prolonging the stimulating effects and tempering the drug's intensity and drastic effects. Advanced heroin addicts may mix cocaine and heroin together. This combination is called a "speedball."

Other drugs belonging to the same family as cocaine (piperidine derivatives) have recently been chemically rearranged in the laboratory into very potent hallucinogenic drugs. The complete group of drugs have some of the effects of hallucinogenics and some of the effects of amphetamines. They are chemically very similar to amphetamines (some authorities classify cocaine as an amphetamine). We have placed it slightly above the hallucinogenics and below the amphetamines on the continuum because of the similarities of its effects.

Amphetamines

The amphetamines are a large group of synthetic drugs that stimulate the nervous system. They exert effects similar to those obtained when the sympathetic nervous system is stimulated (see Chapter 3). Thus they "mimic" the actions of dopamine and norepinephrine (noradrenalin) on the sympathetic nervous system. This action is produced because amphetamines cause

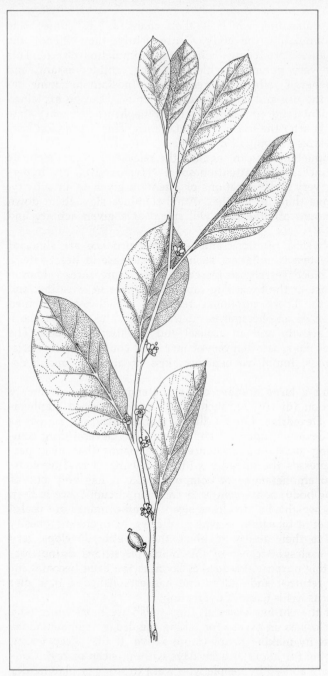

Figure 4.10   A flowering branch of the coca plant, *Erythroxylon coca,* a shrub or small tree that grows to 12 or 15 feet. The drug cocaine is extracted from the leaves.

the release of stored dopamine, which is then changed into epinephrine and norepinephrine, stimulating the body. Consequently, they "flood" the brain with these substances, producing their drastic stimulating effects. This helps to explain their very potent psychic-energizing, antidepressant, and sympathomimetic (adrenergic) effects. Moreover, the "postamphetamine depression," common in the use and abuse of amphetamines, can be explained by the dopamine-deficient (and consequently norepinephrine-deficient) state in which the brain is left after the use of amphetamines. This depression lasts until the body resynthesizes a supply of dopamine.

Small doses of amphetamines can regulate the release of norepinephrine in the brain and help increase the attention span. "Hyperactive" or "hyperkinetic" children show very short durations of attention given to an activity, and they jump from one thing to another. Amphetamines slow them down by lengthening the amount of time they will spend at a given activity and remain interested.

In general, the physical reactions amphetamines produce are signs of sympathetic-nervous-system stimulation, such as an increase in heart rate, a constriction of certain blood vessels, an increase in blood pressure, a dilation of the pupils, an increase in the breathing rate, an increase in sweating, and a dryness in the mouth. These autonomic reactions are always combined with the primary action of amphetamines on the brain. The user has both an increase in bodily activity and an arousal and elevation of mood. The arousal and elevation of mood is often one of increased confidence, euphoria, fearlessness, talkativeness, impulsive behavior, loss of appetite, and a decrease in fatigue.

On the market are a large number of amphetamine drugs commonly used for weight reduction (diet pills), such as the widely abused amphetamines Benzedrine and Dexedrine. On the illegal market they are known as "whites," "bennies," "dexies," "uppers," and "pep pills." Several drug companies, without showing substantial evidence, make claims that their particular compound suppresses the appetite without causing central-nervous-system stimulation. No amphetamine or compound like it has only one of these two actions in the body; consequently, a common circumstance is that, although the user loses weight, he also loses sleep. Amphetamines are useful for depressing the appetite of someone who is dieting to overcome obesity at first, but tolerance to their ability to block the appetite develops very quickly, making them useless. Because of this many physicians do not recommend their use for this purpose, because as soon as the drug becomes ineffective, the appetite returns, and unless one has established a new diet pattern, he usually returns to his habit of overeating.

Actually, many of the chronic users of "pep pills" are housewives who use a desire for weight loss as an excuse for taking the drugs. Amphetamines produce the weight loss by making people more active. If they keep taking more, they can keep going for hours or even days without sleep or rest. Consequently, these drugs are abused by people who want to work or play harder or longer than their normal capacities allow.

Young people often use them with barbiturates or alcohol for "kicks." Such abuse is physically dangerous; it can cause death or lead to impulsive acts of poor judgment and to accidents. Especially abused is the amphetamine compound *Methedrine* or *Desoxyn* (methamphetamine hydrochloride), commonly called "speed" or "meth." Some people swallow "meth" pills or inject the compound into a muscle ("skin pop") or vein ("mainline") to get a quick euphoric "flash," or "rush." With continued injections the users stay awake for days and eat very little, until their bodies become completely exhausted ("strung out"). Then the worst part of a "speed trip" comes, the withdrawal ("crashing") from the effects of the drugs. Heavy users stop their injections, slip between coma and sleep for days, then awaken and start their injections again. The lack of food, sleep, and rest can ruin the physical health of a long-time user. Figure 4.11 clearly illustrates this point: three photographs of the same person taken six months apart show marked physical deterioration. Because of the "crashing" effects of withdrawal some authorities classify amphetamines as addictive drugs. We do not classify them as addicting, because a classic withdrawal syndrome is not produced. "Crashing" seems to be caused by the massive accumulated fatigue built up in the individual and the lack of dopamine and norephinephrine storage for normal nerve function. Amphetamines produce a strong tolerance, and usually those who suddenly stop taking amphetamines go through a rather prolonged period of lethargy, deep psychological depression, nightmares, periods of restlessness, and long, exhausted sleep. This condition, "crashing," is called *post-amphetamine depression*. When post-amphetamine depression passes,

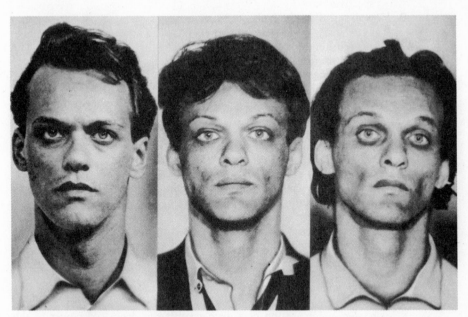

Figure 4.11   The changes in physical characteristics of one amphetamine user; the photographs were taken at six-month intervals. (From Chicago American Publishing Co.)

the tolerance diminishes, and the chronic amphetamine user is apt to start injecting again.

Often the stimulating effect of amphetamines is relied upon by criminals to increase their "nerve." Barbiturate addicts take amphetamines and barbiturates together because the amphetamines counteract the hypnotic action of the barbiturates.

Possibly the greatest danger to the largest number of people from amphetamines is the effect they have on automobile and truck drivers. If a number of pills are taken at one time, or if they are used for a long period of time without rest or sleep, they may produce hallucinations or delusions. Users may feel that someone or something in another automobile is following them and trying to get them, or they may "black out" suddenly while driving at high speeds. These effects are so dangerous that many states have made it a felony offense to drive while under the influence of amphetamines.

SUMMARY

I. Use of drugs
- A. In the last twenty-five years scores of new drugs have been introduced —many are abused.
  1. Decisions on drug use should be left in the hands of trained physicians and dentists.
  2. Understanding how drugs act may help put drugs in proper perspective.
- B. How drugs affect the body
  1. Drugs may be classified in various ways:
     - a. according to their source.
     - b. according to their chemical composition.
     - c. according to their actions and effects.
     - d. according to their medical use.
  2. In this chapter drugs are classified on the basis of their actions and effects.
- C. How drugs work
  1. A drug may act:
     - a. on the surface of cells.
     - b. within the cell.
     - c. in the extracellular fluids of the body.
  2. In most cases the action is within a cell.
- D. Major actions and effects of drugs
  1. Local drug action: action of a drug only at its site of application.
  2. Systemic drug action: the drug is absorbed into the body and distributed throughout the body. The following terms are used to describe the actions and effects of drugs with systemic actions:
     - a. *stimulation*: action of a drug resulting in increased activity of the cell.
     - b. *depression*: action of a drug resulting in decreased power of the cell to function.

    c. *selective action:* ability of a drug to produce a greater effect on some tissue or organ than on others.

    d. *therapeutic action:* action of a drug on diseased tissues or in a sick individual.

    e. *side effect* (side action): any effect or action other than the one for which the drug is administered.

    f. *untoward effect* (untoward action): A *side effect* regarded as harmful to the individual.

    g. *cumulative action:* effect or action produced when drugs accumulate in the body without being destroyed or excreted.

    h. *synergism, potentiation, and additive effects:* ways in which drugs may work together.

       (1) Drugs are *synergistic* when drugs that produce the same general effect are given together and cause an exaggerated effect out of proportion to that of each drug given separately.

       (2) *Potentiation* occurs when two drugs are given together and one intensifies the action of the other.

       (3) When drugs are given together and their combined effects represent the action of one plus the action of the others they are said to be *additive* drugs.

    i. *antagonistic drugs:* drugs that have an opposite effect in the body.

    j. *idiosyncrasy:* any "individualized" abnormal response of a person to a drug.

    k. *hypersensitivity:* an allergic response to a drug.

  3. Drug interactions occur when two drugs are taken at once or close enough in time to alter the expected action of either drug.

  E. Drug dosages

    1. Dosage is the amount of drug which is given or taken at one time.

    2. As shown by Fig. 4.1, a number of terms are used to describe the amount of drug in a dose.

II. How drugs are administered

  A. Most drugs are distributed throughout the body and delivered to the tissues by the bloodstream.

  B. Drugs can be administered in a number of ways.

    1. Drugs can enter the bloodstream by being taken orally.

    2. Drugs may be *inhaled.*

    3. Drugs may be administered by *injection.*

III. Treatment of diseases and conditions

  A. A physician should not prescribe until he knows what he is treating.

  B. Only after he makes a diagnosis can a physician prescribe an appropriate form of treatment.

  C. What a patient can do: follow the instructions of the physician.

IV. Definitions of drug abuse

  A. A drug is any substance other than food that alters the body or its functions.

  B. Forms of drug dependence

    1. *Drug habituation* (see Table 4.1) exists when a person seeks out a drug and has a desire to continue taking the drug in question.

    2. *Drug addiction* is produced by some drugs that evoke biochemical and physiological adaptations in the user (known as tolerance and physical dependence).

3. *Habit-forming drugs* are drugs that have the potential of becoming either habituating or addicting with continued use.

C. Abuse of drugs that modify mood and behavior

1. A drug is being abused when it is self-administered in toxic doses and damages an individual, a society, or both.

2. Drugs considered dangerous and unacceptable to society, when abused, create problems within society by causing personality changes, euphoria, or abnormal social behavior.

3. The abuse of these drugs is always associated with an abnormal personality; whether this personality distortion is the cause or the result of the drug abuse is not known.

4. The person who does not find a pleasurable experience in drug abuse or who is subject to strong social pressures when first experimenting with a drug does not usually continue to abuse drugs—that is, his personality does not lack, or seek, what the drug has to offer, and he tends to reject it.

V. Physical aspects of drug abuse

A. Drug-induced effects on the nervous system

1. The overall actions and effects of mood-modifying drugs are mainly those of either a *stimulant* or a *depressant*, acting directly upon the nervous system so as to increase or decrease the activity of nerve centers and their conducting pathways.

a. A nervous-system stimulant is a drug that temporarily increases body function or nerve activity.

b. Depressant drugs have the ability to decrease temporarily a body function or nerve activity.

2. Drugs that act on the nervous system do not act on all parts of it with the same degree of intensity.

3. The specific response of an individual to a specific drug depends to a large extent on the personality of the individual, on the nature of the drug itself, and on a number of other factors.

B. Spectrum and continuum of drug action

1. The degrees of depression and stimulation of drugs are not discrete.

2. The spectrum of drug actions can be set into a continuum of effects and actions.

3. The continuum of drug effects extends from

a. overstimulation to death at one extreme.

b. to severe depression to death at the other.

4. The central or "neutral area" of this continuum is the degree of stimulation and depression usually encountered in everyday living.

5. The drugs are started on the continuum according to the actions or effects they produce when therapeutic (minimal) doses are consumed by the individual.

6. The weaker groups of drugs end nearest the center; the most powerful drugs, at the two extremes.

7. If doses are increased from minimal, to maximal, to toxic, to abusive, to lethal, any drug group is able to produce the complete range of effects.

VI. General classification

The following is the general classification of commonly abused drugs, based on the continuum of actions associated with their use.

A. Narcotics
   1. The most widely abused drugs throughout the world.
   2. Narcotics are chiefly used for their ability to produce a marked insensibility to pain without producing excessive drowsiness, muscular weakness, confusion, or loss of consciousness.
   3. When abusive doses are used, during the depression of the nervous system there is a temporary elevation of mood, euphoria, relief from fear and apprehension, and feelings of peace and tranquility:
      a. this state usually considered chief reason for abuse of narcotics.
      b. after a short time this state passes, and the individual becomes apathetic, slows, and falls asleep.
   4. Drugs classified at narcotics:
      a. opium—juice obtained by cutting the unripe capsule of the Oriental poppy (*Papaver somniferum*); seldom used in the United States; American narcotics abusers use its derivatives: heroin, morphine, codeine.
      b. morphine—the chief derivative of opium.
      c. heroin—considered the most dangerous of the narcotic drugs.
      d. codeine—not widely used as a narcotic because of its mild effects.
      e. synthetic narcotics—produced synthetically in the laboratory.
B. Volatile solvents
   1. Abuse results from deliberate inhalation of solvent vapors from plastic cement to induce:
      a. euphoria.
      b. exhilaration.
   2. Have a depressant action on the central nervous system similar to that of barbiturates and narcotics.
   3. Produce:
      a. strong drug dependence.
      b. psychotoxic effects (during administration).
      c. strong tolerance.
      d. necessity to increase the dose.
   4. Characterized as addicting drugs in abusive doses.
C. Hypnotic-sedative drugs
   1. Able to depress the central nervous system into a condition resembling normal sleep.
   2. Are characterized by their broad range of suppression of brain functions:
      a. when given in minimal doses to reduce excitement, called sedatives.
      b. when given in moderate to maximal doses to produce sleep, called hypnotics.
   3. When abused, they greatly reduce anxiety and produce a mild euphoria as a relief for people who tend to live in an uncomfortable, painful, or hyperaroused state.
   4. Drugs classified as hypnotic-sedatives:
      a. bromides—are highly dangerous because of extreme toxicity.
      b. alcohol and alcohol derivatives—the oldest hypnotic-sedatives used in modern medicine were alcohol and its major derivatives, chloral hydrate and paraldehyde.
      c. barbiturates—the most widely used and abused as hypnotics or sedatives.

    d. nonbarbiturate hypnotic-sedatives—drugs not related to barbiturates but producing actions very similar to them; are starting to be abused very widely.

  5. Sudden removal forces an addict into withdrawal-producing seizures resembling epileptic convulsions, often severe enough to cause death.

D. Antihistamines
  1. Not abused.
  2. Used in the relief of allergic responses in an individual.
  3. Are included in this discussion of drugs because of some of their side actions—drowsiness, sedation, and sleep when used in increasing doses.

E. Tranquilizers
  1. Can suppress anxiety, diminish abnormal behavior, and calm individuals at dose levels that do not produce sleep.
  2. Deaths from overdoses are rare.

F. Cannabinol drug family (marijuana)
  1. Separate drug family—cannot be discussed without specifying dose levels, amount, or "potency" of drug being used:
    a. most potent forms: charas, hashish, or natural THC.
    b. marijuana probably mildest form of drug.
  2. Drug placed across neutral area of continuum of drug actions, because effects overlap both stimulant and depressant areas.
  3. Compulsive, chronic use of cannabinol does occur.
  4. Controlled research into effects of cannabinol is being conducted.

G. Hallucinogenic drugs
  1. Drugs which create vivid distortions in the senses without disturbing the user's consciousness.
  2. Many individuals under the influence of these drugs exhibit behavior that resembles the disturbances seen in the psychotic or severely mentally ill.
  3. The hallucinogenic drugs are placed only slightly above the neutral area on the continuum of drug effects because, in what would be considered therapeutic or minimal doses, all members of the group produce rather mild stimulation of the individual.
  4. Drugs classified as hallucinogens
    a. phenethylamine drug family. The most significant drug abused in this group is mescaline, a drug derived from a small, spineless cactus called peyote.
    b. indole alkaloids—a number of separate drugs in this group; they are found occurring naturally in plants and animals and have been synthesized in the laboratory; the most widely abused are LSD, psilocybin, and DMT.

H. Cocaine
  1. Its systemic effect on the body is to stimulate and induce excitement.
  2. Extracted from the leaves of the coca shrub, *Erythroxylon coca*.

I. Amphetamines
  1. Central-nervous-system stimulants.
  2. Produce feelings of:
    a. elation.
    b. excitement.
    c. relief of fatigue.

  d. extreme nervousness, tremors.
  e. anxiety, palpitations.
3. One of the most dangerous drugs abused today.

Glossary

If you cannot find the word you wish in this glossary, check the index for text and glossary references.

abstinence syndrome (ab'sti nəns sin'drōm) (L. *abstinere,* to abstain; G. *syndrome,* concurrence). A set of symptoms that occur together, resulting from withdrawal of alcohol, depressants, and opiates.

abuse (ə būz') (ME. *ab-,* away, from + *uto,* to use). To use wrongly or improperly; misuse.

addict (ad'ikt) (L. *addicere,* to consent). To form a habit, as for the use of a drug or alcohol.

addiction (ə dik'shən). Condition resulting from repeated use of a drug in which physical dependence is established because of biochemical and physiological adaptations to the drug.

amine (ə mēn', am'in) (ammonia + -ine). The chemical group NH_2; as a prefix (amino-) indicates the presence in a compound of the group NH_2.

amphetamine (am fet'ə mēn). A central-nervous-system stimulant.

analgesic (an'al je'zik, an'al je'sik) (G. *an-,* without + *algesia,* pain). A chemical or drug which has the ability to relieve pain.

anesthetic (an əs thet'ik) (G. *anaisthesia,* insensibility). Agent that produces insensibility to pain or touch.

antagonistic (an tag'ə nis'tik) (Gr. *antagonizesthai,* to struggle against). Opposing or counteracting.

antidepressant (an ti di pres'ənt) (L. *anti-* against + *deprimere,* to press down). A drug which counteracts the feelings of depression (absence of cheerfulness or hope, with reduction of the functional activity of the body).

barbiturates (bahr bit'yoor its) (L. *barbatus,* bearded; G. *ourikos,* pertaining to urine). Drugs used in medicine as hypnotic and sedative drugs.

Benzedrine (ben'zə drēn). A trade name for an amphetamine.

benzene (ben'zēn). Colorless liquid used as a solvent for fats, resins, and other substances.

bromide (brō'mīd) (G. *bromos,* starch). Central-nervous-system depressant.

carbon tetrachloride (kahr'bən tetrə klōr'īd). Colorless, clear, heavy liquid with a characteristic odor; used in fire extinquishers, as a cleaning agent, and for exterminating destructive insects.

charas (Hindi word) (chär'əs'). The unadulterated resin exuded by the flowering tops of the female hemp plant *Cannabis sativa.*

chemotherapy (kem'ō ther'ə pi) (*chemo-* having to do with chemicals, + *therapy,* the art of treatment). The treatment of disease by the administration of chemicals, medicines, or drugs.

chloral hydrate (klōr'əl hīdrāt). Narcotic drug used as a sedative, hypnotic, and anticonvulsant.

cocaine (kō'kān) (Quechua, *coca, cuca,* a South American plant). Drug used in medicine as a narcotic or local anesthetic; a stimulant to the central nervous system.

codeine (kō′dēn) (G. *kodeia*, poppy head). Analgesic, hypnotic sedative derived from opium; effects resemble those of morphine but are less narcotic than morphine.

coma (kō′mə) (G. *koma*, lethargy). An abnormal deep stupor.

convulsions (kon vul′shənz) (L. *con-*, with + *vellere*, to pull). Contortions of the body caused by violent involuntary muscular contractions.

delirium tremens (də lēr′ē əm trē′mənz) (L. *de-*, off; *lira*, track, thus, "off the track"; *tremere*, to shake). A psychic disorder involving hallucinations, both visual and auditory, delusions, incoherence, anxiety, and trembling; found in habitual users of alcoholic beverages and some drugs.

Demerol (dem′ə rol). An analgesic producing effects similar to those of morphine; it is addicting.

dependence (də pend′əns) (L. *de*, from, away; *pendere*, to hang). The total psychophysical state of an addict, in which the usual or increasing doses of the drug are required to prevent the onset of withdrawal symptoms.

depressant (di pres′ənt) (L. *deprimere*, to press down). Chemical, substance, or agent which has the ability to reduce the functional activity of the body.

Dexedrine (dek′sə drēn). A central-nervous-system stimulant, one of the amphetamines (a trade name).

dosage (dō′sij) (G. *dosis*, a portion). Amount of a medicinal preparation to be taken at one time.

drug dependence (drug di pen′dəns). Condition resulting from repeated use of a drug in which individual must continue to take drug to avoid abstinence syndrome (physical dependence) or to satisfy strong emotional need (psychic dependence).

epileptic (ep i lep′tik) (G. *epilepsia*, seizure). A person affected with epilepsy; a disturbance showing generalized convulsions.

epinephrine (ep′ə nef′rin) (*epi-* word, G. *nephros*, kidney; + *-ine*, having the nature of). Monoamine hormone secreted by the adrenal medulla, most powerful vasopressor substance known; used medically as a sympathomimetic.

euphoric (yoo for′ik) (G. *eu*, well; *pherein*, to bear). Characterized by a feeling of well-being; in psychiatry, exhibiting an abnormal or exaggerated sense of well-being.

gratification (grat′ə fi ka′shən) (L. *gratus*, pleasing, agreeable + *facere*, to make). A source of pleasure or satisfaction.

habituation (hə bich′oo ā′shən) (L. *habituatus*, to bring into a condition or habit of the body). In this context, a condition resulting from repeated use of a drug in which a psychic, not physical, dependence is established.

hallucinogen (hə loo′si nə jen). An agent producing hallucinations; examples of hallucinogenic drugs are LSD, mescaline, and DMT.

hallucinogenic (hə loo′sə na jen′ik) (L. *hallucinoatus*, to wander mentally). Chemical, substance, or agent capable of producing distortions of the senses which may include hallucinations.

hashish (hash′esh, hash′ish) (Fr. *hasher*, to chop, mince) (Ar. *hashish*, an assassin). A powdered and sifted form of the unadulterated resin exuded by the flowering tops of the female hemp plant, *Cannabis sativa*.

hypnotic (hip not′ik) (G. *hypnotikos*, sleep). A drug that acts to induce sleep.

intoxication (in tok si kā′shən) (L. *in-*, intensive; G. *toxikon*, poison). State of being poisoned; condition produced by excessive use of alcohol.

intravenous (in tra vē′nəs) (L. *intra*, within; *vena*, vein). Into a vein, as an intravenous injection.

irritability (ir i tə bil′i tē) (L. *irritare*, to tease). The ability to respond to stimuli.

lactose (lak′tōs) (L. *lac*, milk). Milk sugar.

latency (lā′t′n si) (ME. *late*, slow, tardy). Period of time between the administration of a drug and the beginning of a response.

length of action. The period of time that a drug is effective.

leukopenia (loo kə pē'nē ə). Reduction of the number of *leukocytes* (white blood cells) in the blood.

marijuana (mar i hwan'ə) (Am. Sp. marihuana). A Mexican name for a poisonous hemp. It is not physiologically addicting but can create psychological dependence.

medicinal (mə dis'i nəl) (L. *medicinalis*). Having healing qualities.

mescaline (mes'kə lin) (Sp. *mexrialli*, to drink). A poisonous oil extracted from peyote (*Lophophora williamsii*). It produces an intoxication with delusions of color and music.

morphine (mor'fēn) (G. *Morpheus*, god of sleep). A widely used analgesic and sedative.

narcotic (när kot'ik) (G. *narkoun*, to benumb). Having the power to produce sleep or drowsiness and to relieve pain.

nausea (naw'zē ə, naw'zhə) (G. *nausia*, seasickness). Inclination to vomit.

opiate (ō'pē it) (G. *opion*, poppy juice). A drug containing, or derived from, opium, a narcotic.

opium (ō'pē əm) (L. fr. G. *opion*, poppy juice). A narcotic drug consisting of the dried juice of the opium poppy (*Papaver somniferum*).

organotropic (ôr'gə no trop'ik) (G. *organon*, organ + *tropikos*, belonging to). Having an attraction for certain organs or tissues of the body.

oxidation (ok'sə da'shən) (G. *oxide*, acid, sour). Combination with oxygen or removal of hydrogen from a compound by the action of oxygen; one means by which body disposes of foreign substances (such as alcohol).

paraldehyde (pə ral'də hīd). A hypnotic having prompt action as a sedative.

peyote (pā ō'tē) (Sp. *pejote*, caterpillar; refers to the downy center of the button). A common name for the cactus *Lophophora williamsii*.

phenobarbital (fē'nō bahr'bi tol). Drug used as a hypnotic in nervous insomnia and states of nervous excitement and as a sedative in epilepsy.

psychogenic (sī kō jen'ik) (G. *psyche*, mind, soul; *genesis*, to produce). Orginating in the mind, as a disease might.

sedative (sed'ə tiv) (L. *sedativus*, calming). A remedy that allays excitement; quieting.

solvent (sol'vənt) (L. *solvens*, to dissolve). Dissolving, producing a solution.

stimulant (stim'yoo lənt) (L. *stimulus*, a goad). Any agent temporarily increasing the functional ability of the body.

strychnine (strik'nin) (G. *strychnos*, nightshade). Alkaloid from seeds of *Strychnos nux-vomica*, an extremely potent stimulant of the central nervous system.

subcutaneous (sub'kū tā'ni əs). Under the skin.

synergism (sin' er jiz'm) (G. *synergos*, working together). A working together, as of drugs that work together to effect more than they can separately.

synthetic (sin thet'ik). Formed by a chemical reaction in a laboratory.

thrombocytopenia (throm'bo si to pē'ne ə). An abnormal increase in blood platelets (circular or oval disks found in the blood, important in the clotting of blood).

tolerance (tol'er əns). Increasing resistance to the usual effects of a drug.

toxicity (tok sis'ə ti) (G. *toxikon*, a poison). Quality of being poisonous.

tranquilizer (tran'kwə lizer) (L. *tranquillus*, calm, quiet, still). Drug that acts to relieve an overactive, anxious, or disturbed emotional state; a central-nervous-system depressant.

volatile solvent (vol'ə t'l sol'vənt) (L. *volatilis*, to fly; *solvere*, to release, free). Easily vaporized substance capable of dissolving something; specifically, chemicals contained in lighter fluid, model-airplane glue, and other common substances which produce a state of intoxication when inhaled.

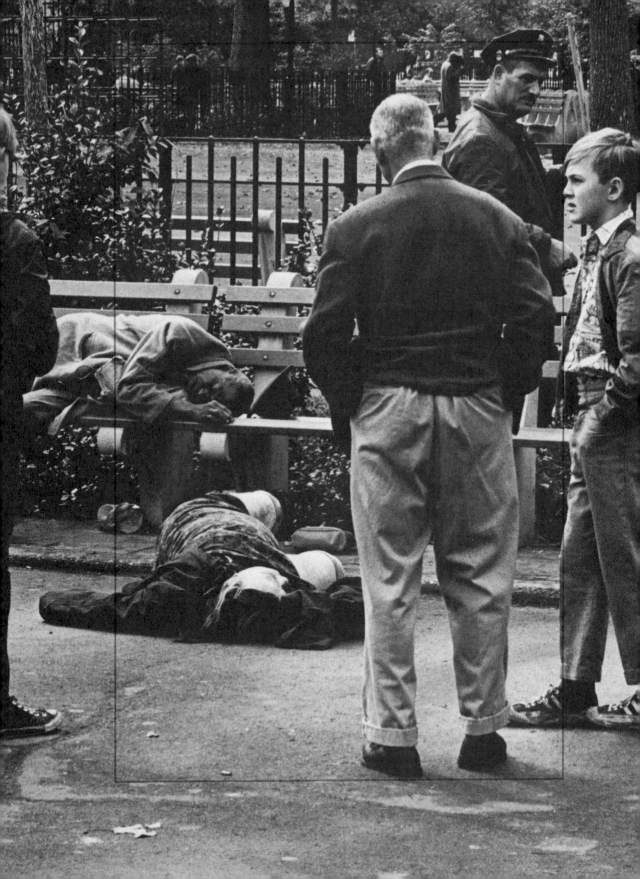

Use and abuse of alcohol

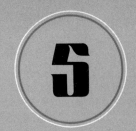

THE SOCIALLY ACCEPTED MOOD-MODIFYING DRUG

The chief distinction between alcohol and the drugs discussed in Chapter 4 is that the moderate use of alcohol is legally and socially accepted. Yet alcohol has a potential for abuse that is as great as that of many of those drugs. In Chapter 4 it was classified as one of the "mood-modifying" drugs, a sedative. It is the most widely used and abused mood-modifying sedative in the United States. About 70 percent of all adults in the United States drink alcoholic beverages. Alcoholic beverages are part of social gatherings, from family meals to public conventions. Because alcohol is so widely used, this complete chapter is devoted to a discussion of alcoholic beverages and alcoholism (compulsive alcohol abuse or alcohol addiction).

ALCOHOLIC BEVERAGES

To understand the effects of alcoholic beverages one needs to know something about their nature. Even among regular drinkers there are many misconceptions regarding alcohol and alcoholic beverages.

121

Types of alcohol

Although there are many kinds of alcohol, the only alcohol in beverages is *ethyl alcohol*, known chemically as *ethanol* and commonly as "grain alcohol." Other common alcohols include *methyl alcohol*, usually referred to as "wood alcohol." Methyl alcohol is used in many products such as antifreeze and fuels. It is a deadly poison; even small amounts can cause blindness or death. "Bootleg" liquor (sold illegally without payment of taxes) is occasionally found to contain methyl alcohol, and it has been the cause of many deaths.

A third common alcohol is *isopropyl alcohol*, the principal ingredient of most "rubbing alcohol." Although it is not as deadly as wood alcohol, rubbing alcohol is definitely too poisonous to be consumed as a beverage.

Throughout the remainder of this chapter the unqualified term "alcohol" will indicate ethyl alcohol. Ethyl alcohol in any alcoholic beverage is produced by the fermentation of sugar by yeast. Each type of alcoholic beverage is produced from a specific source of sugar; see Table 5.1. Beer and ale, for example, are made by fermenting malted (sprouted) barley. Wine is fermented grape juice. The "hard" liquors are made from the distilled product of the fermentation of grains and other sugar sources. Distillation greatly concentrates the alcohol content of a beverage, so that distilled liquors are usually diluted with water, soft drinks, fruit juices, or other mixes instead of being consumed "straight." The alcohol content of distilled beverages is expressed as *proof*, which in the United States is the percentage of alcohol multiplied by 2; for example, 100 proof means 50 percent alcohol.

Table 5.1 *Some common alcoholic beverages*

beverage	product fermented	distilled?	percent of alcohol by volume
Beer	Malted barley	No	4–6
Ale	Malted barley	No	6–8
Wines			
dry (dinner)	Grape juice	No	12–14
sweet (dessert)	Grape juice[a]	No	19–21
Whisky	Malted grains	Yes	40–50
Brandy	Grape juice	Yes	40–50
Rum	Molasses	Yes	40–50
Vodka	Potatoes and other sources[b]	Yes	40–50
Gin	Various sources[c]	Yes	40–50

[a] The sweet wines have sugar added after fermentation and are fortified by the addition of brandy to kill the yeast and prevent fermentation of the sugar.
[b] Vodka is essentially just alcohol and water, without other flavoring agents.
[c] Gin is flavored with extracts from juniper berries and other sources.

Table 5.2 *Nutritional values of alcoholic beverages*

	amount contained		
nutrient	beer, 12 ounces	whiskey, 2 ounces	wine, 8 ounces
Calories	171	140	275
Calories from alcohol	114	140	240
Protein, grams	2	0	0
Fat, grams	0	0	0
Carbohydrate, grams	12	0	8.5
Thiamine (B_1), milligrams	0.1	0	0
Nicotinic acid (niacin), milligrams	0.75	0	0
Riboflavin (B_2)	10	0	0
Ascorbic acid (C), milligrams	0	0	0
Folic acid	0	0	0

Ingredients of alcoholic beverages

Besides alcohol and water alcoholic beverages contain flavoring and coloring agents. Alcoholic beverages have almost no food value; for there are no vitamins, minerals, fats, proteins, or usable carbohydrates in alcoholic beverages; see Table 5.2. The one exception is beer, and the amounts present in beer are nutritionally insignificant.

Calories, however, are abundant in all alcoholic beverages. Most of the calories are derived from the alcohol itself, and they are "empty" calories: that is, they provide no nutrition and displace nutritious foods in the diet. Chronic alcoholics often suffer from malnutrition, and many of their physical ailments are believed to result from faulty nutritional patterns due to their abuse of alcohol.

PHYSIOLOGICAL EFFECTS OF ALCOHOL

All alcoholic beverages have basically the same effects on the body. The only important difference among them is the amount of alcohol they contain. Any two drinks containing the same amount of alcohol will produce the same effect. Table 5.3 and Fig. 5.1 compare the amounts of several different drinks which would contain similar quantities of alcohol.

Effect on the brain

The most important effect of alcohol is its depressant or "sedative" or, in high concentrations, "anesthetic" action on the brain (Fig. 4.3). Alcohol is a mood-modifying drug and can temporarily produce a state of mild euphoria

Table 5.3 *Amounts of different alcoholic beverages yielding similar quantities of alcohol*

beverage	alcohol content (percent)	approximate amount yielding 0.5 ounce of alcohol (ounces)
Beer	4	12
Dinner wine	12	4
Dessert wine	21	2.5
80 proof liquor	40	1.25
100 proof liquor	50	1

and an apparent stimulation. This, undoubtedly, is the basis of its attraction for the "social" drinker (occasional user). The deeper depression, which lets a person "escape" from cares, pressures, tensions and anxieties, that occurs at higher concentrations of alcohol in the blood is what the "heavy" drinker is seeking (Table 5.4). Many people feel an apparent stimulation from one

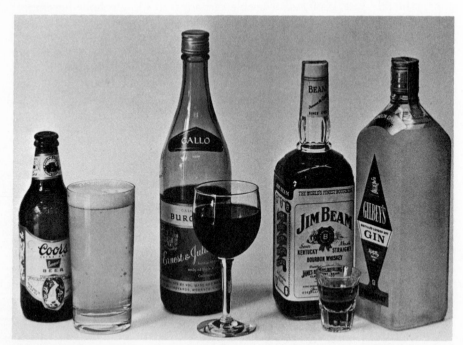

Figure 5.1   The three drinks shown are roughly equivalent in their alcohol content: 12 ounces of beer, 4 ounces of dry wine, and 1 to 1.25 ounces of distilled liquor.

Table 5.4 *Relationships of alcoholic intoxication and concentration of alcohol in the blood*

stage	blood alcohol level (percent)	observations of alcoholic intoxication
No apparent change	0.0–0.11	Normal by ordinary observations; slight changes detectable by special tests
Emotional instability	0.09–0.21	Decreased inhibitions; emotional instability; slight muscular incoordination; slowing of muscular responses to stimuli
Confusion	0.18–0.33	Disturbance of sensations; decreased pain sense; staggering gait; slurred speech
Stupor	0.27–0.43	Marked decrease in response to stimuli; muscular incoordination approaching paralysis
Coma	0.36–0.56	Complete unconsciousness; depressed reflexes; subnormal temperature; anesthesia; impairment of circulation; death possible for some persons
Death	<over 0.44>	Death possible when blood alcohol concentration reaches this level.

SOURCE: Adapted from B. S. Bergersen et al., *Pharmacology in Nursing*, St. Louis, C. V. Mosby.

or two drinks, but this comes about indirectly. As shown by Table 5.4, small amounts of alcohol depress the parts of the brain that function in judgment, self-control, and inhibition. When these parts of the brain are depressed, a person feels an apparent stimulation due to this release from inhibitions.

Research has shown, however, that alcohol starts to be a factor in accidents at blood levels as low as 0.03 percent. Table 5.5 shows the blood alcohol levels that are produced by different amounts of alcohol. It is recommended that the person who plans to drive keep his blood alcohol level below 0.05 percent.

The drinking driver seldom realizes how much his driving ability has deteriorated, because the same effects on the brain that cause him to be a dangerous driver also make him unaware of how poor his driving has become. Thus the person who drinks must plan ahead, while he is still sober, in order to have some means of transportation home other than his driving a car.

At low blood alcohol levels the chief effects on driving are a reduction

Table 5.5 *Blood alcohol levels*

body weight (pounds)	drinks[a]											
	1	2	3	4	5	6	7	8	9	10	11	12
100	0.038	0.075	0.113	0.150	0.188	0.225	0.263	0.300	0.338	0.375	0.413	0.450
120	.031	.063	.094	.125	.156	.188	.219	.250	.281	.313	.344	.375
140	.027	.054	.080	.107	.134	.161	.188	.214	.241	.268	.295	.321
160	.023	.047	.070	.094	.117	.141	.164	.188	.211	.234	.258	.281
180	.021	.042	.063	.083	.104	.125	.146	.167	.188	.208	.229	.250
200	.019	.038	.056	.075	.094	.113	.131	.150	.169	.188	.206	.225
220	.017	.034	.051	.068	.085	.102	.119	.136	.153	.170	.188	.205
240	.016	.031	.047	.063	.078	.094	.109	.125	.141	.156	.172	.188

Under 0.05	0.05 to 0.10	0.10 to 0.15	Over 0.15
Driving is not seriously impaired.	Driving is increasingly dangerous. At 0.08, legally drunk in Utah.	Driving is dangerous. Legally drunk in most states.	Driving is *very* dangerous. Legally drunk in any state.

SOURCE: Reprinted through the courtesy of the New Jersey Department of Law and Public Safety, Division of Motor Vehicles, Trenton, New Jersey.
[a] One drink equals 1 ounce of 100 proof liquor or 12 ounces of beer.

in the level of judgment, the care he takes, and peripheral (side) vision. The person can still drive straight enough, but he may take chances he might otherwise not. At higher blood alcohol levels there are the additional factors of poor vision and slowed muscular reactions. Many states have lowered the blood alcohol level for a drunken-driving conviction from 0.15 percent to 0.10 percent. The federal government has made part of its payment of highway construction funds dependent upon conformance to this standard. In one state, Utah, a blood alcohol level of 0.08 makes a driver legally drunk. Alcohol is believed to be a contributing factor in 25 to 50 percent of all fatal traffic accidents. Although alcohol is not officially listed as the actual cause in many of these cases, it is thought that many accidents blamed on "high speed" or "failure to negotiate a curve" are actually the result of drinking.

At extremely high blood alcohol levels the respiratory and circulatory centers of the brain are depressed, resulting in death (Table 5.4). Such high alcohol levels are not reached in normal drinking, because a person would vomit or pass out first.

The degree of intoxication produced by a given amount of alcohol varies considerably among different individuals. One factor is the body weight. Alcohol is diluted fairly uniformly throughout the body, so the blood alcohol level produced by any given amount of alcohol is in approximate inverse proportion to the body weight of the individual. A lighter person becomes more intoxicated than a heavier person by the same amount of alcohol. Even with two people at the same blood alcohol level there may be a great difference in their degree of intoxication. It has been demonstrated that a *tolerance* for alcohol develops in the frequent and heavy drinker, resulting in a lower degree of intoxication than that reached by the moderate or occasional drinker.

Sensory perception is dulled. The sense first affected is sight; at the higher blood alcohol levels there is also an impairment in the senses of hearing, equilibrium, taste, smell, and touch. Alcohol intoxication impairs both the storage and retrieval of information. The learning ability is decreased, as is the ability to recall past events and learned knowledge. The problem-solving ability also is reduced by alcohol; simple problems become difficult, and difficult problems become impossible.

Many people worry about possible permanent effects on the brain as a result of drinking. Light or moderate drinking has little known permanent effect on the brain; however, if a person drinks long enough and in sufficient quantity he can permanently damage his brain. This damage is discussed in the section on alcoholism.

Effects on other organs

In addition to its effect on the brain alcohol directly and indirectly affects some of the other body organs. One easily noticed effect is the dilation of the small blood vessels of the skin. As a result the face and neck appear red, and the person feels warm. There may also be a slight drop in blood pressure as a result of this dilation.

The problems of muscular coordination experienced by the intoxicated person are not the result of a direct action of alcohol upon the muscles but reflect the action of alcohol on the portions of the nervous system that control the muscles.

There are several possible effects of alcohol upon digestion and the digestive system. Moderate drinkers sometimes notice an improvement in their digestion when they drink before or with a meal. One explanation of this is that alcohol can indirectly improve digestion by relieving nervous tension that may interfere with digestion, and it may also aid digestion by stimulating the production of stomach acid. But large amounts of alcohol irritate the stomach lining and, along with the increased amount of acid, may cause gastritis and other stomach conditions. High concentrations of alcohol in the stomach may cause enough irritation to trigger the reflex action of vomiting, intended to remove the irritant.

Liver disorders are common among alcoholics. About 75 percent of all alcoholics show some degree of loss of liver function. About 8 percent eventually develop cirrhosis of the liver, an often fatal condition. This is 6 times the incidence of cirrhosis among the general population. It is not definitely known how much of this liver damage is due to the direct effects of alcohol and how much is due to malnutrition; it is likely that both are factors.

ELIMINATION OF ALCOHOL BY THE BODY

Although small amounts of alcohol are lost from the body with the breath, sweat, and urine, more than 90 percent of the alcohol taken into the body is disposed of by oxidation in carbon dioxide and water. The oxidation takes place through several steps, the first of which occurs almost exclusively in the liver. Although the remaining steps take place rapidly in various body tissues, it is the liver that governs the speed of the total process, since the second step cannot take place until the liver completes the first step.

Although the rate of alcohol oxidation varies slightly among individuals, it is remarkably constant for any one individual. It remains constant whether the blood alcohol level is high or low. The average person can oxidize in each hour the amount of alcohol contained in 0.5 to 1 ounce of distilled liquor or 6 to 12 ounces of beer. Experiments have shown that little can be done to speed up this rate.

This information has practical application in that a person can estimate how soon he should drive after drinking. A waiting period of one hour per drink consumed is a minimum for most individuals.

PROPER USE OF ALCOHOL

Some people argue that any consumption of alcoholic beverages is improper, but most Americans find no medical, moral, legal, or religious reason for not making moderate use of alcoholic beverages. We shall therefore offer some suggestions that may help a person avoid problems in his drinking.

Even those who fully approve of drinking and themselves drink regularly usually disapprove of certain types of drinking behavior as, for example, drunken driving or such antisocial behavior as physical or verbal violence. Almost all of those who approve of drinking do feel that there are times and places where drinking is not appropriate. Any time that a person needs his fullest mental faculties, such as when he is driving or operating any machinery, is obviously a poor time to have been drinking. Many employers make drinking or being drunk on the job ground for immediate dismissal.

It is very poor policy to drink for courage, such as in preparation for a job interview or sales conference. This is using alcohol as a crutch and is a step in the direction of alcoholism.

There is, of course, no set answer to the question of how much to drink. While drinking is acceptable in our society, getting drunk is definitely not. The person who drinks is expected to drink in moderation, without serious impairment of his physical or mental functions.

The moderate drinker learns to drink slowly and to pace his drinking so that he does not build up a high blood alcohol level. If a person who can oxidize the alcohol from one drink each hour spaces four drinks over the span of a four-hour party, he will not reach an excessively high blood alcohol level.

The host or hostess of a party where drinks are served should feel a certain responsibility for the amount of alcohol the guests drink. He must ask himself how he would feel if someone were involved in a fatal accident on the way home from his party. There should be nonalcoholic drinks available for those who would prefer them, and the person who prefers not to drink should not be pressed or ridiculed. No pressure should be put on any guest to drink more than he wants. If he wants to stop at one drink, let him. During the last hour or so of a party coffee should be served. This serves several purposes. Coffee does not counteract alcohol, but the caffeine may help overcome the drowsiness that can be as much a cause of accidents as intoxication, and the time spent drinking coffee serves as a sobering-up period. Finally, the serving of coffee is accepted by most guests as a signal that the party is almost over, so the host can bring a party to a close when he wishes to. Anyone who is obviously in no condition to drive home should be strongly encouraged to stay over, take a taxi, share a ride, or do something other than drive.

ALCOHOLISM (THE ABUSE OF ALCOHOL)

Even among recognized authorities there are various concepts of what constitutes an alcoholic. Some authorities use a highly restrictive definition of alcoholism; others define it in a very general way. An example of a relatively restrictive definition is that of Chafetz and Demone, who view alcoholism as

> . . . a chronic behavioral disorder manifested by undue preoccupation with alcohol to the detriment of physical and mental health, by a loss of control when drinking has begun, although it may not be carried to the point of intoxication, and by a self-destructive attitude in dealing with relationships and life situations.[1]

An example of a more general definition of alcoholism is that of Diethelm, who considers an alcoholic to be anyone who

> . . . uses alcohol to such an extent that it interferes with a successful life (including physical, personality, and social aspects) and is either not able to recognize this effect or is not able to control his alcohol consumption, although he knows its disastrous results.[2]

It can be seen that both definitions emphasize, not how much a person drinks, but the effects of his drinking. There are some persons who cannot be classified as alcoholics who actually drink more than others who can so be classified.

There is no established system for reporting the incidence of alcoholism in the United States; thus any figures given for the prevalence of alcoholism are estimates. Since much alcoholism escapes medical or legal detection, and since there are various definitions of "alcoholism," it is to be expected that a wide range occurs among published estimates as to the extent of alcoholism in the United States. Alcoholism is America's number one "hidden" health problem.

Theories of alcoholism

Many theories regarding the causes of alcoholism have been proposed, yet none has gained widespread acceptance. Alcoholism has been related to physiological, psychological, and sociological factors. Among the physiological causes that have been proposed are nutritional deficiencies, such metabolic defects as abnormal enzyme levels, disturbed glandular functions, abnormal levels of various body chemicals, and allergic reactions. The proposed psychological causes have included oral cravings, repressed homosexual traits, pleasure fixation, unconscious urges to destroy oneself or to dominate others, feelings of inferiority or insecurity, and many others. Certain personality traits are commonly found among alcoholics. One is low self-esteem. Having little sense of his own worth, he feels insecure and isolated from other people. These feelings cause him emotional pain, and he drinks to wipe

---

[1] M. E. Chafetz and H. W. Demone, Jr., *Alcoholism and Society*, New York, Oxford University Press, 1962.

[2] O. Diethelm, *Etiology of Chronic Alcoholism*, Springfield, Ill., C. C Thomas, 1955.

out this pain. These feelings are also found among abusers of other drugs and overeaters.

Today alcoholism is often recognized as being one of several complex emotional problems. However, a vicious circle often develops, in which personal and family problems lead to excessive drinking, which leads to further family problems, which leads to the eventual destruction of the family unit.

At least some research evidence has been presented to support each of the possible causes of alcoholism, but no single theory of causation has been adequately proved. In fact, there probably is no single cause of all alcoholism. More likely, alcoholism is the result of many complex factors acting together.

The concept of alcoholism as a disease is widely accepted today and is well within the medical definition of disease. The alcoholic is regarded as a sick person rather than as a weak or sinful person.

Phases of alcoholism

Since at least 1 in every 14 drinkers eventually becomes an alcoholic, it is important that anyone who uses alcoholic beverages be able to recognize the signs and symptoms of impending and early alcoholism. Hopefully, if a person noticed these symptoms in himself and knew what they meant, he might have the good judgment to cease drinking before he reached a more advanced stage of alcoholism.

A classic research project in which the late Dr. E. M. Jellinek interviewed more than 2,000 alcoholics revealed that most alcoholics pass through definite progressive stages with characteristic symptoms. The progression is graphically represented in Fig. 5.2, which will be referred to in the following paragraphs. On this graph time proceeds from left to right. There can be no fixed scale of months or years, since some alcoholics make the entire progression in a matter of months and others may take many years to reach the same point. Jellinek pointed out that the development of alcoholism in women is frequently more rapid than in men, and the stages are less clear-cut. The vertical line on the graph indicates the relative degree of alcohol tolerance or, in other words, the amount of alcohol required to reach a given degree of intoxication.

Prealcoholic phases   During the course of social drinking most people learn the feeling of escape from everyday cares that alcohol can provide (Phase I on Fig. 5.2). When an individual occasionally drinks for the specific purpose of escape from tensions, he has progressed to the second prealcoholic phase (Phase II); about 20 percent of all drinkers fall into this category. In the person destined for alcoholism, this escape drinking gradually becomes more and more frequent (Phase III). As his drinking becomes more frequent, he develops a tolerance for alcohol: that is, he must drink more in order to achieve the same effect. At first tolerance increases gradually; then it often takes a sudden jump.

Early alcoholic phase   Soon after his increase in tolerance, the frequent drinker may experience his first *alcoholic blackout* (Phase IV). A blackout is a period of temporary amnesia occurring when a person is drinking. In contrast to passing out, which results in unconsciousness, a person in an alcoholic blackout is still conscious of what he is doing at the time and may be doing all the things he might normally do. But after he comes out of his blackout, he has no memory of anything that took place during the blackout. Anyone who drinks too much will pass out, but only the alcoholic or near-alcoholic blacks out. The mechanism of the blackout is not yet definitely known. It may have a physiological origin or it may be a psychological ego-defense mechanism.

True alcoholic phase   Another major milestone in the development of alcoholism is *loss of control* (Phase V). This means the loss of the ability to drink in a moderate, controlled manner. It does not mean that the individual feels compelled to start drinking, but when he does start, he cannot stop after a predetermined, moderate amount of alcohol. He may continue to drink until he becomes quite intoxicated or gets sick. The period of drinking may last for a few hours or become a binge, lasting for days or weeks. The individual

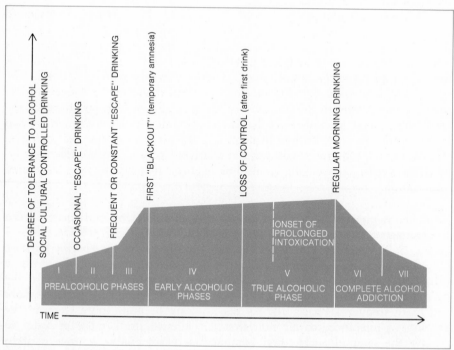

Figure 5.2   The phases of alcoholism.

can choose when he starts his drinking, but not when he stops it. By any definition of alcoholism, this individual is now an alcoholic.

It may be seen on the chart that a high level of tolerance is maintained through both Phases IV and V, until in late alcohol addiction there is a marked loss of tolerance.

Many other symptoms are characteristic of the alcoholic during these phases. These symptoms are arranged in sequence from the characteristics of early alcoholism to those of late alcoholism. In a given individual they may not occur exactly in this order, but they are usually in about this sequence.

1. *Secret drinking.* The alcoholic often "sneaks" his drinks, so that others will not know how much he is drinking.

2. *Preoccupation with alcohol.* The personal aspects of social functions become secondary to the opportunity for drinking. For example, when an alcoholic is invited to a party, he is more interested in the fact that drinks will be available than in who will be there.

3. *Gulping the first few drinks.* The alcoholic drinks for the quickest possible effect.

4. *Guilt feelings about drinking.* As the alcoholic begins to realize that his drinking habits are not normal, he develops vague conscious or subconscious feelings of guilt. These feelings of guilt may lead to several outward symptoms.

    a. *Avoids talking about alcohol.* The person who eagerly talks about his drinking is seldom a problem drinker. The alcoholic, by contrast, does not like to discuss drinking because he is afraid he will be criticized for his excessive drinking.

    b. *Rationalizes his drinking behavior.* The alcoholic always has a "reason" for drinking, which is actually an excuse, a rationalization. It never occurs to the normal drinker to offer a reason for his drinking. For the alcoholic good news and bad news are both valid reasons for drinking. He drinks to celebrate his accomplishments or to drown his sorrows. These rationalizations are needed primarily for the protection of his own ego and only secondarily as alibis to his family and associates.

    c. *Exhibits grandiose behavior.* The alcoholic often goes through overly extravagant and generous periods, during which he throws money around in a showy way. He may buy drinks for perfect strangers and leave unusually large tips. The purpose of such display is not so much to impress others as it is to reassure himself that he is really not such a bad guy after all. This is part of the system of rationalization which strongly influences the life of the alcoholic and serves to protect his ego.

    d. *Has periods of remorse.* Often the guilt feelings of the alcoholic lead to periods of persistent remorse, which may have the unfortunate effect of leading him on to still more drinking.

5. *Periods of total abstinence.* As a result of social pressures or his own concern the alcoholic may go "on the wagon." For several weeks or months he does not take a drink. Then he usually resumes drinking with renewed vigor, because he is satisfied that he can still live without alcohol. Hence the oft-repeated reassurance "I can take it or leave it" becomes the theme song of the alcoholic.

6. *Changing drinking patterns.* The alcoholic feels that there must be some way in which he can drink without loss of control. In attempting to drink in a normal and controlled manner he frequently varies his drinking pattern, trying different types of liquor, different mixes, or different times or places. Of course, none of these changes help.

7. *Behavior becomes alcohol-centered.* This symptom is characterized by a marked loss of interest in anything other than alcohol. Personal appearance is neglected, as is the maintenance of living quarters and possessions. There is a deterioration in interpersonal relationships. Instead of worrying about how his drinking is affecting his activities, the alcoholic avoids activities that might interfere with his drinking. The alcoholic becomes increasingly egocentric.

8. *Effects on the family.* The family members of the alcoholic often change their habits. They may withdraw into the home for fear of embarrassment or else become very active in outside interests as a means of escape from the home environment. Financial problems are usually a way of life for the family of the alcoholic.

9. *Unreasonable resentments.* The alcoholic often builds up tremendous feelings of resentment and self-pity. He spends much time brooding over minor or imaginary injustices he has suffered.

10. *Hiding bottles.* The many jokes and cartoons about alcoholics hiding (and losing) their bottles have a factual basis. The alcoholic often takes elaborate precautions to avoid running out of liquor.

11. *Neglect of proper nutrition.* The alcoholic typically, while drinking, has little interest in food; he derives most of his calories from alcoholic beverages, which are very poor sources of vitamins, minerals, and proteins. He may suffer from serious malnutrition, which may actually cause more physical damage than the toxic effect of alcohol.

12. *Decrease in sexual drive.* As a result of his deteriorating physical and emotional condition the alcoholic may suffer a decrease in sexual drive. This decrease often leads to *alcoholic jealousy,* in which the spouse of the alcoholic is accused of having extramarital affairs. The marriage which has managed to survive to this point is often shattered by such jealousy.

Phases VI and VII of alcohol addiction (compulsive alcohol abuse)

Phase VI is the beginning of true physical alcohol addiction. Alcoholism and narcotic addiction are similar processes; the major differences are the length of time and the dosage required for the development of physical dependence. In 1970 the Expert Committee on Alcohol and Alcoholism of the World Health Organization stated:

. . . recent evidence makes it appear that there is more resemblance between the responses of the withdrawal from alcohol and from opiates than was previously realized . . . when serious symptoms follow the withdrawal of alcohol they persist almost as long as do those following the withdrawal of opiates.

1. *Regular morning drinking.* Alcohol is an addictive drug. After years of heavy drinking a level of addiction may be reached which requires the constant presence of alcohol in the body to prevent withdrawal symptoms. This level of dependence indicates *chronic alcohol addiction* (Phase VI). The alcoholic must now start his day with a drink; see Fig. 5.3. If the fully addicted alcoholic is deprived of alcohol, his first withdrawal symptom is usually a shaking of the hands, arms, and body. His mood may be one of apprehension or fear, and he may suffer hallucinations. The alcoholic at this stage should not be forced to sober up without medical assistance, as there is a chance he will go into convulsions and perhaps even die.

2. *Intoxication during working hours.* Another result of the addiction aspect of alcoholism occurs when the alcoholic finds himself intoxicated in

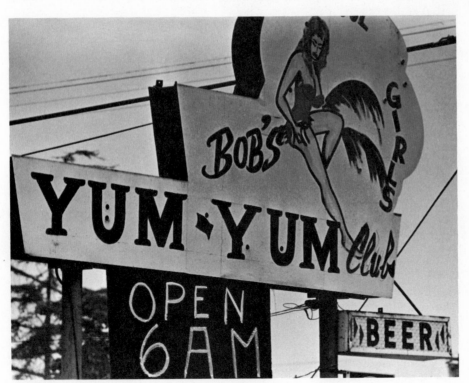

Figure 5.3 "Open 6 A.M." This sign is typical of the bars that cater to early-morning drinkers.

the morning on a working day and either misses work or sneaks drinks while on the job. This is the "beginning of the end" of his job.

3. *Loss of tolerance.* After a long term of heavy drinking the alcoholic loses the tolerance to alcohol he previously had acquired. This loss is possibly connected with a decrease in the ability of the liver to oxidize alcohol. After this loss of tolerance he becomes intoxicated on less liquor than before and sobers up much more slowly. He is able to remain intoxicated at all times with only a moderate total consumption of alcohol.

4. *Mental impairment.* Many alcoholics eventually suffer a severe disintegration of personality. If drinking continues after this symptom appears, there may be permanent brain damage. It is believed that this brain damage is due to the combined effect of severe dietary deficiency plus the direct effect of alcohol.

A type of psychosis that commonly appears in late alcoholics is *delirium tremens,* the "DTs." This is a temporary condition, lasting only from two to ten days, but there may be repeated attacks. An attack may be triggered by injury, illness, or withdrawal from alcohol. The symptoms may include confusion, vivid visual hallucinations, fear, apprehension, restlessness, and sleeplessness. There may even be convulsions similar to epileptic seizures. This is the *alcohol-barbiturate abstinence syndrome.* The attack ends with a period of deep sleep.

5. *Termination of alcoholism.* There are several ways in which a case of alcoholism may terminate. They include the following:

   a. *Failure of the rationalization system.* Eventually the elaborate system of rationalization that has sustained the alcoholic breaks down, usually in response to some serious crisis. If the alcoholic can admit defeat, he becomes accessible to treatment and often successfully regains his sobriety.

   b. *Wet brain.* After several attacks of delirium tremens a more serious condition, known as "wet brain," develops. This is a chronic condition that is seldom curable and may even be fatal. The thought processes are completely disrupted, and all other functions of the nervous system are impaired. This is permanent brain damage, and the alcoholic who reaches this stage either dies or spends the rest of his life in an institution.

Fortunately, it is not necessary for an alcoholic to go through the entire course of the disease of alcoholism. An alcoholic can be successfully treated at any stage, if he is willing to admit that he has a drinking problem and if he really wants to do something about it.

SUMMARY

    I. Socially accepted mood-modifying drug
   II. Alcoholic beverages
      A. Types of alcohol
         1. Ethyl alcohol, only alcohol in alcoholic beverages.

2. Methyl alcohol, a deadly poison.

3. Isopropyl alcohol, too poisonous to be consumed as a beverage.

   B. Other ingredients of alcoholic beverages

     1. Water.

     2. Flavoring.

     3. Coloring agents.

     4. Calories—7 calories per gram.

III. Physiological effects of alcohol—all alcoholic beverages have basically the same effects on the body.

   A. Effects on the brain

     1. Depressant or sedative effect.

     2. Apparent feeling of stimulation due to loss of inhibition.

     3. Degree of intoxication depends upon:

       a. given amount of alcohol consumed.

       b. body weight.

       c. degree of tolerance for alcohol.

     4. Intoxication often includes a state of euphoria.

     5. Sensory perception is dulled.

     6. The storage and retrieval of information is impaired.

     7. Heavy drinking over long periods of time can produce permanent damage.

   B. Effects on other organs

     1. Produces dilation of blood vessels of the skin.

     2. Liver disorders are common among alcoholics.

IV. Elimination of alcohol by the body

   A. Primarily through oxidation to carbon dioxide and water.

   B. Rate of oxidation determined by liver.

     1. Rate remains constant whether the blood alcohol level is high or low.

     2. Average person can oxidize in each hour the amount of alcohol in:

       a. 0.5 to 1 ounce of distilled liquor.

       b. 6 to 12 ounces of beer.

V. Proper use of alcohol

   A. Some suggestions that may help a person avoid problems in his drinking.

     1. There are times and places where drinking is not appropriate.

     2. Using alcohol as a crutch is a step in the direction of alcoholism.

     3. A person who drinks is expected to drink in moderation.

     4. One should learn to drink slowly and to pace drinking so that he does not build up a high blood alcohol level.

   B. The host or hostess of a party where drinks are served should feel a certain responsibility for the amount of alcohol the guests drink.

     1. Nonalcoholic drinks should be available for those who would prefer them.

     2. Persons who prefer not to drink should not be pressed or ridiculed.

     3. Some nonalcoholic drinks (such as coffee) should be served during the last hour of a party to provide a sobering-up period.

VI. Alcoholism (the abuse of alcohol)

   A. Several definitions of alcoholism exist.

     1. Restrictive definition based upon the concept of loss of control and inability to stop at a predetermined number of drinks.

     2. More general definition is that of a person whose drinking interferes with a successful life.

B. Theories of alcoholism.
  1. Alcoholism is the result of many complex factors acting together.
  2. Alcoholism is a disease.
C. Phases of alcoholism—it is important that anyone who uses alcoholic beverages be able to recognize the signs and symptoms of impending and early alcoholism.
  1. Prealcoholic phases:
    a. drinking as an escape from tensions.
    b. drinking more and more to achieve the same effect; *tolerance* to alcohol is developing.
  2. Early alcoholic phase—*alcoholic blackout* (a period of temporary amnesia occurring when a person is drinking).
  3. True alcoholic phase:
    a. *loss of control:* loss of the ability to drink in a moderate, controlled manner.
    b. when someone starts drinking he cannot stop after a predetermined, moderate amount of alcohol is consumed.
    c. by any definition of alcoholism, this individual is now an alcoholic.
  4. Many other signs of alcoholism—usually appear in a certain order.
D. Alcohol and narcotic addiction.
  1. Alcohol-induced addiction is similar to opiate addiction.
  2. Symptoms of withdrawal from alcohol persist almost as long as those of withdrawal from opiates.

Glossary

If you cannot find the word you wish in this glossary, check the index for text and glossary references.

abstinence syndrome (L. *abstinere,* to abstain; G. *syndrome,* concurrence). Set of symptoms resulting from withdrawal from alcohol, opiates, and specific depressants.

abuse (ə būz') (ME. *ab-,* away, from + *uto,* to use). To use wrongly or improperly; misuse.

amnesia (am nē'zē ə, or am nē'zhə) (G. *amnesia,* forgetfulness). Inability to recall past experiences.

blackout (blak'out). A period of temporary amnesia occurring while drinking, usually associated with alcoholism.

cirrhosis (G. *kirrhos,* orange-yellow). Disease of the liver involving progressive destruction of liver cells accompanied by regeneration and increase in connective tissue.

depressant (L. *depressio,* down; *de,* down; *premere,* to press). Chemical, substance, or agent which has the ability to reduce the functional activity of the body.

depression (di presh'ən). Reduction of the functional activity of the body.

euphoria (G. *eu,* well; *pherein,* to bear). Feeling of well-being; in psychiatry, exhibiting an abnormal or exaggerated sense of well-being.

hypnotic (G. *hypnotikos,* sleep). A drug that acts to induce sleep.

intoxication (L. *in-,* intensive; G. *toxikon,* poison). Literally, state of being poisoned or drugged; condition produced by excessive use (abuse) of toxic drugs, alcohol, barbiturates, etc.

oxidation (ok'sə dā'shən). Combination with oxygen or removal of hydrogen from a compound by the action of oxygen; one means by which body disposes of foreign substances (such as alcohol).

sedative (sed'a tiv) (L. *sedativus,* calming). Depressant drug that allays excitement; quieting.

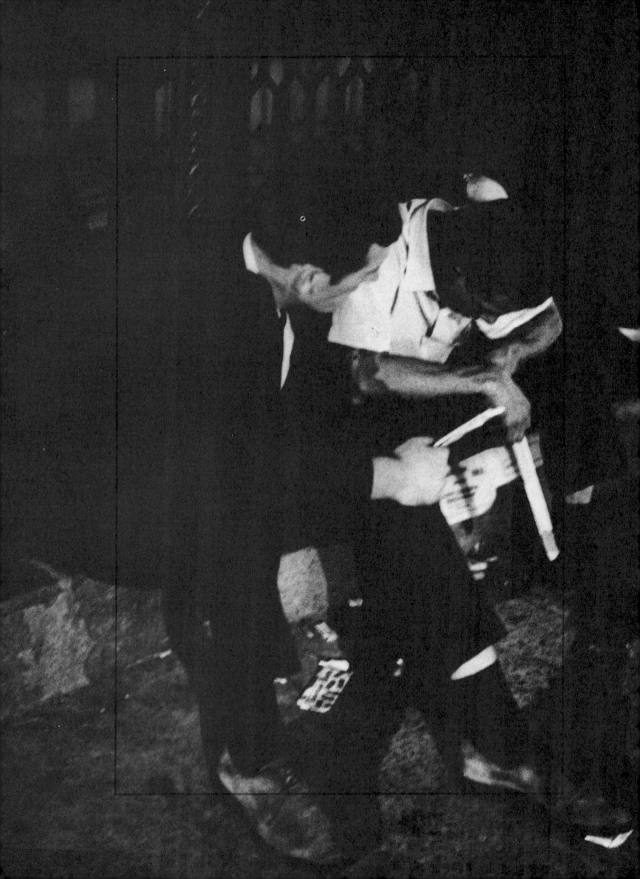

Psychosocial aspects of drug abuse

It is becoming increasingly evident that people with problems—emotional, social, and intellectual—abuse drugs. Individuals do not continue to do something that does not provide them with at least some satisfaction. The reasons for abusing drugs are complex and exist whether the drugs are socially acceptable or not. The reasons are basically the same whether the person uses marijuana, alcohol, hallucinogens, narcotics, barbiturates, amphetamines, tranquilizers, nicotine, or caffeine. They center about wanting to change the pace, to modify moods, to reduce anxiety, to achieve increased activity, to relieve tension, to relieve boredom, to facilitate social interaction, to sleep, or just to have "fun."

SOCIOLOGICAL ASPECTS OF DRUG ABUSE

In previous chapters the biological aspects of drugs and drug abuse have been discussed. Drug use and abuse itself is a social problem. This is being shown by the increasing number of individuals who (1) use drugs *regularly*, (2) use them *occasionally*, (3) try them at some time, or (4) vigorously defend the personal right of those who abuse drugs to do so. This is not a simple problem, and a dialogue among all strata of society must continue.

Helen H. Nowlis, Professor of Psychology, University of Rochester, has outlined nine points that focus upon individuals and the abuse of drugs. Drug abuse is a problem of the following.

1. *Ignorance.* There is a lack of knowledge about the actions of chemical substances upon the complex, delicately balanced chemical system that is the living person. There is also a lack of knowledge about the relationship of variations in human behavior and human behavior itself. Here drug abuse is a problem of opinion, attitudes, and belief without knowledge.

2. *Semantics.* Talking, thinking, acting rationally in an area in which every term is entangled in myth, emotions, assumptions, beliefs, and attitudes that too often turn the dialogue into a futile argument.

3. *Communications.* Scientists in different areas often lack communication among themselves. These individuals are also largely unable to communicate their ideas and findings to laymen. A communication problem also exists between a generation brought up before and during the development of automation, television, jet travel, nuclear energy (and the hydrogen bomb), large urban centers, cramped schools, and an affluent social order and a generation that has known no other conditions.

4. *Lack of understanding of scientific method and concepts.* This is a lack of understanding that there are no simple relationships between cause and effect. Human behavior has many facets, and there is a difference between correlation and causation. The design and execution of experiments may be open to "bias," and a consequent "conclusion" based on *an* experiment has no meaning except in terms of an almost infinite number of dimensions. Statements about these results, even at a biological level, are in terms of averages and probabilities.

5. *Living and learning and growing.* Change is always taking place and the future is increasingly unpredictable.

6. *Philosophy of social control.* In a complex society the individual's relationship to social values is expressed in law. When these laws impinge upon an individual they react directly to the law.

7. *Education.* This becomes a problem of the relationship of the institution both to current social values and to the needs of society.

8. A *"pill society."* This well-advertised proposition states that there is a chemical solution for any problem of unpleasantness and discomfort. The "pill society" spends more on alcohol, tranquilizers, and sleeping pills than it does on education or the social and economic ills of the nation.

9. *Increasing retreat in the face of complex and difficult problems.* The biggest "cop out" of all time is the insistence that everything is all good or all bad, and that good is "not bad" and bad is "not good."

The abnormal social behavior of drug-influenced individuals is an increasingly prominent sociological, medical, and legal problem. The problem actually involves the issue of personal responsibility during times of drug-induced behavioral changes, mood modifications, or personality dysorganization (see Chapter 2). Clearly, the prohibition of drugs is not the answer. The proper control of drug abuse lies in answering the above-listed nine problems. The real problem is not drugs but the people who use drugs.

Social problems resulting from regular and compulsive drug abuse

The relationship between drug abuse and society is complex, each influencing the other. Much of the effects of drug abuse is intangible, but there are certain readily apparent costs to society. The most obvious costs are those that can be measured in dollars, such as those of crimes, hospitalization, and law enforcement. Some doctors in high-abuse areas will see as many as 7000 drug users in one year. There are specialized state and private hospitals treating alcoholics and drug addicts. Many large corporations have special programs, costing thousands of dollars, to help their employees who have drinking problems.

Other, less measurable, costs are broken homes, premature deaths, and the loss of creativity and productivity. The role of alcohol in a family has been studied for many years. It is influenced by the religious, ethnic, and social affiliations of that family. As long as the drinking practices of family members are in accord with those of the social groups to which the family belongs, drinking is usually not associated with family problems. But when drinking or any other type of drug abuse becomes associated with family problems, it is of prime importance to determine whether the abuse is the cause of the family problems or a symptom of a deeper social, family, or personal problem. In the past alcohol was automatically held responsible for family poverty, divorce, child neglect, juvenile delinquency, and most other family problems. Today problem-drinking behavior is recognized as often being just one symptom of a deeper emotional problem.

Drug behavior

Not everyone who explores the effects of mood-modifying drugs will follow the same predictable pattern of behavior. But the behavior of all individuals introduced to drugs will fall within one or more of the following categories.

Experimenters   Well over half of all individuals reported to be "drug users" turn out to have "used" drugs—often not more than three times—and have no intentions of using illicit drugs again. Such people, in reality, are *drug experimenters* or *tasters*. They have no place in a discussion of drug abuse, because they have already made their decision not to use drugs.

Occasional users   Many experimenters find they need the social or personal gratification that mood-modifying drugs give them. They continue their experimentation with drugs and may be called *occasional users*. These individuals are extremely "socially conscious" and use the current "in" drug or drugs. When applied to alcohol use, these individuals are called "social drinkers." There is a very fine line that divides this occasional user from the next group, the regular user.

Regular users   Some individuals use drugs regularly—one or more times per week. They often experiment with a variety of different drugs and are "in-drug" users. They function within society, but drug abuse is a central focus of their life. Drugs to them are part of a more general "turned-on" ideology and a membership card in a "life style" or "subculture." Regular users are called "heads," "pot heads," "coke heads," "acid heads," "weekend drunks," "periodic alcoholics," or "problem drinkers."

These individuals do not seek help from clinics, consulting rooms, or "hot lines," and the physician may never see them. They usually "recover" from their "drug experience," none the worse for wear, often proclaiming loudly that they have gained a profound and valuable insight into themselves, nature, or religion. They are often the greatest defenders of the personal right to use drugs. They have very closed minds concerning drugs because of *street experimentation:* "I know, because I have been there." Judged by mental health criteria—ability to function within society—they are neither less nor more effective after their use of drugs.

The most dangerous aspect of regular drug use is the danger of lapsing into an enduring form of *personal dysorganization* (Chapter 2) and an apparently self-destructive immersion in a drug-using life style that results in *personality deficiencies* and *emotional problems* that may restrict the individual's ability to deal constructively with life. Such drug dependence would be considered compulsive drug abuse.

Compulsive users   Addiction of any kind is always associated with an abnormal personality (Chapter 2). The personality changes are best shown during the actual periods of drug use. Whether the behavioral distortion is a cause or a result of the abuse is not always apparent. Whether there are predisposing physiological factors, inherited by the individual, is also unknown. But the abnormal social behavior, the mood modifications, and the *personality problems* of such individuals are more of a problem to society than the drug abuse itself. The actions of a compulsive drug abuser label him as being *mentally ill*.

PSYCHOLOGICAL CAUSES OF DRUG ABUSE

The adjustment of humans to living is much more complicated than that of simpler animals. We have the ability to *reason* and make decisions based on learned behavior and on physiological and emotional needs. All of us are frustrated to some extent in our attempts to satisfy all our emotional needs. Why do we do the things we do? Why do we feel the way we do? As explained in Chapter 2, the answers come largely from our understanding and reaction to *basic human needs*, how these needs are fulfilled, and how we react to the frustration of unfulfilled needs.

Relationship of drug behavior to normal needs

The paragraphs that follow contain a discussion of the relationships between drug behavior, basic human needs, and emotional dysorganization (see Chapter 2).

Curiosity, or the *need to know and understand*, is often a major reason for a first drug experimentation—too often, it may be with little prior knowledge of drugs or drug effects. This is dangerous, because an individual's knowledge is *street knowledge:* "I know because I have tried it." No two people are exactly alike, and such knowledge can produce either the thrills a curious young person is looking for in an extremely structured society or death. Drug education can be instrumental in reducing this reason for drug experimentation.

The *need of love and belonging* is very important, and young people feel a strong need for friends, companionship, and acceptance by a group. Belonging is very important in the first experimentation with drugs, and if group acceptance is derived from drug abuse, a person may progress from an occasional user into the drug subculture as a regular or compulsive drug user.

Opportunities for group involvement without drugs helps a person to keep from becoming involved with drugs. It also helps him to relinquish an involvement with drugs. Belonging is the basis of therapeutic communities.

Every person needs *self-esteem*, a feeling of personal value or worth. An inability to satisfy the self-esteem need produces feelings of dependence, inferiority, weakness, helplessness, and despair. Such feelings may be both the cause and the outcome of drug abuse. Something has to be done to break a drug abuser's feeling of insignificance and begin the building of self-esteem, an important part of any successful drug-abuse treatment program. Sincere praise is basic to good interpersonal relationships, and giving someone tasks (duties or jobs) that he can perform well can bring the sincere praise and self-esteem needed to break the drug behavior cycle. This is one of the hardest needs to satisfy in a drug abuser, and the frustration of it keeps putting drug abusers back "on the street."

The most basic of human needs are the *physiological needs* of food, water, sleep, and sexual satisfaction. The compulsive drug user, addict, and alcoholic substitutes the drug he is abusing for a fulfillment of his physiological needs. He eats only the food and water needed to keep him alive. The decrease in sexual drive in drug addicts and alcoholics is well documented. Fulfillment of the physiological needs is the basis of methadone maintenance therapy. To a drug addict Utopia is seen as an unlimited supply of drugs. "If I were guaranteed drugs [heroin or, often, replacement by methadone] for the rest of my life, I would never want anything else." This is not so, and when this need is satisfied (as in methadone maintenance), the emotional needs of the individual emerge and can be dealt with through the many forms of psychotherapy.

Emotional maturity and drug abuse

As explained in Chapter 2, pioneer psychoanalyst Sigmund Freud conceived of the *personality* as being divided into three "control processes": the id processes (personal pleasure and gratification), the ego processes (mature, appropriate behavior), and the superego processes (self-ideal and personal judgment of right and wrong, a person's "conscience" or sense of "acceptable behavior"). There is constant interaction, through the ego processes, of the id and superego processes. The ego processes act as regulators, controlling and balancing the needs of the id and the demands of the superego. The regulating responses of the ego develop gradually and gain strength as an individual matures and responds to the emotional, social, and environmental pressures around him.

Aggression is seen by many authorities as a fundamental, inherent, human id process capable of being expressed in both harmful and beneficial ways. Drug abuse is a self-inflicted form of aggression, especially when someone is injecting drugs and needs the "needle itself" for full enjoyment. Competition in business, politics, and sports is seen as acceptable expression of basic human aggression. The need in extreme "hedonistic personalities" for pleasure, regardless of the physical, social, or legal consequences, is seen as an expression of exaggerated id control. The release of aggression or the extreme pleasure many find in drugs are expressions of such id control and show a lack of emotional maturity. Emotional maturity is the ability of an individual to control the id processes adequately. Regular and compulsive drug abusers do not have this maturity and still operate at the id, or "child role," level.

As explained in Chapter 2, Menninger has described increased id control as five levels of *emotional dysorganization*, ranging from mild to severe; see Fig. 2.1. These levels are points on a continuum, and most emotionally ill individuals fall somewhere between them.

The person entering the continuum of emotional dysorganization experiences a somewhat more than normal amount of tension and shows it through "nervousness." The *occasional drug user* or *social drinker* starts to establish a pattern of using drugs either to "block out" these feelings or to provide himself with experiences that make them seem insignificant. When not under the influence of drugs, he starts to be increasingly alert or "hyperalert": sounds are exaggerated, lights are more intense, and his perception seems keener. He looks for possible danger—refuses to relax during sleep; displays restlessness—walks the floor or drives aimlessly about in his car; suffers touchiness, tearfulness, irritability, nervous laughter, moodiness, or depression. He may worry obsessively and daydream excessively. All of this impairs realistic thinking and effective action, and he begins to be overzealous in identifying with some cause—often drugs and the use of drugs. By this time he has moved from being an occasional user to a regular user and into the second level of dysorganization.

An individual at the second level of emotional dysorganization abuses drugs as a means of coping with the stress of his environment and is now a regular user or "periodic" alcoholic. During prolonged periods between drug use (when "straight" or "on the wagon") he is normal and functions within society, but when stresses are placed upon him, his ego cannot find any other means of control, and he turns to a drug (possibly alcohol). The changes in personality of one under the influence are often very dramatic. This is why the second level is called the level of "personality disorders."

The *compulsive drug user, addict,* or *chronic alcoholic* makes drug use a permanent part of his personality and functions at the second level whenever under the influence of drugs. Such an individual has a *personality deformity* often referred to as the "addictive personality" and is *mentally ill.* Compulsive drug abusers periodically dip into the third level (level of open and direct aggression) and the fourth level ("classic mental disorders"). Such dips are observable when the alcoholic beats or abuses members of the family or can always find a fight and when extreme psychotic states are produced by hallucinogenic drugs, especially by LSD and mescaline.

In light of the millions of Americans who are addicted to alcohol or narcotics or who chronically abuse other drugs, drug abuse represents the largest single symptom of psychiatric affliction in the United States.

LEGAL CONTROLS OF DRUGS

Any review of drug use and abuse must include a description of the laws that have been enacted in an attempt to protect society. Throughout history legal controls such as quarantines and isolation have been invoked in an attempt to stop the spread of disease.

Actually, law enforcement is a means of control only until research gives us the knowledge we need to prevent drug abuse. At the moment our best promise of control is education based on the knowledge that has accumulated until now. Laws are preventive measures, but the controls now available are far from meeting the present needs.

A compulsive drug abuser is a sick person, but he is often quite willing to transmit the sickness to others. Therefore, to prevent the transmission drug laws have been established that are concerned with the illegal possession, manufacture, and sale of drugs rather than with their use (which is a medical problem).

Federal controls

In 1970 a new trend in drug control was established when Congress passed the Comprehensive Drug Abuse Prevention and Control Act. This law completely redesigned and updated older drug laws to fit the drug-abuse problems of the 1970s. It divides all drugs into five classes, whose illegal manufacture, distribution, possession, and possession for sale are controlled by the federal government. An outline of the five classes and the penalties for violations are shown in Table 6.1.

Class I drugs have the highest potential for being abused because of their mood-modifying properties. They carry the most severe penalties, are regarded as the most dangerous, and are outlawed from being used medically in the United States. Class II drugs have the same potential for abuse as Class I drugs but are used in medicine. Class III drugs are considered to have a potential for abuse but one not as high as those of Classes I and II. Class IV drugs have a lower potential for abuse; their penalties are further

Table 6.1 *Drug schedules and penalties for violation of the Comprehensive Drug Abuse Prevention and Control Act*[1]

drug schedule	potential for abuse	medical use?	production controls?	examples of drugs in each class	maximum penalties for manufacturing, distribution, and sales	maximum penalties for simple illegal possession
Class I	High	No	Yes	Opium derivatives and hallucinogenic drugs: heroin, marijuana, THC, LSD, mescaline	Narcotics: 1st offense, 3 to 15 years, $15,000 fine / 2nd and subsequent offenses, 6 to 30 years, $50,000 fine	1st offense, 1 year, $5,000 fine and probation may be given / 2nd offense, 2 years and $10,000 fine
Class II	High	Yes	Yes	Medically used narcotics and injectable metamphetamine: morphine, cocaine, methadone	Nonnarcotics: 1st offense, 2 to 5 years, $15,000 fine / 2nd and subsequent offenses, 4 to 10 years, $30,000 fine	
Class III	High but less than classes I and II	Yes	No	"Mild" narcotics: codeine, amphetamines, barbiturates	1st offense, 2 to 5 years, $15,000 fine / 2nd and subsequent offenses, 4 to 10 years, $20,000 fine	
Class IV	Low	Yes	No	"Mild" barbiturates, chloral hydrate, meprobamate	1st offense, 1 to 3 years, $10,000 fine / 2nd and subsequent offenses, 2 to 6 years, $20,000 fine	
Class V	Low, less than class IV	Yes	No	"Low-percentage" narcotic mixtures, tranquilizers	1st offense, up to 1 year, $5,000 fine / 2nd and subsequent offenses, up to 2 years, $10,000 fine	

[1] The schedules and penalties may be changed by the U.S. Attorney General at any time.

reduced. Class V drugs have the lowest potential for abuse, and the penalties are the mildest.

This law gives the U.S. Attorney General the power to decide which class a drug belongs to on the basis of its "potential for abuse." He may move a drug up or down the schedule or add new drugs. Before doing so he must consult a scientific panel appointed by the President.

A controversial aspect of this federal act is the "no-knock" provision, which allows police to enter and search a home or room without the ordinary warrant and without knocking—if there is a reason to believe that drugs are on the premises.

Under the law marijuana has been reclassified as a dangerous drug and is handled under the "nonnarcotic" penalty structure of Class I drugs; individual possession of marijuana is now a misdemeanor.

The maximum penalty for possession of any drug (first offense) is one year; for a first offense an individual under twenty-one years of age, convicted of possession, may be placed on probation (without sentencing), and if he successfully completes the probation, the official arrest, trial, and conviction can be erased from his record.

The enforcement of federal drug laws is the responsibility of the Bureau of Narcotics and Dangerous Drugs (BNDD) of the United States Justice Department.

State controls

In drug control there is usually cooperation between federal, state, and local law-enforcement officers. Until a few years ago the problem of enforcement was left largely to the Federal Bureau of Narcotics. Now there are separate "narcotics" units in local police departments of all large cities, and a large proportion of the narcotics cases are prosecuted in local and state courts.

In 1932 a model, uniform, state narcotics law was submitted to several state legislatures. Since that time this law, with minor changes in some states, has been enacted by the state legislatures of most of the states, by Puerto Rico, and by Congress for the District of Columbia. Some states, such as Ohio and Minnesota, have enacted even heavier penalties. For instance, in 1955 Ohio enacted legislation providing for a 20-year minimum penalty for the unlawful sale of narcotics. In many other states the penalties range from 2 to 10 years of imprisonment for a first offense of unlawful possession to 5 to 20 years for the unlawful sale of narcotics.

Since most states have no clinics or laboratories in which to evaluate possible dangerous drugs or narcotics, they depend upon the recommendations made by the federal government. States usually enact laws against the abuse of those drugs that federal laws have declared to be *dangerous drugs* or *narcotics*. Nevada and California reversed this procedure by enacting laws governing LSD prior to the enactment of federal regulations.

States are constantly reexamining their laws and making extensive changes. Prosecution to the limit of the law is rare. Judges now have greater flexibility in interpreting and applying state laws. In the past the practice of most states was to remodel old laws. This trend may have been broken in 1972 by California, when the state legislature established five classifications for narcotics and restricted dangerous drugs, bringing California law into conformity with the federal Comprehensive Drug Abuse Prevention and Control Act of 1970.

If you would like to know more about the drug laws of your state contact your local district attorney's office, and it will gladly answer any of your questions.

LEGAL CONTROLS OF DRUG ABUSE AND DRUG ABUSERS

Most drug-control laws are directed toward the criminality of the individual, not toward his illness. They do not attack the actual drug problem but simply jail the offender. Since it is obvious that the misuse of drugs is a medical problem that has legal consequences, the abuse of drugs should be attacked as such. We should study those persons who become compulsive users and addicts for common traits, so as to find the conditions, both social and psychological, that produce drug abuse. Then, possibly, we can arrive at workable methods of prevention or of treatment, rehabilitation, and control.

Actually, law enforcement is the means of control we must use until research gives us the knowledge we need for preventing drug abuse. Then law enforcement would be treated as a remedial action. Our governments are justified in applying preventive measures, but the controls until now are far from meeting the present needs. Some type of control is needed in the treatment of drug abuse. This may be legal or social or a self-control, but it must be present. More control than is necessary is actual punishment, but less control than is necessary is useless.

Two kinds of agency are available for the treatment of drug abuse: private and public. The private programs mainly control the individual by either family or social control through peer populations. Individuals who lack the personal self-control to stay within the framework of a private program, and who would leave it against medical advice, will always be the ones who are placed within the legal controls of public programs. However, too often we commit people to public treatment programs when we are angry and vindictive rather than concerned.

As shown by the penalties for drug possession, the predominant method of dealing with drug abuse has been to place the individual in jail. After his release he generally resumes using drugs. We still do not have effective methods of treatment for this kind of abuser.

There are different kinds of drug abusers, who need different kinds of treatment and differing amounts of control. A drug user should voluntarily enter a treatment program that offers the amount of control he needs, before laws are invoked against him.

Federal hospitals

There are two U.S. Public Health Service hospitals that are research centers for drug abuse. One, at Lexington, Kentucky, was established in 1935; the other, in Fort Worth, Texas, was established in 1938. They were originally set up to treat federal prisoners. Today voluntary patients are admitted and make up about half the individuals under treatment. The program consists of withdrawal treatment, psychiatric examinations, and a range of personal services. Many leave against medical advice, and there is no effective after-care program except when a prisoner-patient is granted parole.

Under the Federal Narcotic Addict Rehabilitation Act of 1966 these hospitals were changed into research facilities. These hospitals are to be used as diagnostic, short-term treatment centers during commitment procedures. As state programs develop, the prisoner-patients will be restricted. Eventually only addicts needed to conduct research will be admitted.

State treatment programs

Few states have proper facilities or adequate treatment programs. A majority of states attempt treatment in state-operated mental or general hospitals, and only a few have posthospital programs. States with a small drug-abuse problem face a special problem themselves. It is prohibitively expensive for such states to establish special rehabilitation facilities and programs. These states should explore with neighboring states the feasibility of establishing regional facilities.

Federal treatment program

The Federal Narcotic Addict Rehabilitation Act of 1966 is a law which helps states and communities to treat drug abusers. Under this law an eligible person charged with a crime may be told by a judge that the criminal charge will be "held in abeyance" if he will submit to a medical examination to determine whether he is an addict and could be rehabilitated through treatment. He has five days in which to make a decision. If he elects to apply for treatment, he then is retained in a hospital for not more than sixty days for examination purposes. Further, he will be placed in a state hospital through a *commitment procedure* if he is found to be a suitable candidate for treatment.

Criminal commitment for drug abuse If a judge believes an eligible, convicted, criminal offender is an addict, he may order him to be examined and then committed to a treatment program for an undetermined period of time. This cannot be more than ten years, but it must be more than six months. He then may be released under the supervision of a probation or parole officer.

An individual related to an addict may volunteer him for commitment (without a criminal record's being established) by filing a petition with the federal district attorney, who may then order the alleged addict to appear for examination. At commitment the process stops being voluntary. The term of treatment cannot exceed three and a half years, but no minimal period of stay in the hospital is required.

Civil commitment for drug abuse The civil commitment is a legal mechanism utilized in lieu of a criminal commitment to ensure control over drug abusers during rehabilitation—first in an institution, later in a "halfway" house, and still later in the community under the close supervision of a probation or parole officer. The significant step in this procedure is that the drug-abuse victim does not establish a criminal record when seeking therapy and help.

An individual is limited to a two-year maximal commitment, unless the judge renews the commitment. If, after release to the community, the individual resumes using drugs, he may be returned for further treatment, or the criminal proceedings may be started again. Should he then be found guilty, any time served in the treatment program will be credited toward the time to be served under the criminal sentence.

DRUG-ABUSE THERAPY

Establishment of self-control

Not everyone who explores the effects of drugs immediately becomes a compulsive user. Some use drugs only occasionally, others use them intermittently or regularly, and others take many months to arrive at compulsive drug abuse. There is no sharp line that divides the regular user from the constant compulsive user. Drug abuse is only an extreme on a *behavioral continuum*. The treatment of drug abuse should not be directed at the drug; it must be aimed at the problems of the individual abusing drugs. Many drug abusers, such as alcoholics, would prefer not to stop using drugs or drinking but to return to controlled, moderate drinking or drug use. Most authorities are convinced, however, that at the present time this is an unrealistic or even impossible goal. Very few, if any, compulsive drug users (including alcoholics) have been able to return to a controlled use of drugs. Abusers also must be aware of the dangers in their medical prescriptions and in certain over-the-counter drugs bought for medicinal purposes.

There are no proven techniques or procedures that can be applied to the total drug-abusing population. The current methods of drug-abuse treatment, used at institutions in the United States, are highly varied in their results. Actually, motivation of the individual is the greatest factor that favors rehabilitation.

Enforcement of the drug laws temporarily takes the user out of his environment and, for the period of his jail sentence, he is forced to do without drugs. Another beneficial effect of a jail sentence is that for the time being the innocent (the "forgotten man" in many of our laws) is at least temporarily protected from the compulsive drug users' need for money.

Most experimenters and occasional users, given adequate supervision, will eventually give up the use of illicit drugs after a period of drug-free living—if only to avoid an involuntary return to an institution. It may be unrealistic to expect every user to reach all of the goals of ideal treatment, but probably the first realistic step in the control of drug abuse is for the individual to perform normally within society. Medical authorities feel that the compulsive drug abuser is a sick person. He is emotionally disturbed and often physiologically ill. He needs treatment for the physical effects of the drug he is abusing, and he needs psychological help, often continuing throughout life, to keep from going back to drug abuse when he leaves the hospital.

Tests for drugs

One of the first tests for drug use was the nalline test. In this test nalline (nalorphine) or levallorphan is injected subcutaneously. If the individual has used an opiate within the last week he will show, according to how much he has used and how recently, a drastic constriction of the pupils, sweating, vomiting, or the full withdrawal symptoms.

In 1970 the U.S. Armed Forces started testing servicemen for drug use. One test, the free-radical assay technique, or FRAT, measures forms of morphine, which are the end products of heroin metabolism in the body, in the urine of heroin users. The thin-layer chromatography test, or TLC, measures barbiturates, amphetamines, opiates, methadone, and many other mood-modifying drugs, depending on how the test is performed. If an individual shows a positive reaction to either of these tests, he is given the gas-liquid chromatography test, or GLC, which is 99 percent accurate in detecting any drug in an individual. As more equipment becomes available, the last two tests will replace all other tests.

"Emergency" therapy

When an individual under the influence of drugs comes to the attention of a hospital staff or a private physician, it is usually an emergency situation. There is certain information a physician needs to know to save someone from death. The first information needed by the physician is the name of the drug or *combination of drugs* the individual has used. This is often difficult to determine, because the user may be unconscious, semicoherent, disoriented, frightened, or unreliable and often behaves as an "acute psychotic." Friends and the contents of the user's pockets and the conditions under which the adverse reactions occurred help the doctor in his evaluation of the situation.

If the patient is conscious, this is the "talk-down" phase. During this time a quiet and "cool" environment and a well-established "rapport" between the physician and the patient become very valuable. Sometimes, little more than acceptance and reassurance are necessary. If definite signs of toxic complications or withdrawal occur, the physician will treat them as they appear, regardless of what the patient has told him. A very important complicating factor in emergency treatment is the fear of legal incrimination. In addition to the unpleasant feelings produced by the drugs the patient fears the introduction of the police into the situation. He will try to cover up potential evidence, will become very wary of doctors' questions, and might have difficulty distinguishing medical from legal personnel. Though this is all very understandable, a doctor is not a law-enforcement official. His goal is to help the patient come out of what is an extremely disturbing and dangerous experience. He needs the patient's greatest possible cooperation in order to succeed, and a patient should be made to realize this.

Most drug prosecutions are based on evidence of possession. If the police obtained such evidence at the time they brought the patient to a health facility, his fears are simply too late. But if they have not obtained such evidence, they will not pursue the search into the examining room.

Withdrawal therapy

When certain groups of drugs, such as opiates or barbiturates, are used several times a day, the user becomes *tolerant* and physically dependent upon the drug. Some cells and body systems become tolerant rapidly and others slowly. When a drug is "withdrawn," the tolerant cells and body systems must return to normal. The symptoms produced while these cells are returning to normal are called *withdrawal* or the *abstinence syndrome*. Withdrawing an individual from the addicting drugs by a gradual reduction in dosage and substitution of less potent drugs is the accepted medical procedure. Abrupt withdrawal, the so-called "cold turkey," is painful and can be fatal. Gradual withdrawal is usually done within a hospital. The American Medical Association states that a physician should not ordinarily try to attempt withdrawal without the individual's being in a hospital.

Someone who is waiting for admission to a hospital for withdrawal from the opiates can be given daily doses of *methadone* to keep from going into withdrawal, until he can be admitted. The withdrawal symptoms are nausea, watering of the eyes, muscle spasms in the stomach and legs, and hot and cold flashes. Methadone may be substituted for the addicting drug, because methadone tends to block the euphoric effects and relieve the craving for such drugs as heroin and morphine. Methadone also can be given orally once daily (instead of four to six "shots" of heroin, for example) and lets the individual perform in a more normal work or school situation. All of this seems to create more responsible behavior toward society in general.

During barbiturate withdrawal, grand mal convulsions and delirium tremens often occur. The drug *pentobarbital* may be used as a substitute drug during withdrawal. Abrupt withdrawal from barbiturates is extremely dangerous and often has been fatal. Consequently, a physician must know what drug an individual has been using before he can attempt withdrawal.

The alcoholic in a late phase of alcoholism (Phase VI) should not suddenly stop drinking, either voluntarily or involuntarily. Doing so involves a risk of serious withdrawal symptoms. He therefore needs medical treatment during his sobering-up period. He may even require hospitalization at this time. He should be treated with consideration and sympathy rather than with contempt. Drugs such as tranquilizers, insulin, and thiamine are often given at this time. A correction of dietary deficiencies is very important in the rehabilitation of the alcoholic, since his thought processes may be impaired by extreme malnutrition. In addition to a balanced diet, vitamin preparations are often given.

Drug therapy (drugs in treatment)

Drug therapy for alcoholism Many drugs have been tried in the treatment of alcoholics, with variable success. The tranquilizing drugs are sometimes effective in decreasing such symptoms as anxiety, tremor, and restlessness, all common among alcoholics.

Maintenance treatment Because of the short-acting ups and downs of psychotropic drug abuse (especially with heroin), a drug user is preoccupied with thoughts of drugs. To establish the first step in treatment—normal social functioning—medical therapy should eliminate the need for psychotropic drugs and at the same time discourage their use. One way this has been done is with *methadone maintenance.* Other drugs with these blocking properties are *acetylmethadol* and *Darvon B.*

Individuals on a methadone program are given one oral dose daily. Acetylmethadol is the longer acting, and a patient needs to take it only two or three times a week. With maintenance compounds individuals have been successful in staying away from psychotropic drugs and have become acceptable citizens by a treatment program that combines methadone blockage with rehabilitation.

The major objections to maintenance programs have been that they work only with highly motivated individuals. Also, many physicians see it as merely substituting one addictive drug for another. The New York Academy of Medicine concedes that methadone management is not the final solution, but it points out that "no other regimen currently available offers so much to the chronic addict."

Narcotics antagonists Another treatment approach is the use of *narcotic antagonists*—drugs chemically and structurally so like narcotics that they can apparently occupy the place in the nervous system where narcotics act without having much, if any, narcotic action. Three of the more important antagonists are *nalline, cyclazocine,* and *naloxine.*

Nalline has been used in testing-control programs for years. True treatment programs are relatively new. Antagonists, when given to a person physically addicted to narcotics, will bring on withdrawal symptoms rather than preventing them. This way a physician can tell whether an individual is currently using narcotics.

While someone is taking several daily doses of cyclazocine he will not feel the effects of a narcotic nor will he become addicted to it. Thus, during a treatment program antagonists may provide a means of "unlearning" drug-using behavior. With these drugs people may keep from becoming physically addicted, making it possible for them to continue working and participating in a rehabilitation program. To be effective these drugs must be part of a broad program of psychological and social rehabilitation.

Therapeutic communities

Another distinct approach involves the establishment of complex social systems that are run almost entirely by ex-addicts. Such organizations as Synanon (California), Daytop Village, Phoenix Houses, Odyssey House (New York), Gateway Houses (Illinois), and the federally sponsored Tacoma Narcotics Center (Washington) are some of the better-known therapeutic communities. Individuals are not required to remain at these centers and are free to leave at any time. However, to stay, they must at all times demonstrate a willingness to participate and conform to community rules. Many of these therapeutic communities now admit alcoholics, and some communities have been set up for alcoholics only.

Many former compulsive drug abusers are able to remain drug-free and function productively while they are in such communities. Here again, motivation is the key to staying drug-free. There is much group and individual interaction, which has as its goal exposing and correcting the immature and exploitative attitudes that underlie the compulsive drug abuser.

The therapeutic community is often criticized for the inability of its residents to reenter the community at large. Some, such as Synanon, no longer encourage addicts to leave the community and reenter society. Experience indicates that addicts often require the permanent support of a therapeutic community to prevent them from returning to drugs. This was first shown to be the situation with alcoholics, who need association with Alcoholics Anonymous throughout life.

Very few therapeutic-community members ever achieve fulltime employment in positions unrelated to addictive programs. Therapeutic communities do not make people independent. They provide a drug-free life in which dependence is transferred from drugs to the "community life style."

Psychotherapy

The success of psychotherapy in treating drug abuse has been variable. As in other psychotherapy, the approach may be either a superficial emotional reinforcement of the individual or a deep exploration of the subconscious mind to uncover underlying emotional conflicts that may be contributing to the addiction. For success the therapist must have an unusually good understanding of the addict. It is very difficult for someone who has never been, for example, an alcoholic to understand what it means to be one. Group psychotherapy seems especially helpful, because drug abusers do tend to understand each other.

Alcoholics Anonymous

The most successful approach to the problem of drug abuse today is probably exemplified by Alcoholics Anonymous (AA). Alcoholics Anonymous is a loosely organized group of individuals whose sole purpose is to help its members stay sober. In a large city there may be groups meeting every night of the week. There are even special groups for young alcoholics and for spouses and children of alcoholics.

The approach taken by AA is a variety of group therapy, in which members find a deep personal, emotional, and spiritual experience through association with other sober alcoholics. Despite popular belief, all but the very newest members at a meeting are sober. At a typical AA meeting several members may stand and informally tell their "stories" of trouble and misery during their drinking years and how AA has helped them. The new member, usually defensive and skeptical, hears experiences similar to his own and often finds that he can identify strongly with a person who has just stood and made the statement "I am an alcoholic." The new member learns to think of alcoholism as an illness and finds encouragement in seeing alcoholics who have remained sober for years. The new member takes an important step when he admits his own alcoholism. He can now feel a part of AA and often finds himself eager to help other alcoholics regain their sobriety.

It should be emphasized that AA does not claim to cure the alcoholic, only to help *control* his illness, much as insulin does not cure diabetes but does enable the diabetic to live a normal life. There have been many cases of AA members' becoming overconfident after many years of sobriety and attempting social drinking, with disastrous results. AA firmly believes that no alcoholic can ever return to moderate social drinking.

Also it must be stressed that AA cannot help the alcoholic who does not fulfill three essential qualifications: a sincere desire to stop drinking, a willingness to admit that he, by himself, is unable to solve his drinking problem and must have help, and the ability to be honest with himself.

The return to society

After an individual has been treated for drug abuse and returns to society, he faces many problems, which may be social, legal, economic, and medical. Often in drug problems the offender and the victim are the same person, and the social pressures that encouraged him to abuse drugs in the first place are present in his environment when he returns.

If there are facilities available for him to be returned in stages, or if he has not established a criminal record (civil commitment) because of drugs, he has a much better chance of adjustment. Short visits home should be made at first, then to a halfway house, a work camp, parish house, or day-night hospital. Any of these settings is useful in providing the abuser with social, therapeutic, and vocational services; they also give him controlled contacts with the community.

Unhappily, too often the individual just leaves the hospital (or, more often, the jail) and literally is "dumped back onto the street." Consequently, it is a very short time before he is again abusing drugs—and back or beyond where he was before treatment was first initiated.

If an individual has been convicted of a "felony," there may be further problems. Such a conviction can mean the loss of voting rights, the loss of the right to hold public office, and the loss of the right to obtain certain state licenses, such as a license to sell liquor or practice law or dispense drugs. A felony conviction can also hamper a person economically. Very often an individual convicted of a felony is required to register with the local police department of a city or area or to register with the Emigration Agency whenever he leaves or enters this and other countries. He also is unable to be "bonded" and cannot hold positions that require a bond. Because of this and his inability to acquire types of security clearances through the government he is also excluded from certain employment, such as in defense establishments or with defense contractors. Further, many employers refuse to hire a person with a felony conviction on his record.

TOWARD THE FUTURE

Drug-treatment programs can succeed only when they correct the basic problem of drug users, which is that compulsive users have inadequate ability to combat the ordinary stresses of life. A user has relied for months, or perhaps years, on the external solace provided by drugs. A cure of his dependency requires him to redirect his attitudes toward his own weaknesses.

The cure of the compulsive drug user is not a reliable prospect. To "arrest his addiction," which would allow him to function within the bounds of society, may be the most practical outcome of treatment. A great deal more research will be necessary in order for our society to maintain a consistent level of cure and rehabilitation. The damage done to the individual and society by drug abuse is so powerful and so widespread that the only practical long-range "cure" is prevention. There is no doubt that rehabilitation and planned prevention hold much greater promise for both the individual and society than do jails and prisons.

The rescue of a person from a possible life of compulsive drug abuse or alcoholism saves society a good deal more than the cost of his rehabilitation or maintenance. The more our nation's policy-makers become convinced that the cost of ambitious, well-planned, humane programs is worthwhile, the more progress in combating drug abuse we may expect to witness.

SUMMARY

I. Sociological aspects of drug abuse
  A. The abnormal social behavior of drug-influenced individuals is an increasingly prominent sociological, medical, and legal problem.
    1. Drug abuse is a problem of:
       a. ignorance.
       b. semantics.
       c. communications.
       d. lack of understanding of scientific method and concepts.
       e. living and learning and growing.
       f. philosophy of social control.
       g. education.
       h. "pill society."
       i. increasing retreat in the face of complex and difficult problems.
    2. Prohibition of drugs is not the answer.
    3. The real problem is not drugs but the people who use them.
  B. Social problems resulting from regular and compulsive drug abuse—complex and highly intangible.
  C. Drug behavior
    1. All individuals introduced to drugs will fall within one or more of the following categories:
       a. *experimenters*—individuals who have tried drugs and have no intention of using them again.
       b. *occasional users*—find they need the social or personal gratification that mood-modifying drugs give them; "socially conscious" and users of "in" drugs; "social drinker."

      c. *regular users*—use drugs one or more times a week; "in-drug" users, "heads," or "weekend drunks"; often great defenders of the personal right to use drugs.

      d. *compulsive users*—addiction; always associated with a deficient personality; actions of compulsive drug abuser label him as mentally ill.

II. Psychological causes of drug abuse

  A. Relationships between drug behavior, basic human needs, and emotional dysorganization.

    1. Need to know and understand is major reason for first drug experimentations.

    2. Need of love and belonging (need for friends, companionship, and acceptance by group) will cause an individual to progress from being an occasional user to being a member of a drug subculture.

    3. Self-esteem, a feeling of personal worth, is one of the hardest and most important needs to satisfy in a drug abuser.

    4. Physiological-need fulfillment is basis of maintenance therapy.

  B. Emotional maturity and drug abuse

    1. Freud conceived of personality as three processes:

      a. id processes—seen by many authorities as expressed in self-inflicted aggression and "hedonistic personalities" of drug users.

      b. ego processes—include maturity and ability of individual to control unrealistic id processes.

      c. superego processes—judgment exercised by a mature individual.

    2. Emotional dysorganization:

      a. continuum of emotional dysorganization entered by occasional drug user or social drinker (Fig. 2.1).

      b. regular user moves into second level of dysorganization.

      c. compulsive drug user, addict, or chronic alcoholic functions at second level whenever under the influence of drugs; he periodically dips into the third and fourth levels.

III. Legal controls of drugs

  A. Federal controls

    1. Current law established in 1970—Comprehensive Drug Abuse Prevention and Control Act.

    2. Law divides all drugs into five classes, whose illegal manufacture, distribution, possession, and possession for sale are controlled by federal government.

    3. Penalties outlined in Table 6.1.

  B. State controls

    1. Model, uniform, state narcotics law has been enacted by numerous states since 1932.

    2. State laws dealing with the dangerous drugs are anything but uniform.

IV. Legal controls of drug abuse and drug abusers

  A. Federal hospitals—mainly research centers.

  B. State treatment programs—being improved with federal help.

  C. Federal treatment program—Federal Narcotic Addict Rehabilitation Act of 1966 helps states and communities to treat drug abusers.

    1. Criminal commitment for drug abuse—a legal mechanism to require a drug abuser to be examined and committed for treatment during criminal proceedings.

2. Civil commitment for drug abuse—a legal mechanism utilized in lieu of a criminal commitment, to control drug abusers and potential addicts without establishing a criminal record.

V. Drug abuse therapy
  A. Drug abuse is a behavioral continuum—therapy is establishment of "self-control" within an individual.
  B. Tests for drugs within the body—a number of tests are available.
  C. "Emergency" therapy—often consists of "talk-down" in a quiet and "cool" environment.
  D. Withdrawal therapy—first stage after an emergency situation has been taken care of.
  E. Drug therapy (drugs in treatment)
    1. Drug therapy for alcoholism—many drugs are used to decrease symptoms of alcoholism.
    2. Maintenance treatment—administration of a drug that can block the psychotropic effects of mood-modifying drugs during psychological treatment.
    3. Narcotics antagonists—drugs that can replace the narcotics in the nervous system and stop their action or cause an individual to go through withdrawal.
  F. Therapeutic communities—complex treatment communities run almost entirely by ex-addicts.
  G. Psychotherapy
    1. Emotional reinforcement of the individual, at least.
    2. Deep exploration of the subconscious mind to uncover underlying emotional conflicts that may be contributing to drug abuse.
  H. Alcoholics Anonymous—most successful approach to control of alcoholism to date.
  I. The return to society
    1. After an individual has been treated for drug abuse and returns to society, he faces many problems.
    2. If there have been facilities available for him to be returned in stages, or if he has not established a criminal record (civil commitment) because of drugs, he has a much better chance of adjustment.
    3. A felony conviction can hamper a person in many ways.

VI. Toward the future
  A. Cure of compulsive drug user is not easy.
  B. Arresting his addiction, which allows him to function within the bounds of society, may be the most practical course of treatment.
  C. The only practical long-range "cure" is prevention.

Glossary

If you cannot find the word you wish in this glossary, check the index for text and glossary references.

abdomen (ab dō′mən, ab′ də mən) (L. possibly from *abdere*, to hide). The area between the diaphragm and the pelvis; the belly.

abstinence syndrome (ab′sti nəns sin′drōm) (L. *abstinere*, to abstain; G. *syndrome*, concurrence). A set of symptoms which occur together, resulting from withdrawal of alcohol, depressants, and opiates.

abuse (ə būz') (ME. *ab-*, away, from + *uti*, to use). To use wrongly or improperly; misuse.

addict (ad'ikt) (L. *addicere*, to consent). To form a habit, as of using a drug or alcohol.

addiction (ə dik'shən). Condition resulting from repeated use of a drug, in which physical dependence is established because of biochemical and physiological adaptations to the drug.

amine (ə mēn', am'in) (ammonia + -ine). The chemical group NH_2; as a prefix (amino-) indicates the presence in a compound of the group NH_2.

amnesia (am nē'zē ə, am nēzhə) (G. *amnesia*, forgetfulness). Loss of memory or loss of a large block of interrelated memories.

blackout (blak'out). A period of temporary amnesia occurring while drinking, usually associated with alcoholism.

chemotherapy (kem'ō ther'ə pi) (*chemo-*, having to do with chemicals, + *therapy*, the art of treatment). The treatment of disease by the administration of chemicals, medicines, or drugs.

cirrhosis (sə ro' səs) (G. *kirrhos*, orange-yellow). Disease of the liver involving progressive destruction of liver cells accompanied by regeneration and increase in connective tissue.

convulsions (kon vul'shənz) (L. *con-*, with + *vellere*, to pull). Contortions of the body caused by violent involuntary muscular contractions.

delirium tremens (də lēr'ē əm trē'mənz) (L. *de-*, off; *lira*, track, thus "off the track"; *tremere*, to shake). A psychic disorder involving hallucinations both visual and auditory, delusions, incoherence, anxiety, and trembling; found in habitual users of alcoholic beverages and some other drugs.

depression (di presh'ən). Reduction of the functional activity of the body.

drug dependence (drug di pen'dəns). Condition resulting from repeated use of a drug, in which individual must continue to take drug to avoid abstinence syndrome (physical dependence) or to satisfy emotional need (psychic dependence).

felony (fel'ə ni) (LL. *felonia*, treason, treachery). Offense punishable by death or imprisonment for more than one year.

gratification (grat'ə fi ka'shən) (L. *gratus*, pleasing, agreeable + *facere*, to make). Source of pleasure or satisfaction.

habituation (hə bich'oo ā'shən) (L. *habituatus*, to bring into a condition or habit of the body). In this context, a condition resulting from repeated use of a drug in which a psychic, not physical, dependence is established.

hypnotic (hip not'ik) (G. *hypnotikos*, sleep). A drug that acts to induce sleep.

intoxication (in tok si kā'shən) (L. *in-*, intensive; G. *toxikon*, poison). State of being poisoned; condition produced by excessive use of alcohol.

medicinal (mə dis'i nəl) (L. *medicinalis*). Having healing qualities.

misdemeanor (mis'di mēn'êr) (ME. *mis-*, wrong, badly, + LL. *minare*, conduct). Offense defined as less serious than a felony; punishable by less than one year in jail.

psychogenic (sī kō jen'ik) (G. *psyche*, mind, soul; *genesis*, to produce). Originating in the mind, as a disease might.

synergism (sin' ẽr jiz'm) (G. *synergos*, working together). Working together; drugs working together.

synthetic (sin thet'ik). Formed by a chemical reaction in a laboratory.

thrombocytopenia (throm'bo si to pe'nē ə). An abnormal increase in blood platelets (circular or oval disks found in the blood, important in the clotting of blood).

tolerance (tol'er əns). Increasing resistance to the usual effects of a drug.

toxicity (tok sis'ə ti) (G. *toxikon*, a poison). Quality of being poisonous.

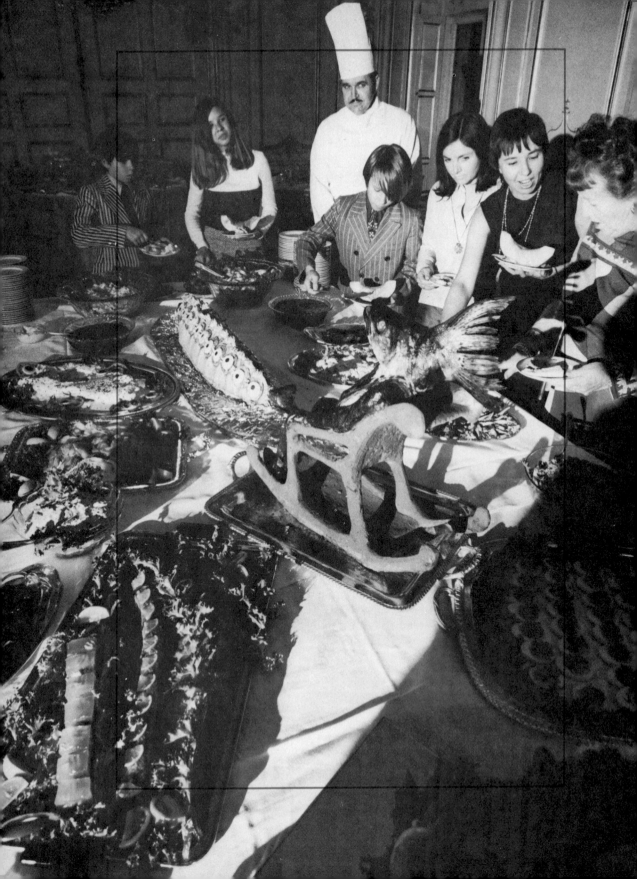

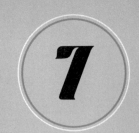

Foods and the digestive system

ENERGY RELATIONSHIPS

The human body acts as a very efficient energy-conversion machine. Energy (defined as the capacity to do work) exists in two basic forms: *potential energy*, such as is found in a sugar cube or a rock perched on the edge of a cliff, and *kinetic energy*, such as heat, motion, light, and electricity. The human body converts potential energy from foods into kinetic energy in the forms of heat and movement. This energy is converted by means of a complex system of *enzymes*, protein substances that cause chemical reactions to take place within us. The normal human body contains some two hundred thousand different enzymes, most of which are within the cells. If only one enzyme is missing, the results may be serious or even fatal.

The calorie

The unit for expressing the energy content of food is the *large calorie*, or *kilocalorie*, abbreviated C. One kilocalorie is the amount of energy required to raise the temperature of one kilogram (2.2 pounds) of water by one centigrade degree. All further references to calories in these chapters will imply the large calorie.

163

Metabolism

The total chemical reactions that go on in a person are *metabolism*. It includes both those reactions in which food is broken down and energy is released (catabolism) and those in which new substances are produced within the body and energy is stored up (anabolism).

A person uses a considerable amount of energy just staying alive. Such basic changes as cell renewal and repair, breathing, heartbeat, and glandular secretions all require energy. This unavoidable energy expenditure is called the *basal metabolic rate* (BMR), which is measured while a person is awake but reclining and completely relaxed. The number of calories required for basal metabolism varies with weight, sex, stature, and hormone production, especially the thyroid hormone level. The basal metabolic rate is highest in childhood and drops gradually throughout life, requiring a gradual adjustment in eating habits in order to avoid excess weight gain. The average adult utilizes about 1,500 to 1,800 calories per day for his basal metabolism. The basal metabolic rate of females typically is lower than that of males. A twenty-five-year-old male requires an average of 1 calorie per hour in a day for each kilogram (2.2 pounds) of body weight; a twenty-five-year-old female requires 0.9. For example, a twenty-five-year-old male of average stature weighing 70 kilograms would require 1,680 calories per day (24 × 70) for basal metabolism, and a female of the same size and age would require 1,512.

Total energy requirements

In addition to the energy needed for basal metabolism a widely varying quantity of energy is needed for everyday activities. The sedentary or inactive person may utilize as few as 500 additional calories, whereas a large man doing heavy manual labor may need several thousand additional calories; thus, the total energy requirement may range from only slightly more than the amount needed for basal metabolism to more than double that amount.

TYPES OF FOOD

Besides their obvious function as sources of energy, foods are necessary for several other important body requirements. Foods must supply materials for growth and replacement of worn or damaged cells and for the manufacture of cellular products such as enzymes and hormones. Other materials (vitamins) are needed in minute amounts for various functions in the body. Some vitamins form a part of vital body chemicals; others act as regulatory agents. Although the hundreds of kinds of food we consume may show little outward similarity, the actual nourishing materials they contain consist of six classes of food, which fall into two major groups, as follows:

Organic food substances:

yielding energy $\left\{ \begin{array}{l} \text{carbohydrates} \\ \text{fats} \\ \text{proteins} \end{array} \right.$

not yielding energy   vitamins

Inorganic food substances:

not yielding energy   minerals
not yielding energy   water

Organic foods

The word *organic*, so often misused by "health food" salesmen, indicates a substance based upon a chain of carbon atoms. See Chapter 14 for further discussion. Organic food substances, except vitamins, yield energy to the body metabolizing them.

Carbohydrates The carbohydrates in the diet consist of the sugars and starches. For the majority of people in the world today the carbohydrates are the most important source of energy. Foods high in carbohydrates are rice, corn, other grains, potatoes, and any sweet food.

Carbohydrates consist of one or more simple-sugar units, called saccharides. Each simple-sugar molecule, called a monosaccharide, contains six carbon atoms plus hydrogen and oxygen atoms. The simple sugars glucose (dextrose) and fructose are found in many fruits and in honey.

Those carbohydrates consisting of two simple-sugar units are called disaccharides. Examples of disaccharides are sucrose, which is table sugar (cane and beet sugars are identical), maltose (produced by germinating grains), and lactose (found only in milk).

The starches are among the polysaccharides, consisting of long chains of simple-sugar units. One polysaccharide, cellulose, although present in most of our foods from plant sources, is not available for conversion into energy by humans, since we lack the digestive enzymes necessary for its breakdown. Cellulose is, however, useful in stimulating intestinal activity through its addition of bulk or roughage to the diet.

It actually matters little whether carbohydrates are consumed as monosaccharides, disaccharides, or polysaccharides, since the process of digestion reduces most of them to their monosaccharide components before there is absorption into the blood. Those monosaccharides other than glucose are further converted by the liver into glucose, which is the only carbohydrate used as a source of energy by the cells of the tissues.

The primary function of carbohydrates in the body is to supply energy. Each gram of carbohydrate consumed yields an average of 4.1 calories of energy. Table 7.1 compares the energy value of the several basic food groups.

Table 7.1 *Energy values of foods*

food type	average calories per gram	average calories per pound
Carbohydrates	4.1	1,860
Fats	9.3	4,220
Proteins	4.1	1,860

If the diet is low in carbohydrates, fats or proteins will be converted into glucose as a source of energy. If there is a surplus of carbohydrates in the diet, these substances are quickly converted first into muscle and liver glycogen (animal starch), and excesses beyond this are converted to human fats in the adipose tissue for future use.

Fats   Fats are abundant in such foods as meat, whole milk, cheese, nuts, and olives. Some food products, such as butter, margarine, oils, and shortenings, are almost pure fat. The oils are fats of low melting points, being liquid at room temperature.

The fats have the highest available energy content of any known foods, yielding 9.3 calories per gram, over twice as much energy as carbohydrates. In addition to being used as a source of energy, fats serve several other functions in the body: they serve as the body's reservoir for the long-term storage of energy, they are important in the membranes of all cells and in the nerve sheaths, and small quantities of them in the diet appear to be necessary for absorption into the blood of the fat-soluble vitamins.

A fat molecule is the result of the union of one glycerol molecule and three fatty-acid molecules; through digestion it is broken down into these components. The human body needs certain fatty acids. In the event a person's body does not include all of them, the body is able to synthesize (produce) some of the needed fatty acids. Fatty acids the body needs but is unable to produce itself are referred to as *essential* fatty acids and must be obtained through food. Fortunately, these substances are widely distributed in foods in abundant quantities, and fat deficiency is virtually unknown in the United States (rather, it is more likely that an excess of fat intake is of concern).

Proteins   Of the three groups of energy-yielding foods the proteins are the most complex in structure and the most essential to life. Protein molecules consist of chains of *amino acids*, organic compounds containing nitrogen, hydrogen, carbon, and oxygen, and sometimes sulfur. Through digestion proteins are broken down into their component amino acids, which are then absorbed into the blood. Although thousands of different proteins occur in foods, no specific protein is an absolute necessity in the human diet. After absorption into the blood the amino acids are reassembled to form human body proteins. Among the twenty commonly occurring amino acids only eight, the *essential* amino acids, *must* be present in the human diet; the body itself has no means of producing them. The remaining amino acids can be obtained either through the diet or be produced within the body.

Proteins containing all eight essential amino acids in significant quantities are of high biological value; proteins low in one or more essential amino acids are of low biological value. Most proteins from animal sources are of high value, but many plant proteins are of low value. This is why it may be difficult for a vegetarian to get proper nutrition.

Since normal growth and maintenance of the human body are based upon amino acids, proteins are of prime importance in the diet. In addition, amino acids may also serve as energy sources. Such is true when the diet is high in protein but low in fats and carbohydrates. As sources of energy the proteins yield 4.1 calories per gram and are thus equivalent to the carbohydrates.

Vitamins Vitamins are organic compounds present in minute amounts in natural foods; they are essential for specific chemical reactions to take place in the body. Some can be synthesized from sources within the body; others must be derived entirely from food sources. Vitamins are not energy sources, but certain specific ones are essential for normal energy metabolism, which in turn supports the proper functioning of the body. The vitamins and their major properties are summarized in Table 7.2.

Table 7.2 cites the recommended daily allowance (RDA) for each vitamin. This is the amount required to maintain optimal health. Vitamins may also be rated by minimal daily requirement (MDR), the amount needed to prevent vitamin-deficiency diseases. MDRs have been established by the Food and Drug Administration as standards for labeling of food and pharmaceutical preparations. MDRs are generally less than RDAs.

The solubility of a vitamin is important in that it influences the source of the vitamin, its absorption into the body, and its fate within the body. In general, the fat-soluble vitamins are the more likely to be stored in the body, which increases the possibility of toxic effects after overdoses. Unlike the carbohydrates, fats, and proteins, the vitamins have no underlying chemical similarity other than their all being organic compounds.

The complete absence of a given vitamin from the diet is referred to as *avitaminosis*, a condition rare in the United States today. However, many Americans suffer from *hypovitaminosis*, the diet falling below the optimal quantity of one or more vitamins. They are not seriously ill, but they lack the health and vitality to enjoy life to its fullest.

Inorganic foods

Minerals In contrast to the complex organic structure of vitamins, the minerals are usually consumed as rather simple compounds. Once in the body, however, they may be incorporated into some very complex organic compounds. Some of these compounds are vital parts of cells, bones, teeth, and blood; others are important parts of body products, such as hormones.

As many as thirteen minerals are now believed by some authorities to

Table 7.2 *Vitamins*

vitamin	rich sources	properties
Fat-soluble vitamins		
A	Cheese, green and yellow vegetables, butter, eggs, milk, fish-liver oils. Converted from carotene in vegetables by the liver.	Lost through oxidation in long cooking in open kettle. Overdose possible.
D	Beef, butter, eggs, milk, fish-liver oils. Produced in the skin on exposure to ultraviolet rays in sunlight. No plant source.	Very stable vitamin. Large doses may cause calcium deposits, poor bone growth in children, congenital defects.
E	Widely distributed in foods. Abundant in vegetable oils, wheat germ.	Lost through oxidation in long cooking in open kettle. Overdose unknown.
K	Eggs, liver, cabbage, spinach, tomatoes. Produced by intestinal bacteria.	Destroyed by light and alkali. Absorption from intestine into blood depends on normal fat absorption.
Water-soluble vitamins[a]		
B_1 (thiamine)	Meat, whole grains, liver, yeast, nuts, eggs, bran, soybeans, potatoes.	Not destroyed by cooking but may dissolve in cooking water. Not stored in body; needed daily.
B_2 (riboflavin)	Milk, cheese, liver, beef, eggs, fish.	Not destroyed by cooking acid foods. Unstable to light and alkali.
Niacin (nicotinic acid)	Bran, eggs, yeast, liver, kidney, fish, whole wheat, potatoes, tomatoes. Synthesized from amino acid tryptophan.	Not destroyed by cooking but may dissolve extensively in cooking water.
B_6 (pyridoxine)	Meat, liver, yeast, whole grains, fish, vegetables.	Stable except to light.

[a] Several other water-soluble vitamins are believed essential to nutrition but are not as well understood, and deficiency is less common.

Table 7.2 (*continued*)

function	deficiency symptoms	recommended daily allowance
Necessary for growth, normal bone development, tooth structure, night vision, healthy skin.	Slow growth, poor teeth and gums, night blindness, dry skin, lack of tears.	5,000–8,000 units, adult. 1,500–5,000 units, child.
Essential for normal intestinal absorption of calcium and body metabolism of calcium and phosphorus and for normal bone and tooth development.	Rickets. Poor tooth and bone structure. Soft bones.	400 units.
Not definitely known for humans.	Not definitely known for humans.	Not established.
Necessary for blood clotting.	Slow blood clotting, anemia.	Not established. Given to pregnant women and newborn infants, since newborns lack bacteria normally producing adequate supply.
Necessary for carbohydrate metabolism, normal nerve function. Promotes growth.	Beriberi. Slow growth, poor nerve function, nervousness, fatigue, heart disease.	0.8–1.6 milligrams, adult. 0.4–1.4 milligrams, child.
Essential for metabolism in all cells.	Fatigue, sore skin and lips, bloodshot eyes, anemia.	1.2–2.0 milligrams, adult. 0.6–2.0 milligrams, child.
Necessary for growth, metabolism, normal skin.	Pellagra. Sore mouth, skin rash, indigestion, diarrhea, headache, mental disturbances.	13–20 milligrams, adult. 6–22 milligrams, child.
Functions in amino acid metabolism.	Dermatitis (rare).	Not established.

Table 7.2 (continued)

vitamin	rich sources	properties
B$_{12}$ (cyanocobalamin)	Meat, liver, eggs, milk, yeast.	Unstable to acid, alkali, light.
C (ascorbic acid)	Citrus fruits, cabbage, tomatoes, potatoes, green peppers, broccoli.	Least stable vitamin. Destroyed by heat, alkali, air. Dissolves in cooking water.

be required for optimal human health. Minerals which are believed to be essential and which are almost never deficient in the American diet include sodium, potassium, chlorine, copper, sulfur, zinc, manganese, and magnesium. Those minerals which are more likely to be deficient in the diet are discussed in Table 7.3.

Water   No other chemical compound serves the body in so many distinct and vital functions as does water. The body weight of man is more than 50 percent water, and many of his tissues are 70 to 90 percent this substance. The importance of water to the body is so great that a loss of only 10 percent of its water results in death.

The great solvent properties of water make it the medium in which all the chemical reactions of metabolism take place. Digestion, absorption, and secretion can take place only in a water medium. Water moistens the surfaces of the lungs to make possible gas diffusion. Water is important in uniformly distributing heat throughout the body and in eliminating excess heat through evaporation. It is the vehicle for transport of many vital substances through the body. It serves as a cushion of the brain and spinal cord. It takes part in many of the chemical reactions of the body, such as digestion.

The daily water requirement depends greatly upon the environmental temperature and the degree of activity. The moderately active person on a cool day might lose only 2½ quarts of water through the four channels of loss—kidneys, lungs, skin, and digestive tract. The same person working vigorously on a hot day might lose several times as much water.

In addition to the water contained in liquids, the average person consumes a considerable amount of water as a part of the solid foods he eats. Many fruits and vegetables are from 80 to 95 percent water; even a seemingly dry piece of bread is 30 to 35 percent water. Other water is produced through metabolism, being one of the end products of the breakdown of carbohydrates to yield energy.

Although thirst is usually an accurate indicator of water needs, it is usually agreed that a water intake (water, tea, coffee, milk, etc.) in slight excess of that dictated by thirst is advantageous for good kidney health.

Table 7.2 (*continued*)

function	deficiency symptoms	recommended daily allowance
Needed for production of red blood cells and growth.	Pernicious anemia.	Not established.
Essential for cellular metabolism; necessary for teeth, gums, bones, blood vessels.	Scurvy. Poor teeth, weak bones, sore and bleeding gums, easy bruising, poor wound healing.	70–100 milligrams, adult. 30–80 milligrams, child.

THE DIGESTIVE SYSTEM

Cells require that their nutrients be dissolved in the tissue fluid that surrounds them. The problem facing the body is to break down complex foods into molecules small enough to pass through tissues, so that they can enter the bloodstream or lymphatic system and be delivered in a soluble form to the various cells that make up the body. This activity is known as *digestion*—the breaking down of insoluble complex food materials into simple, soluble, absorbable forms. The passage of substances through the tissue lining the stomach and small intestine into the blood and lymph is known as *absorption*.

Anatomy and physiology of the digestive system

The general design of the human digestive tract (also called the alimentary canal or gastrointestinal tract) is a long muscular tube (up to twenty-five feet in length), which begins at the mouth and ends at the anus. The digestive tract consists of the mouth, pharynx, esophagus, stomach, small intestine, and large intestine; see Fig. 7.1. The wall of the tract takes its general form in the lower part of the esophagus and extends as such to the lower end of the large intestine.

The overall function of the digestive system is digestion and absorption. This digestive action involves the splitting of large, complex molecules of food substances—such as carbohydrates, fats, and proteins—into smaller and simpler molecules which can be absorbed. This process involves the action of many enzymes and several specific areas of the digestive tract: salivary digestion occurs in the mouth, gastric digestion in the stomach, and intestinal digestion in the small intestine. In the last section of the digestive tract, the large intestine, no digestion takes place. Here water is absorbed, bacteria flourish, and the unabsorbed solid residue is excreted as feces. This complex process is shown as a continuous flow chart of digestion in Fig. 7.2.

Salivary digestion

The oral cavity begins at the lips and extends into the pharynx. The cavity of the mouth is bounded on the sides by the cheeks, its roof is the palate, and the

Table 7.3 *Minerals*

mineral	rich sources	characteristics
Calcium	Dairy products, leafy vegetables.	Element most likely to be deficient in diet. Lack of vitamin D prevents use of calcium.
Phosphorus	Milk, liver, meat, beans, whole grains, cottage cheese, broccoli	Most functions of any mineral in body. Widespread among foods we consume, thus deficiencies rare.
Iron	Liver, meat, shellfish, egg yolk, legumes, dried fruits.	Very little in milk; infant or child must have other source.
Iodine	Iodized salt.	Integral part of thyroid hormones which have metabolic roles in body.
Fluorine	Drinking water in some areas of U.S.	Excess causes mottling of teeth.

greater part of its floor is formed by the tongue. The mouth contains the teeth, which reduce food to smaller pieces and thoroughly mix it with the saliva by the action of chewing (*mastication*), so that it may be swallowed as a premoistened, soft, round *bolus* (lump) of material. Surrounding the mouth are three pairs of salivary glands, named according to their location: parotid, submaxillary, and sublingual (Fig. 7.1). These glands secrete a fluid known as *saliva*, which contains *mucin* and an enzyme known as *salivary amylase* (ptyalin).

The enzyme functions to change cooked starch into sugar. The food remains in the mouth too short a time for the digestion of starch to be fully completed. This will be accomplished later.

The mucin contained in saliva lubricates the food and assists swallowing. Saliva also serves to put certain food materials into solution, thus serving the sense of taste. One can taste only materials that are in solution. Saliva also aids in keeping the mouth and teeth clean.

Continuing on from the mouth is the *pharynx* (throat area), which also opens into the nasal cavity. The nose and mouth are separated from one an-

Table 7.3 (*continued*)

function	deficiency symptoms	recommended daily allowance
Building material for bones and teeth. Necessary for blood clotting and nerve function.	Rickets. Poor bone and tooth structure. Stunted growth. Cramps, twitching, and other symptoms of increased nerve irritability.	0.8–1.0 gram, adult, 0.8–1.4 grams, child, up to 2 grams during pregnancy and nursing.
Essential in cell metabolism. Building material for bones and teeth. Serves as buffer to maintain proper pH of blood. Important in many enzyme systems including energy release.	Poorly developed teeth and bones, stunted growth, rickets, weakness, loss of weight.	1.5 grams, adult; 1.0 gram, child. Ratio of phosphorus to calcium should be 1.5:1 for adult and 1:1 for child.
Ingredient of hemoglobin, the oxygen-carrying pigment in red blood cells. Necessary for enzymes of cellular respiration.	Anemia (low oxygen-carrying capacity of blood).	10–15 milligrams for adult, 8–15 milligrams for child.
Basis of thyroid hormone.	Low metabolic rate. Goiter.	0.15–0.30 milligram
Strengthens bones and teeth.	Tooth decay.	1 part per million in drinking water.

other by the *palate,* which is hard in the front roof of the mouth and soft in the back. The soft palate projects backward and reaches almost to the back wall of the pharynx. When a person swallows, the soft palate elevates, preventing foods from being pushed up into the nasal cavity.

At its lower end the pharynx leads into both the *trachea* (windpipe) and the *esophagus* (food tube). Thus both air and food pass through the pharynx.

The esophagus is a collapsed, muscular tube about 10 inches long (Fig. 7.1). It is located in the center of the body with its upper 2 inches in the neck and lower 8 inches in the chest cavity (thorax). The esophagus transports foodstuffs from the pharynx to the stomach. Food is moved through the esophagus by muscular, wavelike contractions called *peristalsis.*

Gastric digestion

The stomach (Fig. 7.1) is an expanded portion of the digestive tract that has an average capacity of about 1 quart. It is usually in the shape of the letter J

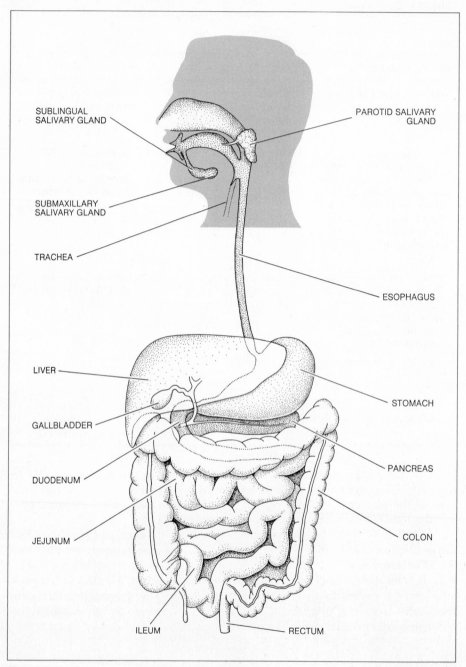

SUBLINGUAL
SALIVARY GLAND

PAROTID SALIVARY
GLAND

SUBMAXILLARY
SALIVARY GLAND

TRACHEA

ESOPHAGUS

LIVER

STOMACH

GALLBLADDER

DUODENUM

PANCREAS

JEJUNUM

COLON

ILEUM

RECTUM

Figure 7.1   General plan of the digestive system.

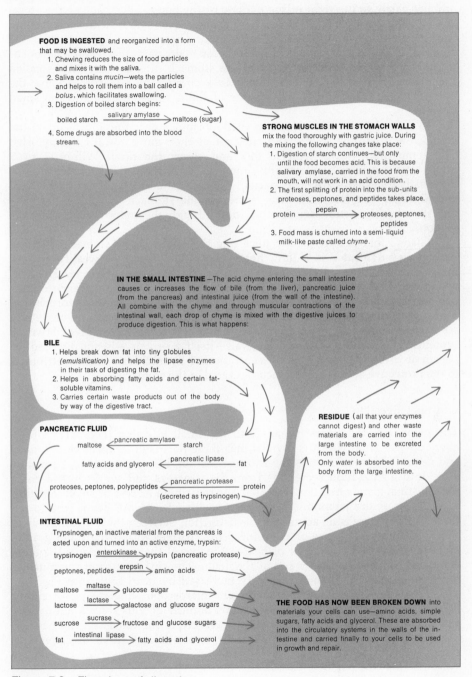

FOOD IS INGESTED and reorganized into a form that may be swallowed.
1. Chewing reduces the size of food particles and mixes it with the saliva.
2. Saliva contains *mucin*—wets the particles and helps to roll them into a ball called a *bolus*, which facilitates swallowing.
3. Digestion of boiled starch begins:

   boiled starch $\xrightarrow{\text{salivary amylase}}$ maltose (sugar)

4. Some drugs are absorbed into the blood stream.

STRONG MUSCLES IN THE STOMACH WALLS mix the food thoroughly with gastric juice. During the mixing the following changes take place:
1. Digestion of starch continues—but only until the food becomes acid. This is because salivary amylase, carried in the food from the mouth, will not work in an acid condition.
2. The first splitting of protein into the sub-units proteoses, peptones, and peptides takes place.

   protein $\xrightarrow{\text{pepsin}}$ proteoses, peptones, peptides

3. Food mass is churned into a semi-liquid milk-like paste called *chyme*.

IN THE SMALL INTESTINE—The acid chyme entering the small intestine causes or increases the flow of bile (from the liver), pancreatic juice (from the pancreas) and intestinal juice (from the wall of the intestine). All combine with the chyme and through muscular contractions of the intestinal wall, each drop of chyme is mixed with the digestive juices to produce digestion. This is what happens:

BILE
1. Helps break down fat into tiny globules (*emulsification*) and helps the lipase enzymes in their task of digesting the fat.
2. Helps in absorbing fatty acids and certain fat-soluble vitamins.
3. Carries certain waste products out of the body by way of the digestive tract.

PANCREATIC FLUID

maltose $\xleftarrow{\text{pancreatic amylase}}$ starch

fatty acids and glycerol $\xleftarrow{\text{pancreatic lipase}}$ fat

proteoses, peptones, polypeptides $\xleftarrow{\text{pancreatic protease}}$ protein
(secreted as trypsinogen)

RESIDUE (all that your enzymes cannot digest) and other waste materials are carried into the large intestine to be excreted from the body.
Only *water* is absorbed into the body from the large intestine.

INTESTINAL FLUID

Trypsinogen, an inactive material from the pancreas is acted upon and turned into an active enzyme, trypsin:

trypsinogen $\xrightarrow{\text{enterokinase}}$ trypsin (pancreatic protease)

peptones, peptides $\xrightarrow{\text{erepsin}}$ amino acids

maltose $\xrightarrow{\text{maltase}}$ glucose sugar

lactose $\xrightarrow{\text{lactase}}$ galactose and glucose sugars

sucrose $\xrightarrow{\text{sucrase}}$ fructose and glucose sugars

fat $\xrightarrow{\text{intestinal lipase}}$ fatty acids and glycerol

THE FOOD HAS NOW BEEN BROKEN DOWN into materials your cells can use—amino acids, simple sugars, fatty acids and glycerol. These are absorbed into the circulatory systems in the walls of the intestine and carried finally to your cells to be used in growth and repair.

Figure 7.2 Flowchart of digestion.

and lies partly to the right of the midline of the body. The shape of the stomach and the position of its lower part changes from time to time, according to the degree to which it is filled with food. The rounded upper part of the stomach is called the *fundus*, the middle or main part, the *body*. The opening through which food passes from the stomach into the intestine is called the *pyloric orifice*. The *pyloric valve* is a circular muscle surrounding the pyloric orifice that controls movements of fluids or semifluids into the small intestine.

Waves of contraction begin as shallow ripples near the upper end of the stomach and become deeper and stronger as they move toward the pylorus. These muscular waves tend to mix and churn the food. Within 2 to 5 hours after a person has eaten, his stomach has reduced much of the food to a partially digested state. This partially liquefied material, consisting of food and digestive enzymes, is called *chyme*. As the stomach completes the mixing, its wavelike action squirts food out through the pylorus into the *duodenum*.

Glands that secrete gastric juice line the walls of the stomach. Normal gastric digestive juice is a thin, light-yellow fluid which is weakly acid in infants and children but increases its acidic concentration with age. The acid condition is due to the presence of *hydrochloric acid*. In addition, gastric juice contains various salts and enzymes. The major function of the hydrochloric acid is to provide a medium in which the enzymes can act most completely.

Pepsin is an enzyme in gastric juice that acts to begin the breakdown of proteins. The fact that the stomach wall—itself a protein—is not digested by pepsin or irritated by the high concentration of hydrochloric acid is attributed to the protective action of the mucus secreted in the stomach.

Intestinal digestion

The pylorus of the stomach leads into the small intestine (Fig. 7.1), a tube about 23 feet long, which is divided into three portions: *duodenum, jejunum,* and *ileum*. The duodenum is the shortest section, being only about 10 inches long. Into it flow fluid secretions from the pancreas and the liver and from the intestinal glands that line its walls. The remaining 22 feet of small intestine is made up of the jejunum (the upper two fifths) and the ileum (the lower three fifths). There is no actual line of distinction between these two; the division is arbitrary. The size of the *lumen* (the channel within the tube) gradually decreases from a diameter of nearly 2 inches at the upper end of the duodenum to 1 inch at the lower end of the ileum. The surface area of the mucous membrane lining the lumen is greatly increased by deep folds; see Fig. 7.3. These folds are lined with *villi*, which are microscopic, fingerlike projections that extend into the lumen. The enormous number of villi gives a nubby appearance to the interior surface, which is velvety to the touch. At the base of the villi are the openings of glands that secrete the intestinal digestive enzymes.

Pancreatic juice   The pancreas is the single most important source of digestive enzymes in the digestive system. It is the second largest gland connected to the digestive tract. In the adult it is approximately 6 inches long and 1 inch wide. The pancreas secretes digestive juices into the duodenum by way of a duct.

The pancreatic juice is a colorless fluid with a strong alkaline reaction. The major enzymes found in it are the following:

pancreatic protease, which acts to split up proteins further
pancreatic amylase, an enzyme similar to salivary amylase in the mouth
pancreatic lipase, the most important fat-splitting enzyme in the digestive tract

Certain cells arranged within the pancreas in definite groups called the *islets of Langerhans* manufacture an endocrine hormone called *insulin.* This hormone plays an important role in the control of carbohydrate metabolism of the body. Insulin increases the rate of passage of glucose through the membranes of most cells in the body. Too little insulin slows down such movement and leads to elevated glucose in the blood. The blood glucose later is passed off with the urine. The sugar-starved cells then resort to an imperfect combustion of fats that may lead to acidosis, and finally coma and perhaps death. Insulin also plays a dominant role in favoring lipogenesis, or the formation of fat in the adipose tissue. In this manner insulin also influences blood glucose levels.

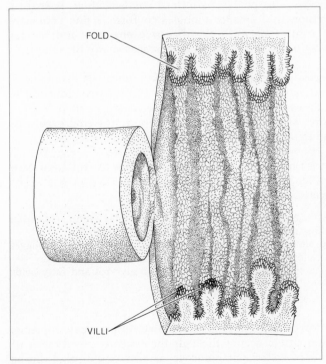

Figure 7.3   Small intestine, showing folds and villi.

An insulin deficiency is known as *diabetes mellitus*. About 2 to 4 percent of Americans eventually develop this extremely common disorder, and about 10 percent carry the trait and pass the tendency on to their children. Insulin deficiency may be treated with hypodermic injections of insulin given on a daily basis. There are also several drugs that can be taken by mouth to stimulate the pancreas to release more insulin. These oral forms are useful only with patients who still have an active pancreas; they are of value only in mild cases.

Bile The liver is one of the largest organs in the body. It is situated mainly on the right side of the abdomen, lying under and protected by the lower ribs. The liver is the great chemical laboratory of the body and is concerned in the metabolism of carbohydrates, proteins, and fats.

The digestive function of the liver is to secrete *bile*, which passes into the intestine after storage in the gallbladder. At mealtime bile flows through a duct from the gallbladder into the duodenum. At other times a muscular valve prevents its passage.

Bile is not an enzyme; it contains many salts and also fatlike substances and pigments. It is a yellow-brown or greenish fluid. The pigments are responsible for the bile's color and producing the color characteristic of *feces* (the body's solid wastes). The bile salts are the active constituents of bile. They act as wetting agents, lowering the surface tension of the fatty film that surrounds fat particles in food. This process is termed *emulsification*. It enables the fats to undergo division into smaller globules to form a fine emulsion, which facilitates closer contact between the digestive enzymes and the fat particles. The digestive action of the enzymes is increased many times by this close contact.

The fatlike substances in bile are *lecithin* and *cholesterol*. The amount of cholesterol in the bile varies with the amount in the blood. Any reduction in the bile-salt concentration causes cholesterol to be deposited in solid form in the gallbladder as *gallstones*. Because the gallbladder is not a vital organ, its removal is often resorted to when gallstones form.

Intestinal juice The intestinal juice has a definite alkaline reaction and contains a large number of enzymes that complete the digestive process. The most important of these enzymes are

> *erepsin,* a very powerful enzyme that separates the individual amino acids from one another and thus carries protein digestion to its final stage
> *maltase, lactase,* and *sucrase,* which finish the breakdown of complex sugars into simple sugar molecules
> *intestinal lipase,* which splits the molecules of fat into glycerol and fatty acids

Intestinal absorption

Nearly all of the absorption of digested foods takes place in the small intestine. The absorption of certain drugs occurs through the mucous membranes of the mouth; small amounts of water, salts, glucose, aspirin, and alcohol can be transferred through the mucous membranes of the stomach into the bloodstream.

The villi (Fig. 7.3) are the structures responsible for the absorption of digested food materials from the lumen of the small intestine. Each of the four or five million villi in an adult contains a central lymph vessel called a *lacteal,* which is surrounded by a network of blood *capillaries.* After food has been digested, it passes through the walls of the intestine into the capillaries and lacteals of the villi.

Simple sugars and amino acids pass into the capillaries. Fatty acids and glycerol may either pass directly into the capillaries or, once they have passed through the wall of the intestine, recombine and pass into the lacteals.

Other significant materials absorbed in the small intestine are vitamins, water, and salts. The fat-soluble vitamins A and D are absorbed along with dietary fats. The water-soluble vitamins are readily absorbable through the capillaries. Water and salts are similarly absorbed.

Control of digestive processes

The digestive processes are controlled both by neural connections and by specific hormones. Salivation is under the control of the autonomic nervous system. The presence in the mouth of food or inert materials (for example, chewing gum) stimulates the flow of saliva. The thought, sight, taste, or smell of food also causes saliva to flow.

The flow of gastric juice in the stomach also is started by the presence of materials in the mouth and by the thought, sight, taste, or smell of food. The arrival of food in the stomach and the release of *gastrin* (a hormone from the pyloric region of the stomach) cause great secretions of gastric juice. The entry of fats into the duodenum causes the intestinal wall to release the hormone *enterogastrone,* which inhibits, or slows, the secretion of gastric juice.

The secretion of pancreatic juice is controlled both by nerves and hormones. The movement of acidic *chyme* from the stomach into the duodenum causes the intestine to release *secretin,* which is carried by the blood to the pancreas, causing large secretions of pancreatic juice; secretin also stimulates the flow of bile from the gallbladder. The movement of fatty foods into the small intestine also causes the release of the hormone *cholecystokinin,* which also helps in the discharging of bile from the gallbladder. The presence of chyme in the small intestine stimulates the flow of intestinal juice. Hormones from the intestinal lining also enhance the secretion of intestinal juice.

Movement through the large intestine (colon)

The small intestine opens into the first part of the large intestine, the *cecum;* see Fig. 7.4. The entrance into the large intestine is guarded by a muscular valve, the *ileocecal valve,* which prevents backflow of the cecal contents into the ileum. Opening into the cecum is a blind sac, the *vermiform appendix,* which ranges in length from 2 to 8 inches. The functions of the appendix are not known; it may become infected and need to be surgically removed.

The large intestine extends up the right side of the abdomen from the cecum as the *ascending colon,* across the abdomen as the *transverse colon,* and down the left side of the abdomen as the *descending colon.* After making an S curve called the *sigmoid colon,* the large intestine terminates as the *rectum* (Fig. 7.1). The rectum is about 6 inches long and opens to the exterior of the body through the *anus.* The retention of rectal contents is controlled by two muscular valves; these muscles are constantly active and contracted except during evacuation of the waste product, the feces. The act of excreting feces from the rectal reservoir is known as *defecation.* Adults on a mixed diet require 20 to 36 hours from ingestion for the passage of food through the alimentary canal.

Although no digestive enzymes are secreted by the large intestine, bacteria present break any unabsorbed amino acids into simpler compounds and gases, many of which have strong odors and may be toxic. The odor of feces is mainly due to this process. The color of fecal material is caused by the

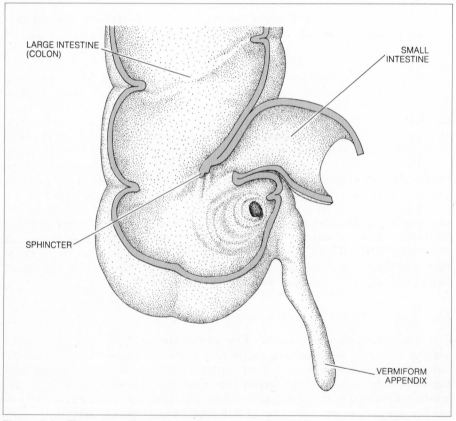

Figure 7.4   The cecum (including the ileocecal sphincter) and the appendix.

action of bacteria on the bile pigments, as indicated earlier. Besides these effects the bacterial action of the intestine performs an important function in nutrition. It synthesizes vitamin K and certain vitamins of the B complex, which are then absorbed into the bloodstream.

One of the principal functions of the large intestine is the absorption of water. Material entering the cecum is fluid, but by the time the undigested wastes have reached the lower portion of the descending and sigmoid colons, their consistency is that of paste, owing to loss of water. Little, if any, digestible food remains in the feces. In other words, almost all the protein, fat, and carbohydrate that is eaten is absorbed; the food residue of the feces consists almost entirely of indigestible substances. Vegetable material, since its framework is composed of indigestible cellulose, contributes more bulk to the feces than do other foods. This indigestible material, or "roughage" as it is commonly called, serves a useful purpose in that it acts as a mechanical stimulus, increasing the mobility of the ingested material as well as the secretions of the intestinal wall. Fecal material consists of bacteria (about 9 percent), solids (mainly nitrogenous wastes), and minerals excreted into the large intestine from the blood, together with loose lining cells and white blood cells shed from the intestinal lining.

THE TEETH

Teeth are essential for preparing solid food for digestion. The most important physical change that foods undergo is through chewing. Four specific benefits are derived from it:

1. The food is broken up into small particles.
2. Proper mixing of saliva and food is facilitated by proper chewing, which enables the digestive juices to work more quickly and thoroughly upon them. Indigestion may be traced to faulty chewing, which in turn may reflect poor teeth.
3. The taste of food is enhanced, and thus increased pleasure is derived from eating. Taste sensations help to stimulate the secretion of gastric juice.
4. Thorough chewing increases blood flow to all the structures of the mouth. In children such increased blood flow, in conjunction with the factors of heredity, nutrition, and proper tooth eruption, helps the development of the jawbones.

Structure of the teeth

Man has two sets of teeth, a temporary and a permanent one. In man the temporary, or deciduous, teeth (commonly called "milk teeth") in each lateral half of each jaw consist of two incisors, one cuspid, and two molars. They begin to erupt at about the sixth to eighth month of life (lower central incisors) and continue erupting to about the twenty-fourth month (second molars). The permanent teeth later begin to erupt and gradually replace and supplement the temporary teeth. This process begins during the fifth or sixth year (first molars) and continues until the seventeenth or even the twenty-fifth year (third molars, or "wisdom teeth"). This permanent set of teeth, shown in Fig. 7.5, consists of two incisors (for biting food), one cuspid (for biting and tearing food), two bicuspids or premolars (for grinding food), and three molars (for crushing food) in each lateral half of each jaw. The total number of teeth contained in the adult mouth is 32.

A tooth is composed of an inner structure known as the *dentin,* a soft bonelike material that forms the frame and substance of the tooth; see Fig. 7.6. The part of the dentin projecting beyond the jawbone is known as the *crown,* which is covered with a very resistant material, the *enamel.* The section of the dentin embedded in the bone is the *root;* it is surrounded by a layer of *cementum.* The cementoenamel junction is the *neck* of the tooth. Inside the dentin is the *pulp cavity,* which consists of a form of connective tissue, blood vessels, and nerves that enter the tooth through the opening at the

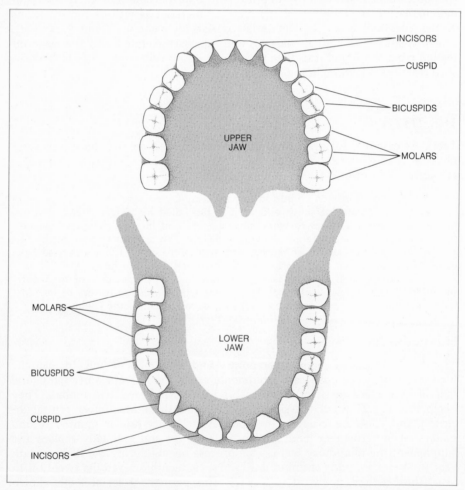

Figure 7.5 The permanent teeth.

apex (tip) of the root. The root, surrounded by the *periodontal membrane,* is situated in an *alveolar socket* in the bone of the jaw. The periodontal membrane, made up of thousands of tiny fibers, attaches the root to the alveolar socket. It helps to support the tooth in its socket, acts as a cushion by taking up the shock of chewing, and allows for some movement of the teeth. This movement is best illustrated in the field of *orthodontia* (straightening of teeth), in which constant but gentle pressure is applied to move the teeth in the direction desired.

Disease conditions associated with the teeth

Dental caries (tooth decay)   Tooth decay is man's most prevalent disease; almost 100 percent of our population is affected by it. In dental caries the insoluble calcium salts of the hard structures of the teeth (enamel and den-

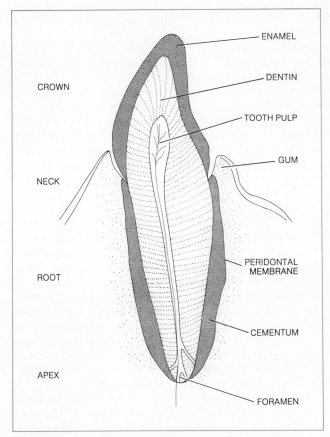

Figure 7.6   Longitudinal section of an incisor tooth in the alveolar socket.

tin) are transformed into soluble materials by chemical action; these soluble materials are washed away, and a *cavity* forms. The destruction is generally attributed to acids formed by bacterial decomposition of food lodged upon and between the teeth. Bacteria (*Lactobacillus* and others) are always present in the mouth. The presence of food residue, other than during meals, is determined by the brushing habits of the individual. In addition to adequate oral hygiene a reduction, in the diet, of fermentable carbohydrates (especially sugar), on which acid-forming bacilli flourish, will help to reduce the conditions required for tooth decay. Whether a tooth can withstand the attacks of these acids depends upon its physical and chemical structure, as determined by heredity and diet. Some teeth are so excellent in their makeup that no external aid is required for their preservation; others are of such poor quality that with the best diet they decay.

The diet of the mother during pregnancy and the diet of the child during his first years are important factors in determining the quality of the teeth and the development of caries. Therefore, during infancy and childhood the diet should be well fortified by foods rich in calcium, phosphorus, and vitamins A, C, and D. These can be best obtained from milk, egg yolk, cod liver oil, and citrus and other fruit juices.

Cavities expose the dentin, causing the nerves in the pulp cavity to register sensitivity to sweets and to temperature (hot and cold). *Pulpitis* (inflammation of the pulp cavity) will occur when the decay of the dentin goes deeper, coming closer to the pulp cavity. Once the caries has eroded the harder enamel, the erosion of the softer dentin usually takes place very quickly.

· FLUORIDATION OF THE TEETH The element fluorine plays an important role in the formation and preservation of teeth. It has been found that when drinking water containing 1 to 2 parts of fluorine per million parts of water is used, dental caries in children are reduced by about 60 percent. Excess levels of fluorine, however, tend to produce *fluorosis* (a mottling or staining of the enamel, which is permanent and cannot be brushed away). Fluorine in 1 to 2 parts per million is not sufficient to produce fluorosis.

The problem is how to get fluorine to the children who should have it. In some areas natural water supplies contain more or less than the fluorine needed. Many towns are now adding fluorine artificially to municipal water. In other towns citizens have voted down such a proposal. Fortunately, there are other ways of obtaining this substance. Many dentists apply solutions of sodium fluoride or stannous fluoride directly to the teeth (topical application). Topical application is of great value to young people who show much tooth decay and to rural families in areas where fluoridation of the water supply is not practicable; there are even indications that such application may reduce tooth decay in adults. Better yet is to take fluorine daily. Soluble fluoride tablets are available by prescription. Bottled drinking water containing fluorides is also available, and some toothpastes contain small amounts.

· PROSTHETIC DEVICES Prosthetic dentistry is the art of dental replacement. This dentistry deals with tooth replacement, restorations, crowns, bridgework, and dentures. Dentistry has developed with remarkable speed in the matter of correcting tooth deformities after they have occurred. Nowhere in the world has restorative dentistry been so energetically and seriously practiced as in the United States. Americans needing prosthetic devices and restorations and who seek treatment without delay may be assured that they will have the best.

Abscesses Abscesses are infections that usually involve the periodontal membrane, cementum, and bone in the area of the apex of the tooth. They are usually caused by dental caries that have extended into the pulp cavity, causing pulpitis. The infections then extend down through the root canal and apical foramen of the tooth into the underlying tissues. An abscess may also be caused by injury to the tooth or by infection in the tissue around the root.

An abscess may be either acute or chronic. If acute, there may be a swelling of the *gingiva* (gums) opposite the apex of the tooth, known as *gum boil*. Severe cases can be dangerous, and swelling may expand to around the eyes and into the cranial cavity. A chronic abscess ordinarily is discovered only by x-ray examination, although it may become evident in pain when adjacent teeth are depressed upon the abscess during chewing. All symptoms of an abscess require immediate attention by a dentist. There are various treatments: draining of the gum boil, cleaning out of the root canal and disinfecting the area (which aids in bone repair), or extraction of the tooth.

Periodontal diseases Periodontal diseases are those showing inflammation or degeneration, or both, of the gingiva and the periosteum, bone, and cementum.

· GINGIVITIS Gingivitis is an inflammation of the gums characterized by congested, red, and swollen gingiva. It is sometimes painless, but the gums tend to bleed easily on pressure. The inflammation may be acute or chronic and generalized throughout the mouth or confined to certain areas. The causes of gingivitis usually are poor oral hygiene, malocclusion of the teeth, an accumulation of *calculus*, also called tartar (a hard, crustlike material on the teeth at or slightly below the gum margin and neck region), or faulty dental restorations. General body conditions which may cause gingivitis are lack of specific vitamins (usually B and C) in the diet, allergic reactions, disturbances of the endocrine system of the body, such as diabetes or those of pregnancy and menstruation, and drug toxicity (alcoholism or other drug addiction). Gingivitis may also be the first sign of such disorders as leukemia.

In the treatment of gingivitis the factors contributing to the condition should be eliminated as soon as possible by a dentist or physician. A thorough cleaning of the teeth under the direction of a dentist is the only manner by which accumulated calculus may be removed. Malocclusion and faulty dental restorations should be remedied. Systemic factors, such as drug toxicity, diabetes, and chronic infections, should be corrected as completely as possible. In the treatment of inflammation of the gingiva a dentist may prescribe vitamins, antibiotics, or the topical application of ointments; in severe cases a portion of the gums may be removed surgically (gingivectomy) to facilitate drainage and healing. More extensive removal may be used in treating periodontitis (pyorrhea).

· VINCENT'S ANGINA Vincent's angina is a severe form of gingivitis which, because of its prevalence among soldiers during World War I, was named "trench mouth." It is a noncommunicable, inflammatory disease of the gingiva resulting from local irritation and the presence of Vincent's organisms. These organisms, which are components of the normal flora of the mouth, invade and destroy the gingival tissue when its resistance is lowered. The symptoms are redness, swelling, ulceration, bleeding, and pain in the gums. If treatment is inadequate, the condition may become chronic. In severe cases there is a fetid odor and foul taste in the mouth. Treatment is by complete elimination of local irritants by scaling and polishing the teeth. Mild medications and antibiotics may be used with thorough prophylactic procedures but are of no use by themselves.

• PERIODONTITIS (PYORRHEA) Periodontitis is characterized by inflammatory tissue changes, resorption of the bone around the teeth, and recession of the gingiva severe enough to cause loosening or loss of the teeth. In periodontitis the changes are usually due to gum irritation caused by calcareous deposits on the teeth, improperly contoured tooth restorations, or incorrectly designed prosthetic devices. In addition, malocclusion may cause foods to be impacted between the teeth, giving rise to bacterial growths that may cause or aggravate the condition.

The bleeding of gums while brushing the teeth, separation of gingiva from the teeth, loose or shifting teeth, and persistent "bad breath" are symptoms which should cause a person to seek early dental care. If not treated, this condition may continue until extreme bone resorption may cause the teeth to fall out.

Malocclusion There are several types of malocclusion; see Fig. 7.7. One is what appears to be protruding upper incisors, commonly referred to as "buck teeth"; another is a protruding lower jaw, which gives the appearance of pugnacity; another type is that in which the palate is so narrow as to cause crowding or protrusion of the cuspid teeth; in still another type the lower teeth bite up into the palate rather than into the tongue (lingual) surfaces of the teeth. Many other types and variations of malocclusion may be recognized by a dentist. The correction of malocclusion and the realignment of teeth is accomplished by a specialist known as an orthodontist.

Not all teeth that look crooked need orthodontic treatment. As the teeth erupt at various ages, the combination of large and small teeth in the same mouth, the development of the jaws, and the usual space between the central incisors all give a youngster an awkward appearance and may alarm the mother. Under such circumstances neighbors and friends are not the people to go to for advice. They will confuse parents with misinformation or smatterings of some other person's experience, and the result will be bewilderment. One's dentist is the person to be consulted in such instances. If the child has been brought to him regularly for care, he will have noticed irregularities long before the parent has.

The guide the orthodontist uses to determine the type of irregularity he has to contend with is the relationship of the upper six-year molars to the lower six-year molars. These teeth are called "the keys to the dental arch."

Generally speaking, orthodontic treatment should begin as soon as an undesirable condition is noticed or as soon as the child is old enough to give

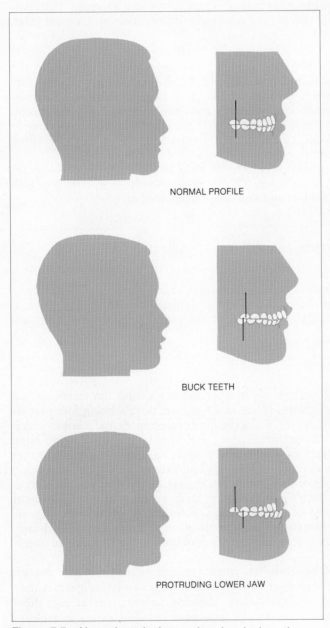

Figure 7.7   Normal occlusion and malocclusion, the six-year molars being used as guides.

the orthodontist the required cooperation. Excellent results have been obtained by orthodontists who make it a rule to begin treatment when the child is about twelve. The primary thing for the parent to consider, regardless of the age at which orthodontic treatment is begun, is that it is a long process, sometimes taking several years, and that it requires regular cooperation by the youngster.

Preventive dental care

People can greatly minimize dental difficulties and resultant expense by caring for their teeth properly throughout life. This begins with good nourishment, plenty of milk, sufficient vitamins and minerals, and a very careful regulation of intake of refined sugars. General body health contributes directly to strong teeth. Equally important is daily dental hygiene or tooth brushing immediately after each meal.

At about age three a child should begin visits to the dentist and a program of regular dental care (see Appendix C). Every six months thereafter his teeth should be cleaned and checked and any decay taken care of.

ABNORMAL CONDITIONS ASSOCIATED WITH DIGESTION

Since the digestive system is one of the largest organ systems of the body, a number of abnormal or diseased conditions associated with it may cause a person considerable discomfort. Several of the more common conditions are described below.

Indigestion

The common causes of indigestion (dyspepsia) are eating too much or too rapidly, inadequate mastication, often as a result of teeth's being lost prematurely and not replaced, severe malocclusion, neglected dental caries, which make chewing painful, eating during emotional upsets, and swallowing large amounts of air. Other factors are excessive smoking, constipation, ingestion of poorly cooked foods or foods rich in fat, and eating the wrong foods.

The major symptoms of indigestion are nausea, heartburn, and flatulence. Nausea may be produced by any condition that increases the tension upon the walls of the lower end of the esophagus, stomach, or duodenum. Distention of any part of the esophagus may result in what is usually called heartburn. Flatulence is an excessive accumulation of gas in the stomach or intestine.

A physician should be consulted whenever indigestion is severe enough to produce pain or excessive discomfort. Generally speaking, indigestion may be prevented by eating a balanced diet, allowing an hour for eating, thoroughly chewing food without haste and, whenever possible, eating in a pleasant, quiet, relaxed environment. After a meal one should avoid excitement or exercise. Smoking immediately before a meal may cause indigestion.

Peptic ulcer

A peptic ulcer is an open sore or lesion produced by an erosion of the lining membrane in one of four places: the lower end of the esophagus, the stomach (gastric ulcer), the duodenum (duodenal ulcer), and the junction of the duodenum and jejunum. The exact causes of peptic ulcers are unknown. Emotional tensions seem to play an important part in the mechanism of ulcer formation in producing an oversecretion of the acid in gastric juice.

Pain is the outstanding symptom of a peptic ulcer. It has four distinctive characteristics: it seems to always appear in the same area, it recurs periodically, with long periods of absence of pain, it may become chronic, and the pain is related to the digestive cycle, usually being absent before breakfast, appearing during the day one to four hours after mealtime, and often being sufficiently severe at night to awaken the individual. The pain is relieved by food and antacids and aggravated by alcohol and spices. Such symptoms may last for a few days, a few weeks, or several months and may leave and reappear during periods of emotional tension.

If an ulcer is not properly treated by a physician, complications such as the following may occur: perforations or holes in the walls of the intestinal tract, which can cause death within a few hours, massive hemorrhaging of the intestinal wall, causing the vomiting of blood, and partial or complete obstruction of the outlet of the stomach.

All peptic ulcers should be treated by physicians. Generally, an individual requires mental and physical rest and an improvement of his diet.

Appendicitis

Appendicitis is an inflammation of the vermiform appendix (Fig. 7.4). The inflammation results from obstruction and from infection of the wall of the appendix by the numerous bacteria in the intestine.

Typically, appendicitis is noticed in pain in the umbilical region, sometimes accompanied by nausea and vomiting. After several hours the pain shifts to the lower right portion of the abdomen, is continuous, may be dull or severe, and is accompanied by coughing or sneezing.

The early diagnosis and treatment of appendicitis are imperative. Because it is safer to operate than to permit an inflammation to proceed to rupture, surgery is common. The operative mortality in early appendicitis is extremely low, in many hospitals being less than 1 percent. But once the disease has progressed to rupture, the prognosis becomes very grave. The use of a laxative, cathartic, purgative or the application of heat can cause early rupture of the appendix in the abdominal cavity, with death as a possible outcome.

Constipation

Constipation is the difficult or infrequent passage of feces, in which large quantities of dry, hard feces accumulate in the descending colon. The most common cause of constipation is irregular bowel habits developed through a lifetime of ignoring defecation reflexes. Newborn children are rarely constipated. A child's early training requires that he learn to control defecation by inhibiting these natural defecation reflexes, but he must also be trained to defecate when these reflexes are excited, for otherwise the reflexes become less and less strong and the muscles controlling the process become progressively less active over a period of time. The early establishment of regular bowel habits in children is important.

One type of constipation is called *inactive colon;* it is commonly found in elderly invalids or in people confined to bed as the result of illness. In these people feces accumulate because the colon does not respond to the usual nerve stimuli prompting defecation. These people often lack normal eating and physical activity.

"Imaginary" constipation is common to people who are excessively "bowel conscious" and harbor fear that their bowel movements are abnormal. This fear promotes the use of laxatives, suppositories, and enemas, with the result that a normal colon becomes irritated, sensitive, and impaired, causing real constipation. Daily bowel movements are not essential for everyone. No real harm comes from the bowel that has not moved for even four days. The bowel itself must be given a chance to work, and laxatives or enemas taken more frequently than once every three days may cause constipation.

Megacolon is an abnormally large colon, congenital or acquired, usually found in children. It is a disorder of the nervous network controlling the large intestine. Because of this condition the sigmoid colon remains contracted instead of relaxing when peristalsis in the transverse and descending colon attempts to fill the rectum. Bowel movements occur infrequently and never evacuate the colon completely. The abdomen enlarges, and the disease usually becomes noticeable within the first year.

Diarrhea

Diarrhea, meaning "a flow through," is a condition in which fecal material is unusually fluid and flows out of the rectum instead of being eliminated in solid form.

It may be caused by irritation of the colon by bacteria or other organisms, or cathartics or laxatives such as castor oil, epsom salts, and magnesium sulfate. The eating of irritating or spoiled foods, emotional upsets, and fevers may be other causes.

Diarrhea may result in dehydration of the body, since the intestinal contents pass through the colon too rapidly to permit the proper resorption of water by the colon's lining. Water loss in severe diarrhea is often great enough to be extremely dangerous.

Hemorrhoids (piles)

The mucous membranes of the anal canal are pleated in vertical folds known as anal columns. They contain veins and arteries. Occasionally the veins become so dilated as to form knoblike projections called *hemorrhoids* or "piles." These blood vessels appear as small, rounded, purplish tumors covered with skin. They may bleed during and after defecation and become quite painful.

They may also create a sensation of needing to defecate. Such protrusions inside the anal canal are spoken of as internal hemorrhoids; those appearing below the junction of the skin and mucous membranes are called external hemorrhoids.

Hemorrhoids can be caused by straining or spending too much time in defecating; staying on the toilet longer than necessary tends to aggravate the condition (usually the act of defecation should take no longer than five minutes). Other causes are obesity, pregnancy, chronic cough, and disorders of the prostate gland. Hemorrhoids occurring during pregnancy usually disappear after delivery.

The severity of hemorrhoids may be reduced by not straining and by defecating *only* when the urge to do so is *real*, even if this means defecating only once every three or four days. Failure to consult a physician in time may allow the condition to become so severe that surgical intervention is required to cut out the protrusions.

SUMMARY

I. Energy relationships
    A. Energy—ability to do work; exists in two forms.
        1. Potential energy.
        2. Kinetic energy.
    B. Calorie (kilocalorie)—amount of energy required to raise the temperature of one kilogram (2.2 pounds) of water by one centigrade degree.
    C. Metabolism—total series of chemical reactions which make up the process of life.
    D. Total energy requirements—the widely varying quantities of energy needed for everyday activities.
II. Types of food
    A. Organic food substances
        1. Substances yielding energy:
            a. carbohydrates—sugars and starches.
            b. fats.
            c. proteins.
        2. Substances not yielding energy are vitamins.
    B. Inorganic food substances not yielding energy
        1. Minerals.
        2. Water.
III. The digestive system
    A. Anatomy and physiology of the digestive system
        1. The digestive tract is a long, muscular tube which begins at the mouth and ends at the anus.
        2. Digestion is the process of breaking down insoluble, complex food materials into simple, soluble, absorbable forms.
        3. Absorption is the passage of substances through the mucous lining of the stomach and small intestine into the blood and lymph.
    B. Salivary digestion
        1. Mouth:
            a. acts as receiver for food and ducts of the salivary glands (which produce *saliva*).

b. contains teeth, which function to reduce food into smaller pieces and thoroughly mix it with saliva.

c. its roof is the palate; its soft extension elevates and prevents the possibility of food's being pushed up into the nasal cavity during swallowing.

2. Pharynx and esophagus:

a. pharynx—downward extension of the mouth, leads into the esophagus and trachea.

b. esophagus—a collapsed, muscular tube leading into the stomach.

C. Gastric digestion—food enters the stomach from the esophagus and undergoes a thorough churning and mixing with the digestive juices, after which the stomach's muscular, wavelike action squirts *chyme* out through the pyloric orifice into the small intestine.

D. Intestinal digestion—small intestine (about 23 feet long) consists of duodenum, jejunum, and ileum.

1. Pancreatic juice produced by pancreas.

2. Bile produced by liver and stored in gallbladder.

3. Intestinal juice produced by glands in wall of intestine.

E. Intestinal absorption

1. Limited absorption in mouth (drugs) and stomach (water, salts, glucose, and alcohol).

2. Primary absorption through villi of small intestine:

a. carbohydrates as simple sugars.

b. proteins as amino acids.

c. fats as fatty acids and glycerol.

F. Control of digestive processes

1. Digestion controlled both by neural connections and specific hormones.

2. Hormones controlling digestion:

a. mouth—saliva flow under neural control.

b. stomach—gastrin stimulates flow of gastric juice; enterogastrone from duodenum slows gastric juice secretion.

c. pancreas—secretin from intestine causes large secretions of pancreatic fluid.

d. gallbladder—cholecystokinin from small intestine stimulates bile secretion from gallbladder.

G. Movement through large intestine (colon)

1. Colon consists of ascending colon, transverse colon, descending colon, sigmoid colon, rectum, and anus.

2. Principal function of the large intestine is absorption of water, leaving an undigested waste material called *feces*.

IV. The teeth

A. Structure of teeth

1. Consist of two sets, 24 temporary teeth and 32 permanent.

2. Each tooth composed of inner *dentin*, covered by very hard *enamel*, with central core of *pulp cavity* (containing nerves and blood vessels).

B. Disease conditions associated with teeth

1. Dental caries (cavities)—most common disease of Americans:

a. fluoridation helps in prevention of tooth decay.

b. prosthetic devices used for tooth replacement, restorations, crowns, bridgework, and dentures.

      2. Abscesses—caused by caries which have extended into the pulp cavity, causing pulpitis; they extend down through the root canal and apical foramen of the tooth into the underlying tissues.

      3. Periodontal diseases—diseases showing inflammation or degeneration, or both, of the gingiva, or soft tissues, and the underlying structures surrounding the teeth:

        a. gingivitis—an inflammation of the gums (gingiva).

        b. Vincent's angina (trench mouth)—severe form of gingivitis caused by local irritation and the presence of specific bacteria.

        c. periodontitis (pyorrhea)—an inflammatory tissue change with resorption of the bone around the teeth and recession of the gingiva severe enough to cause loosening or loss of the teeth.

      4. Malocclusion—the incorrect or irregular alignment of the teeth.

    C. Preventive dental care—care of the teeth in adolescence is guide to minimizing adult dental troubles.

  V. Abnormal conditions associated with digestion

    A. Indigestion—characterized by nausea, heartburn, and flatulence.

    B. Peptic ulcer—an open sore (lesion) produced by an erosion of the mucous membrane in one of four places

      1. Lower end of the esophagus.

      2. Stomach (gastric ulcer).

      3. Duodenum (duodenal ulcer).

      4. Junction of the duodenum and jejunum.

    C. Appendicitis—inflammation of the vermiform appendix.

    D. Constipation—difficult or infrequent passage of feces, causing large quantities of dry, hard feces to accumulate in the descending colon. Caused by

      1. Inactive colon.

      2. Megacolon—an abnormally large colon, a disorder of the nervous network controlling the large intestine.

    E. Diarrhea—unusually watery passage of feces.

      1. Caused by bacteria, cathartics, spoiled foods, emotional upsets, and fever.

      2. May result in excessive, sometimes fatal, dehydration of the tissues.

    F. Hemorrhoids (piles)—dilation of the veins in the mucous membranes of the tissues.

Glossary

If you cannot find the word you wish in this glossary, check the index for text and glossary references.

abscess (ab'ses) (L. *abscessus,* from *ab,* away; *cedere,* to go). A localized collection of pus in a cavity formed by the disintegration of tissues.

absorption (ab sorp'shən) (L. *absorptio,* from *absorbere,* to suck in). The taking up of a liquid or gas through the mucous membrane, skin, or vessels.

alveolar socket (al vē'ə lər sok'it) (L. *alveolaris,* a cavity). The socket of a tooth.

amino acid (ə mē'nō as'id) One of about thirty-three different compounds containing the amino (NH_2) group and the carboxyl (COOH) group; the building blocks of protein and the end products of protein digestion.

anabolism (ə nab'ə lizum) (G. *anabole*, a building up). The building up of the body substance; constructive metabolism.

avitaminosis (ā vī'tə mi nō'sis) (G. *a-*, without; L. *vita*, life). Condition due to a lack or deficiency of vitamins.

bile (bīl) (L. *bilis*, bile). The yellow or greenish fluid secreted by the liver; used in the digestion of fats.

bolus (bō'ləs) (G. *bolos*, lump). A mass of food ready to be swallowed or a mass passing along the intestines.

calorie (kal'ə rē) (L. *calor*, heat). The calorie used in the study of metabolism is the *large* calorie, or *kilocalorie*, and is the amount of heat required to raise the temperature of 1 kilogram (2.2 pounds) of water by 1 centigrade degree.

carbohydrate (kahr'bō hī'drāt) (L. *carbo*, coal; G. *hydro*, water or liquid). A group of compounds containing carbon, hydrogen, and oxygen, and including the sugars, starches, and celluloses.

caries (kair'ēz) (L. rottenness). Disease of the calcified external portions of the teeth, causing their disintegration and the formation of cavities.

catabolism (kə tab'ə lizm) (G. *katabole*, a throwing down). Destructive metabolism. Any destructive process by which complex substances are converted by living cells into more simple compounds.

cathartic (kə thahr'tik) (G. *kathartikos*, a cleansing agent). A medicine that quickens and increases evacuation from the bowels.

cecum (sē'kəm) (L. *calcum*, blind). The intestinal pouch into which the ileum, colon, and vermiform appendix open.

cementum (sə men'təm) (L. *caementum*, rough, unhewn stone). The layer of bony tissue covering the root of a tooth.

cholesterol (kə les'tə rol) (G. *chole*, bile, anger; *stereos*, solid). A white, fatty, crystalline substance, tasteless and odorless. Found in bile, blood, gallstones, egg yolk, etc.

chyme (kīm) (G. *chymos*, juice). The semifluid, creamy material produced by gastric digestion of food.

crown (kroun) (L. *corona*, a crown). The portion of a tooth which is covered with enamel.

defecation (def ə kā'shən) (L. *defaecare*, to deprive of dregs). The discharge of fecal material from the bowel.

dentin (den'tin) (L. *dens*, tooth). The chief substance or tissue of the teeth which surrounds the tooth pulp and is covered by enamel.

diarrhea (di ah re'ah) (G. *dia*, through; *rhein*, to flow). Abnormal frequency and liquidity of fecal discharges.

digestion (di jes'chən) (L. *digestio*, from *dis-*, apart; *gerere*, to carry). The process of converting food into materials able to be absorbed and assimilated.

duodenum (doo ə dē'nem, doo od'ə nəm) (L. *duodeni*, twelve). The first 10 to 12 inches of small intestine.

dyspepsia (dis pep'shə) (G. *dys-*, difficult or painful; *peptein*, to digest). See *indigestion*.

emulsification (i mul si fi kā'shən). Conversion into an emulsion, a preparation of one liquid distributed in globules, throughout a second liquid.

enamel (i nam'əl) (ME. *enameler, enamayller*, to coat with enamel). The white, calcareous, very hard substance that covers and protects the softer layers of the tooth.

endocrine (en'də krin) (G. *endon*, within; *krinein*, to separate). Pertaining to internal secretion; producing internal secretions.

enema (en'ə mə) (G. *enema*, send in). Injection of a liquid into the rectum.

enzyme (en'zīm) (G. *en*, in; *zyme*, leaven). A complex organic compound that accelerates or catalyzes chemical change.

erepsin (i rep'sin) (G. *ereptesthai*, to feed on). An enzyme of the intestinal juice, capable of decomposing proteoses and peptones to produce amino acids.

esophagus (i sof'əgəs) (G. *oisen*, to carry; *phagema*, food). A canal extending from the pharynx to the stomach.

fat (fat) (AS. *faett*, firm). Whitish animal or plant substance, also called *adipose tissue.*

feces (fē'sēs) (L. *faeces*, refuse). The discharge from the intestine, consisting chiefly of food residues, bacteria, and intestinal excretions.

flatulence (flat'yə ləns) (L. *flatulentia*, a blowing). Distention of the stomach or intestines with air or gases.

fluoridation (floor i dā'shən). Treatment with fluorides; specifically, addition of fluoride to water to reduce the incidence of dental caries.

fundus (fun'dəs) (L. *fundi*, the bottom). The base or part of a hollow organ remotest from its mouth.

gallbladder (gawl'blad ər) (AS. *gealla*, bile; *blaedre*, a sac). The pear-shaped reservoir for the bile on the undersurface of the liver.

gallstone (gawl'stōn). A concretion formed in the gallbladder or bile duct.

gastric digestion (gas'trik di jes'chən) (G. *gaster*, stomach). That part of digestion which takes place in the stomach.

gingiva (jin jī'və) (L. *gingiva*, gums). The gums. The tissue which covers the alveolar processes of the upper and lower jaws and surrounds the necks of the teeth.

gingivitis (jin ji'vī'tis) (L. *gingiva*, the gums; G. *-itis*, inflammation). Inflammation of the gums.

globule (glob'yool) (L. *globulus*, a small globe). Any small spherical mass of material.

glycerol (glis'ə rol) (G. *glykys*, sweet). A clear, colorless, syrupy liquid compounded of various fats and oils.

heartburn (hahrt'burn). A burning sensation in the esophagus, a symptom of indigestion.

hemorrhoids (hem'ə roidz) (G. *haimorrhois*, from *haima*, blood). A swelling of the veins in the mucous membranes of the anal canal and rectum.

hypovitaminosis (hī'pō vī'tə mi nō'sis) (G. *hypo*, under; L. *vita*, life; *osis*, a condition of). A condition due to a deficiency of one or more essential vitamins.

ileum (il'ē əm) (L. *ilium*, groin). The last division of the small intestine, the part between the jejunum and large intestine.

indigestion (in di jes'chən). Lack or failure of digestion.

insulin (in'sə lin) (L. *insula*, island; *in*, ending indicating a chemical compound). A protein hormone formed by the islets of Langerhans in the pancreas and secreted into the blood, where it regulates carbohydrate (sugar) metabolism.

jejunum (ji joo'nəm) (L. *jejuno*, "empty"). That portion of the small intestine which extends from the duodenum to the ileum.

kinetic energy (ki net'ik en'ər jē) (G. *kinetikos*, from *kinetos*, movable). Energy engaged in producing work or motion.

lactase (lak'tās) (L. *lac*, milk; *-ase*, enzyme). An intestinal enzyme that splits lactose into glucose and galactose.

lacteals (lak'tē əl[z]) (L. *lacteus*, milky). The intestinal lymphatics that take up fats.

laxative (lak'sə tiv) (L. *laxare*, to unloose). A medicine causing defecation.

lipase (lī pās, lip'āz) (G. *lipos*, fat; *-ase*, enzyme). A fat-splitting enzyme.

lumen (loo'mən) (L. *lumen*, light). The cavity or channel within a tube or tubular organ.

malocclusion (mal ə kloo'zhən) (L. *malum*, ill; *occlusio*, to close). Failure of the jaws to close properly, a result of poor placement of the teeth.

maltase (mawl′tās) (L. *malt*, grain; *-ase*, enzyme). An enzyme which breaks down maltose into dextrose.

mastication (mas ti kā′shən) (L. *masticare*, to chew). The chewing of food.

metabolism (me tab′ə lizm) (G. *metaballein*, to change). The sum of all the physical and chemical processes of the body.

mineral (min′ə rəl) (L. *minerale*, mineral). An inorganic element or compound occurring in nature.

mucin (myoo′sin) (L. *mucus*, mucus). The chief constituent of mucus.

mucous membrane (myoo′kəs mem′brān) (L. *mucosus*, pertaining to mucus; *membrana*, membrane). The lining membrane of the body cavities and canals which are connected with the outside.

mucus (myoo′kəs) (L. *mucus*, mucus). The viscid, slippery secretion produced by mucous membranes, which it moistens and protects.

nausea (naw′zē ə, naw′zhə) (G. *nausia*, seasickness). An uncomfortable sensation related to the alimentary system, with a desire to vomit.

orthodontia (or thə don′shə) (G. *orthos*, straight; *odous*, tooth). The branch of dentistry which deals with the prevention and correction of irregularities of the teeth and malocclusion.

palate (pal′ət) (L. *palatum*, palate). The roof of the mouth.

pancreas (pan′krē əs) (G. *pan*, all; *kreas*, flesh). A large gland located behind the stomach; its secretion (pancreatic juice) is used in digestion.

pepsin (pep′sin) (G. *pepsis*, digestion). The chief enzyme of gastric juice, which acts upon proteins (protease).

peptic ulcer (pep′tik ul′sər) (G. *peptikos*, pertaining to digestion; L. *ulcus*, ulcer). An opening lesion occurring in the lower esophagus, stomach, or duodenum.

perforation (pur fə rā′shən) (L. *perforare*, to pierce through). Act of piercing through a part.

periodontal membrane (per ē ə don′təl mem′brān) (G. *peri*, around; *odous*, tooth; L. *membrana*, membrane). The tissue that connects the cementum of a tooth to the surrounding structures.

periodontitis (per ē ədon tī′tis) (G. *peri*, around; *odous*, tooth; *-itis*, inflammation). Inflammatory reaction of periodontal tissues.

peristalsis (per i stal′sis) (G. *peri*, around; *stalsis*, contraction). Progressive wavelike contractions by which muscles of the alimentary canal propel their contents.

pharynx (far′inks) (G. *pharynx*, pharynx). The part of the digestive canal between the cavity of the mouth and the esophagus.

potential energy (pə ten′shəl en′ər jē) (L. *potentia*, power). Existing energy, ready for action but not yet active.

prosthetics (pros thet′iks) (G. "a putting to"). A branch of surgery involved with replacement of an absent part of the body by an artificial one as, for example, dentures.

protein (prō′tēn, prō′tē in) (G. *protos*, first). Any of a class of complex organic combinations of amino acids which are essential constituents of all living cells.

ptyalin (tī′ə lin) (G. *ptyalon*, spittle). An enzyme occurring in the saliva which converts starch into maltose and dextrose.

pulp cavity. Inner portion of the tooth which contains the connective tissue, capillaries, lymph vessels, and nerve endings.

purgative (pur′gə tiv) (L. *purgare*, to cleanse). Cathartic, causing evacuations from the bowels (defecation).

pylorus (pī lor′əs) (G. *pyloros*, from *pyle*, gate; *ouros*, guard). The opening between the stomach and the duodenum.

pyorrhea (pī ə rē'ə) (G. *pyo*, pus; *rhoia*, flow). A discharge of pus; pus-filled inflammation of the sockets of the teeth.

rectum (rek'təm) (L. "straight"). The last few inches of the large intestine, terminating the anus.

saliva (sə lī'və) (L. *saliva*, saliva). The first digestive secretion, emitted from the salivary glands into the mouth.

salivary glands (sal'i ver ē gland[z]) (L. *saliva*, saliva; *glans*, acorn). The three pairs of glands which secrete saliva.

sigmoid (colon) (sig'moid) (G. *sigmoeides*, shaped like the letter s). The lower part of the descending colon, shaped like the letter s.

sublingual gland (sub ling'gwəl) (L. *sub*, under; *lingua*, tongue). Salivary gland in floor of mouth.

submaxillary gland (sub mak'si ler'ē) (L. *sub*, under; *maxilla*, the jaw). Salivary gland in floor of mouth.

sucrase (soo'krās) (Fr. *sucre*, sugar). An enzyme in intestinal juice that begins digestion of sugar (amylase).

suppository (sə poz'i tor ē) (L. *suppositorium*, that which is placed underneath). A medicated preparation for introduction into rectum, vagina, or urethra.

tartar (tahr'tər) (G. *tartaron*, dregs). Material deposited on the teeth; consists of lime.

vermiform appendix (vur'mi form ə pen'diks) (L. *vermis*, worm; *forma*, shape; *appendere*, to hang upon). A worm-shaped process projecting from the cecum.

villi (vi'lī) (L. *villus*, tuft of hair). Short, fingerlike projections found on certain membranous surfaces, mainly in the digestive system.

Vincent's angina (vin'sənts an jī'nə). Painful ulcerative disease of the gingiva which may affect the tonsils and pharynx, commonly called "trench mouth."

vitamin (vī'tə min) (L. *vita*, life). A general term for a number of organic substances that are necessary for the normal functioning of the body.

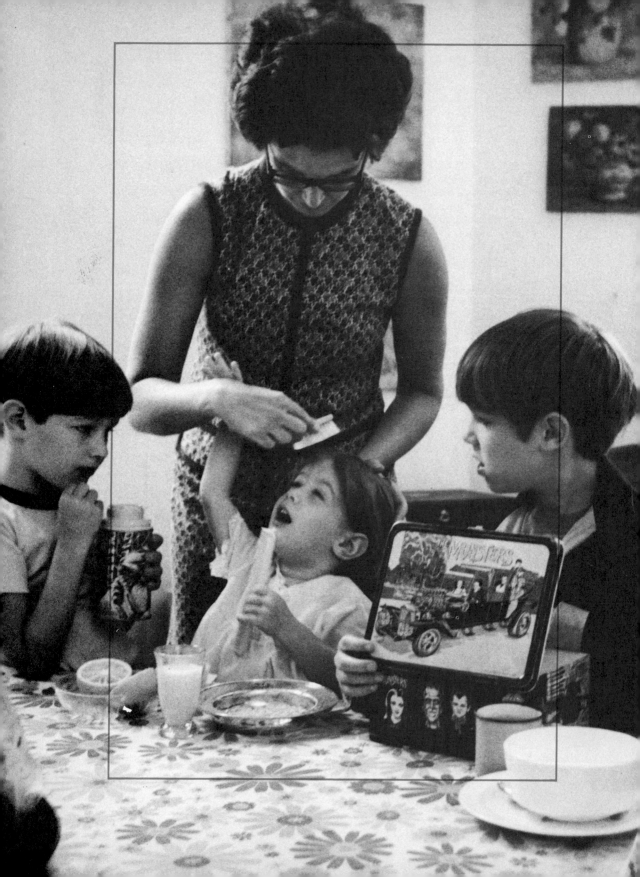

Diet and weight control

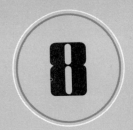

8

There are many paradoxes in this world. Not the least of them is that, while many of the world's people are fighting starvation, approximately 20 percent of the people in the United States are overweight because of excessive eating. The preoccupation that Americans have over the problem of weight control is shown by the quarter- to half-billion dollars a year that they pay "fat doctors" for help in overcoming this problem. Such concern is not only a reflection on the importance we attach to proper weight but also a frank commentary on the failure many people encounter in their attempts to maintain a satisfactory weight.

APPETITE CONTROL

Appetite and hunger control relate to one's ability to control his weight. They are known to be regulated by a small area in the brain called the "appetite center," or *appestat*; see Fig. 8.1. This center consists of two parts, or *nuclei* (small groups of cells). When one set is stimulated, you want to eat; when the other set is stimulated, you feel satisfied. Thus the appestat operates something like a thermostat in controlling the temperature in a room.

As to what activates the appestat, there is still some question. It may be the glucose level in the blood (blood sugar level), body temperature changes, or the level of amino acids in the blood. But it is known that the appetite center has nerve connections with the cortex of the brain and may also be consciously controlled. This would mean that emotional factors, as well as chemical ones, appear to control appetite. Worry, tension, frustration, and conflicts in interpersonal relations can influence a person's appetite. Other research has shown that appestats vary in different individuals; thus, a person may inherit a "higher setting" in his appestat than another person and require more food before he feels satisfied. Consequently, we can say that one's appetite is regulated by his emotions, body chemistry, and inheritance. All these factors influence the ability to control weight.

DETERMINING DESIRABLE WEIGHT

To determine the ideal weight for an individual is difficult, if not impossible. Body weight varies with sex, age, height, skeletal structure, rate of basal metabolism, and endocrine peculiarities. Since the so-called "ideal" or "average" individual does not exist, it is neither realistic nor possible to suggest an "ideal weight" that could be applied to all adults. Consequently, in trying to arrive at a reasonable weight recommendation for adults the Food and Nutrition Board of the National Research Council has had to take a number of factors into consideration. Life insurance actuarial tables have indicated that the most favorable health expectation is associated with the weight normally achieved

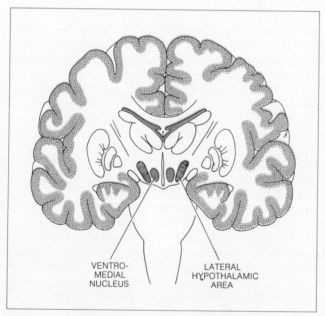

Figure 8.1 The two sets of bilateral nuclei which form the appetite center, or appestat.

Table 8.1 *Desirable weights according to height*

height without clothing (inches)	weight without clothing (pounds)					
	men			women		
	small frame	medium frame	large frame	small frame	medium frame	large frame
60				100	109	118
62				106	115	124
64	122	133	144	112	122	132
66	130	142	154	119	129	139
68	137	151	165	126	136	146
70	145	159	173	133	144	155
72	152	167	182	140	152	164
74	160	175	190			
76	166	182	198			

SOURCE: Food and Nutrition Board, National Research Council.

at age 22. It is accordingly recommended that the desirable weight for this age is a proper weight to maintain throughout adult life. Maximal body development in either sex usually is attained several years earlier: at 18 in the female and at 20 in the male. In Table 8.1 adjustments in recommended weights are made for sex, height, and body build. An individual with a smaller than average frame would be expected to weigh somewhat less than the weight recommended for his given height, whereas an individual with a larger than average frame would usually weigh more. The adjustments on the table provide for this variation. A general ideal to keep in mind for maintaining a desirable weight is summarized in Fig. 8.2.

OVERWEIGHT AND OBESITY

A distinction should be made between the terms *obesity* and *overweight*. *Obesity* is defined as "an excessive deposition of fat beyond what is considered normal for a given age, sex, and build." Weight, on the other hand, is

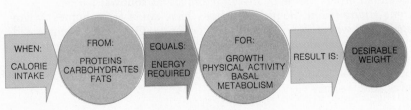

Figure 8.2   Rule for achieving a desirable weight.

defined as "a quantity of heaviness." *Overweight*, then, is simply "over-heaviness" without any regard to fatness. Overweight can be defined also as any weight in excess of that recommended for a given person according to a desirable weight.

Body weight is affected by fat, muscle, and bone. If fat or muscle development is greater than normal, one can be overweight. It is unlikely that large bone structure per se would render one overweight. One may be overweight because of heavy muscular development and still not be obese. It is also possible that one may be of average weight and yet excessively fat, if he has relatively small muscular and bony structure.

The problem is that there is no easy way to measure body fat in relation to the person's total weight. A weight lifter or football player may have developed his muscle mass to a point where his weight is excessive, and yet he has only minimal amounts of body fat. Generally speaking, however, if a nonathletic person is 20 percent above his desirable weight, he can be rather sure he is obese.

One indicator of fatness is the "ruler test." When one is lying flat on his back and is relaxed, the surface of the abdomen between the flare of the ribs and the pubis (bone below the navel) is normally flat or slightly concave. A ruler placed on the abdomen parallel with the vertical axis should touch both ribs and pubis. Another guide is the "pinch test." With your finger and thumb gently pull on the loose skin at the back of your upper arm or at your waist and measure the thickness. It should be between a half-inch and an inch thick. If it's thicker, you're too fat.

In the United States 20 to 25 percent of the population weigh more than they should. Further studies point out that 23 percent of male college freshmen and almost 36 percent of female college freshmen are overweight.[1] The problem generally increases with age. As a person ages his basal metabolic rate drops, but he tends to eat as much as he did when he was younger. In the United States 60 percent of men in their fifties are considered overweight.

Causes of overweight

The accumulation of excess fat leading to eventual overweight and obesity may be attributed to an excess intake of calories, a deficiency of calorie expenditure through sedentary behavior, or to a combination of these two factors. Not all people have the same metabolic rate; thus each individual must develop eating habits which maintain his best weight.

Certain factors affect a person's eating habits. Some contribute to overweight more than others. Some of these factors are as follows:

1. *Home environment.* Some individuals have come from homes where meals are rich and where excessive eating is common. Others are accustomed to heavy between-meal eating, particularly of sweets, such as soft drinks, candy, ice cream, and pastries. Still others have been accustomed to too little exercise because of available transportation, lack of organized sports, modern conveniences, and laziness.

[1] S. Grollman, *The Human Body*, New York, Macmillan, 1969, p. 417.

2. *Poverty.* Some families, because of limited finances, buy cheap foods, which tend to be high in carbohydrates (sugars and starches).

3. *Occupation.* Housewives who are often around food sometimes become habitual samplers and nibblers. The same holds true of people who work in food industries, such as candy shops, restaurants, and bakeries.

4. *Emotional factors.* Some people find eating a pleasant break from a monotonous routine. Others find it a satisfying compensation for domestic troubles, financial problems, illness in the family, social upsets, or anxiety over schoolwork or a pending business deal.

5. *Age and disease.* As a person grows older, his dietary needs change, but he may have difficulty in diminishing long-established eating patterns. Disabilities may reduce the previous amount of activity and make a change in earlier eating habits necessary; see Fig. 8.3.

Regardless of the underlying causes of obesity, the basic problem is simply one of taking in *more* calories than are needed for one's total activities, or basal metabolism, heat loss, work, and exercise. Unused calories from any source are stored in the body as fat, each pound of stored fat representing about 3,500 calories. We either use the calories or we store them, regardless

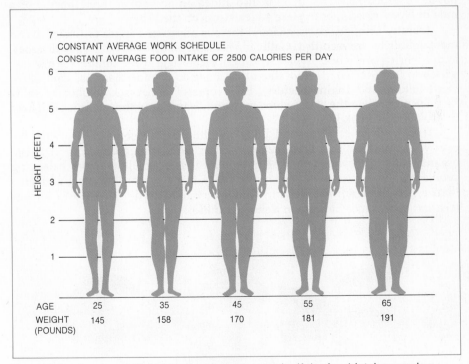

Figure 8.3 Age in relation to reduced dietary needs. If the food intake remains the same over the decades, a person gains weight; to maintain a given weight, it is necessary to reduce the food intake.

of where they come from. The more of stored calories, the greater the obesity; see Fig. 8.4.

Effects of overweight

There are various reasons why overweight is undesirable. Life insurance records show that overweight individuals, for several reasons, are poorer risks than those who have normal weight. Their life expectancy is less: the prevalence of certain diseases and the danger of death increase in direct proportion to the amount of overweight.

Respiratory difficulties are common. With more weight in the chest wall, more work is required in breathing. Obese people have less tolerance of exercise. They show a higher frequency of respiratory infections than do people of normal weight. Reduced ventilation results in a buildup of carbon dioxide in the blood.

Blood pressure generally goes up with weight increase (and often returns to normal with comparable weight loss). An obese person with high blood pressure (hypertension) runs a greater risk of coronary heart disease than does a nonobese person with hypertension. Grossly obese persons have 1.5 to 3.5 times as many fatal heart attacks and strokes as do others. With every pound of added fat tissue there is also added an additional three fourths of a mile of blood vessels; both place added stress on the heart.

Obesity complicates pregnancy: there is a greater danger of toxemia, and more stillbirths are recorded. Gallbladder diseases, diabetes, digestive diseases, and nephritis are more prevalent. Obesity can aggravate conditions such as varicose veins, osteoarthritis and other bone and joint diseases, congestive heart failure, and angina pectoris. Fat people of either sex frequently show "stretch marks" on the skin (which may not disappear with weight loss). There is also increased risk in surgery.

It is work to carry around body weight that is not needed, giving the overweight person "that tired feeling." Fat accumulating around internal vital organs tends to crowd them. The individual is less agile, has more balancing problems, and moves more slowly; he tends to have more physical accidents than a person of normal weight. Thus overweight leads not only to an unpleasant appearance but also to a shortened life.

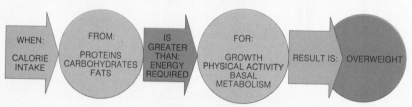

Figure 8.4   Process of becoming overweight.

Reducing

The problem of reducing weight is a personal one. An overweight person must *want* to lose weight badly enough to go through the rigors of ignoring the sight and smell of appealing food within his reach. He must have intention plus willpower. Motivation can be created in various ways. Young people may be strongly motivated by the desire for a pleasing appearance; older people may require other reasons, such as the advice of a doctor or the prospect of living longer and possibly avoiding certain bodily disorders.

The next thing the overweight person must do is to admit that his obesity in all likelihood was caused by overnutrition, that his intake of food has exceeded his output of energy. If food intake is reduced to energy output, a person should be successful in "holding his own." The overweight person needs to go one step further: his intake must be reduced to the point at which it will be less than his output. Accordingly, as the body uses more energy than is being taken in, the fat will be reduced and the weight diminish. This assumption is the basis of most reducing programs.

How can this reversal be achieved? One of several methods or combinations of them may be followed. First of all, food intake can be cut by going on a reducing diet. Second, the body's use of calories can be increased through increased exercise. The best choice combines reduced food intake and increased exercise to improve muscle tone and body regulation mechanisms. Third, a method recommended by physicians only in very extreme cases, is *lipectomy*. This is a surgical removal of some excessive fat from those parts of the body which are quite accessible and which tend to receive the largest accumulations of stored fat. Such removal usually is from the abdomen, breasts, arms, or legs. Lipectomy may be a *beginning* in selected, severe cases; it needs to be followed by the first or second plan if the patient is to reach and maintain desirable body weight.

Reducing diets Today we find an incredible number of suggestions for losing weight. They range all the way from the "miracle diets" that will take off ten pounds in two weeks, the prescribed pills, oils, tablets, seeds, juices, extracts, and high-fat or high-protein diets, and the prepared formulas one can buy in the form of cookies or prepared drinks, to simply eating less of whatever food one normally chooses to eat. Some of these devices have value, and some are medically considered to be dangerous. Although it is not our intention to enumerate the many products advertised to help lose weight, a few general statements are necessary.

The basic problem is in readjusting the regular diet. Whatever is taken or done to accomplish weight loss must be viewed in terms of the total picture. Although various aids may be helpful temporarily, one does not want to use them the rest of his life and, besides, some of them are expensive. At best they may help the overweight person change his eating habits. They are not magical in solving the problem. There just is no easy way to lose weight.

Generally, no reducing diet is decidedly better than another. Any one of them faithfully followed should help a person to lose weight successfully.

Several guidelines should be observed in deciding on a reducing diet. The following should be considered:

1. *See a physician.* Let him decide whether it is safe to lose weight, how much weight to lose, and how long the reduction should take.

2. *Choose a practical diet.* The problem of dieting will be life-long. Therefore a person should choose a type of reducing diet he will be able to follow without undue regimentation. It should be compatible with the eating habits he is accustomed to and likes. It is not necessary to stop eating the foods he cherishes, but he may have to cut out some things or govern the amount he eats. This regulation is true not only for *losing* extra pounds but also for *maintaining* a desirable weight. Unless he can successfully readjust his old diet, which allowed him to become fat, he probably will end up with the overweight problem all over again, and all the discomfort of reducing will have been in vain.

3. *Reduce the calories taken in.* Some studies indicate that calorie reduction can be done best by limiting the carbohydrate intake; some, by reducing fats eaten; and others, by limiting protein intake. Regardless of the method, calories *do* count (even if one refuses to count them). Many kinds of food that don't look "rich" (high in calories) are actually abundant in them. The same could be said for certain drinks. Table 8.2 is a listing of the calories in some favorite foods and drinks, based on a usual restaurant serving.

4. *Plan a diet.* A reducing diet should contain the basic food groups: meat, milk, vegetables and fruits, and cereals. During the reducing period the body still will be functioning. It will need not only proteins, minerals, and vitamins, but also limited calories. Generally, a reducing diet should provide at least 1,200 to 1,800 calories a day. Some commercial reducing formulas allow a minimum of 900 calories per day. This minimum is acceptable when such products are supplemented by certain nutrients such as vitamins and minerals. Table 8.3 suggests a pattern for a reducing diet of 1,200 calories per day. Generally, however, a person should not try to account for all calories in foods eaten, because it is almost impossible to be accurate. The calorie charts do not and could not list all foods. Besides such counting unnecessarily regiments eating, so that many people give up the whole idea of weight reduction.

5. *Know what the goal is.* To lose 1 pound of stored fat in a week a person should reduce his calorie intake by at least 3,500 calories a week, or 500 calories a day. To lose 2 pounds a week he should reduce his intake by 1,000 calories a day. Nutritionists suggest that a good reducing regimen should work toward a loss of 1 to 2 pounds of weight a week. A more rapid rate of loss may result in deficiencies in essential dietary elements and, therefore, be less likely to result in a permanent improvement in eating habits. The reducer should weigh himself daily on a good bathroom scale. He should do it at the same time each day and under similar conditions. He should consider each pound lost a reduction of 3,500 calories of stored fat. (A "crash" diet aimed at taking off 10 pounds in two weeks would mean a calorie reduction of 2,500 calories a day, which is more calories than most women normally get in their food. Such a reducing suggestion represents starvation and is therefore preposterous.)

Table 8.2 *Calories in some favorite foods and drinks*

breakfast	calories	drinks	calories
1 scrambled egg	110	Whole milk, 1 cup	160
2 slices fried bacon	100	Nonfat milk, 1 cup	90
Ham, slice, lean and fat	245	Malted milk, 1 cup	280
1 wheat pancake	60	Cocoa, 1 cup	235
1 waffle	210	Orange juice frozen,	
Grapefruit, ½ whole	55	1 cup diluted	110
Cantaloupe, ½ melon	60	Apple juice, 1 cup	120
Corn flakes, 1 oz.	110	Grape juice, canned, 1 cup	165
Oatmeal, 1 cup	130	Yoghurt, 1 cup	120
White bread, 1 slice	160	Cola drink, 1 cup	95
Butter, 1 pat	50	Ginger ale, 1 cup	70
Jam, 1 tablespoon	55	Beer, 1 cup	100

lunch or dinner		snacks	
Tomato soup, 1 cup	90	Cheddar cheese, 1-inch cube	70
Spaghetti, meat balls and		Bologna, 1 slice	85
tomato sauce, 1 cup	335	Peanut butter, 1 tablespoon	95
Pork chop, 1 slice lean	130	Peanuts, roasted, 1 cup	840
Roast beef, 1 slice lean	125	10 potato chips	115
Hamburger, meat only, 3 oz.	245	Raisins, dried, 1 cup	460
1 frankfurter, cooked	155	1 apple	70
Chicken, ½ breast	155	1 banana	85
Mashed potatoes, buttered,		1 orange, navel	60
1 cup	185	1 peach	35
Pizza, 1 section	185	Watermelon, 1 wedge	115
Cottage cheese, creamed,		Popcorn, 1 cup	65
1 cup	240	2 graham crackers	55
Custard, 1 cup	285	1 doughnut, cake type	125
Angelfood cake, 1 section	110	Candy, milk chocolate, 1 oz.	150
Iced chocolate cake, 1 section	445	Marshmallows, 1 oz.	90
Apple pie, 1 section	345	Pretzels, 5 small sticks	20
Ice cream, 1 cup	285	1 fig bar	55
Sherbet, orange, 1 cup	260	1 cookie, 3-inch	120
Corn starch pudding, 1 cup	275		

SOURCE: *Nutritive Value of Foods*, Home and Garden Bulletin No. 72, rev. September 1964, Washington, D.C., U.S. Department of Agriculture.

6. *Graph the progress.* A person gains weight gradually; ideally, he should lose it the same way. Because gradual reducing programs can be discouraging, he might lose sight of his initial goal. A good psychological crutch to use in keeping track of progress is a simple graph set up at the beginning of the program. One should plan his weight loss according to how many pounds he needs to lose. He should aim at 1 to 2 pounds of weight loss per week, and then construct a graph. The graph shown in Fig. 8.5 is set up on the basis of 1 pound of weight loss per week. A straight line can be drawn from

Table 8.3 *Diet pattern for 1,200 calories per day*

breakfast

Fruit—1 medium serving, fresh, frozen, or canned.

Egg—1, poached or boiled.

Toast—1 slice with 1 teaspoon butter or margarine *or*

Cereal—½ cup with ¼ cup milk, no sugar.

Coffee or tea—no cream or sugar.

midmorning snack

Nonfat milk or buttermilk—1 glass.

luncheon

Meat or cheese—1 3-oz. portion.

Vegetable—1 medium serving; may be raw, as a salad such as lettuce and tomato, or cooked; use lemon or vinegar for seasoning rather than butter or salad dressings.

Fruit—1 medium serving, fresh or unsweetened canned.

Bread—1 slice.

Butter or margarine—1 teaspoon or 1 pat.

Tea or coffee—no cream or sugar.

midafternoon

Iced tea, lemonade, or a soft drink.

dinner

Bouillon or consommé or vegetable-juice cocktail—1 serving.

Meat—1 3-oz. portion.

Potato or a substitute for potato—1 small serving of mashed or baked potato, steamed rice, corn, lima beans, or macaroni; or 1 slice bread.

Vegetable—1 serving, raw, as a salad, or cooked; one vegetable a day should be a green, leafy one.

Butter or margarine—1 teaspoon, for potato.

Fruit—1 medium serving, fresh or unsweetened canned.

Tea or coffee—no cream or sugar.

evening or bedtime

Nonfat milk, buttermilk, soft drink, or glass of beer.

Crackers or pretzels—2.

where one's weight is when he began to diet to where he wants it to be when he finishes. Weight is measured each morning. A dot is put at the point at which his weight is each day. The line of dots will tell him how close he is to his plan of weight loss on any particular day during the reducing time. The idea is not to allow his weight to stray too far from the suggested weight in any given week. The graph will serve as a daily reminder of progress. This method has been used with success as a help during a reducing regimen.

7. *Exercise regularly.* A reasonable program of regular physical exercise helps a person resist weight gain through expenditure of energy. It also improves muscle tone and contributes toward a general feeling of well-being, both physical and mental. However, the reducer must be careful not to look upon physical exercise as a substitute for controlled calorie intake. Only about 100 calories are used by walking a mile. Vigorous sports activities, such as tennis or active swimming, use up as many as 1,000 calories an hour. Too strenuous an exercise, however, is apt to result in an increased appetite. Moderate and regular periods of exercise will help to use up stored energy without increasing the appetite.

As a person becomes older, his calorie requirements decline. The National

Research Council suggests that an individual's calorie allowance should be reduced by 5 percent per decade between the ages of 35 and 55 and an additional 8 percent per decade between the ages of 55 and 75. A further reduction of 10 percent is recommended for people 75 and older.

As the American "way of life" becomes less strenuous, the calorie requirements for the average American decrease as well. The National Research Council has found that it takes fewer calories today to maintain an adult at the desirable "age-22" weight than it did a decade ago. Consequently, the Recommended Dietary Allowances of the Food and Nutrition Board of the National Research Council have been reduced. It becomes important for an adult to be guided in his diet by his weight rather than by the eating habits he may have learned before life became as automated and leisurely as it is in this country today.

Pharmaceutical aids Another approach in the management of overweight has been through the use of drugs. Viewed by some physicians as a controversial method of weight reduction, drugs nonetheless have been found to assist some individuals in achieving a negative caloric balance, according to a report by the Council on Drugs of the American Medical Association. Different compounds, affecting the body in different ways, have been used. Generally, these drugs serve to decrease or distract the appetite, increase metabolism, tranquilize the body, or speed up loss of body fluids. Most of them

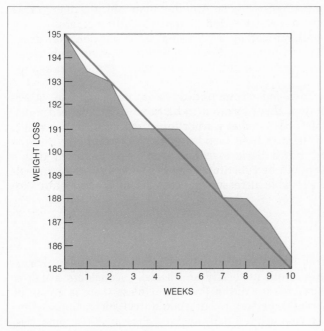

Figure 8.5 A reducing graph.

are potentially dangerous and should never be used unless medically prescribed. Any of them may have undesirable side effects. At best they are aids in restricting caloric intake. They cannot be considered an easy road to reducing.

Several further precautions are in order. There is no magic in the dietary pills or drugs. First, any diet pills one buys in a drugstore or supermarket without a prescription contain little medicine and have very limited effectiveness. Second, pills a physician prescribes are almost always only chemical crutches for desperate dieters to lean on. The amphetamines, or "pep pills," which stimulate a person physically while curbing his diet, can be habit-forming; the danger of drug dependency is a greater hazard than being overweight. Third, some physicians, known as "diet doctors," push "miracle drugs," which may be pep pills containing thyroid extract for boosting the metabolic rate and digitalis for stimulating the heart; such a combination may involve serious risk.

Reducing don'ts   In addition to the specific reducing dangers already pointed out in the text several general things should be mentioned.

1. *Don't blame overweight problems on inheritance.* Although there are surely a few cases of faulty heredity that tend to make overweight more of a problem for some people than others, most cases can be traced to either a personal or a cultural problem. Even though an overweight problem can be traced to a physical problem of some kind, many physical problems can be successfully treated. Be careful not to misconstrue faulty home practice in matters of overeating as being a hereditary problem.

2. *Don't be tempted by "crash" diets.* Any diet plan which claims to take off any number of pounds in a short period of time should be carefully scrutinized. It may be a case of misleading advertising, or it may be that drugs that can cause organic damage to the body are to be used. Seeing a physician before going on any reducing diet should give one ample protection against such plans.

3. *Don't follow the food fads.* Some fad diets are not palatable, others are monotonous, and many of them turn out to be expensive. Balanced nutrition calls for a variety of foods. A diet purporting to succeed with a single food could well result in malnutrition. Good nutrition for the body is to be considered, not a luxury, but a basic essential. Don't be convinced that a so-called "perfect" food should be substituted for the wide variety of appealing and nutritious foods available at reasonable cost in our grocery stores today.

UNDERWEIGHT

The underweight person is the exception in the United States today. Fortunately for him, our culture, both medically and socially, considers a lighter weight more desirable today than it did in the past. Unless there is a case of malnutrition, the underweight person today should feel increasingly comfortable socially. As the recommended daily dietary allowances become less, the individual who once was considered underweight comes closer to what is now held to be a normal weight. And not to be overlooked is the prospect that the underweight person may live longer than his overnourished friends. If he is feeling well and appears to be healthy, he doesn't carry the known liability of obesity. Being underweight with good health is a favorable state.

An individual may be underweight for various reasons, including malnutrition, disease, endocrine disorders, lack of appetite, overactivity, or nervousness. Underweight frequently is the result of faulty nutrition; see Fig. 8.6. Symptoms may include anemia, chronic digestive disturbances, low resistance to disease, and mental and physical slowness. In severe forms malnutrition can lead to various deficiency diseases brought on by inadequate amounts of vitamins or minerals. In selected cases malnutrition may result from the inability of the body to digest or use certain foods it needs. This inability may be due to faulty enzyme action. In any case, malnutrition can lead to additional problems—increased susceptibility to diseases (such as tuberculosis), injury to certain body organs (such as the heart or kidneys), or, in severe cases, death.

For the underweight person who is apprehensive over his condition the first step is to decide what he can change. If underweight is being caused by some emotional problem—brought on by unpleasant working conditions, family problems, worry—the underweight person should try to change the situation or remove himself from it. If underweight is due to physical ailments such as infected body organs (tonsils, teeth), or the use of drugs, the family physician should be consulted.

One method of gaining weight is to increase the intake of food from the basic food groups, by taking either larger helpings or more helpings in a balanced food plan. There can be danger in greatly increasing the intake of certain kinds of high-calorie foods. Some recommend increasing the intake of butter, eggs, and cream or cream products (malted milks, milk shakes, ice cream). Such foods may result in weight gain, but they are suspected in the development of atherosclerotic plaques within the circulatory system, with the increased hazard of premature heart disease.

FOOD FADS AND FALLACIES

Although the food faddist may be sincere in his beliefs about food and honestly concerned about his health, he frequently turns into a disciple attempting

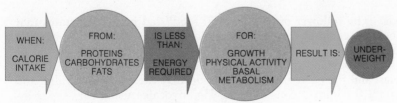

Figure 8.6   Process of becoming underweight.

to convert his friends to his particular beliefs regarding food. He finds it easier to believe the bizarre and spectacular claims of a quack than the more moderate, but realistic, statements of proper authorities.

All kinds of food faddism may be found—for example, for molasses, yoghurt, oysters, cottage cheese, wheat germ, seaweed extracts. Some people believe that fish is a brain food or that carrots will make hair curly. Some warn against drinking milk and eating acid fruits together because the acid will curdle the milk in the stomach (curdling occurs naturally as a result of the normal activity of stomach acids) or against eating ice cream with rhubarb or buttermilk with cabbage. A few warn against drinking milk for fear of cancer, constipation, or indigestion. The following are some foods and the disorders they are falsely claimed to cure:

> Honey and vinegar—constipation, high blood pressure, asthma, tooth decay, corns, pyelitis
> Wheat germ oil—arthritis, gallstones, gangrene, cirrhosis of the liver, epilepsy, shingles, ulcers
> Carrot juice—varicose veins, gout, cystitis, Addison's disease

Usually promoted for a commercial purpose, fad diets offer promises in five general areas:

> Cure of a specific malady, such as arthritis, cancer, circulatory disease
> Prevention of a specific malady, such as the common cold
> Treatment for sexual inadequacy, real or imagined
> General panacea for unending good health and longevity
> Sure cure for obesity

Food faddism can be serious and dangerous for several reasons. It is usually a waste of money, it tends to give the faddist a false sense of security, and it may keep him from seeing a doctor in time to prevent disease. The federal courts have forced some producers of certain quack products either to relabel their products or to destroy them.

Food faddism may concern substances that are harmful or that can lead to malnutrition because they have replaced too much of the normal diet. It also tends to undermine public confidence in the scientific study and practice of nutrition.

Forms of faddism

Although food faddism is practiced in many forms today, we shall discuss only a few forms that have large followings and particularly vocal supporters.

Natural foods   The follower of the "natural food" fad implies or states that all foods should be eaten in their natural states. He may cook, wash, or treat his food, but not process it specially. He is convinced that the processing of grains into white flour and milled and enriched cereals, the canning of fruit and vegetables, and the pasteurizing of milk destroy their nutritive value and make them unfit for human consumption. He advocates using raw sugar instead of refined sugar, sea salt for regular table salt, lemon juice for vinegar, and whole grains instead of enriched bread. Although there is no harm in eating natural foods, most nutritionists are convinced that processing foods does not destroy their value.

Raw foods   Raw-food faddists contend that raw foods are best, since cooking or heating of natural foods destroys much of their nutritive value; they also are opposed to the pasteurization of milk. Pasteurization, while protecting the consumer against certain bacteria, *does not* destroy the nutritive value of the milk. And vegetables and other foods, if properly cooked, retain most of their nutritive value. In addition, cooking makes them more palatable and more easily digested.

A new line put forth by raw-food faddists is that "liquefied vegetables" have marvelous properties. They contend that by drinking vegetable juices or purées the consumer will be cured of rheumatism and indigestion, relieved of high blood pressure and gallbladder ailments, and improved in his complexion. Although there is certainly nothing wrong with vegetable juice, it has no more nutritive value than the vegetable it came from. Usually the promoter of the fad is also selling juicing devices at a favorable profit.

Miracle foods and food supplements   Some special foods, along with special food combinations, are supposed to have unique nutritive and therapeutic value. They are supposed to cure "subclinical deficiencies," "hidden hunger," and "that tired feeling." They are special supplements that have "miracle ingredients" or that remedy "devitalized food." The list includes blackstrap molasses, wheat germ, yeast, honey and vinegar, sunflower seeds, alfalfa extract, and kelp. One of them, royal jelly ("the miracle food of the queen bee"), was purported to have the ability to beautify the face and bring back the "joy of life," not to mention being beneficial for cataracts, drunkenness, and other unwanted conditions. One minor sidelight: it was available at $140 an ounce.

It is easy to see how a sufferer from painful arthritis, high blood pressure, gallstones, ulcers, or any of many other conditions might be tempted to believe that his condition was due to a lack of essential nutrients and that this lack could be supplied by some food or supplement available at a special price. It is important to scrutinize carefully all claims of "miracle substances" that purport to cure these ancient diseases and to recognize that modern medicine and the nutrition sciences are the surest road to any kind of remedy that is or will be available to treat and prevent disease.

Sources of reliable information

Where can a person obtain reliable information on foods and nutrition? He may check with his personal physician or nurse or write the Council on Drugs and Nutrition of the American Medical Association. Occasionally there are articles dealing with nutrition in *Today's Health,* the *American Journal of Nursing,* the *American Journal of Public Health, Science News Letter,* and *Medical World News. Nutrition Reviews* is a professional nutritional journal containing technical reports of research being conducted in nutrition. Publications such as *Food for Us All: The Yearbook of Agriculture* (1969) or *Nutri-*

tive Value of Foods (Home and Garden Bulletin No. 72) are available from the U.S. Department of Agriculture. *Recommended Dietary Allowances* (latest edition) is available from the National Research Council. Material dealing with proper nutrition is also generally available from state departments of agriculture or state universities. Many libraries have books that contain good information on this subject.

MEAL PLANNING

The preceding chapter and sections within this chapter have emphasized the importance of adequate intake of various foods for the maintenance of good nutrition and health. The next problem, then, is the proper correlation of this information for the planning of a satisfactory daily diet. Meal planning is not a mere counting of calories or grams of protein. It is impossible to obtain good nutrition without the daily inclusion of the necessary nutrients; it is impractical to consider feeding from the standpoint of essentials alone. Such factors as digestibility, palatability, and economy determine whether a food supplied will be eaten.

A good way to keep away from stereotyped meals is to include in the meal plan at least one different food or one new recipe each week. This innovation should give satisfaction to the homemaker who is preparing the meal and also extend the tastes of the children and the family. Foreign foods may suggest new combinations for menus, as will recipes from neighbors, recipe books, food articles in magazines and newspapers, and food advertisements.

THE FIVE BASIC FOOD GROUPS

Foods may be grouped according to the nutrients they provide. They have traditionally been divided for this purpose into four groups: dairy foods, meats, fruits and vegetables, and bread and cereals. The authors of this text have chosen to separate the fruits and vegetables, creating *five* basic food groups. We believe that this change will give added insurance of adequate amounts of vitamin C and other vitamins and minerals. Even though this guide is general, it is specific in that it stresses foods of preeminent value— those foods that when left out of the diet cause deficiencies. Table 8.4 is a useful food guide that the student may refer to in reading the remainder of this chapter.

The Basic Five, as they may be called, when drawn from daily recommended amounts, will supply all the essential nutrients except vitamin D. This vitamin is obtained in sufficient amounts by a person's direct exposure to sunlight and from fish-liver oils and milk to which vitamin D has been added. Vitamin D should be supplemented in the diets of infants, children, expectant mothers, nursing mothers, and adults who work inside and receive little exposure to sunlight.

There are no foods which in themselves are nutritional necessities. Any one food may be high in a variety of nutrients or make no essential contribution to the diet. No food is actually bad or harmful, except perhaps when illness forces strict dietary regulation. No food is especially beneficial; people who believe certain foods possess unusual curative or cosmetic properties have been badly misled. In the long run more benefits come from eating a well-balanced diet regularly than from consuming any one food, tonic, or dietary supplement.

Group 1: dairy foods

The dairy foods are milk, cheese, ice cream, and other foods made with milk, such as soups, beverages, desserts, and sauces. Milk and its many products are our main source of calcium; they also contribute protein, riboflavin, and vitamins A and D. Butter and cream products supply flavorful fat and vitamins A and D, but they do not contain the protein, riboflavin, and calcium of milk. (Evidence now links animal fats to high serum-cholesterol levels and to artery plaque formation in atherosclerosis. It is now recommended that growing children and adults limit their intake of butter and cream products and of soft cheese. For those who are obese, butter, cheese, and ice cream are all too high in calories.) Skim milk and buttermilk supply all the nutrients of whole milk except vitamins A and D and fat, which have been removed together. The nutritional value of cereals and breads are enhanced when they are combined with the protein of dairy foods. Thus traditional combinations of cereal and milk or macaroni and cheese provide good nutrition.

Group 2: meat, fish, poultry, and eggs

The meat group includes all foods that supply nutrients similar to those in meat—fish, poultry, eggs, dried beans, nuts, and peanut butter. These last three contain some incomplete proteins and are best consumed with cheese, meat, milk, or eggs to make their proteins complete and useful to the body. For example, a peanut-butter sandwich could be eaten with a glass of milk, or pork and beans with cheese. Foods in the meat group are rich sources of protein. Eggs and meat, especially liver, are important sources of iron, B vitamins, and vitamin A. Pork is an especially good source of vitamin B_1 (thiamine). Dried beans, peas, and nuts are good sources of thiamine and iron.

Again, it is well to remember that the consumption of animal fats in excess may contribute to the development of cardiovascular problems. Thus it is recommended that excess fat in meats be removed before eating and that egg consumption be limited to two or three eggs weekly. However, it is not recommended that these products be removed from the diet, since the protein is of high biological value. Any one of the foods in the meat group has great potentialities for injecting variety into family meals.

Group 3: vegetables

Vegetables are important sources of minerals and vitamins when they are prepared correctly. Overcooking or cooking at high temperatures or in large

Table 8.4 *Daily food guide according to the Basic Five food groups: number of servings per person per day*

	group 1 dairy food (milk)	group 2 meat, fish, poultry, and eggs
Preschool children	1 pint	2 ounces of lean meat, fish, or poultry; 2 or 3 eggs per week
Elementary school children	1 cup 3 times daily	6 ounces of protein foods; 2 or 3 eggs per week
Adolescents: Boys	4 cups	6 ounces of protein foods; 2 or 3 eggs per week
Girls	3 cups	6 ounces of protein foods; 2 or 3 eggs per week
Adults: Men and women	2 cups	2 servings of meat, poultry, fish; 2 or 3 eggs per week
Pregnant women	3 cups	2 servings of meat, poultry, fish; 2 or 3 eggs per week
Nursing mothers	4 cups	2 servings of meat, poultry, fish; 3 eggs per week

amounts of water decreases the amounts of water-soluble vitamins present in this group. Vegetables also supply the needed bulk and roughage and give a variety of interesting colors and flavors to daily meals. The recommended two or more servings a day are easy to plan in the form of cooked or raw vegetables and salads. A dark-green leafy vegetable or a deep-yellow fruit or vegetable should be eaten daily for vitamin A. Because water will absorb the nutrients, vitamins, and flavors of vegetables, it is nutritionally sound to use the water in which vegetables have been cooked to make soups, gravies, and sauces.

Group 4: fruits

Two servings of fruit each day is the recommendation. At least one of them should be a citrus fruit or tomato or other food high in vitamin C. Since vitamin C is believed by some to be stored somewhat in the body, the absence of the vitamin from the diet should not affect a person for several days. Although not technically needed each day, the daily intake of vitamin C is

Table 8.4 (*continued*)

group 3 vegetables	group 4 fruits	group 5 breads and cereals
½ cup of cooked yellow or green leafy vegetables	½ cup of orange juice or other source of vitamin C	2 slices of enriched bread or other cereal
1½ cups of two or more vegetables or fruits or both	½ cup of two or more vegetables or fruits or both	1 slice of enriched or whole-grain bread
½ cup of green or yellow vegetables	½ to 1 cup of orange juice; other fruits as desired	4 slices of enriched or whole-grain bread
½ cup of green or yellow vegetables	½ to 1 cup of orange juice; other fruits as desired	4 slices of enriched or whole-grain bread
½ cup of green or yellow vegetables	½ to 1 cup of orange juice; other fruits as desired	4 slices of enriched or whole-grain bread
2 green or other vegetables	1 or more fruits	4 slices of enriched or whole-grain bread
2 green or other vegetables	1 or more fruits	4 slices of enriched or whole-grain bread

SOURCE: *Food for Us All, Yearbook of Agriculture*, Washington, D.C., U.S. Department of Agriculture, 1969, pp. 294–303.

considered desirable. Fruits are easily included in the diet as fresh, frozen, or canned whole fruits or juices, fruit desserts, or snacks. Fruits and vegetables and their juices supply approximately the same nutrients whether they are fresh, frozen, or canned. Children should be encouraged to enjoy fruits in place of other sweets for desserts and snacks.

Group 5: breads and cereals

This group contains a wide variety of foods, including breads; cereals, both cooked and ready to eat; cornmeal; grits; rice; spaghetti; macaroni; noodles; and all baked products made with whole-grain or enriched flours. The foods in this group are the body's most valuable sources of carbohydrate energy; they also provide thiamine, riboflavin, niacin, and iron. A combination of bread or cereal and protein from the dairy or meat group makes the most satisfying meal and will delay hunger longer than any other combination of nutrients.

SIMPLE NUTRITION FOR STUDENTS

Studies have shown that many Americans of college age are suffering from nutritional deficiencies. If a person tires easily, or if his physical appearance, as indicated by the luster of his hair and the texture of his skin, is not what it should be, he may be suffering from a nutritional deficiency. The only person able to tell an individual specifically what he is deficient in is a physician. But the average individual should first check his overall diet by writing down everything eaten in seven days and comparing this list with the recommended nutritional amounts needed by the body, shown in Table 8.4. If his overall nutrition is not what it should be, he should put himself on a *two-week demonstration diet*. If such a course is followed for two weeks, the person may see a marked improvement in his energy and appearance; if not, he should consult a physician for an extensive examination of his specific body needs.

When students are attending college, especially if they are living away from home, the free time they have is limited. If they are doing their own cooking, they do not have time to plan meals days ahead. Because of this the authors have secured a simple nutrition plan which will provide an adequate diet without lengthy planning. This diet is known as the Four-Five-Five Plan.

The Four-Five-Five Plan stresses adequate amounts of every substance known to be nutritionally necessary by putting emphasis on the five basic food groups. One simple way of incorporating the required foods in a diet and have it come out correct each day is to count these groups after each meal; see Fig. 8.7. Whenever a person is about to order something to eat, he should think back to the last meal or snack and count off which of the groups were covered by that snack and which should be covered by this meal. After breakfast (or mid-morning snack, if the morning meal is split) he should be able to count off *four* groups. After lunch or a mid-afternoon snack he should count off all *five*. After dinner he could count off all *five* once more. Without the advance menu planning assumed by the Basic Five and other popular plans of nutrition instruction (almost impossible for most college students) he can still achieve a sound nutrition by this portion-counting technique, counting four-five-five every day to keep energy and resistance to illness at a well-nourished peak.

There is no need to worry about proportions with this scheme, because the average individual will eat the amount that satisfies his hunger; this will probably be more than enough in total amount of food consumed. The main nutritional problem with college students is in the lack of *variety* of foods needed for a proper nutritional diet.

APPLYING THE BASIC FIVE IN FAMILY MEALS

A person cannot trust chance or a spur-of-the-moment selecting of foods consistently to provide good meals. A plan is needed. This "planning" may not involve writing down menus and keeping tedious records, but the results should be good nutritious meals, achieved through an informal, relaxed approach to the job of menu-making as a pleasurable task.

Most families tend to buy by the week, to take advantage of lower sale and bulk prices (the economy of buying will be discussed later) and the changing needs and desires of the family; thus a plan should usually be made by the week. Unless the planning is done on a weekly or longer basis, a balanced diet is difficult to maintain.

The basis of the plan is the selection of the amount of food needed for the family from each of the food groups. Watching the local food advertisements can become a habit for the homemaker's planning of meals containing the correct amounts of the basic five food groups.

Planning should include all the meals and between-meal items eaten at home and elsewhere. Planning for extra items, or at least being aware of them, makes it easier for the family to pick the foods that are best for them. It must reflect the interests of the family, or it will not work. Such planning for a family group may become fairly complex unless one adheres to certain basic rules.

Step 1: the menus

The first step is to decide which foods and amounts of foods are needed to make a nutritionally adequate and pleasant diet for each person in the family. A sensible rule to follow is to select foods that give the most nutritional value for the calories present. Each person in the family will have different caloric needs (explained in the preceding chapter). A tense, active, underweight

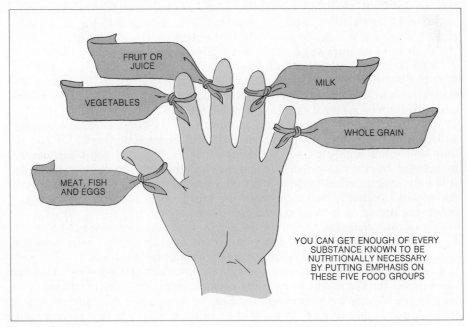

Figure 8.7   Count 4-5-5 diet.

youngster needs additional food allowances; a placid, less energetic individual needs a smaller caloric intake. A man doing heavy outdoor labor or a college athlete may need as many as 3,000 to 3,500 or more calories daily; he can eat all the essential foods plus a number of extra high-calorie foods to fill his great energy requirement. Other people must budget their calories more strictly. A homemaker, a business person, or a coed who does not exert a great deal of physical effort may need only 1,600 to 2,500 calories a day. But *the lower the calorie requirement, the greater the need to find satisfaction and variety in the essential foods.*

Step 2: budgeting the food bill

Apportioning money for meals eaten at home or away is not a problem that is limited to any one income group. Considering the large percentage of family income that goes for food, it is amazing how often it is spent with little or no thought.

Careful planning of the family meals will make shopping easier and more economical. A shopping list, made according to the meal plan for a week, will be a real help in buying the right foods in the right amounts. The fact that changes will be made during shopping need not detract from the value of the list. Flexibility and substitution are badges of an informed shopper, but without a list a person's purchasing is likely to be unorganized and expensive.

The smart shopper will make careful preparation before starting to the market. In addition to thoughtful meal planning, she will read the food advertisements before making her shopping list. The advertisements will provide tips on seasonal availability, supply, price, grades, and brands. With this background information, combined with the shopping list, the shopper is alerted to particular items to watch for in the store.

The following are suggestions for economy that have been found to be valuable in lowering the food bill:

1. *Plan menus for one week at a time at the very least,* to meet the nutritional needs of the family. These menus should be sufficiently flexible so that advantage can be taken of sales and leftover food.

2. *Select the most economical method of marketing.* Weekly shopping will cut down shopping time and the time and expense of travel. Of course, milk and other highly perishable items must be obtained more frequently. In-between buying can usually be tied in with other trips to avoid extra costs. It is very uneconomical to drive a car on a special trip to buy a loaf of bread; the trip will probably cost more than the bread. Also, home delivery usually boosts the cost of an item by several cents.

3. *Know what constitutes a good purchase.* A knowledge of cuts of meat, for example, will help one to determine when a cheap cut is a wise selection or when the waste is so great that buying it becomes false economy.

4. *Be familiar with the grades and brands of foods* and know what grades can be used for the meal planned. For example, broken pieces of canned fruit may be just as satisfactory in fruit salad as the more expensive, perfect, whole fruit. A not highly advertised product is often as good as one with a well-known brand name. Reading labels and comparing prices are important in

careful shopping. Great variations occur in style of pack, ingredients, size and weight, and the number of servings obtainable from canned, frozen, or packaged food. Substituting one food for another, one variety for another, or one can or package for another within the shopping plan can save money.

5. *Buy foods that are in season* and in abundance on the market, since their cost should be less. Meats, for example, go up and down in price from year to year and season to season. The choice, more expensive, quick-cooking cuts vary more in price than those in less demand. It pays to watch for pork bargains in the late fall and beef bargains in late winter; that is when prices are usually lowest for the year. If a family eats more of the expensive cuts in the low-price season, it can balance this off by using more of the less expensive cuts in the high-price season. Very pronounced seasonal price changes occur with fresh fruits and vegetables; see Table 8.5. Prices tend to be lowest for the year when individual produce items can be secured from local producing areas. The substitution of one fresh fruit or vegetable for another according to the ups and downs of supplies and prices offers a real opportunity for savings with little or no sacrifice in quality, nutritive value, or variety.

6. *Buy foods in bulk,* if they are sold under sanitary conditions, since they are less expensive than boxed products.

7. *Buy foods in quantities,* if there is adequate storage space and if the food can be used without waste through spoilage. The time to fill the freezer is when prices are low. On poultry and fish, whether for immediate use or for stocking the freezer, money can be saved by taking advantage of low seasonal prices. When fresh vegetables and fruits are in season, the canned and frozen counterparts decline in price; this is the time to buy quantities for use during the off season. It pays to stock up when there are bargains.

8. *Compare weights and prices* of packaged and canned goods.

9. *Buy the less expensive forms of food* whenever possible. Margarine fortified with vitamin A is a good substitute for butter. Lard, suet, and vegetable oils are less expensive than hydrogenated fats and olive oil. Bread is more economical than fancy rolls. The color and grade of eggs do not reflect their food value. In some places canned or powdered milk is more economical than fresh milk.

10. *Store foods properly* after their purchase to avoid loss of vitamin values and to prevent spoilage. Suggested storage methods and times for different kinds of food are given in Table 8.6. Newly purchased food should always be placed so that the older food will be used first.

Canned or frozen foods purchased by the case may provide real savings, if there is space to store them. With canned foods it is a question of space. If one has a freezer, frozen foods can be stored for the periods of time shown in Table 8.7. The only question is the cost of the freezer: does it more than offset the savings on the food stored in it? The combined ice tray and freezing compartment of the refrigerator usually stays at 15 to 24° F; frozen foods can be kept at this temperature for a few days, but they cannot be kept for long periods of time as they can in a separate freezing compartment of a refrigerator or in a freezer. Most refrigerators maintain a temperature of 35 to 45° F; this is fine for keeping refrigerated foods for a few days, but not for longer periods of time.

11. *Do not let pride and prejudice dictate* the buying habits of the fam-

Table 8.5 *Usual availability of fresh fruit in season*

G = Good supply / F = Fair supply / S = Small supply	Jan.	Feb.	Mar.	Apr.	May	June	July	Aug.	Sept.	Oct.	Nov.	Dec.
Apples	G	G	G	G	F	S	S	G	G	G	G	G
Apricots					S	G	S	S	G			
Avocados	G	G	G	G	S	F	F	F	F	F	G	G
Bananas	G	G	G	G	G	G	G	G	G	G	G	G
Berries (misc.)					S	G	G	G	S	S	S	
Blueberries					S	G	G	G	S			
Cantaloupes		S	S	S	F	G	G	G	G	S	S	
Cherries				S	G	G	S	S				
Cranberries	S								F	F	G	G
Dates	G	F	F	S	S	S	S	S	S	G	G	G
Figs						F	G	G	F			
Grapefruit	G	G	G	G	G	F	S	S	S	G	G	G
Grapes	S	S	S	S	S	F	G	G	G	G	G	F
Honeydews		F	G	F	F	G	G	G	G	G	S	S
Lemons	G	G	G	G	G	G	G	G	G	G	G	G
Limes	S	S	S	S	G	G	G	F	F	F	S	G
Mangoes		S	S	F	G	G	G	F	S			
Nectarines	S	S				F	G	G	G	S		
Oranges	G	G	G	G	G	F	S	S	S	F	G	G
Papayas	S	S	S	S	F	S	S	S	S	F	S	S
Peaches					S	G	G	G	G	S		
Pears	F	F	F	F	F	S	S	G	G	G	G	F
Pineapples	S	F	G	G	G	G	F	F	S	F	F	F
Plums, prunes						G	G	G	G	S		
Strawberries	S	S	F	G	G	G	G	S	S	S	S	S
Tangelos	F	S							S	F	G	G
Tangerines	G	S	S	S	S	S				S	G	G
Watermelons	S	S	S	S	F	G	G	G	S	S	S	S

SOURCE: *Food for Us All, Yearbook of Agriculture*, Washington, D.C., U.S. Department of Agriculture, 1969.

ily. Food misconceptions are frequently passed along in family lines; they are difficult to dissipate.

Some foods cannot be frozen. The following is a list of the general foods affected and the problems associated with each kind.

Raw clams—lose texture, become tough

Hard-cooked eggs—become tough and rubbery

Milk custard—curdles

Mayonnaise—curdles

Salad greens—lose crisp texture

Table 8.6 *Suggested methods and times of storing common foods*

food and method of storage	max. time (days)
In the refrigerator (35–40° F)	
Steaks, chops, roasts[a]	3
Freshly ground meat[a]	2
Liver, heart, other variety meats[a]	2
Table-ready meats—frankfurters, bologna, liver sausage, etc.[a]	7
Fish[a]	2
Chicken[a]	2
Turkey[a]	3
Eggs—large end up and covered	14
Milk—covered	5
Cheese	
Cottage—covered	7
Cream—covered	7
Cheddar—tightly wrapped	until used
Processed—tightly wrapped	until used
Butter—tightly wrapped or covered	14
Margarine, lard, oil—tightly covered	until used
Fresh fruits—lightly covered	7
Fresh vegetables—in hydrator	7
In the ice-tray compartment of the refrigerator (15–24° F)	
All fruits, juices, vegetables, meats, and other items purchased in the frozen state	up to 2 weeks
In the home freezer or freezing compartment of the refrigerator (0° F)	
Meats and frozen foods bought on special sale	up to 3 months
Bread supply	1 to 2 weeks
In unrefrigerated storage at room temperature (70° F)	
Potatoes, onions, bananas, hydrogenated cooking oils and fats, staples such as flour, sugar, coffee	until used

SOURCE: Lola T. Dudgeon, *Buying Food for Your Family*, Food Marketing Leaflet 13, p. 3 (New York State College of Agriculture and Home Economics, Cornell University, Ithaca, N.Y.). Reprinted from Carton E. Wright, *Food Buying: Marketing Information for Consumers*, New York, The Macmillan Company.
[a] Wrap loosely and store in coldest part of refrigerator. Signs of deterioration are drying, discoloration, slickness, and off odor.

MEAL-PLANNING PROBLEMS OF WORKING WIVES

When both adult members of a family work outside the home, the meals served are often not adequate, although the expenses for feeding the family may be extremely high. The ideas in this section have been found helpful in bringing better nutrition to a working family, releasing the working wife from excessive weekly meal preparation and lowering the family's food costs.

The chief problem with general meal planning during the working week is the daily time involved in preparation of the meals. Tired adults do not con-

Table 8.7 *Storage life of home-frozen foods at 0 °F*

food	max. storage period (months)	
Fruit	8	to 12
Vegetables	8	to 12
French-fried potatoes	2	to 6
Meats		
Beef	6	to 12
Lamb and veal	6	to 9
Pork	3	to 6
Sausage and ground meat	1	to 3
Cooked meat—not covered with gravy or other sauces	1	
Meat sandwiches	1	
Poultry		
Chicken	6	to 12
Turkeys	3	to 6
Giblets	3	
Cooked poultry meat	1	
Cooked poultry dishes	3	to 6
Precooked combination dishes	2	to 6
Baked goods		
Cakes		
Prebaked	4	to 9
Batter	3	to 4
Fruit pies, baked or unbaked	3	to 4
Pie shells, baked or unbaked	$1\frac{1}{2}$	to 2
Cookies	6	to 12
Yeast breads and rolls		
Prebaked	3	to 9
Dough	1	to $1\frac{1}{2}$

sistently prepare planned, nutritious meals. The key to such a preparation is precooked frozen meals.

During hours of relaxation the wife may plan the following week's meals. With the aids established in previous sections of this chapter she can make out a menu and shopping list. After she has completed the shopping, one free morning of the weekend may be set aside to prepare and freeze the following week's meals. After this an average of half an hour each night is needed to thaw, warm, and prepare the previously cooked meal and produce a delicious, well-planned, nutritious meal.

Instructions found in booklets which are given to an individual with purchase of a new freezer have been found to be valuable for organized weekly planned frozen meals. Not all foods freeze equally well; some of the problems that occur in freezing precooked foods are listed in Table 8.8. Also —and this is vitally important with meat and fish dishes—the additional cooking time necessary to reheat the frozen dish must be calculated in the

Table 8.8 *Problems that occur in freezing foods*

food	problem	solution
Potatoes, cooked	Lose texture.	Do not add to stews or other cooked dishes before freezing; add when reheating.
Rice, noodles, and macaroni, cooked	Lose texture.	Freeze only if in sauce or gravy, or add when reheating dish.
Creamed soups	Separate or curdle.	Add milk or cream when reheating.
Creamed foods	Become rancid.	Use as little fat as possible; reheat at very low temperature.
Chicken dishes, cooked	Meat separates or shreds.	Freeze when chicken is partially cooked.
Poultry or meat cut in small pieces, cooked	Lose flavor.	Cover with sauce or gravy before freezing.
Fatty meats, cooked	Become rancid.	Cut away excess fat before freezing.
Rich sauces	Curdle, separate, or become runny.	When reheating, mix almost constantly until very smooth.
Garlic	Develops an off flavor.	Add when reheating.

original cooking time. For example, it generally takes about one half hour to reheat the average meal, so this time must be subtracted from the original cooking time wherever possible. If it normally takes one and one half hours to cook something for immediate consumption, the original cooking time should not be one and one half hours but one hour, when it is to be frozen, or the reheated dish will be overcooked.

As another timesaver, the homemaker will find it almost as easy to prepare enough of a given dish for several additional meals. When the dish is half an hour from completion, she should remove all but what is required for that evening's meal and freeze the rest in portions suitable for one meal each.

Too much stress cannot be placed upon the proper protection of foods to be frozen. Whether the food is raw or cooked, it must be wrapped so that as much air as possible is excluded from the package. Pointers on packaging of food for freezing are given in Table 8.9.

Specific instructions are set forth in individual recipes; the following are the *basic* rules:

1. For storage longer than one week, food should be placed in a moistureproof, vaporproof wrap. When foods are frozen quickly, they should be covered with foil or

Table 8.9 *Pointers on packaging foods for freezing*

food	method of packaging
Egg whites	Freeze each egg white in individual ice-cube trays, wrap, and seal. Larger numbers can be frozen in covered containers (label with the number of egg whites). Remove and thaw 4 hours before using.
Egg yolks	Stir lightly and add 1 teaspoon of salt for each cup of yolks and freeze. One tablespoon of sugar may be added instead of the salt, but then the egg yolks can only be used for sweet dishes.
Whole eggs	Follow the instructions for yolks.
Broths and stocks	Freeze in ice-cube trays, then remove and wrap, seal, label, and return to freezer. A cube added to soup or stew is a marvelous supplement.
Stews and casseroles	Line a casserole with foil, freeze stew in it, and then lift out. Wrap, seal, label, and return to freezer. Heat in original casserole when ready to use.
Herbs	Chives, dill, parsley, and all herbs may be frozen ready for use. Wash and dry thoroughly; then chop. Pack into small freezer containers, or wrap in foil, Saran, or freezer paper. Use from the frozen state without thawing.

plastic wrap first. After quick-freezing they should be overwrapped and returned to the freezer for storage. When thawing, foods should be kept wrapped unless otherwise specified in the recipe.

2. Undercook foods by approximately one half hour (this is the average length of time required to reheat in most cases).

3. Cool as quickly as possible by placing the pot or dish in ice water, over ice, or in the refrigerator.

4. Skim as much fat as possible from the dish (this may be readded when reheating).

5. Do not overfill containers; leave about 1 inch at the top to allow for expansion.

6. Label each package with the name, number of servings, and date (for example, "Roast duck with cherry sauce, 4, October 8").

7. Place the freshly prepared dishes in the back of the freezer and bring the older ones gradually to the top and front, so they will not be overlooked.

8. Do not keep foods longer than the time specified under the individual categories.

These ideas and suggestions, when worked into the overall picture of meal planning, may very readily offer a substantial nutritional basis for any family.

FOOD-PROCESSING GUIDELINES

A recurring question is "What basic guidelines should govern the relations between consumers and the food processors?" Put more simply, "What does the consumer want?"

Regardless of regional preferences and variations, there is a high degree of similarity shown around the country with respect to selection, purchasing, and the consumption of food. Yet food consumers are not consulted about the foods that are being produced and marketed. People have little control over what is available for them to eat. This places great responsibility on food processors, government regulating agencies, and food researchers. As they establish and regulate our tastes, we have every right to expect them to take our health into consideration and to act on our behalf. They must ensure that all foods offered for sale are nutritious, safe, and appetizing.

The following are some guidelines directed at those who produce our foods:

1. A given food must be what it claims to be.
2. A given food must be produced under sanitary conditions and must be safe to eat.
3. The nutrient composition of a food, as far as it is known, should be information available to the prospective buyer.
4. Changes in or modifications of foods from their natural state should be based on public need, not sales expediency.
5. Factual information on the safety and nutritional losses inherent in various cooking, storage, and manufacturing procedures should be given the consumers.

FOOD STANDARDS AND GRADES

An increasing number of foods are being processed, packaged, or prepared in such a way as to make it difficult to know what actually goes into a product in terms of quality, quantity, condition, or cleanliness. Thus it has become important over the years to establish standards for certain foods.

Several federal agencies have authority to establish standards for foods in interstate commerce. Some standards are mandatory—they must be met unless the product is clearly labeled with a *substandard* legend, including the reason it is substandard. Other standards are optional; the manufacturer or distributor can decide whether to label products according to these voluntary standards. If he chooses to use such standards, the product so labeled must comply with them.

The basic types of standard are *identity standards*, *quality standards*, *fill-of-container standards* (all established and administered by the U.S. Food and Drug Administration), and *grade standards*, which were established and are administered by the U.S. Department of Agriculture and the U.S. Department of the Interior (Bureau of Commercial Fisheries).

Identity standards

Identity standards describe the nature and character of a given product or specify the kinds and amounts of various ingredients that must or may go into a product. Such standards are *mandatory;* they have been established for about two hundred products. An example is the standard of identity for fruit preserves and jellies; this standard requires not less than 45 parts of fruit or fruit juice to each 55 parts of sugar. Substandard or low-fruit jam can be legally marketed, but the label on such foods must be clearly marked "Imitation."

After a standard of identity has been established for a food product, such as mayonnaise, catsup, or mustard, only the name of the food and any optional ingredients added (such as mustard *and* horseradish) must be listed on the label. For this reason the labels of some foods do not have a complete list of ingredients.

Quality standards

Quality standards are mandatory. They apply chiefly to canned fruits and vegetables and describe the condition of the ingredients of a product. Canned foods falling below standard in appearance must be labeled "Substandard," "Below Standard in Quality," or "Good Food—Not High Grade" with the reason, such as "excess peeling." These foods are wholesome and entirely suitable for some uses, particularly in prepared dishes in which the original appearance and texture of the food is lost.

Fill-of-container standards

Some standards regulate the quantity of food in the container. In general, standards of fill require packages to contain the maximal quantity of food that can be sealed in the container and processed without damaging the food. These standards apply mainly to products that may shake down or settle after filling or that are made up of a number of units or pieces packed in a liquid. For example, a canner is not allowed to fill a can half way with peas and the rest with water. Fill-of-container standards apply only to food such as canned fruits and vegetables, tomato products, and shellfish.

Grade standards

Grading standards have been established for many agricultural and fishery products. The U.S. Department of Agriculture establishes the grade standards for agricultural products; grades for fish and seafood products are established by the Bureau of Fisheries, U.S. Department of the Interior.

The standards of grading are based primarily on quality and appearance, not on food value. Federal and state grading systems exist for foods which represent more than half of the nation's food bill: milk, butter, cheese, meat, poultry, and fresh, canned, and frozen fruits and vegetables. Most of these systems of grading are optional or voluntary and may or may not be followed; a few are mandatory.

The food shopper may find federal or state grade shields on many of the foods seen in the market. If the foods are graded, the grade shields will be clear. If the grade shields are not there, the food probably is not graded. The ungraded foods may be just as good as those with grade shields, but the purchaser must depend on a personal judgment of quality. Unless the prefix "U.S." appears on the grade shield, the item has not been certified by a federal grader. As a reference for the shopper, a list of U.S. grades is shown in Table 8.10.

Meat grades   Meat grades depend on the appearance of the food, including the color of the meat and fat, the amount and distribution of the fat, and the conformation or build of the live animal. To the homemaker these grades can be clues to appropriate uses of the meat.

The top grades of meat come from well-fed animals; they have more fat and consequently can be aged to develop more flavor than lower grades. More cuts of top-grade meat are suited for oven roasting and broiling than are cuts of low-grade meats. The meats of lower grades, with a higher proportion of lean meat to bone, are more economical and, with skillful cooking to increase flavor, are tender, tasty, and nutritious. Ground meat, stewing meat, and pot roasts are among the popular choices from the lower grades.

Meat grading is voluntary. Only meat which has first passed a strict *inspection* for wholesomeness may be graded; see Fig. 8.8. All meat processed in plants that sell their products across state lines must, under federal law, be inspected for wholesomeness. Thus one can be sure, when he sees the grade mark, that the meat came from a healthy animal and was processed in a sanitary plant.

There are eight official government grades of beef, as shown in Table 8.10. The first five may be found in retail stores; the last three—ordinarily used in processed, precooked, and canned meat products—are rarely sold in

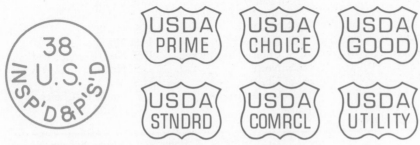

Figure 8.8   Federal inspection mark for wholesomeness of meat (U.S. Department of Agriculture), indicating "inspected and processed," and federal grade shields for beef (U.S. Department of Agriculture).

retail stores. U.S.D.A. Prime (top grade) is used chiefly by restaurants and is rarely found in retail stores. If the beef has been federally graded, it will carry one of the United States grade stamps, in the shape of a shield, as shown in Fig. 8.8.

Veal, calf, lamb, and mutton also are federally graded and carry grade shields similar to that for beef. In addition, the kind of meat will be indicated by a stamp on the surface of the animal, as the words "veal," "calf," "yearling mutton," or "mutton." For veal, if the animal was under three months old, the stamp will read "veal"; if over three months old, it will read "calf."

Poultry grades Poultry grades are based on appearance and freedom from skin cuts, tears, bruises, broken bones, and pinfeathers. The federal grades for ready-to-cook poultry, found in Table 8.10, are voluntary. The official grade shield may indicate the words "Federal-State Graded" if done in cooperation with a state; see Fig. 8.9. The grade shields may be used only if the poultry was first inspected for wholesomeness and was processed in an

Table 8.10 *United States food grades at a glance*

	first grade	*second grade*
Beef	USDA Prime	USDA Choice
Veal	USDA Prime	USDA Choice
Calf	USDA Prime	USDA Choice
Lamb	USDA Prime	USDA Choice
Yearling mutton	USDA Prime	USDA Choice
Mutton		USDA Choice
Butter	U.S. Grade AA (U.S. 93 Score)	U.S. Grade A (U.S. 92 Score)
Cheddar cheese	U.S. Grade AA	U.S. Grade A
Swiss cheese	U.S. Grade A	U.S. Grade B
Nonfat dry milk	U.S. Extra Grade	U.S. Standard Grade
Cottage cheese		No grades—may be marked
Poultry	U.S. Grade A	U.S. Grade B
Eggs	Fresh Fancy or U.S. Grade AA	U.S. Grade A
Milled rice	U.S. No. 1	U.S. No. 2
Brown rice	U.S. No. 1	U.S. No. 2
Dried beans	U.S. Choice Handpicked U.S. No. 1	U.S. No. 1 Handpicked U.S. No. 2
Dried peas	U.S. No. 1	U.S. No. 2
Processed fruit and vegetables (and related products)ᵃ	U.S. Grade A (Fancy)	U.S. Grade B (Choice or Est. Std.)

SOURCE: *Shopper's Guide for U.S. Grades for Food, Home and Garden*, Bulletin No. 58, revised January 1961. Washington: U.S. Department of Agriculture. Reprinted with permission of The Macmillan Company from C. E. Wright, *Food Buying*. Copyright © 1962 by C. E. Wright.

approved plant under sanitary conditions. The federal inspection mark for wholesomeness of poultry also is seen in Fig. 8.9. The grade of the poultry does not indicate how tender the bird is; the age (class) of the bird determines that. Young birds are more tender than old ones. If the poultry is not young, the label will carry the words "mature," "old," or some such, as follows.

1. Young tender-meated classes are most suitable for barbecuing, frying, broiling, or roasting:

Young chickens may be labeled "young chicken," "Rock Cornish game hen," "broiler," "fryer," "roaster," or "capon."

Young turkeys may be labeled "young turkey," "fryer-roaster," "young hen," or "young tom."

Young ducks may be labeled "duckling," "young duckling," "broiler duckling," "fryer duckling," or "roaster duckling."

2. Mature, less tender-meated classes may be preferred for stewing, baking, soups, or salads:

Mature chickens may be labeled "mature chicken," "old chicken," "hen," "stewing chicken," or "fowl."

Table 8.10 (*continued*)

third grade	fourth grade	fifth grade
USDA Good	USDA Standard	USDA Commercial[a]
USDA Good	USDA Standard	USDA Utility[b]
USDA Good	USDA Standard	USDA Utility[b]
USDA Good	USDA Utility	USDA Cull
USDA Good	USDA Utility	USDA Cull
USDA Good	USDA Utility	USDA Cull
U.S. Grade B (U.S. 90 Score)		
U.S. Grade B	U.S. Grade C	
U.S. Grade C	U.S. Grade D	
USDA "Quality Approved"		
U.S. Grade C		
U.S. Grade B	U.S. Grade C	
U.S. No. 3	U.S. No. 4	U.S. No. 5
U.S. No. 3	U.S. No. 4	
U.S. No. 2 Handpicked	U.S. No. 3 Handpicked	
U.S. No. 3		
U.S. No. 3		
U.S. Grade C (Standard)		

Table 8.10 (*continued*)

| | consumer grades | |
	first grade	second grade
Beet greens	U.S. Grade A	
Potatoes	U.S. Grade A Large	U.S. Grade B Large
	U.S. Grade A Medium to Large	U.S. Grade B Large
	U.S. Grade A Medium	U.S. Grade B Medium
	U.S. Grade A Small	U.S. Grade B Small
Brussels sprouts	U.S. Grade A	U.S. Grade B
Carrots	U.S. Grade A	U.S. Grade B
Corn, husked (on the cob)	U.S. Grade A	U.S. Grade B
Cranberries	U.S. Grade A	
Kale	U.S. Grade A	U.S. Grade B
Parsnips	U.S. Grade A	U.S. Grade B
Spinach leaves	U.S. Grade A	U.S. Grade B
Tomatoes	U.S. Grade A	U.S. Grade B
Turnips	U.S. Grade A	
Celery	U.S. Grade AA	U.S. Grade A (3rd Grade— U.S. Grade B)
Apples	None	None

Mature turkeys may be labeled "mature turkey," "yearling turkey," or "old turkey."

Mature ducks, geese, and guineas may be labeled "mature" or "old."

The wing-tag on processed poultry may include the class name as well as the grade shield and inspection mark; see again Fig. 8.9.

Egg grades   Eggs are graded by quality and according to weight classes. The federal grades are often adopted by states as their official grades. The grades shown in Table 8.10 are based on interior quality and condition of the shell. All grades, AA to C, may be found in the markets.

There are six separate United States weight classes for eggs, based on the weight of a dozen eggs: Jumbo, 30 ounces; Extra Large, 27 ounces; Large, 24 ounces; Medium, 21 ounces; Small, 18 ounces; and Peewee, 15 ounces. The "jumbo" and "peewee" are not usually seen in retail stores.

The grade letters indicate quality only; the weight classes indicate size only; grade AA eggs will have the same quality whether they are "large," "medium," or "peewee." The color of the shell determines neither size nor

Table 8.10 (*continued*)

wholesale grades[d]			
first grade	*second grade*	*third grade*	*fourth grade*
U.S. No. 1			
U.S. Fancy	U.S. No. 1	U.S. Commercial	U.S. No. 2
U.S. No. 1	U.S. No. 2		
(Topped carrots)	U.S. No. 1	U.S. No. 2	
U.S. Extra No. 1			
(Green corn)	U.S. No. 1	U.S. No. 2	
U.S. Fancy			
U.S. No. 1	U.S. Commercial		
U.S. No. 1	U.S. No. 2		
U.S. Extra No. 1	U.S. No. 1	U.S. Commercial	
U.S. No. 1	U.S. Combination	U.S. No. 2	U.S. No. 3
(Topped turnips)	U.S. No. 2		
U.S. No. 1			
U.S. Extra No. 1	U.S. No. 1	U.S. No. 2	
U.S. Extra Fancy	U.S. Fancy	U.S. No. 1	
		U.S. No. 1 Cookers[e]	U.S. Utility
		U.S. No. 1 Early[f]	
		U.S. Hail Grade[g]	

[a] The three lowest grades are USDA Utility, Cutter, and Canner.
[b] Lowest grade is USDA Cull.
[c] Grades used for these products are usually as listed here, but there are some exceptions.
[d] Partial listing of commodities for which there are wholesale grades, to show how these grades compare with consumer grades.
[e] Same as U.S. No. 1 except for color.
[f] Same as U.S. No. 1 except for color, maturity, and size.
[g] Same as U.S. No. 1 except for hail injury.

quality. Cracked eggs should be avoided, since they may harbor *Salmonella* bacteria, which cause intestinal infections.

Generally speaking, if there is less than a 10-cent price spread per dozen eggs between one size and the next smallest size in the same grade, you get more for your money by buying the larger size. When large eggs sell for 80 cents per dozen, that's the equivalent of 53 cents per pound—a very reasonable cost for a pound of high-protein food.

Dairy-product grades   Of dairy products butter is the item most commonly sold by federal grade, although cheese and nonfat dry milk also have federal grades; see Fig. 8.10. The federal grades of cheese and nonfat dry milk are shown in Table 8.10. The "score" legend need not appear on the grade label.

Many states have butter grades, which usually conform to the federal grades. Many butter distributors will use the letters or the score on their packages without the federal or state designation. In such case the buyer must depend on the distributor's statement of the quality of the butter.

Whole milk and other dairy products are not covered under federal grade inspection and usually are controlled locally by the county, city, or state.

Fruit and vegetable grades   Federal standards and grades exist for a large number of fresh and processed fruits and vegetables. Most of these are wholesale grades for use by growers and shippers, but they may be used in advertising or in the market. Also, some strictly consumer grades are optional. Their use might spread if more consumers knew the grades and sought this kind of information.

Commonly, the wholesale grades for fresh fruits and vegetables follow the numbering pattern shown in Table 8.10. Consumer grades for fresh fruits and vegetables use letters for quality and further designations of words or numbers to show size.

Among the factors that determine the grade into which fruits and vegetables may fall are size, color, and freedom from defects. Workmanship in peeling and cutting fruits and vegetables for canning and freezing also affects the grades of these items.

Fruit and vegetable grades can help a discriminating shopper choose them with specific uses in mind. Top grades of fruits and vegetables are attractive when the plan is to use them whole or in large pieces. The lower grades, which may be smaller and less perfect in shape and have more blemishes, are very satisfactory in many cooked dishes. The commercially canned

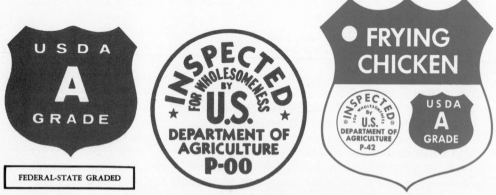

Figure 8.9   Grade shield for poultry in conjunction with federal-state grading programs, inspection mark for wholesomeness of poultry, and wing tag on poultry showing class, inspection, and grade marks; all three labels are from the U.S. Department of Agriculture.

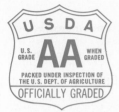 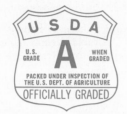 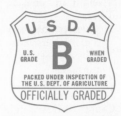

Figure 8.10   Federal grade shields for butter and cheese, U.S. Department of Agriculture.

products usually use low grades. Some defects just mar appearance; others cause waste.

Seafood grades   Fish and other sea foods carry seals for inspection and grade, authorized by the U.S. Department of the Interior. The use of a shield on frozen fishery products indicates that the product was prepared, according to approved specifications, from wholesome raw fish or seafood in a plant where a trained government inspector was continuously present.

Signs, seals, and grade marks

Many food products bear seals or statements of approval from either government or private agencies. The seals have meaning only when what they stand for is known.

The grade marks for food that has been federally graded usually appear in the form of a *shield*. Unless the number or letter grades are official federal or state grades, the consumer may be fooled. "Grade A" may be a meaningless term unless it has the letters "U.S." in front of it. Many foods are sold as "choice," "1st quality," "top grade," and so on, when the term has no connection with grade at all. Private brands are only as meaningful as one's understanding of them. The shopper should not be confused by meaningless designs or words. He should look for official government sponsorship (federal, state, or local); it is the best guide to true meaning.

SUMMARY

    I. Appetite control
   II. Determining desirable weight
      A. Determination of ideal weight for an individual is difficult.
      B. Factors to consider
        1. Sex.
        2. Age.

        3. Height.

        4. Body build.

III. Overweight and obesity

  A. Terms

    1. Overweight—any weight in excess of the weight recommended for a given person by the Desirable Weight table.

    2. Obesity—excessive deposition of fat beyond what is considered normal.

    3. Usage of either term in the text implies a condition of overweight due to obesity.

  B. Causes of overweight

    1. Faulty metabolism (rare).

    2. Faulty regulation of diet (usual).

  C. Effects of overweight—lessened life expectancy

  D. Reducing—need of adequate motivation

IV. Underweight—many factors responsible

V. Food fads and fallacies

  A. Natural foods

  B. Raw foods

  C. Miracle foods

  D. Food supplements

VI. Meal planning

VII. Five basic food groups

  A. Dairy foods—milk, cheese, ice cream, and other foods made from milk

  B. Meat, fish, poultry, and eggs

  C. Vegetables—dark-green or deep-yellow

  D. Fruits—fresh, frozen, or canned

  E. Breads and cereals

VIII. Simple nutrition for students—four-five-five plan devised for college students stresses the five basic groups.

  A. Breakfast and mid-morning snack should together include items from four groups.

  B. Lunch and mid-afternoon snack should together include items from five groups.

  C. Dinner and the evening should together include items from five groups.

IX. Applying the basic five in family meals

  A. Menus

  B. Budgeting the food bill

X. Meal-planning problems of working wives

XI. Food-processing guidelines

XII. Food standards and grades

  A. Identity standards have been established for about 200 products which need not have ingredients listed on label.

  B. Quality standards are mandatory and must be met or labeled as substandard.

  C. Fill-of-container standards do not apply to all foods.

  D. Grade standards—most are optional, a few mandatory.

    1. Meat grades—based on appearance.

    2. Poultry grades—based on appearance and freedom from blemishes.

    3. Eggs—graded by quality and put into weight classes.

    4. Dairy products—most covered by state or local, rather than federal, inspection.

5. Fruit and vegetable grades—primarily used in wholesale transactions.
6. Seafood grades—under standards of the U.S. Department of the Interior.
E. Signs, seals, and grade marks
1. Many products bear seals of approval from either government or private agencies.
2. Private seals or grades may have little significance.

Glossary

If you cannot find the word you wish in this glossary, check the index for text and glossary references.

diet (dī′ət) (G. *diaita,* way of living). The customary allowance of food and drink taken by a person from day to day.

lipectomy (li pek′tə mē) (G. *lipos,* fat; *ektome,* excision). Cutting out of fatty tissue from fatty areas of the body.

malnutrition (mal nyoo trish′ən) (L. *malus,* bad; *nutritio,* to nourish). Any disorder of nutrition.

minimum daily requirements. The amounts of each nutrient which are regarded as necessary in the diet for the prevention of deficiency diseases.

nutrient (nyoo′trē ənt) (L. *nutriens,* nourishment). A substance which provides nourishment to the body.

nutrition (nyoo trish′ən) (L. *nutritio,* to nourish). The process of assimilating food into the body for nourishment.

obesity (ō bē′si tē) (L. *obesus,* that has eaten itself fat). An increase in body weight beyond skeletal and physical requirements, as the result of an excessive accumulation of fat.

osteoarthritis (os′tē ō ahr thrī′tis) (G. *osteon,* bone; *arthron,* joint; *itis,* inflammation). A chronic joint disease which is degenerative.

overweight (ō′vər wāt′). An excess of more than 10 percent above the desirable weight.

recommended daily allowances. The amounts of nutrients which are considered adequate for the maintenance of good nutrition in healthy persons in the United States.

underweight (un′dər wāt′). A deficiency of more than 10 percent under the desirable weight.

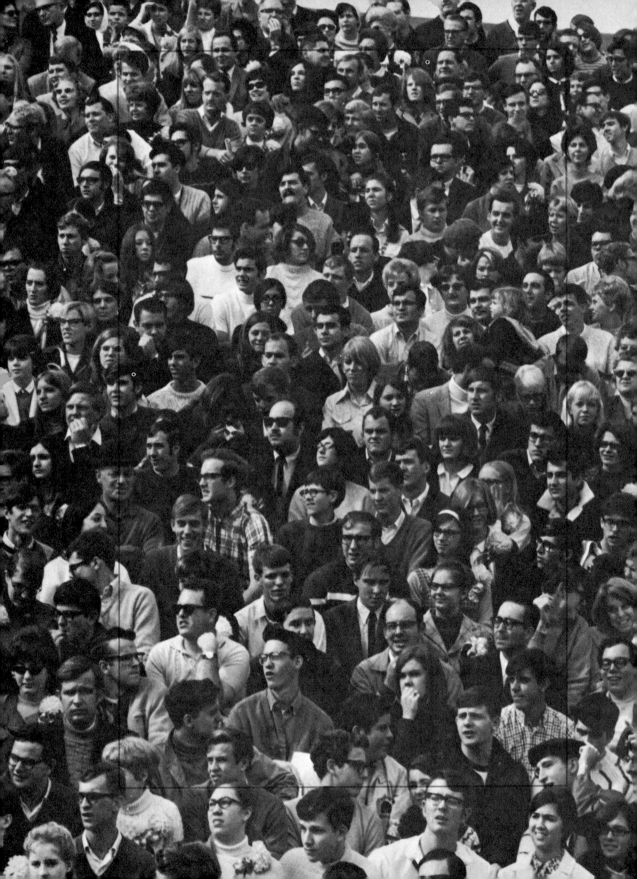

Population

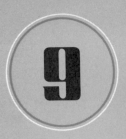

Evaluation of man's current status on earth and of his likely future prospects reveals many paradoxes and enough danger signs to give anyone other than the most extreme optimist cause for grave concern. The world picture today shows some countries enjoying a standard of living never before reached, while other countries suffer from mass starvation. Countries whose people are already hungry are increasing in population at an alarming rate, with no comparable increase in food supply. Thus the disparity in standard of living between the "haves" and the "have-nots" grows with every passing day.

At the same time many of the forces that have contributed to the high quality of living enjoyed by the "haves" seem to be turning against us. We find that the reduction in infant death rate and the conquering of many traditional causes of death are resulting in population levels that tax the resources of even the most fortunate nations. The same factors are also creating populations with increasing numbers of persons at the two extremes of age (very young and very old), both age groups having high levels of dependence upon persons of intermediate age.

The adequate food supply of the "haves" is largely the result of the intensive use of pesticides, agents that we now find are polluting our environment, with disastrous effects on certain birds, fishes, and other animals, and perhaps even on man himself. The same industrial developments that have given the "haves" an abundance of free time have so modified and polluted recreational resources—such as lakes, rivers, and ocean beaches—that our free time often becomes a burden rather than a joy. New industrial processes are introducing several hundred *new chemical pollutants* into our air and water each year—pollutants about whose long-term effects upon man and his environment are little known. This subject will be expanded in Chapter 10; let us now concentrate on population itself.

POPULATION AND WORLD RESOURCES

We are currently living in a world in which a rapidly increasing number of people must share a fixed or, in some cases, decreasing abundance of natural resources. In reality the world population problem is the total of all the widely differing population problems in the major regions and countries of the world. Through modern modes of transportation and communication the world has become so "small" that a population problem in any one country may have serious effects in other countries.

Discussion of the population problem often centers on two issues, *space* and *food,* as though resolution of this problem depends only on finding enough standing room and enough food per person to allow survival. Such oversimplification obscures the seriousness of the problem for the following reasons.

1. Most of the world's people already live so poorly that it is not enough that food production merely keep pace with population growth. A great increase in food production would be necessary just to feed the current population properly.

2. Many of the methods that have been proposed to increase food production (such as use of insecticides and fertilizers and land reclamation) are, even at their current level of application, proving harmful to the total environment.

3. World production of many commodities, not only food, must be increased sharply to meet the reasonable needs and demands of people for living adequately.

4. The production of waste products (pollutants) increases with the population. The ability of the environment to "absorb" pollutants is limited. Even the disposal of human wastes becomes a serious problem at high population levels.

5. Frustration of the growing desire among all people for decent living conditions, education, and economic opportunity is creating tremendous political and social tensions throughout the world.

6. The world is *not* one big, unified reservoir of space, skills, resources, knowledge, and capital, from which nations can procure their respective needs.

7. There is a wide gap between what is technologically or theoretically possible and the practical application of these principles.

It can be seen that the bases of the population problem are limited resources and the *alarming differentials in consumption of these resources* among different regions and nations of the world. Furthermore, a society devoted to supporting maximal numbers of people at a bare subsistence level is incompatible with the values of modern civilization. To what extent are we willing to sacrifice *quality* of life in order to attain *quantity* of life?

Population and health

Public health agencies have been highly successful in their battle against long-established infectious diseases. Through measures such as antimalarial programs it has been possible (for example, in Ceylon) to open huge areas for habitation and cultivation that were formerly uninhabitable. Public concern over health problems has resulted in improved sanitation, purer and more adequate water supplies, and the prevention and control of communicable diseases through immunization, insecticides, antibiotics, and increased attention to nutritional disorders. These improvements have contributed to a lowered death rate and an increased life expectancy.

It is mistakenly assumed by some that the present world population problem is due to the great efficiency of health programs. It is true that, as countries develop economically, better living conditions and improved nutrition usually result and that these in turn lead to a drop in death rates. In addition, however, after a lag of several generations of better conditions the birth rate also tends to decline. In the past, owing to infant mortality, parents conceived more children than they expected to raise to maturity. For example, parents conceived six children in order to raise four to maturity. As available medical services improve, infant mortality drops. It takes time for parents to realize that they can be assured of survival of most, if not all, of their children. If this lag could be reduced from several generations to a single generation, the total population growth in economically developing countries would be lessened.

Health programs, therefore, provide the *best* rather than the worst prospects for solving the population problem. Family planning might well be decided upon and practiced when parents feel secure about the health of their children. As a result of this logical relationship between health programs and population control national family-planning programs are commonly assigned to health services. Such programs have been pioneered in Japan, India, Korea, Taiwan, Pakistan, Egypt, Turkey, Tunisia, Czechoslovakia, and Poland. The success of these measures, however, lies in sufficiently motivating the entire population.

Various factors influence motivation: religious scruples, traditions, family relationships, and a family's view of its socioeconomic condition. Some families have to realize they are living below subsistence levels before they are willing to limit family size. Unfortunately, some families realize their economic limitations only after the number of their children has exceeded their resources.

Ample instruction for obtaining and using contraceptive devices needs to be promoted. Among the better devices in recent years have been the oral contraceptives, "the pill." Women in some parts of the world, however, have trouble in remembering when to take the pills, cannot count, or are unable to afford them; further, the safety of long-term pill use remains to be absolutely established. A method that has high contraceptive effectiveness—although less than the pill—is the intrauterine device. Acceptance of sterilization is growing in many areas. Research is continuing on many new approaches to birth control; such research may provide the kind of technical breakthrough needed to control world population.

Population and food

The majority of people living on the earth today do not have enough food to eat. More than half of the people in the world today live on less than 2,200 calories per person per day, although the Food and Agricultural Organization (FAO) of the United Nations recommends a daily minimum of 2,650 calories. The amount of calories in food is only one consideration; equally important is how well the diet is balanced with the various kinds of foods. Generally the low-calorie diets of the world consist primarily of plant foods, which cannot be considered balanced diets. Though the majority of Americans enjoy adequate diets, millions of people even in this wealthy country suffer from diets deficient in quantity, quality, or both.

Most of the world's population increase is occurring in areas that are already short of food and are poorly developed: Asia, Africa, and Latin America. To believe *blindly* that God will "provide for His flock" regardless of how large it becomes is a form of utopianism. This argument is unsatisfactory because it overlooks the fact that more than a billion people already in the world today are not provided with even the minimal dietary standards; in other words, they are *starving*.

The basis of most food production is land. But an increasing population itself requires ever more land for housing, industries, businesses, roads, schools, and all the other services necessary to maintain a satisfactory standard of living. In too many places the choicest agricultural land is being taken out of production to provide for increasing populations. As a result, farming operations must move onto less suitable land, where the production of adequate crops requires greatly increased expenditures for land leveling, irrigation, and fertilization. While in the United States this adjustment usually can be made with relative ease, the more limited economies of most of the world's countries simply cannot absorb a greatly increased cost of producing food.

The more important techniques for increased food production have included intensive use of insecticides and mineral fertilizers. Only through their use is the world being fed as well as it is, though that is not universally very well, as we have indicated. However, insecticides cannot be used haphazardly without inflicting severe damage to man's environment and perhaps to man himself. Moreover, some evidence now indicates that excessive nitrates from fertilizer applications are present in food and water supplies at levels that may be harmful to human infants and are probably contributing to the pollution of rivers and lakes.

Thus it seems that the cost of greatly increased food production to feed our exploding population will be much higher than has been predicted and that this cost will be measured, not only in economic terms, but also in damage to the environment.

Population and energy-mineral resources

The earth's capacity to provide raw materials and land is limited. Many minerals and most of the sources of energy in current use are nonrenewable. In some places the scarcity of forest stands is limiting the use of wood and wood products. More and more cities are having to curtail their water service or find new and more remote sources of fresh water.

If the entire world is to develop industrially on a level comparable to that of the United States and Europe, our known reserves of coal, petroleum, and natural gas will not be able to provide sufficient energy. It has been forecast that the high point in petroleum production will be reached in the relatively near future—sometime before the year 2000. The fossil fuels—natural gas, petroleum, and coal—are expected to provide the world's energy needs for no more than several hundred years.

Our traditional sources of energy are water (for about 10 percent of our electrical power), coal, gas, and oil. By fulfilling an ever-increasing demand for power by burning these fossil fuels we are depleting stores which are not being replaced. These are nonrenewable natural resources and, in time (an alarmingly short time if the demand grows as it has for the past quarter of a century), these fuels will be gone. However, there are two energy sources that may replace fossil fuels: one is radiation from the sun (solar energy) and the other is nuclear energy—that derived from the fission of heavy atoms and the fusion of light ones.

It would seem that capturing solar energy directly would be preferable to utilizing atomic energy, with all its inherent dangers. However, the practical utilization of solar energy at present is restricted to rather small solar batteries. It is possible that this source of energy will be developed, but at the moment atomic energy is far in the lead.

The adoption of fission power will be slow, and its rate will depend ultimately on the exhaustion of fossil fuel reserves. Fusion power, while potentially having many advantages over fission power, including an inexhaustible fuel supply of negligible cost, has not yet been established as feasible, and its costs cannot be readily assessed.

Since in the past the most easily obtained minerals and sources of energy have been used, the continued mining of less accessible deposits will cost this country increasingly more than they have in the past. Yet even this low-yield extraction has its limits. Each of the acts mentioned above represents an unnecessary *borrowing on the future.*

Borrowing on the future is being done with the resources in the United States as well as with those elsewhere in the world. Although North Americans constitute only about 6 percent of the world's population, they consume half of the world's production of major minerals; they consume twice as much commercial energy per person as the British and four times as much as the people of India. It is estimated that each year the average American utilizes an amount of natural resources equal to that used by twenty-five or thirty Indians. In these terms the increase in *this country's population* appears frightening. In light of the aspirations of many parts of the world for better living standards it can be questioned whether it will be justifiable for the 6 percent of the world's population in North America to continue consuming 40 to 50 percent of the world's resources.

Population and pollution

In our great concern over environmental deterioration we have tended to blame technology, profiteering industrialists, oil companies, auto manufacturers—in fact, anyone but ourselves. We too often overlook the fact that the auto makers, oil companies, and other industries produce only such quantities of their products as are purchased by people; and the more of us there are, the greater this demand becomes. Thus any discussion of pollution must revolve around population.

The quantity of every pollutant released into the environment relates directly to population. A larger population results in more air pollution, more water pollution, more sound pollution, more pollution of every kind. While some pollutants—such as those in auto exhausts—probably could be reduced through improved technology, others—such as sewage—may not. There is certainly no way to reduce the quantity of body wastes a person produces. More and more of our water supplies are being contaminated by sewage, both treated and untreated. Even sewage that has been treated to eliminate all dangerous bacteria (though many viruses seem to survive sewage treatment) still contains minerals such as nitrates and phosphates, which lower the quality of the water for drinking and for most other purposes. These minerals also stimulate the growth of algae in lakes and streams to undesirable levels, killing fish and turning once-clear bodies of water into murky, stinking cesspools.

A larger population needs more electricity. The use of electricity in the United States is now doubling every six to ten years. Electricity is often mentioned as a "clean" source of energy, but most of the future increase in electricity production must come from turbines driven by steam derived from either fossil fuels or nuclear reactors, rather than from the waterpower of dams. All steam-turbine water plants are inefficient, releasing some of their heat into the environment instead of converting all of it into electricity. This excess heat is usually taken up by cooling water, which is then exhausted into a river, lake, or ocean. This hot exhaust water drastically changes (or eliminates) the organisms living in the body of water, even when the body is as large as the ocean. In addition to such *thermal pollution* from generating plants there is the problem either of air pollution from burning fossil fuels or of radiation that enters the environment from nuclear reactor plants.

Many other examples of population-related pollution could be cited, but the basic point is that an environment suitable for man's continued survival cannot be maintained by merely attacking specific sources of pollutants. The real heart of the problem is man's irresponsible proliferation in numbers. There is certainly some population size that the environment could support indefinitely without serious deterioration, but people do not even want to consider what that population might be. Many authorities believe that world population has already exceeded that size.[1]

[1] LaMont C. Cole, "Thermal pollution," *BioScience, 19*, 11:989–992, November, 1969.

Population pressure

The poorer populations of the world, whose expectations are not fulfilled, form the core of an increasingly larger group. They feel today the hardships of their low level of living more keenly than ever before, even though they may actually be living at a better level than they did in the past.

Table 9.1 shows the disparities between populations and industrial output of the world. Of the world's population 30 percent enjoy 90 percent of the industrial output. The remaining 70 percent of the population uses only 10 percent of the world's industrial products. There is a per capita ratio of the developed to the developing areas of 21:1. From such differences it is clear that even in the absence of population growth the emerging areas face enormous problems of economic development.

From the standpoint of creating tensions between nations it is not absolute poverty that provides people with the strongest motives to support political aggression; it is the feeling that they do not have enough land or other resources to use so that they can live as well as other people. People must have some standard of comparison before they are aware of their own poverty and before they begin to feel the pressure of population as a motive for supporting national action to relieve this pressure. It requires only a little imagination and some knowledge of the actual living conditions in most of the developing countries of the world to make one realize that the growing feelings of deprivation can be a ready-made weapon for aggressive ideologies.

WORLD POPULATION PROBLEMS

During the past centuries man's increase in numbers has been governed by three regulators: *disease, war,* and *starvation.* Man's increasing control of disease has greatly freed him from one of these controls. War and famine, however, still act as biological checks upon populations in those parts of the world where they occur.

Table 9.1 *Population and industrial production as percent of world total*

	industrialized areas (percent)	nonindustrialized areas (percent)
Population	30	70
Industrial production	90	10
Mining	75	25
Manufacturing	91	9
Light	87	13
Heavy	93	7
Electricity	91	9

SOURCE: D. L. Nortman, *The Population Problem,* New York, National Educational Television, 1965, p. 9.

At the same time man is gradually learning how to separate sexual gratification from reproduction through employing effective forms of contraception, or voluntary fertility control. And for the first time in history modern man has the means of directing the course of his own population. Need of birth-control information is clear. Most animal species, including man, are endowed with the capacity to produce offspring in numbers far in excess of available supplies of food, natural resources, and space. As man continues to gain control over the operation of the traditional biological checks—war, disease, and starvation—he must demonstrate his ability to control his reproductive potential.

Although the means are at hand, mankind is still having trouble facing the realities of an important biological law: *any species that multiplies without limit eventually faces stark shortages of food.* Man must choose one of the two biological checks upon increase in number, *higher mortality* or *lowered fertility.*

The past

Only fragmentary data are available to indicate the past rate of growth of the population of the world. A regular census of population was not conducted before 1800, although registers had been maintained for small population groups before then. The commonly accepted population figures of the world prior to 1800 are only informed guesses. Nevertheless, it is possible to piece together a consistent series of estimates of the world's population during the past two centuries. This information, supplemented by rough guesses of the number of persons alive at selected earlier periods, is the background of Fig. 9.1, which contains estimates of the population of the world from A.D. 1 to A.D. 2000. This graph reveals a spectacular spurt during recent decades in the increase of the world's population.

The world's population is estimated to have first reached one billion some time between 1810 and 1850. The second billion was reached in 1925 and the third in 1960; the world population now stands at about four billion. Thus the time spans required for *each increase of one billion* are as follows:

1st billion	several hundred thousand years
2nd billion	about 75 or 100 years
3rd billion	35 years
4th billion	15 years
5th billion	???

The present

The world population continues to grow at a rapid rate, now estimated to be about 2 percent per year. At this rate the world population doubles in about 35 years; see Table 9.2. On the basis of the current population this represents an increase of about 1.5 million people *per week*. If this current 2 percent growth rate persisted, it would result in a world population of over 7 billion by the year 2000. Current United Nations population estimates, based on a

Table 9.2 *Population increases at various rates of growth*

annual increase rate (percent)	number of years to double population	number of millions each 10 million becomes in 100 years
0.5	139	16
1.0	70	27
1.5	47	44
2.0[a]	35	72
2.5	28	118
3.0	23	192
3.5	20	312
4.0	18	505

SOURCE: Information Service, Population Reference Bureau, 1755 Massachusetts Avenue, N.W., Washington, D.C., 20036.
[a] Current world rate.

slightly lower projected growth rate, are for a world population of about 6.5 billion in 2000, now only about 25 years distant.

In general, the fastest-growing countries now are those with the lowest standard of living, the "have-not" nations. The growth rate of many of these countries averages more than 3 percent per year, in contrast with an average of less than 1 percent in the wealthier countries (such as those of Europe and

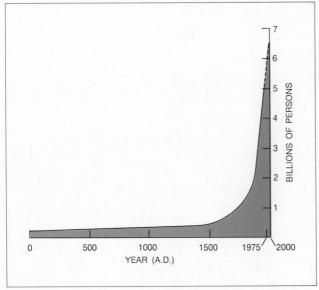

Figure 9.1 Estimated population of the world from A.D. 1 to A.D. 2000, compiled from various sources.

North America). Of the babies being born each day now more than 85 percent are born in Asia, Africa, and South America; see Fig. 9.2. In case a 3 percent annual population growth rate does not sound very high, let us point out that such a rate results in the *doubling* of a population in just 23 years.

According to two well-known authors on world demography (Carr-Saunders and Wilcox), the growth rates of Asia and Europe prior to 1900 were quite different. The population of Europe increased more than fourfold between 1650 and 1900, whereas Asia's population increased only about two and a half times. Moreover, the population in the area of European settlement (including Europe and the Americas) increased about five times. As a result of these differential rates of growth in Asia and Europe the proportion of the world's population living in Asia declined from about 60 percent in 1650 to about 55 percent in 1900. Since 1900 the proportion of the world's population living in Asia has been increasing and, according to Population Reference Bureau figures (Table 9.3), by 1972 it had climbed to almost 57 percent; the proportion living in Europe and North America has been declining, and by 1972 it constituted less than 19 percent of the world's total.

During the past decade 6 out of every 10 persons added to the world's

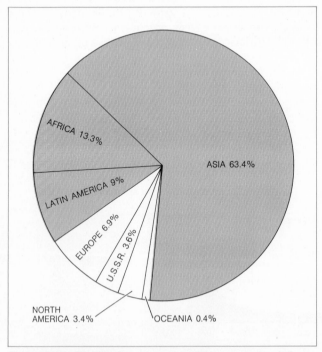

Figure 9.2   Distribution of world births per year. Asia, Africa, and South America account for more than 85 percent of births. (From Population Reference Bureau, *1972 Population Data Sheet.*)

Table 9.3 *World and regional populations*

region	A.D. 1972 population (in millions)	A.D. 2000 population[a] (in millions)	increase (percent)
World	3,782	6,494	72
North America	231	333	44
Europe	469	568	21
U.S.S.R.	248	330	33
Asia	2,154	3,777	76
Africa	364	818	125
Latin America	300	652	117

SOURCE: **Population Reference Bureau,** *1972 World Population Data.*
[a] Based on United Nations estimates.

population live in Asia; another 2 out of 10 live in Latin America and Africa. Undoubtedly this increase will change the world's balance of power and influence world affairs in coming years. Everywhere there seems to be growing impatience with the conditions that limit improvement in the standards of living. This impatience can result only in political unrest and change. The results of human reproduction are no longer the concern only of the country where the people are citizens. Such a problem in one part of the world affects in some manner the health and welfare of those in even the wealthiest nations.

In the past each major upward step in population followed some major discovery or invention, such as agricultural advances, the initiation of urban life and trade, the harnessing of nonhuman power, or the technological revolution. As a more sophisticated and economically responsible society was achieved, the ability to maintain a higher population became a reality. But in the present century the decline in mortality is not only independent of economic development but is a positive obstacle to it. The most decisive factor in increasing population during this time is of a different sort—the application of scientific medicine, or what may be called "death control."

The discoveries of sulfa drugs and especially of the antibiotics, insecticides, and other means of combating disease-carrying organisms radically altered the situation of population dynamics. It became possible to lower mortality irrespective of economic development. This was man's first major victory over death. Within a few years this victory was to be responsible for the rapid population explosion that jeopardizes the economic growth of all developing areas and the world itself.

In the Western world the reduction of the death rate came gradually, and its effect on population growth was buffered by factors that tended at the same time to reduce the birth rate—namely, a rising standard of living and industrialization, which made children no longer an economic asset. The death rates in these advanced countries have gradually been reduced from the traditional 35 or 40 per thousand to less than 10 per thousand. The average life span (life expectancy at birth) has almost doubled in the Western world since the mid-nineteenth century; see Table 9.4. It now stands at more

Table 9.4 *Life expectancy at birth*

year	life expectancy at birth[a] (years)
1840	41.0
1850	41.5
1860	42.2
1870	43.5
1880	45.2
1890	47.1
1900	50.5
1910	54.3
1920	58.3
1930	61.7
1940	64.6
1955 to present	71.0+

SOURCE: *Population Bulletin of the United Nations*, No. 6, United Nations Publication Sales No. 62. XVII.2, Table IV.I.
[a] The average of six European countries and one state in the United States. The countries are Denmark, England and Wales, France, the Netherlands, Norway, and Sweden; the state in the United States is Massachusetts.

than 70 years in Europe and North America, and this process of lengthening life has begun to get under way in the developing areas of the world.

The reduction of the death rate has been a different matter in the developing countries of the world. Here death control was introduced with startling speed. Ancient diseases were brought under control or totally abolished in the space of a few decades or even a few years. Consequently, all are now in a stage of explosive population expansion. As shown in Table 9.5, the developing countries at the present time are showing an annual population increase of 2 to 3 percent.

Just as Thomas Malthus, at the end of the eighteenth century, could not foresee the tremendous changes that have taken place in Europe, we today cannot clearly foresee the final effects of an unprecedented rapid increase in population.

The rate of human reproduction in any part of the globe directly or indirectly affects the health and welfare of the rest of the human race. The increase in the world's population at the present time is occurring far more rapidly in some places than in others. This population increase intensifies the existing imbalance between the distribution of the world's population and the distribution of wealth, resources, and the use of nonhuman energy. It seems inevitable that the breaking up of world domination by northwestern Europeans and their descendants will continue and that the centers of power and influence will shift toward the population centers of the world.

Probably for the first time in human history there is universal aspiration

Table 9.5 *World birth and death rates, 1972*

region	birth rate[a]	death rate[a]	current annual growth rate (percent)	number of years to double population
World	33	13	2.0	35
United States	16	9.4	0.8	87
Europe	16	10	0.7	99
U.S.S.R.	17.4	8.2	0.9	77
Asia	37	14	2.3	30
Africa	47	21	2.6	27
Latin America	38	10	2.8	25

SOURCE: Population Reference Bureau, *1972 World Population Data Sheet* and United States Census Bureau.
[a] Per 1,000 of population.

for rapid improvement in the standard of living and a growing impatience with conditions that appear to stand in the way of its attainment. Millions of persons in Asia, Africa, and Latin America now are aware of the standard of living enjoyed by Europeans and North Americans. They are demanding the opportunity to attain the same standard and resisting the idea that they must be permanently content with less. But continuation of the present high rate of human multiplication in these areas will act as a brake on the already painfully slow improvement in the level of living. This will increase political unrest and possibly bring about changes in governments.

The capital and technological skills that the nations of Africa, Asia, and Latin America require to produce enough food for a rapidly growing population and simultaneously to raise per capita income exceed their existing national resources and ability. An immediate supply of capital in the amounts required is available only from the wealthier nations, which do not have the desire to extend such large amounts of capital to support the economic development of the less advanced nations. Even if such support should be accepted, it is not yet clear how long the wealthier nations would be able to support the uncontrolled breeding of the populations receiving assistance. General acceptance of such a foreign-aid program will only postpone for a few decades the inevitable reckoning with the results of uncontrolled human multiplication.

The future

When looking toward the future we must wonder about the present. Is this present spurt in population growth a temporary phenomenon that will shortly cease, the birth rate falling to near the level of the death rate, or will it continue until the former biological regulators—war, disease, and famine—once again take control?

The future populations of individual nations or of regions, or even of the entire world, cannot be predicted more than a few decades ahead with any degree of certainty. There are just too many unforeseeable influences upon population. Unfortunately, the historical tendency of population predictions has been that of seriously underestimating population growth. There is currently no reason not to expect future populations of a magnitude that will create problems that may be beyond the ability of the nations concerned to solve.

A situation equally favorable to a rapid improvement in the level of living and to a sharp increase in population does not appear likely for the people now inhabiting Latin America, Africa, and Asia. Although there are many thinly populated areas in the world, their existence is testimony to the fact that until now they have been regarded as undesirable living places. The expansion of population to the remaining open areas would require large expenditures of capital for irrigation, drainage, transportation facilities, control of insects and parasites, and other purposes—capital which the rapidly increasing populations that will need these areas do not possess.

The future may witness a dramatic increase in man's attempts to control his environment. Man has been able to modify or control many natural phenomena, but he has not yet discovered how to evade the consequences of biological laws. No species has ever been able to multiply without limit. There are two biological checks upon a rapid increase in number—high mortality and low fertility. Unlike other biological organisms, man can choose which of these checks shall be applied, but one of them *must* be. Whether we use scientific knowledge to guide the future more wisely than the blind forces of nature, only the future can reveal.

UNITED STATES POPULATION

Does overpopulation threaten the United States?

It is clear that overpopulation is already a reality in many of the world's countries and is a threat to many more. But does the United States, with its powerful economy and vast resources, need to concern itself with its own increasing population? In the opinion of the authors the answer is a resounding *yes*.

Let us briefly consider some of the arguments given by those who maintain that the United States is *not* threatened by overpopulation. One such argument hinges upon food supply and reminds us that in the United States farmers are often paid for not growing certain crops. Our answer to this argument is that, although the margin between surplus and shortage of food is more narrow than many people realize, we do not believe that food supply alone should determine the optimal population level in a highly developed country. Other factors are likely to begin to interfere with human welfare before the food supply becomes critical.

Another argument heard is that a vigorous rate of population growth is essential in order to maintain a prosperous national economy. Theoretically, greater population should mean greater demand for the products and services of industries and, therefore, greater profit and prosperity for all. Seldom considered by those who make this argument are the following factors. First, the highest birth rate occurs in the lowest-income families, and additional births in these families result in little additional expenditure for goods and services. In fact, births in these families often result in larger welfare checks, putting a greater drain on the economy rather than having a stimulating effect. Children born into such circumstances are likely to receive inadequate education and to remain an economic burden, possibly for life. Another commonly overlooked factor is that as the population increases, there are more individuals present to share in any increased prosperity. Since many of our national resources are fixed in abundance, there would actually be *less* prosperity per individual.

In further discussion of possible United States overpopulation let us not concentrate on the threat of starvation, since it is likely that other population pressures would curtail the birth rate before the point of starvation was reached in this country. But it is quite possible that our population would grow until the *quality* of living was greatly reduced.

As the country becomes more crowded, life will gradually become less and less pleasant. Technical advances promise us more free time in the future, but population pressures threaten to eliminate much land from possible recreational use and vastly overtax the recreational facilities that do remain. The miles of shoreline, lakefront, and rivers available for recreational use are fixed, but the need for these facilities is increasing. It will become increasingly difficult to "get away from the crowd" as the population increases.

Stress will play an ever larger role in our lives. The more we are crowded, the more we feel stress. The result will be more emotional illness, accompanied by the many physical problems that stress causes or aggravates.

As is discussed in the following chapter, the problem of pollution of the environment is directly related to population. The greater the level of population, the less the right of the individual to pollute his environment. For example, as the number of automobiles in the country continues to increase, the individual owner finds increasing restrictions of his "right" to pollute the air. In the future we may find ourselves restricted in many of our current "rights."

The population of the United States still fits the country fairly comfortably, but the threat of overpopulation does exist. Let us now consider the nature of the population in the past and the present and as it may be in the future.

The past

During the early years of the United States the rate of population growth was a source of great pride. With seemingly limitless resources and room for westward expansion the fertility rate reached levels seldom exceeded anywhere on earth. During the colonial period the average family included about eight children. Even with the high death rate the population more than doubled in every generation. At this time a large family was considered a definite asset. The more children a family produced, the more land could it clear and cultivate.

In addition to this high fertility rate the United States for many years had an open-door immigration policy. Prior to the 1921 Immigration Act about 35 million immigrants entered the country, accounting for about one third of the population growth to that time. Since 1921 immigration has accounted for less than 10 percent of the population growth.

But long before 1921 the women of the United States slowly began to limit the size of their families. Actually, neither the government nor the women had yet become concerned about the threat of overpopulation. The government restricted immigration because of the diminishing need for unskilled labor. The women restricted their family size because their interests were beginning to extend beyond the farm, kitchen, and nursery toward the city, school, and labor force. By the middle 1920s the average family size had dropped to 2.5 children.

During the decade of the 1930s the birth rate dropped still further toward a low of just over 2 children per family. Although the low birth rate of the 1930s is commonly attributed to the economic depression that characterized those years, a study of Table 9.6 shows this rate to be the culmination of a trend that began in 1880. Actually, then (as now) poor economic conditions have been a slight deterrent to large families since, traditionally, the poorest families have the most children. At what point the birth rate might have leveled off without the depression is purely a matter of speculation. In any event, even at this low birth rate the population of the country continued to grow significantly.

After World War II a temporary surge in the birth rate was expected to make up for births "postponed" during the war years, but the birth rate, rather than rising and then returning to "normal," continued to rise year after year, until in 1957 it reached a peak that resulted in an average family of almost 3.8 children. Station wagons and four-bedroom houses suddenly became very popular. After 1957 the birth rate started dropping, at first slowly, then sharply during the 1960s and early 1970s; see Table 9.7.

The present

A real milestone in United States population history was reached during 1972 when, for the first time in the history of the country, the fertility rate dropped to a point which, if continued long enough, could result in a stable population. A hypothetical lifetime birth rate of 2.1 babies per woman will achieve population stability, taking into account that slightly more males than females are born and that some girls die before reaching child-bearing age. During 1972 the fertility rate dropped below this level.

Table 9.6 *History of population growth in the United States*

year	fertility rate[a]	birth rate[b]	death rate[c]	natural increase[d]	immigrants in preceding decade (in millions)	total U.S. population (in millions)	persons per square mile[e]	annual population growth (percent)
1790	—	—	—	—	—	3.9	4.5	—
1800	278	—	—	—	—	5.3	6.1	3.0
1810	274	55.2	—	—	—	7.2	4.3	3.1
1820	260	—	—	—	—	9.6	5.6	2.9
1830	240	51.8	—	—	0.1	12.9	7.4	2.9
1840	222	—	—	—	0.6	17.1	9.8	2.8
1850	194	44.3	—	—	1.7	23.2	7.9	3.1
1860	184	—	—	—	2.6	31.4	10.6	3.0
1870	167	39.8	—	—	2.3	38.6	13.4	2.0
1880	155	—	—	—	2.8	50.2	16.9	2.6
1890	137	—	—	—	5.2	63.0	21.2	2.3
1900	130	32.2	17.2	15.0	3.7	76.2	25.6	1.9
1910	126.8	30.1	14.7	15.4	8.8	92.2	31.0	1.9
1920	117.9	23.7	13.0	10.7	5.7	106.0	35.6	1.4
1930	89.2	18.9	11.3	7.6	4.1	123.2	41.2	1.5
1940	79.9	19.4	10.8	8.6	0.5	132.2	44.2	0.7
1950	106.2	24.1	9.6	14.5	1.0	151.3	50.7	1.4
1960	118.0	23.7	9.5	14.2	2.5	179.3	60.1	1.7
1970	85.7	17.6	9.6	8.0	3.3	205.0	67.8	1.0

SOURCE: Various U.S. Census Bureau Reports.
[a] Fertility rate is the number of births per 1,000 women ages 15 through 44; figures prior to 1900 for white population only, 1900 and subsequent for all races.
[b] Birth rate is the number of births per 1,000 total population.
[c] Death rate is the number of deaths per 1,000 total population; few states registered deaths prior to 1900.
[d] Natural increase is the number of births less the number of deaths per 1,000 population.
[e] Exclusive of Alaska and Hawaii. Major land acquisitions completed by 1850.

Table 9.7 *Recent population growth in the United States*

year	fertility rate[a]	birth rate[b]	death rate[c]	total U.S. population on July 1 (in millions)	annual population growth (percent)
1960	118.0	23.7	9.5	179.3	1.8
1961	117.2	23.3	9.3	183.1	1.7
1962	112.1	22.4	9.5	185.9	1.5
1963	108.0	21.6	9.6	188.7	1.4
1964	105.6	21.2	9.4	191.4	1.4
1965	96.7	19.4	9.4	193.6	1.3
1966	93.2	19.1	9.5	195.7	1.1
1967	87.0	17.9	9.3	198.8	1.1
1968	85.7	17.5	9.5	201.2	1.0
1969	85.4	17.6	9.6	203.1	1.0
1970	87.0	17.9	9.5	205.0	1.0
1971	82.3	17.3	9.3	207.4	1.0
1972[d]	73.4	15.6	9.4	208.9	0.8
1973[d]	71.9	15.0	9.4	210.5	0.7

SOURCE: U.S. Public Health Service and Bureau of Census Reports.
[a] Fertility rate is the number of births per 1,000 women ages 15 through 44.
[b] Birth rate is the number of births per 1,000 total population.
[c] Death rate is the number of deaths per 1,000 total population.
[d] Figures for years 1972 and 1973 are provisional.

There are many possible explanations of the current low birth rate. Women want to take jobs rather than stay home with small children, contraceptive methods have become more effective and more widely available, abortion laws have been liberalized, enabling thousands of women to terminate unwanted pregnancies, and there has been much public discussion of the dangers of overpopulation, leading to increasing social disapproval of large families.

While the fertility rate has dropped to a replacement level, the actual United States population will continue to grow for some years. This is due to the age structure of the current population. The "baby boom" of 1945 to 1960 resulted in a bulge in the population age pyramid; see Fig. 9.3. So the population will continue to increase, until the females in this bulge, and their daughters in turn, pass through their reproductive years. According to current projections, the numbers of births and deaths probably will not balance until about the year 2050.

Within the total United States population there are significant differences in the relative birth rates of various segments of the population. These differences are summarized in Table 9.8. Of course, direct cause-and-effect relationships are obscured, because the poorly educated, the low-income, and the nonwhite women are often one and the same. In addition, a multitude of psychological, sociological, and economic factors influence family size.

In addition to growth in total numbers, several significant changes are taking place in the geographic distribution of the population. Most of these trends began many years ago, but they are now assuming greater importance in light of the increasing total population and the speed with which these changes are occurring. Professor Donald Bogue of the University of Chicago considers the following trends to be important.

1. *Rapid depopulation of rural areas.* Farming areas and small towns are losing population, while the total population grows. Hundreds of small towns are dead or slowly dying.

2. *Heavy movement toward metropolitan areas.* It has been predicted that half of the nation's population will be concentrated into three "strip cities," one extending from San Francisco to San Diego, one from Chicago to Buffalo, and one from Boston through Washington, D.C.

3. *Extensive migration from low-income areas to regions of greater economic opportunity.* Among the results of this move is loss of the economically vital and dynamic younger portion of the population from these depressed areas, leaving only the older persons and those lacking the ambition to move to more prosperous regions. Another problem is the readjustment of those who do migrate.

4. *A flow of middle- and upper-income population from the North and East into the South.* Bogue sees this as a very beneficial trend, weakening the caste system and improving the political and economic conditions of the South.

5. *A great migration to the Pacific Coast of people from all strata and all regions.* Bogue suggests that the economy of California may be based upon a rather weak foundation of population growth and government contracts.

6. *The dying central city and the suburban sprawl.* Almost all the population growth of the metropolitan areas has been concentrated at their suburban edges. The suburbs of one metropolitan area often meet back-to-back with the suburbs of an adjacent metropolitan area. Simultaneously, the middle-class population of the central city has moved out to the suburbs in search of space, privacy, newer housing, and neighbors of similar interests. In the central city housing deteriorates into slums, major business follows the money to the suburbs, and crime rises.

Table 9.8 *Relative birth rates within segments of the U.S. population*

relatively low birth rates	relatively high birth rates
White women	Nonwhite women
Higher-income families	Lower-income families
Better educated women	Less educated women

SOURCE: Various U.S. Census Bureau reports.

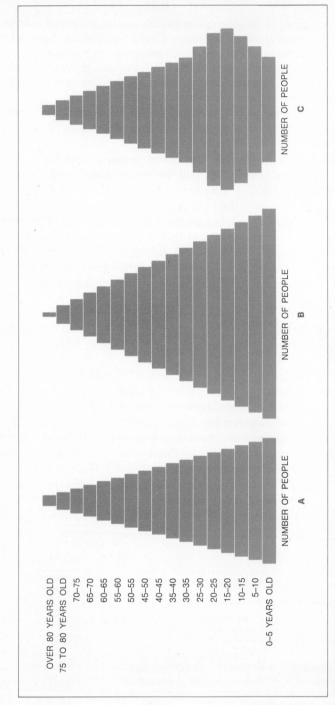

Figure 9.3 Population age-structure pyramids: (A) a stable population, (B) a rapidly growing population, (C) the current United States population (notice the bulge representing the "baby boom" of 1945 to 1960).

258

7. *Concentration of the black population in the deteriorated central portions of the cities.* In less than thirty years, as the need for farm labor has decreased, the black population has shifted from being primarily rural to being primarily urban. Today, more than three quarters of the black population are concentrated in cities, and this move from rural areas still continues. For most of the migrating blacks the move is advantageous, leading to higher income, better housing, better health, and better schools. But for many it is merely a change from rural exploitation to even worse exploitation in the city. Pay is low, rent is high, and commodities and services are priced well above similar goods or services in the suburbs.

The future

As we have seen, even if the current low fertility rate is maintained, the population of the United States will continue to increase for some years. By current estimates the population will stabilize by about the year 2050 at somewhere between 250 and 300 million people *if* the fertility rate remains low.

Our most immediate population concern lies in the "boom babies," born between 1945 and 1960 and now entering their prime reproductive years. In 1980 there will be 20 million women in the prime reproductive age group of twenty to thirty years. This statistic is not just a guess or a rough speculation—these girls have already been born, and the only question remaining is the rate at which they will reproduce. Will the current trend toward smaller families continue, or will a larger family again become fashionable? If the latter takes place, the baby boom of the 1950s will compare to the baby boom of the 1980s as a cap gun compares to a cannon.

Effective contraceptive methods will certainly not be lacking in 1980. The better contraceptive methods of today, such as oral hormones and intra-uterine devices, are already adequate for the maintenance of population growth at an acceptable level. It is likely that even more effective methods will be available in 1980, perhaps based upon entirely new principles. It is also likely that by 1980 family-planning information will be so widely available in the United States that any woman with a desire to control her fertility will find the means to do so readily at a cost she can easily afford to pay.

It would seem that in 1980 the only factor determining the average family size will be the attitudes of the parents regarding the ideal number of children. As the suburbs become increasingly crowded, and as the cost of raising and educating a child continues to rise, the trend toward smaller families may definitely continue. Indeed, as more women are better educated and are interested in careers outside the home, many more married couples may decide to remain childless. The feeling that children are needed to insure security in the parents' old age has largely disappeared through improved pension plans and government programs for the health and other needs of elderly persons.

Thus it is possible that a stable population may be reached through the voluntary decisions of married couples to limit their family sizes. If individuals do not control the birth rate voluntarily, it may eventually become controlled through legal regulation. A first step might be the revision of tax laws to favor the small family rather than the large family, which currently receives tax relief. If the population reached a high enough level, measures such as compulsory sterilization, which seem repulsive today, might find widespread support. It is hoped that voluntary family limitation will preclude the need for more radical means of population control in future years.

MOTIVATIONS FOR CHILDBEARING

The success of any effort at population stabilization depends on the successful motivation of the people to limit their family size. This, in turn, requires a knowledge of the various factors that motivate people to have babies. The importance of each particular factor varies from couple to couple, but every pregnancy is motivated by one or more of these factors.[2]

1. To have sex relations, to have a fetus in the uterus, to go through childbirth, to breast-feed a baby, or to cuddle a baby (innate, or unlearned, motivations).

2. To prove virility of the father.

3. To prove femininity of the mother.

4. To out-do one's parents or prove independence from them.

5. To serve as punishment for sex (for those with sexual inhibitions and guilt complexes).

6. To extend the ego: narcissism, empire building, immortality; for men, to carry on the family name.

7. To prove normality or to conform to cultural expectations, in accordance with cultural or social pressures.

8. To enjoy the action, stimulation, entertainment, and feeling of accomplishment and pleasure in watching children develop.

9. To have a dependent, as a means of building one's sense of personal importance or worth.

10. To insure old-age security.

11. To provide a role in life for a woman; to continue that role after other children have started growing up; to create a role that will pass the test of the work ethic.

12. To share in procreation with a loved one (in a happy marriage), to try to keep an unhappy marriage together, to combat loneliness of ignored wife, to dominate the wife by keeping her "tied down," to have an excuse to pay less attention to the husband.

13. To avoid an "only child."

14. To produce a child of the desired sex—a man may want a son as

---

[2] "After ZPG," National Reporter, November–December, 1972.

proof of his virility (no true connection, of course), and a woman may want a daughter with whom she can identify.

15. To relive the happy memories of one's own childhood.

16. To abide by religious beliefs (for instance, that of reincarnation, which encourages large families).

17. To force marriage upon an unwilling partner.

18. To have revenge upon parents, society, sex partner, or ex-partner.

19. To experience parenthood.

20. To maintain the strength of an ethnic group.

21. The belief that contraception is "not romantic."

22. In emotional conflict over sexual relationship. Obtaining contraceptives requires the conscious acceptance of the fact that intercourse is going to occur. Many people, especially young, unmarried people, are unable or unwilling to take this step. If sex "just happens," there is less guilt produced. Sexual inhibition may prevent open discussion of contraception with a new sexual partner.

Many of these motivations contain glaring errors in logic. Many mean that a child is born to satisfy the needs of his parents, with little or no concern for the needs of the child himself. The child in such cases is merely a "pawn" in his parents' "game."

SUMMARY

Current trends in population growth and environmental deterioration are seen as grave danger signs with regard to the quality of human life in the near future.

    I. Population and world resources
        A. World population problem—extends beyond shortage of food and space.
            1. Differential in consumption of resources between "haves" and "have-nots."
            2. Concept of quality of life versus quantity of life.
        B. Population and health—must be concerned with birth rate as well as with death rate. World health programs must include population control.
        C. Population and food
            1. Majority of world's people subsist on diets deficient in both calories and essential food elements.
            2. Food production is increasing more slowly than population.
        D. Population and energy-mineral resources
            1. Earth's capacity to provide raw materials and land is limited.
            2. Nuclear power offers no cure-all for world's energy problems.
        E. Population and pollution
            1. The quantity of every pollutant relates directly to population.
            2. Many authorities believe world population is already beyond that which environment can support without serious deterioration.
        F. Population pressure—differences in standards of living create tension between nations.

II. World population problems
   A. Past regulators of population have been disease, war, and starvation.
   B. Man must choose one of two checks upon his numbers: higher mortality or lower fertility.
   C. The past—population grew very slowly until recently.
   D. The present—world population now about 4 billion and growing at a rapid rate.
   E. The future—current trends may result in population of more than 6 billion by year 2000. Population problems may be beyond solution.
III. United States population
   A. As population increases, the quality of living decreases.
   B. Past situation
      1. Rate of population growth was once a source of pride.
      2. Prior to 1921 the United States practiced open-door immigration policy.
      3. Long before overpopulation became a concern, women of the United States began limiting family size.
   C. Present situation
      1. Birth rate now at a stabilization level, but population will continue to grow for many years.
      2. Birth rate higher among nonwhite, poor, and poorly educated women.
      3. Other population changes include:
         a. rapid depopulation of rural areas.
         b. heavy movement toward metropolitan areas.
         c. migration to regions of greater economic opportunity.
         d. flow of middle- and upper-income groups from North and East to South.
         e. great migration to Pacific Coast.
         f. dying central city and birth of suburban sprawl.
         g. concentration of blacks in deteriorated central portions of cities.
   D. The future
      1. At current birth rates population would stabilize at 250 to 300 million by about year 2050.
      2. Success of population stabilization depends on motivation of people.
IV. Motivations for childbearing
   A. Listed are 22 motives.
   B. Many contain errors in logic.
   C. Child often is conceived to satisfy needs of parents.

Glossary

If you cannot find the word you wish in this glossary, check the index for text and glossary references.

demography (dē mog′rə fē) (G. *demos*, people; *graphien*, to write). The statistical study of populations.
environment (in vī′ rən mənt) (L. *in*, in; *viron*, circle). The complex of all factors that act upon an organism or an ecological community and ultimately determine its form.

intrauterine contraceptive device (in'trə yoo'tə rin kon trə sep'tiv) (IUD) (L. *intra*, within; *uterus*, womb). A mechanical device placed within the uterus to prevent conception or impregnation.

pollutant (pə lut'ənt) (L. *pollutio*, to defile). Something that pollutes or unfavorably alters the environment.

pollution (pə loo'shən) (L. *pollutio*, to defile). Act of defiling or making impure.

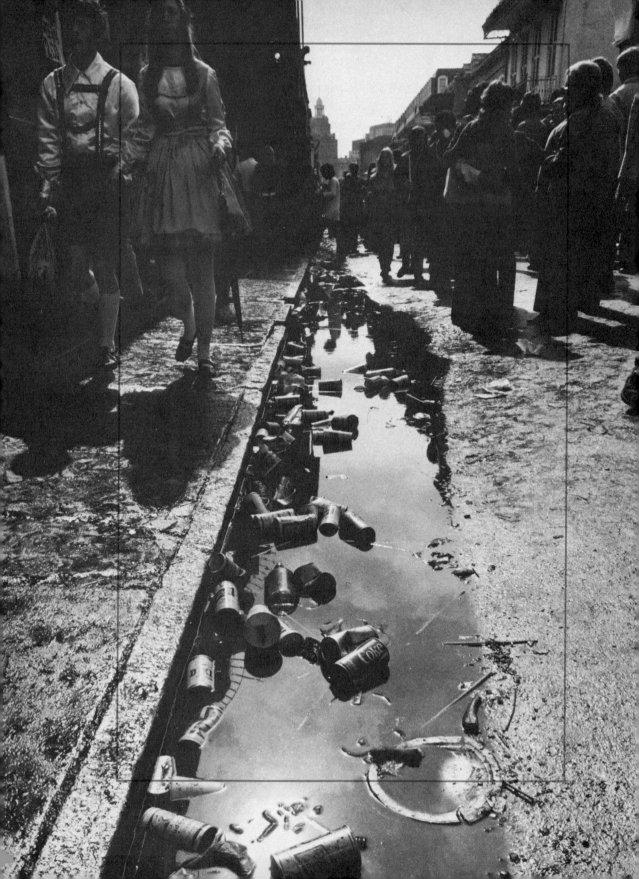

Man and his environment

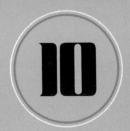

Within the past few years man has, somewhat belatedly, become aware of his intimate relationship with his environment—his total dependence upon that same environment which he has so casually and recklessly altered and despoiled. He is now beginning to take seriously the warnings of the ecologists and conservationists who for so many years were often brusquely dismissed as "crackpots."

For centuries man was impressed with the seeming vastness of the earth and the apparently unlimited resources it possessed. If one area became too populated or despoiled, there were always new frontiers to "conquer." The very word "conquer" was indicative of man's attitude toward his environment. The natural environment was seen as a hostile force, which had to be overcome at any cost.

We are now becoming painfully aware of the cost of abusing our environment. It is now clear that the resources of the earth are not at all unlimited; they are indeed finite. The air and water cannot absorb unlimited amounts of pollutants without those pollutants' accumulating to levels that threaten the continued existence of man on this planet. The earth cannot feed an unlimited population. Man, for all his technical sophistication, cannot suspend the basic laws of nature.

POLLUTION

Pollutants are substances that unfavorably alter our environment. They are the byproducts of man's actions, the residues of things he makes, uses, and throws away. They include the excretory wastes from humans and farm animals, industrial sewage and gases, pesticides, automobile exhausts, empty cans and bottles, radiation, and even heat and noise.

Since most of these wastes have been present with us for many years, why has pollution only recently been recognized as a major problem? One important reason is the recent, explosive increase in human population. An environment that could easily assimilate the byproducts from fewer people can be completely befouled by the proportionately increased byproducts of an increased population. In addition, new pollutants are constantly being introduced into our environment as a result of our continuing technical advancement. An estimated 400 to 500 new chemical substances are being created for our use each year. The long-term effects of these new chemicals upon our environment is virtually unknown.

It must be borne in mind that many pollutants are in fact unavoidable byproducts of man as a biological organism and as a creative social being. They are the wastes from his own metabolic processes and of his efforts to feed, house, clothe, and transport himself. Pollutants will always be with us. They will increase as our population and living standard increase. They will become more concentrated as the process of urbanization continues and more people live in smaller areas.

The answer to our pollution problems cannot lie in attempting to eliminate all production of pollutants, because as long as man exists he will produce such byproducts. Rather, the goal should be to *minimize* the production of pollutants (particularly those with serious environmental consequences) and to *manage* the disposal of pollutants so that they can be effectively assimilated into the environment.

Pollution of the air

A person can live without food for weeks and without water for days, but he can live without air only for a few minutes. Thus, safe air is the most immediately vital of the natural resources.

For many years people have been treating the atmosphere as if it were a sewer, letting different kinds of waste products into it—gases, dusts, fumes, vapors, and smoke. Since the atmosphere is relatively vast, and since until recent years the amount of contamination had been small in terms of the amount of atmosphere, little real trouble was created. Now, however, this contamination is proving harmful to man, animals, and plants.

Air pollution involves different air contaminants in different areas. By general definition, air pollution is the introduction of materials into the air as a result of man's activity. This definition would exclude from our discussion pollutants from such natural sources as volcanoes, hot springs, and dust storms. There are other pollutants, such as smoke from forest fires, which may have started from either natural or human causes. Pollution, as discussed here, will imply the *possibility of control.*

Based upon their physical state, air pollutants may be considered in two categories: the aerosols and the gases.

Gaseous pollutants   Gaseous pollutants exist as individual molecules and behave like the air itself. They do not settle out. Principally the product of industrial and domestic combustion, they arise from two general sources: the combustion of fuels and the handling and processing of chemicals.

1. *Sulfur oxides.* These are widely prevalent and in some concentrations are harmful. Low concentrations of sulfur dioxide (SO_2), for instance, cause irritation of the nose and throat. Sulfur dioxide has been the suspected cause in several air-pollution disasters, among them those of Donora, Pennsylvania, and London, England. Most fuels contain small amounts of sulfur, which is converted into sulfur dioxide during combustion. The sulfur oxides also result from smelting and other metallurgical operations.

2. *Nitrogen oxides.* Of the nitrogen oxides, nitrogen dioxide and nitric oxide appear to be of greatest health importance as air pollutants. Health effects are usually noticeable only when comparatively high concentrations are found in enclosed areas. In addition, these oxides contribute to the nuisance effects of photochemical smog (smog conditions resulting from the action of sunlight on certain chemicals in the air) under certain weather conditions. The most important sources of nitrogen oxides in the atmosphere are the combustion of fuels and certain chemical manufacturing operations. When anything is burned, some of the nitrogen in the air combines with some of the oxygen to form nitric oxide (NO), which will combine with more oxygen to form nitrogen dioxide (NO_2). The actions of nitrogen dioxide and olefinic hydrocarbons produce eye-irritating products, vegetation damage and, under intense sunlight, ozone.

3. *Ozone.* Ozone is formed from the photochemical reaction of nitrogen dioxide and olefinic hydrocarbons in the air. It is very eye-irritating and is also thought to produce pulmonary fibrosis after long exposure.

4. *Carbon monoxide.* Carbon monoxide (CO) is a highly poisonous gas produced by the incomplete combustion of carbon and its compounds. Because of its strong power of combining with hemoglobin in the blood it has caused many deaths in homes and garages, where it has been released in closed spaces. Auto exhaust, smoking, and defective heating systems are the most important sources.

5. *Other gases.* Many gaseous air pollutants exist, such as alcohols and esters, halogens, oxides, and aldehydes. Some of these substances may be strong eye irritants and rather toxic.

Aerosols   Aerosols are finely divided solid or liquid droplets, the larger of which will settle out of a gas. The finer particles can be buoyed up by the slightest air movement and may never settle out. Aerosols may consist of many things, but they commonly include dusts (silica, iron, coal, uranium), fumes, mists, and smoke.

Dusts are solid particles of natural or industrial origin. *Fumes* are solid particles generated by the condensation of vapors in various ways. *Mists* are liquid particles which may arise from vapor condensation or chemical reactions.

The sources of aerosols are many. Fuel burning, incineration, agricultural operations, crushing and grinding operations, construction, mining, spraying, and sandblasting represent some common sources.

A new and very serious type of pollution to the atmosphere is radioactive aerosols. These materials are a source of concern, because they cannot be detected by taste, smell, or the other human senses, and also because there is no way of neutralizing their radioactivity. It is important that they be kept out of the air. Possible sources include uranium mining operations, atomic laboratories, nuclear reactors, and radioactive waste disposal. The greatest concern has been shown over radioactive dusts and gases from atomic bomb tests, particularly strontium 90, which has a half-life of 28 years.

Temperature inversion layers   The problem of air pollution is further complicated by the existence of *inversion layers* over many of the world's major cities. An inversion layer is a layer of warm air overlying a cooler layer of surface air; see Fig. 10.1. It results from an area's topographical character and is especially common along seacoasts. An inversion layer acts as a "lid," which prevents air pollutants from mixing with upper layers of air. Thus, instead of pollutants' being mixed through some twelve miles of atmosphere, they are held within several hundred feet of the ground. In some western cities, such as Los Angeles, inversion layers may be present on as many as 340 days of the year.

Photochemical smog   The word *smog* is coined from *smoke* and *fog*. Smog is a common phenomenon in many metropolitan areas, especially those along seacoasts; see Fig. 10.2. Photochemical smog results when air pollutants trapped under an inversion layer are changed to more harmful chemicals by the action of sunlight.

The basic ingredients of photochemical smog include nitrogen dioxide and incompletely burned hydrocarbons from auto exhausts. Carbon monoxide is not involved in this problem. When nitrogen dioxide, NO_2, absorbs energy from sunlight, it separates into nitric oxide, NO, and atomic oxygen, O. The normal atmospheric oxygen is in the form of molecular oxygen, O_2. The atomic oxygen then unites with the atmospheric oxygen to form ozone, O_3, with its above-mentioned harmful effects. Ozone also reacts with other air pollutants, especially hydrocarbons, to form, literally, hundreds of undesirable compounds. Among the worst offenders in photochemical smog are PAN (peroxyacetyl nitrate) and various aldehydes. Both PAN and the aldehydes are highly irritating to the eyes and respiratory tract and are harmful to vegetation as well. In the mountain ranges of Southern California thousands of acres of prime forest are currently being killed by photochemical smog.

Effects of air pollution   The effects of air pollution may be considered in several rather broad categories: (1) property damage, (2) damage to plants and animals, (3) soiling of surfaces, (4) sky-darkening, (5) limited visibility, (6) annoyance to human senses, and (7) damage to health. The effects on plants, though economically important, is not often dramatic. Air pollution can cause leaf lesions and reduced productivity. Air pollution is of major concern to animal owners. Arsenic from smelting operations, for instance, may settle on vegetation and poison grazing cattle. Excessive absorption of fluorides may cause fluorosis in animals.

Of primary concern to us is the effect of air pollutants on man. This effect is not completely clear, but some things are known. The unburnt substances found in smoke are of particular importance; benzpyrene, one of them, may play a role in cancer. The aerosols are so fine they may easily penetrate the lungs. And, besides being harmful themselves, they may act as carriers of microbes and viruses. Mass attacks by air contaminants on people may be triggered by accidental escapes of large quantities of gases or dust. Although

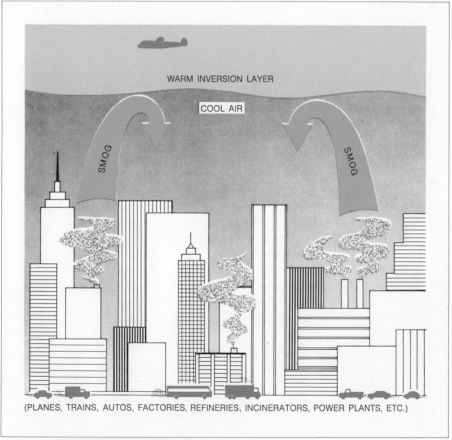

Figure 10.1   Inversion layer: a layer of warm air acting as a "ceiling" over the cooler surface air; it holds air pollutants close to the ground.

such acute episodes may be disastrous, as was the London attack in 1952 in which 4,000 people died as the result of air pollution, these tragic situations reflect highly unusual meteorological conditions. More common are the noxious gases that are more or less chronically present in the air of some urban areas. Some of the known or suspected effects of air pollution on human health are summarized in Table 10.1.

In addition to its more obvious effects, such as eye and throat irritation, air pollution is believed to cause more serious harm to the respiratory system and heart. Air pollution levels can be correlated with chronic bronchitis, asthma, emphysema, lung cancer, and (through impaired lung function) to heart diseases. Air pollution is particularly harmful to infants, the elderly, and those suffering from chronic respiratory disorders.

There is enough definite evidence of the harmful effects of air pollution for many public health authorities now to recommend curtailing vigorous outdoor activities during intense smog attacks. In Los Angeles County, where ozone levels are monitored daily as indicators of photochemical smog levels, schools are advised to keep pupils indoors during recess and lunch periods

Figure 10.2   Air pollution: view of Los Angeles, California, on a typically smoggy day.

Table 10.1 *Effects of air pollution on human health*

pollutant	known or suspected effect
Oxides of sulfur	Aggravation of existing respiratory diseases and contribution to their development; impairment of lung function; eye and throat irritation.
Oxides of nitrogen	Eye and throat irritation; contribute to development of photo-chemical smog.
Ozone	Considerable eye and throat irritation; possible association with asthmatic attacks; possible lung damage (pulmonary fibrosis).
Carbon monoxide	By combining with hemoglobin, reduces oxygen-carrying capacity of blood, deprives tissues of oxygen; low concentrations may cause severe impairment of mental abilities; higher concentrations cause death.
Lead	Intake through air adds to burden through food and water; may result in lead poisoning.
Asbestos	Particles inhaled into lungs remain permanently, irritate lung tissues, cause cancer and other lung diseases; extreme care must be taken to avoid asbestos inhalation.
Beryllium	Causes bronchitis and systemic poisoning; has poisoned people living three quarters of a mile from a processing plant.

when ozone levels exceed 0.35 parts per million, a level reached several days each year.

Control of air pollution   The control or prevention of air contamination is a complex problem and often expensive. Some authorities believe it is now possible to achieve almost the complete elimination of such pollution, but each locality must decide how clean its air must be and how much its people are willing to pay for smog control. At the present time the toleration levels for only a few contaminants are known and can be specified. Ideally, however, pollution should be eliminated at the source.

In some places the answer lies in reducing the source of pollution by substituting certain heating procedures with nonpolluting methods. In other cases, as of motor vehicles, the problem is to ensure proper combustion by regulating the operating conditions of vehicles. In all places the problem involves whether control measures are feasible both economically and practically.

Also involved are the legal and regulatory aspects. A person must be free to use his property, yet at the same time he must be prevented from doing harm to others. The atmosphere must be kept clean enough for humans to breathe safely and for the growth of food crops. Conflicts of interest must be overcome. The "right" to discharge waste products into the atmosphere must be made subordinate to the "right" to breathe safe air. This will require the modification of certain practices by both corporations and individuals. Does anyone really have the "right" to pollute the air that others must breathe to live?

Pollution of water

Water in its natural state is never 100 percent pure. As soon as it condenses as rain, it begins gathering impurities, which it carries until it is purified or until it evaporates. Much of this impurity is not sufficient to spoil the usefulness of water; some materials and substances, however, do limit its usefulness.

By definition, "water pollution" means the presence in water of any substance that impairs any of its legitimate uses—for public water supplies, recreation, agriculture, industry, the preservation of fish and wildlife, and esthetic purposes; see Fig. 10.3.

The principal forms of pollution are domestic wastes, industrial wastes, and silt. Domestic wastes include everything that goes down the drains of a city into its sewer system: used water from toilets, bathtubs, and sinks, and washings from restaurants, laundries, hospitals, hotels, and other businesses.

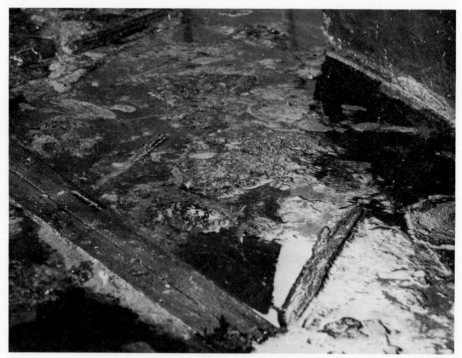

Figure 10.3   Water pollution: beneath the layer of floating scum lies the "water" of Los Angeles Harbor.

Industrial wastes are the acids, chemicals, oils, greases, and animal and vegetable matter discharged by factories; they are discharged either through some sewer system or through separate outlets directly into waterways. Silt is the soil that is washed into streams, which muddies waters and fills up reservoirs and waterways. In addition to these principal forms of pollution there can be other pollutants, such as heat, radioactive substances, pesticides, and detergents.

Effects of water pollution   Almost every use to which water is put may be affected by pollution. Foremost, we want safe water for drinking and other domestic purposes. Some of the effects of water pollution on human health are summarized in Table 10.2.

Water is the most used of all raw materials in industry. The availability of pure water determines the location of many industries. Since its lack discourages many industries from locating in that area, pure water becomes an economic asset for most communities.

There are other economic considerations. Crops irrigated with polluted water may well transmit disease. Certain forms of industrial pollution in irrigation waters can damage crops. Fish often cannot survive in excessively polluted waters. Because of polluted water beaches are closed to swimmers, boating is made undesirable, and outdoor water recreation is limited—all of which restricts certain forms of income in those localities, altering the economy.

The future demands on our country's water may well outstrip the sup-

Table 10.2 *Effects of water pollution on human health*

pollutant	effect
Human wastes	Contains pathogens of many diseases, such as typhoid, cholera, shigellosis, salmonellosis, hepatitis, amebic dysentery, parasitic worms.
Mercury	Methyl mercury poisoning through concentration through food chains.[a]
Lead	Lead poisoning.
Cadmium	Cadmium poisoning when concentrated through food chains.
Arsenic	Arsenic poisoning.
Fluorides	Mottling of teeth when present in excess.
Nitrates	Converted to nitrites in digestive tract. Nitrites combine with hemoglobin to form methemoglobin, which is incapable of carrying oxygen. Causes severe anemia in infants, elderly people, and people with heart or respiratory disorders.
Other chemicals	Oils and phenols, for example, may make water toxic or unpleasant to drink.

[a] A food chain is the transfer of mass and energy from one organism to another by eating and being eaten.

ply. It is believed that only by the reuse of water will future needs be supplied. This reuse cannot occur, however, if polluted water cannot be reclaimed. Thus it becomes of utmost importance that answers be found to cope with the present pollution problem.

Purification processes   There are two primary methods of purifying water: by natural processes and by the specific treatment of domestic and industrial sewage.

· NATURAL PROCESSES   Water can purify itself by natural means up to the point at which a stream cannot handle the pollution load. The self-purification can be brought about by chemical, physical, and biological factors. The rate of self-purification will depend upon the water body's local features.

The time required will depend upon both the degree of pollution and the character of the water. Organic wastes are broken down by the action of aerobic bacteria present in the water. Their action in turn depends upon the amount of dissolved oxygen in the water. This is available either from direct absorption from the air over the surface of the water or from the oxygen given off by respiring water plants. But the more oxygen used up in this purification process, the less is available for fish and other aquatic life. In addition to the presence of aquatic plants as an oxygen source, the nature of the water body will largely determine the amount of oxygen present: for example, oxygen replenishment will take place rapidly in a fast-flowing active stream, the splashing of which allows for more air contact; and the more motionless and sluggish a stream or the greater its depth, the longer the time required to replenish its oxygen supply.

Because sunlight is restricted in polluted water, few water plants will grow in it; thus its oxygen supply is reduced. This reduction in turn leads to fewer aerobic bacteria in the water and an increased pollution problem, resulting in foul-smelling, unattractive water that cannot support fish or other aquatic life. The solution here is reduction of incoming wastes to a point where the stream can handle them through self-purification. This level will differ from stream to stream, depending upon the stream's characteristics.

· SEWAGE TREATMENT   One of the worst sources of water pollution is the dumping of untreated or incompletely treated municipal sewage. There are many different degrees to which sewage may be treated. At one extreme, raw sewage is merely collected and dumped, without any treatment, into the most convenient river, lake, or ocean; at the other, the finished product is pure enough to be used for drinking or almost any other purpose. As the world's population and degree of industrialization continue to grow, the luxury of using fresh water just once before "discarding" it is one which we can no longer afford. More and more sewage must be treated and recycled as fresh water, or in addition to the problem of polluted lakes and streams the world will be plagued by increasingly severe water shortages.

Radiation in the environment

Since entering the "atomic age" some years ago we have all felt concern about the effects of excessive radiation in our environment. Actually, however, there has always been some radiation, referred to as *natural background radiation*. All forms of life have been subjected to low levels of radiation from natural sources throughout their evolution. In fact, such natural radiation is believed to be important in producing the mutations upon which evolution is based. This background radiation comes from naturally occurring radioactive substances in the ground, air, and water, and as cosmic radiation from space.

In recent decades man has also been subject to his own *man-made radiation*. The intensity of man-made radiation varies from high doses such as might result from a nuclear weapon, reactor accident, or radiotherapy, down to low doses comparable to those from natural background radiation. Some of the major man-made radiation sources are outlined below.

Radiotherapy is the use of radiation (usually x-rays and gamma radiation) for diagnosis and treatment in medicine and dentistry. It is the major source of man-made radiation in the world today.

Radioactive isotopes are atoms of radioactive elements used in research, in medical diagnosis and treatment, and in industry.

Industrial x-rays are x-rays used in industry for radiography of welds, castings, and products in which flaws could impair quality.

Radioactive fallout is the result of the explosion of nuclear devices, as in the testing or use of nuclear weapons.

Radioactive wastes are the products of the use and processing of radioactive materials, fission products, and the possible accidental release of radioactive substances. Some of these affect only individuals who are subjected to radiation because of their occupation; others constitute a hazard to the whole population by pollution of the environment.

Effects of radiation on the body tissues   Large doses of all types of radiation will kill cells. With smaller doses of radiation a recovery of the cells can take place, and they can continue to function. However, recovery may not be complete, and there may be later malignant changes. In general, certain cells are more readily affected by radiation than are others, and tissues which are actively regenerating, with constant cell division and multiplication—such as embryonic tissue, intestinal mucosa, blood-forming tissue, gonadal germ cells, and skin—are the more vulnerable. These types of tissue damage may be divided into two main classes, as follows:

Somatic tissue effects. Somatic tissue is the general tissue of the body. Large doses of radiation destroy somatic tissue, leading to the death of the individual. Lesser doses of radiation may show no immediate effect, but they may accumulate until cell function is altered, possibly causing leukemia or another form of cancer.

Genetic effects. Genetic effects are effects upon the germ, or reproductive, cells. No damage will appear in the individual who receives the radiation, but the effects of the radiation will appear in his descendants as abnormalities of form and function. Such genetic effects may be caused by small doses of radiation; therefore, *all* radiation must be considered deleterious to a greater or lesser degree.

Radioactive fallout Fallout is the return to earth of radioactive material which had been carried up into the atmosphere by the detonation of a nuclear device. It also is any contamination of food, drink, soil, air, or building materials resulting from such return to earth. Environmental contamination produced by the worldwide dispersion of radioactivity from nuclear-weapons tests has been a source of both internal and external radiation.

Distribution of a fallout pattern is determined by yield, height, and location of the detonation and by meteorological conditions. The dose rate and the accumulated dose from fallout depend not only upon the amount of radioactive fallout but also upon the ionization effects of the radiation products.

In the process of detonation of a nuclear device, for every 1 megaton of fission, the yield will be about 110 pounds of intensely radioactive substances. Fortunately, many of the substances formed have extremely short radioactive half-lives and thus have little significance other than in local fallout. Isotopes remaining 1 hour after detonation will decay by a factor of approximately 10 for every 7-fold increase in time after detonation time plus 1 hour. As shown in Table 10.3, 7 hours after a nuclear explosion the radioactivity has decreased to $\frac{1}{10}$ of what it was at 1 hour; in 49 hours it is only $\frac{1}{100}$ of what it was at 1 hour; in two weeks it is only $\frac{1}{1000}$ and in three months only $\frac{1}{10,000}$ of its level at 1 hour.

It has been shown that the total dose in bone marrow from artificial sources of radiation in technically advanced countries is approximately equal to the typical natural-background dose. In children under five fallout probably accounts for some 5 to 10 percent of the artificial dose in bone marrow. With the advent of a test-ban treaty this may decrease in younger children. The genetically significant dose from artificial sources probably is annually about 3 percent of the amount of natural-background dose. Fallout during atmospheric testing was responsible for about 20 percent of the total artificial dose.

Disposal of radioactive waste Radioactive wastes from industry vary so much that there is no single solution to their management or disposal. The solution depends upon such factors as the *specific nature* (radioactive half-life or type of radiation), *concentration* (quantity of radioactive material in-

Table 10.3 *Fading radiation hazard*

contamination from radioactive material (curies)	time after formation of fission products	radiation intensity from fission products (roentgens per hour)
1,000	1 hour	10,000
100	7 hours	1,000
10	49 hours (2 days)	100
1	14 days (2 weeks)	10
0.1	14 weeks (3 months)	1

SOURCE: Adapted from C. W. Shilling, *Atomic Energy Encyclopedia*, Philadelphia, W. B. Saunders Company, 1964.

volved), and the *specific environment* in which disposal is being considered. The problem of disposal of radioactive wastes is that there is no way to destroy the radioactivity immediately; time alone, with its radioactive decay, serves to render the waste stable and harmless or of very low radioactivity and, therefore, nontoxic.

The magnitude of the waste-disposal problem far outweighs the problems of fallout, or operation of a reactor. Waste disposal is potentially the greatest hazard to public safety. And the time of this danger is *now!* Many reactors are not currently in use or are being run at reduced capacity because of the many tons of high-level radioactive waste *already* stored. Yet no satisfactory method of disposal has been developed. As the nuclear-power program builds up, the disposal of fission products in a manner that will not be injurious to health will need to have particular attention.

Spent-fuel elements are now removed from reactors and shipped to one of the major United States Atomic Energy Commission processing sites. Here they are "cooled" for ninety days to allow decay of radioactive isotopes with short half-lives. They are classified as to energy level (high, medium, or low) and disposed of in the following manners:

High-level radioactive wastes must be handled by containment in tank storage to allow time for radioactive decay. Suggestions for the final disposal of high-level wastes include the conversion of liquid wastes to solids and their permanent storage in geological strata, the major sites being salt beds. Or liquids could be put directly into geological strata, either in deep wells or salt beds. Or both solids and liquids could be disposed of in the sea.

Medium-level radioactive wastes are usually held in trenches, in artificial ponds, or in tanks to allow for radioactive decay to a level at which they may be discharged into the environment. Some wastes with radioisotopes of reasonably short half-lives (weeks or months) are discharged directly into the ground. Some medium-activity wastes have been incorporated in concrete in steel drums, which have been buried in trenches or dumped at sea.

Low-level radioactive wastes, defined as having a radioactivity concentration in the range of one microcurie per gallon, are usually disposed of by dilution with water and released directly into the environment—in air, land, or sea. These wastes include things such as the reactor cooling water used in nuclear-powered ships and submarines.

Various other forms of waste processing, including chemical processing, are being used or experimented with, in an attempt to find a more economical and satisfactory method of waste disposal.

Pollutants in food

One of the favorite topics of discussion today among people concerned with maintaining health is the matter of substances added to food. On one side are people who claim that all types of chemical substance are being added to food without due regard to the consequences. On the other, food industry spokesmen are quick to point out that purposely added substances (additives) are used with justification: they retard spoilage, enhance flavor, improve color, improve consistency, retard drying, or help to retain crispness, and some are added as nutritional supplements, such as thiamine in bread, iodine in salt, fluoride in water, or vitamins A and D in milk.

Some substances gain entrance into foods accidentally: they may be insecticides, hormones, antibiotics, or disinfectants. Some of these are substances which get into the food from the wrappers or containers where packaging materials touch the food.

Great efforts are made on the part of certain federal agencies to protect the consumer against injurious substances. Before we point out these areas of concern, however, we should define several terms as they will be used here. A *food additive* is a substance, other than a basic foodstuff, which is intentionally put into food as a result of any aspect of production, processing, storage, or packaging. This definition does not include chance contaminants. *Toxicity* is the capacity of a substance to produce injury. *Safety* is the practical certainty that injury will not result from use of a substance in a proposed quantity and manner. *Hazard* is the probability that injury will result from use of a substance in a proposed quantity and manner. An *adulterant* is a foreign or inferior substance added to a food product in place of a more valuable substance. The adulterant might be actually harmful when consumed or merely deceptive, such as the inclusion of horsemeat or cereal in hamburger. A *residue* is a quantity of a pesticide or other contaminant remaining on a food product from treatments made during its growing or processing.

Pesticide residues in foods   Modern food-production practices include the use of hundreds of pesticide chemicals such as insecticides, fungicides, and herbicides. In fact, it is doubtful whether the current population of the United States could be fed without at least some use of chemical pesticides. There is, however, mounting concern regarding possible immediate and long-term adverse effects from the consumption of foods containing residual traces of various pesticides (pesticide residues).

All pesticides must be registered with the Environmental Protection Agency (EPA) before application to crops is allowed. Such registration is granted only after extensive safety testing—including such phases as feeding the pesticide in measured quantities to test animals over long periods of time and analysis of treated crops for the amount of pesticide residue. Pesticide registrations may be granted on the basis of a "zero tolerance"—no trace of residue permitted—or on the basis of minute amounts of residue allowed. In the latter case the Food and Drug Administration (FDA) insists upon a residue safety margin of a hundredfold; in other words, only 1 percent of the presumed safety level of residue is allowed in consumer foods.

Some authorities now question the wisdom of allowing any pesticide residues in foods; they fear the possibility of yet unknown effects of long-term consumption of even small amounts of pesticides. They often cite possible genetic damage, cancer, and metabolic disorders as effects that might show up after many years of exposure.

A more immediate danger lies in the occasional cases of the improper use of pesticides. Excessively heavy or frequent application, improper formulation, or application too close to harvest are examples of practices that may result in residues above the legal tolerance. While many of such cases are detected by FDA inspectors with the subsequent destruction of the contaminated food, much food carrying illegal residues must be assumed to be reaching the consumer.

Some, though not all, of the pesticide residues can be removed from foods by thorough washing and peeling and removing of outer leaves and similar procedures. Foods showing visible residues or having unusual smells should not be purchased.

Intentional food additives Shifting our attention now to chemicals that are purposely added to foods, we find that some of the highly prepared "convenience" food products contain up to a dozen or more chemical additives. Like pesticides, new food additives must undergo intensive testing before their use is approved by the FDA. However, many additives that were introduced prior to 1958 did not receive the safety testing now required and have been permitted to remain in use. The 1969 withdrawal of cyclamates from general use illustrated that some of the older additives may not be as safe as had been presumed.

Increasing numbers of authorities are questioning the wisdom of our consumption of ever-increasing quantities of food additives. While it is unlikely that the amount contained in any one food product presents any great threat to health, the individual or family who relies heavily on "convenience" foods potentially could consume quantities and combinations of additives that might disturb the metabolism or result in genetic damage, cancer, or other serious disorders. It seems only sensible to minimize the intake of additives by selecting simple, basic food ingredients rather than premixed, additive-laden "convenience" foods.

Radioactive pollution of foods The problem of man-made contamination of foods with radioactivity is rather new. So far the responsible governmental agencies have made studies when they have seemed necessary. Large-scale studies have not yet been conducted, because so far the present and potential hazard, according to the National Research Council, has not warranted the expenditure of money and effort. However, some studies are starting to show an order of hazard which may be much greater than was previously believed possible.

Other food contaminants Outbreaks of food-borne diseases continue to be reported. By prompt inquiry into the circumstances in each particular case Public Health Service epidemiologists are often able to pin down the particular disease organisms causing the outbreak, the food involved, and the way in which the food became contaminated. Causes of food-borne infections include species of *Salmonella* and *Clostridium*. Ways to prevent this contamination include elimination of flies (*Salmonella*), high-temperature sterilization (*Clostridium*), and the freezing, washing, and proper cooking of food. All these safeguards will reduce the bacterial count.

Noise pollution

One of the more recently "discovered" pollutants in the modern environment is noise. For the city dweller noise may be the most significant environmental pollutant. He may be constantly buffeted by the noise of aircraft, trains, motorcycles, buses, sirens, machinery at home and at work, his neighbor's stereo, and his neighbor's toilet flushing. One study showed that the average noise level in residential areas rose as much as 9 decibels between 1954 and 1967. The decibel scale is logarithmic: an increase of 10 decibels indicates a tenfold increase in noise intensity.[1]

Some of the effects of noise have been known or suspected for years. Fatigue, emotional stress, and permanent loss of hearing acuity are well documented effects of excess noise. Other studies have shown that noise, either prolonged or sudden, produces involuntary responses by the circulatory, digestive, and nervous systems. Adrenalin is shot into the blood, as during stress and anxiety. The heart beats rapidly, the blood vessels constrict, the pupils dilate, and the stomach, esophagus, and intestines are seized by spasms. A three-year study of university students showed that noise of only 70 decibels consistently caused constriction of the coronary arteries, which supply oxygen to the heart muscle. Permanent hearing loss occurs with prolonged exposure to sounds of over 90 decibles. Table 10.4 compares the intensity of some common sounds.

Highly amplified music, pleasant as it may be, has been implicated as an important source of hearing loss among young people. Live performances, radio, tapes, and records may all reach loudness levels that cause permanent hearing loss. Stereo headphones are especially capable of damaging hearing. A study in Sweden in 1970 showed that 19.5 percent of persons aged fifteen to twenty showed hearing losses attributed to noise.[2] A similar survey in 1956 showed only 9 percent with such loss.

Probably the most damaging effect of noise on the quality of human life is its disruption of our psychic balance. Loud, harsh, or persistent noise robs us of our peace of mind, puts our nerves "on edge" so that our personal relationships are strained and even explosive, interferes with our concentration, and impairs the efficient functioning of our minds. Noise must be regarded as far more than just an annoyance: it is a serious threat to the quality of our lives.

Land pollution

Man alters the surface of the earth in countless ways. In his efforts to feed, house, and transport himself he has cleared much of its surface of its native vegetation. He has drained swamps, built dams and irrigation projects, logged forests, dredged and filled bays, and in a thousand other obvious or subtle ways modified his earth's physical condition.

Many of these changes have been necessary in order to feed a constantly

---

[1] "How Today's Noise Hurts Body and Mind," *Medical World News, 10,* 24:42–47, June 13, 1969.

[2] Martine Allain-Regnault, "The Decibel Inferno," *World Health* (May, 1972), 12–15.

Table 10.4 *Intensity of some common sounds*

sound source	intensity decibels[a]
Human whisper	30
Normal conversation	60
City traffic	80
Garbage disposal unit	80
Alarm clock	80
Domestic quarrel	80
Vacuum cleaner	85
Garbage truck	85
Food blender	93
Subway train	95
Jackhammer	95
Power lawnmower	96
Printing press	97
Farm tractor	98
Punch press	105
Boiler shop	105
Textile looms	106
Motorcycle	110
Riveting gun	110
Rock band (amplified)	114 to 140
Drop hammer	130
Jet airplane	135 to 150
Siren	150
Rocket	170

SOURCE: Compiled from *Medical World News*, 10, 24:42–47, June 13, 1969, and other sources.
[a] A decibel is the smallest difference in intensity of sound that the human ear can detect. The scale is logarithmic; a difference of 10 db represents a tenfold increase in sound intensity.

growing population. Others have been purely for the benefit of land speculators or other special-interest groups. Sometimes the results of carelessly changing the nature of the land are drastic and unpredictable. Many former forests and grasslands have been converted first to farmland and then, through poor farming practices, to sterile deserts or gully-riddled, eroded wastelands. In the building of cities the planning has often been so poor that the quality of life is almost intolerable.

In much of the world, and especially in the United States, very little land remains in its original state. Great care must be taken in the development of this irreplaceable natural resource. Enough land must be left in its natural state to allow for the survival of wildlife and for the enjoyment of man. That land which must be developed must not be blighted by the haphazard or selfish development which now characterizes so much of the earth's surface. Greater concern must be shown for the quality of life. No generation has the right to deprive future generations of a decent place to live.

ROLE OF THE GOVERNMENT IN POLLUTION CONTROL

Traditionally, the regulation of pollution has been left to state and local governments, but it has become increasingly clear that such regulation is often not adequate. State and local governments are often reluctant to pass or to enforce regulations that would restrict the activities of large corporations, which contribute significantly to the employment and tax rolls within their jurisdiction. Similarly, the citizens within an area are often reluctant to push for pollution control when it might affect their "bread and butter."

Unfortunately, pollution does not confine itself to the political jurisdiction in which it originates. Polluted air drifts freely from county to county and state to state. A polluted river may flow through many states. Several states may share the shoreline of a polluted lake or ocean. Thus the control of pollution rightfully becomes an interstate problem, subject to federal control.

Federal control of pollution has evolved slowly, over a period of many years. Until recently federal efforts were often ineffective, as responsibilities were fragmented among many different agencies. There have even been instances in which the policies of two federal agencies were directly contradictory.

In a move to coordinate and strengthen the environmental control activities of the federal government President Nixon in 1970 authorized the formation of the Environmental Protection Agency (EPA). This agency consists of units transferred from other federal agencies, including the Department of the Interior, the Department of Agriculture, the Department of Health, Education and Welfare, and the Atomic Energy Commission. Thus, the federal agencies dealing with air and water pollution, the regulation of pesticides, atomic radiation, and solid waste control were brought under one "roof," with a budget in excess of $2 billion per year. Among the specific activities and powers of the EPA are the setting of air-quality standards for all sources of air pollutants, with authority to assess penalties up to $25,000 per day for first violations and up to $50,000 per day and up to 2 years in prison for second offenses.

Other EPA activities include control over all industrial waste discharged into bodies of water, though the total elimination of such discharges will be a gradual process. Local government agencies are being given financial and technical aid in the construction of sewage treatment facilities. Another goal is the closing down of more than five thousand open dumps scattered across the country.

SUMMARY

Man has finally become more aware of his intimate relationship with his environment.

    I. Pollution

        A. Pollutants are substances which unfavorably alter our environment.

        B. Pollutants include excretory wastes from humans and animals, industrial sewage and gases, pesticides, auto exhausts, radiation, heat, noise, and empty containers.

II. Pollution of the air
  A. Gaseous pollutants—sulfur oxides, nitrogen oxides, ozone, and carbon monoxide
  B. Aerosols—dusts, fumes, and mists
  C. Temperature-inversion layers—trap pollutants near ground
  D. Photochemical smog—produced by effect of sunlight on pollutants trapped under inversion layer
  E. Effects
    1. Property damage.
    2. Vegetation damage.
    3. Soiling of surfaces.
    4. Sky-darkening.
    5. Limiting of visibility.
    6. Annoyance to human senses.
    7. Damage to health.
  F. Control—complex; legal regulation of emission of pollutants
III. Pollution of water
  A. Includes domestic wastes, industrial wastes, silt, heat, radioactive substances, pesticides, and detergents
  B. Affects every use of water
  C. Purification processes
    1. Natural processes.
    2. Sewage treatment—must be upgraded in many areas.
IV. Radiation in the environment
  A. Some natural background radiation has always been present
  B. Sources of man-made radiation
    1. Radiotherapy.
    2. Radioactive isotopes.
    3. Industrial x-rays.
    4. Radioactive fallout.
    5. Radioactive wastes.
  C. Effects of radiation
    1. Death or damage of body tissues.
    2. Genetic changes affecting future generations.
  D. Radioactive fallout—source of both internal and external radiation.
  E. Disposal of radioactive wastes is a major problem.
V. Pollutants in food
  A. Pesticide residues
  B. Intentional additives
  C. Radioactive pollution
  D. Other contaminants
VI. Noise pollution
  A. Full significance just being realized.
  B. Many physical and emotional effects.
VII. Land pollution
  A. Much of the earth's surface has been blighted by careless development.
  B. Remaining natural areas must be preserved or developed with greater concern for the quality of life.
VIII. Role of government in pollution control
  A. Control by state and local agencies is often inadequate.

B. Pollution is an interstate problem, subject to federal control.

C. The federal Environmental Protection Agency (EPA) was formed in 1970 from units transferred from other agencies.

Glossary

If you cannot find the word you wish in this glossary, check the index for text and glossary references.

adulterant (ə dul'ter ant) (L. *alter*, other, different). A foreign or inferior substance added to a food product in place of a more valuable substance.

aerosol (air'ə sol) (G. *aer*, air or gas; (*hydro*)*sol*, a suspension of a solid in a liquid). A system consisting of solid particles dispersed in a gas; a smoke, or fog.

atom (at'əm) (G. *atomos*, indivisible). Any one of the ultimate particles of a molecule or of any matter.

decibel (des'ə bel, des'ə bəl) (L. *decimus*, tenth; Alexander Graham *Bell*). A unit for measuring the relative loudness of sounds on a scale beginning with 1 for the faintest audible sound.

electron (i lek'tron). Unit of negative electricity.

element (el'ə mənt) (L. *elementum*, element). Any one of the simple substances that make up all compounds.

environment (in vī' rən mənt) (L. *in*, in; *viron*, circle). The complex of all factors that act upon an organism or an ecological community and ultimately determine its form and survival.

fission (fish'ən) (L. *fissio*, to cleave). The splitting of the nucleus of an atom, releasing a great quantity of energy.

food chain. The transfer of mass and energy from one organism to another by eating and being eaten.

fusion (fyoo'zhən) (L. *fusio*, from *fundere*, to pour). The union of material into one body or mass.

genetic dose (jə net'ik). The amount of irradiation needed to affect the gonads, germ cells, or embryos produced by an individual.

half-life. The time in which the radioactivity originally associated with an isotope will be reduced by one half through radioactive decay.

isotope (ī'sə tōp) (G. *isos*, equal; *topos*, place). An element of a chemical character identical with that of another element, occupying the same place in the periodic table, but differing from it in other characteristics, as in radioactivity or in the mass of its atoms.

megaton (meg'ə tun) (G. *megas*, large). A million tons.

nucleus (nyoo'klē əs) (L. *nucleus*, a kernel). In nuclear technology, that part of an atom in which the total positive electric charge resides. It contains the protons and neutrons.

pesticide residue (rez' i dū) (L. *residuus*, remaining). A quantity of a pesticide remaining on a food product from treatments given it during its growing or processing.

photochemical (fō'tō kem'i kəl) (G. *photos*, light; chemistry). Pertaining to the effect of radiant energy in producing chemical changes.

pollutant (pə lut'ənt) (L. *pollutio*, to defile). Something that pollutes or unfavorably alters the environment.

pollution (pə loo'shən) (L. *pollutio*, to defile). Act of defiling or making impure.

radiation (rā dē ā'shən) (L. *radiatio*, to emit rays). The emission and propagation of energy through space or through a material medium in the form of waves or particles.

radiotherapy (rā dē ō ther'ə pē) (L. *radio,* ray; *therapeia,* cure). The treatment of disease by x-ray, radium rays, etc.

toxicity (tok sis'i tē) (G. *toxikon,* a poison). Quality, state, or degree of being toxic or poisonous.

x-ray (Named by German physicist Wilhelm Conrad Roentgen in 1895 because he did not know the nature of the rays). Also called *roentgen rays.* Penetrating electromagnetic waves of radiation.

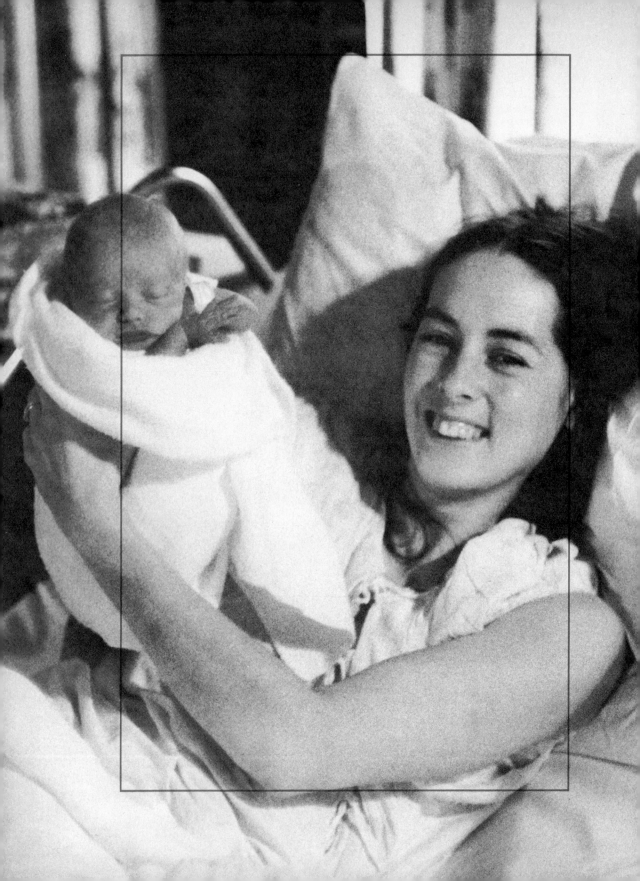

Human reproduction

Like almost all of the familiar plants and animals human beings reproduce by a *sexual* process, involving the fusion of specially produced sexual cells, the sperm and the egg. These mature sex cells are called *gametes*. The major biological importance of sexual reproduction is that it allows new genetic combinations each generation; throughout the course of evolution this has been an important means of bringing together favorable mutations in the offspring. Even some of the most primitive plant and animal forms, which ordinarily reproduce by such *asexual* means as merely dividing into two smaller but similar halves, can also reproduce sexually.

Why such a basic and universal process should have become a source of prudery and embarrassment to many individuals is a matter of speculation. Perhaps the very fact that sexual intercourse is a source of great human pleasure has contributed to some of these attitudes about sex. If sex were still viewed in light of the concept that pleasure is evil, then some of the remaining puritanical attitudes about sex might be justified, but today's enlightened individual considers sex not only important in reproduction but also very legitimate and an important source of pleasure in marriage. That person gives his children a thorough and factual understanding of the reproductive processes and, because his child lives with well-adjusted, loving parents, that child gains a healthful attitude toward sex and the total relationship between man and wife.

HUMAN REPRODUCTIVE SYSTEMS

The differences between the outward anatomical structures of the male and female are quite simple compared with the internal differences; see Fig. 11.1. In this section we shall examine the major physiological processes of reproduction in human beings.

The male reproductive system

The male reproductive system, described in the paragraphs below, is illustrated by Figs. 11.2 to 11.5.

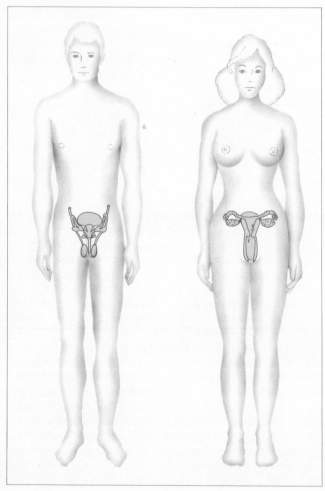

Figure 11.1   The male and female human bodies.

Testis The primary reproductive organs of either sex are called the *gonads*. The gonads of the male consist of a pair of *testes*, often called *testicles*. The testes serve a dual function, producing both *sperm* (the male gametes) and the male sex hormone *testosterone*. Human sperm cells, or *spermatozoa*, are microscopically small, each measuring about 50 microns (thousandths of a millimeter) in length. Each sperm consists of a *head*, which contains the genetic material, a *neck*, a *middle piece*, and a *tail* with which it swims. Sperm cells secrete the enzyme *hyaluronidase*, required for penetration of the egg. Although only one sperm actually will penetrate and fertilize an egg, many millions of sperms are required to secrete enough hyaluronidase for fertilization to occur. This important requirement will be discussed further in the discussion of fertility problems.

Each testis is composed of about eight hundred narrow, twisted tubes called *seminiferous tubules*. In the inner lining of each tubule the spermatozoa are produced by a special type of cell division, *meiosis* (also to be discussed later in this chapter). The production of sperm cells continues at a constant rate from puberty (the time of sexual maturity) often until a very advanced age. There is no definite cessation of sexual activity in the male, although the sexual *processes* gradually decline with age.

Between the seminiferous tubules lie the *interstitial cells*, which produce testosterone. Testosterone production begins in adolescence in response to the production of *gonadotropic hormone* by the anterior lobe of the pituitary gland, located at the base of the brain. Testosterone stimulates the development of the male reproductive system and the secondary masculine charac-

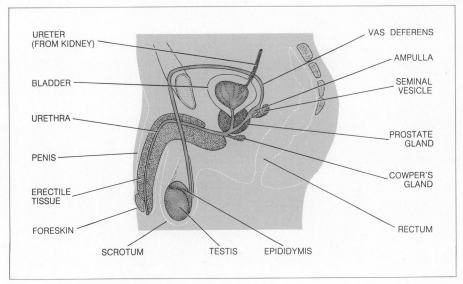

Figure 11.2 Male reproductive system, side view.

teristics, such as the beard, body hair, and muscle formation. The production of testosterone continues throughout life.

In the human being, as in most mammals, the production of spermatozoa cannot occur at the temperature found within the body cavity. For this reason just prior to birth the testes descend from the abdomen into the *scrotum*, a saclike structure suspended at the base of the abdomen. The temperature within the scrotum is maintained at 3 to 4 degrees below body temperature by muscles within the scrotum, which draw the testes up tight against the body in response to cold or relax, allowing the testes to fall away from the body in response to high temperature. Occasionally one or both of the testes fails to descend into the scrotum, a condition which results in partial or total *sterility* caused by a lack of sperm production, although the production of the hormone testosterone is not affected. An undescended testis usually can be corrected surgically, with resulting normal fertility.

Epididymis   Attached to each testis is a long (18 to 20 feet), tightly coiled tube, the *epididymis*. The epididymis is a storage structure that holds the maturing sperm cells until they are discharged from the body. The sperm cells remain alive for 30 to 60 days, after which they die and disintegrate.

Vas deferens   The vas deferens are small ducts carrying sperm upward from each epididymis into the abdomen. Constriction of the vas deferens is a common cause of sterility in the male. Surgical sterilization of the male usually consists of cutting or tying off each vas deferens. Near the end of each

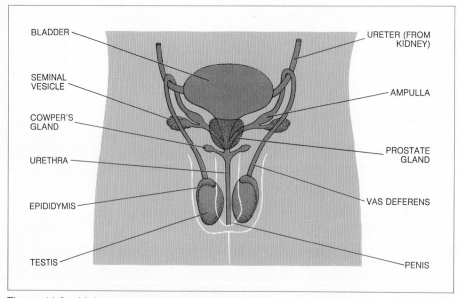

Figure 11.3   Male reproductive system, front view.

vas deferens is an enlarged section called the *ampulla*, which, like the epididymis, serves for storage of sperm.

Fluid-producing glands Sperm cells make up only a small portion of the male ejaculate, or *semen*, which is composed of sperm cells plus the fluid secretions of several glands. The most important fluid-producing glands are the *seminal vesicles*, one of which empties into the upper end of each vas deferens at the ampulla. The second source of fluid is the single *prostate gland*. The two vas deferens and the duct carrying urine from the urinary bladder unite within the prostate gland. The single duct, which now carries both semen and urine from the prostate to the tip of the penis, is called the *urethra*. Emptying by ducts into the urethra near the base of the penis are a pair of small glands, *Cowper's glands*. In response to sexual stimulation Cowper's glands produce a few drops of a clear, lubricating fluid, which prepares the urethra for ejaculation and is of some slight importance in lubricating during intercourse.

External genitalia The male organ of intercourse is the penis, so adapted as to deposit semen within the vagina of the female. In order that intercourse may occur, it is necessary that the penis become hard and erect. *Erection* is made possible because the penis is made of a special spongy, erectile tissue, highly supplied with blood vessels. In response to sexual stimulation the veins carrying blood away from the penis are constricted, causing the spongy tissue to become engorged with blood. Thus, it is the blood pressure of the male which is responsible for erection. The inability to attain erection is called

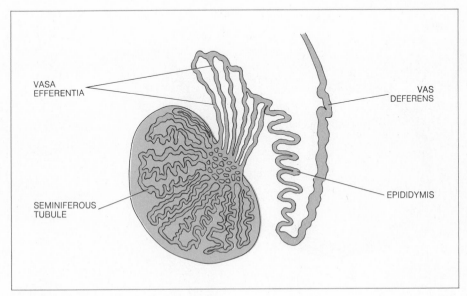

Figure 11.4 Structure of human testis.

impotence or *impotency;* it may be the result of either physical or psychological factors. Impotency, the inability to carry out sexual intercourse, must not be confused with *sterility,* a deficiency of sperm cells in the semen. A man can be sterile yet fully potent.

Sexual intercourse   The climax of sexual intercourse in the male consists of *ejaculation,* accompanied by *orgasm.* Ejaculation is the expulsion of semen, brought about by muscular contractions of the ampullae, seminal vesicles, and urethra. Orgasm in both the male and female is the intensely pleasant sensation which comes at the peak, or *climax,* of intercourse.

The average male tends to come to orgasm more rapidly than the female. By restricting motion the male can delay orgasm so that it occurs about the same time for both. Achieving simultaneous orgasm is really not necessary for the enjoyment of orgasm. Although some couples are more successful than others, most of the time it does not happen this way. If it does, it can be a spectacular highlight of intercourse. But more important is that both achieve orgasm if possible. After orgasm the male generally is fatigued, loses his sexual desires, and his penis usually loses its erection. The female, on the other hand, is capable of multiple orgasms over a short period of time.

Nocturnal emissions   A normal, virile male with limited sex experience may find periodic, involuntary sexual release in nocturnal emissions, or "wet dreams." These are releases of seminal fluid and are usually accompanied by dreams relating to sex. They result from the natural accumulation of the fluid in the seminal vesicles. A normal occurrence, they are typically marked with pleasurable sensations.

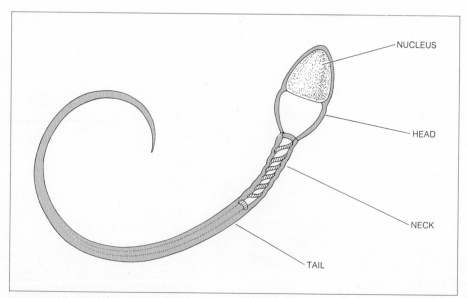

Figure 11.5   Human sperm cell.

The female reproductive system

The female reproductive system, described in the paragraphs below, is illustrated by Figs. 11.6 to 11.8.

Ovary   The primary reproductive organs, or gonads, of the female consist of a pair of *ovaries*. Unlike the testes, the ovaries function at the internal abdominal temperature and are carried in the abdomen, but like the testes, they serve a dual function, producing both eggs and hormones. Both these functions will be discussed in the section of this chapter that covers the menstrual cycle.

Fallopian tube   The duct that carries the egg from each ovary to the uterus is called the *fallopian tube*, or *oviduct*. As may be seen in Fig. 11.7, the fallopian tube does not make a closed connection with the ovary but is flared open near the ovary, with numerous fingerlike projections called *fimbria*. The inner lining of the fallopian tube is covered with countless microscopic hairlike

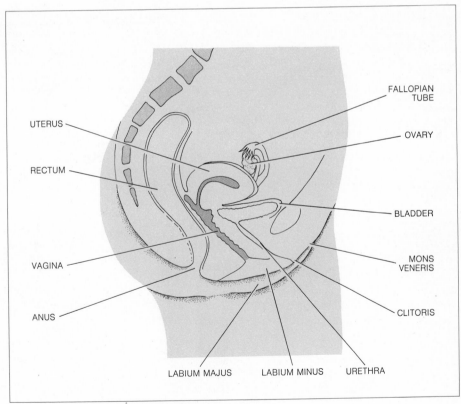

Figure 11.6   Female reproductive system, side view.

projections called *cilia*. When an egg bursts forth from the ovary (*ovulation*) it is caught by the fimbria and slowly carried down the oviduct by the cilia. One of the more common causes of sterility in the female is obstruction of the fallopian tube.

Uterus The *uterus*, sometimes called the *womb*, is specialized for the growth and protection of the unborn child. The nonpregnant uterus is about the size and shape of a pear, with thick muscular walls. Its necklike portion, which extends down to the vagina, is called the *cervix*, which means *neck*. The inner lining of the uterus, heavily supplied with blood vessels, is the *endometrium*; it is shed at each menstrual period.

Vagina The *vagina* is the female organ of sexual intercourse and also the *birth canal*. It is a very flexible muscular tube, 4 to 6 inches long, lined with mucous membrane. The vagina is provided with numerous small mucus-producing glands, which upon sexual arousal provide lubricating materials for intercourse. A few women produce insufficient lubricating material and require the use of additional lubricant for intercourse.

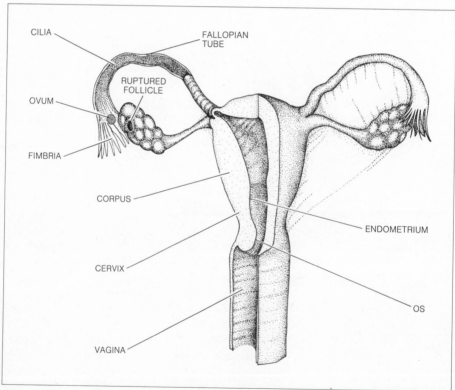

Figure 11.7 Female reproductive system, front view.

External genitalia The opening of the vagina is surrounded by two pairs of *labia* (lips), also called *vulva:* the outer, and larger, *labia majora* and the inner *labia minora* (Fig. 11.7). The external opening of the urethra lies forward of the vaginal opening, between the right and left labia minora, about halfway between the vaginal opening and the clitoris; the clitoris, about the size of a pea, is a small, erectile structure located above the urethral opening, at the junction of the right and left labia majora. Somewhat analogous to the male penis, it is highly supplied with sensory nerve endings and erectile tissue and is the most intense center of sexual sensation in the female. It rarely exceeds one inch in length.

A partial membrane, the *hymen* ("maidenhead"), may be present around the opening of the vagina. The hymen varies in size and thickness and may remain intact until the first mating. It may, however, be greatly reduced in size before mating by the use of tampons (a vaginal insertion used during menstrual discharge), by a physician as a part of a medical examination, or through participation in active sports. During a premarital examination the physician can determine whether the hymen will present a barrier to inter-

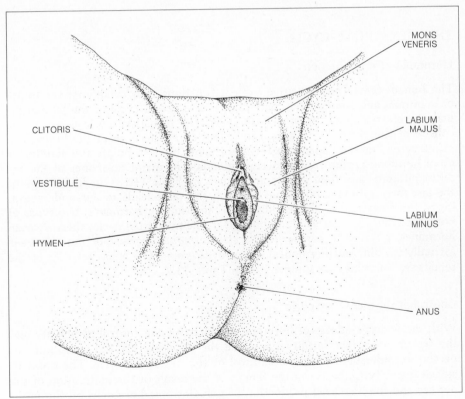

Figure 11.8 Female external genital organs.

course and, if so, surgically cut it. The presence or absence of the hymen should not be regarded as proof or lack of virginity.

Sexual intercourse The enlightened female expects to receive and does receive pleasure through intercourse that is at least equal to that of the male. For her to receive maximal pleasure skill and consideration are required on the part of her husband. He must understand that the female is often more slowly aroused than the male and requires time prior to penetration to prevent pain and often a longer duration of intercourse to achieve orgasm. Erotic response in the female can originate in almost any part of the body, especially the breasts; it is the husband's duty to find and stimulate responsive areas of the wife. The length of the penis does not influence the degree of pleasure in the female, since the nerve endings which respond during intercourse are most concentrated in the clitoris, abundant in the labia and lower vagina, but absent higher in the vagina.

Orgasm in the female involves no release of fluids but consists of rhythmic contractions of the muscles of the vagina and highly pleasant diffuse sensations. Unlike the male, females can achieve *multiple orgasm,* or orgasm several times in rapid succession.

THE MENSTRUAL CYCLE

Hormones of reproduction

The human female reproductive system functions in a cyclic manner found only in man and some of the higher apes. The sexual cycle of the human female is referred to as the *menstrual cycle.* The menstrual cycle is under the control of the *anterior pituitary gland,* located at the base of the brain. The pituitary or "master" gland secretes hormones that stimulate the activity of other hormone-producing (endocrine) glands. The major hormones of the anterior pituitary and their effects are shown in Table 11.1. Our knowledge of the last three pituitary hormones listed in the table leads to our understanding of the menstrual cycle. In addition to the pituitary hormones, two types of hormone from the ovaries are important in the menstrual cycle; these ovarian hormones, referred to as the *female sex hormones,* consist of the *estrogens* (actually six different hormones) and *progesterone.* The characteristics of the female sex hormones are summarized in Table 11.2.

Control of the menstrual cycle

With the widespread use of hormone products for the control of fertility and the treatment of low fertility has come the necessity for the well-informed person to understand hormonal control of the menstrual cycle. The onset of sexual maturity (puberty) in the female is the result of the maturation of the ovaries and the increased production of gonadotropic hormones by the pituitary gland. The first menstrual period, called the *menarche,* usually occurs

Table 11.1 *Anterior pituitary hormones*

hormone		effect
Somatotropic hormone (STH)		Stimulates growth of bones and muscles.
Thyrotropic hormone (TSH)		Stimulates the thyroid gland to produce thyroxin.
Adrenocorticotropic hormone (ACTH)		Stimulates adrenal cortex to produce its hormones.
Follicle-stimulating hormone (FSH)[a]	*Ovary:*	Stimulates growth of egg follicle and production of *estrogens*.
	Testis:	Promotes sperm production.
Luteinizing hormone (LH), also called interstitial cell-stimulating hormone (ICSH) in male[a]	*Ovary:*	Causes ovulation; causes a ruptured follicle to become *corpus luteum* and produce the hormone *progesterone*.
	Testis:	Stimulates production of the hormone *testosterone*.
Luteotropic hormone (LTH), also called *prolactin*[a]	*Ovary:*	Causes corpus luteum to secrete increased amounts of both estrogens and progesterone during latter half of menstrual cycle.
	Testis:	Function unknown.
	Breast:	Promotes secretion of milk after birth of child.

[a] Called a gonadtropic hormone because it stimulates the ovaries or testes.

between ages eleven and fifteen in American girls, the average age being about thirteen. Menarche occurs earlier in the United States than in most other countries, perhaps as a result of good nutrition.

Menstrual cycles take place, except during pregnancies, from puberty until their cessation at about the age of forty-seven. The cause of this cessation, called *menopause,* is not fully understood but seems to be due to a "burning out" of the ovaries rather than a change in the pituitary. At the time of birth the ovaries of the average woman contain about four thousand immature *egg* (or *Graafian*) *follicles.* During her reproductive years a woman will mature one egg follicle per menstrual cycle for a total lifetime production of about four hundred mature eggs (*ova*). The remainder of the immature follicles gradually degenerate, until by the time a woman is forty-five or fifty none remain to respond at a very high level to the gonadotropic hormones, since the production of estrogens by the ovaries drops to almost nothing. This loss of estrogens causes the characteristic complications of menopause, such as "hot flashes," irritability, anxiety, and fatigue. Such symptoms are often treated today through hormone therapy and also psychotherapy, since they are often partially psychosomatic.

The events of the menstrual cycle are presented graphically in Figs. 11.9 and 11.10. The average menstrual cycle is 28 days in length, although there

Table 11.2 *Characteristics of the female sex hormones*

hormone	source	function
Estrogens	Ovary (egg follicle); placenta during pregnancy	Growth of the female sexual organs and promotion of secondary sexual characteristics of the female, such as breasts, hair distribution, voice, bone structure. Growth of the endometrium; inhibits production of FSH, increases production of LH.
Progesterone	Ovary (corpus luteum, the ruptured egg follicle); placenta during pregnancy	Primary function is to maintain endometrium of uterus for fertilized egg. Causes swelling of breasts, but not milk production. Causes salt and water retention in body. Inhibits production of LH.

is great variation between different women and sometimes between different cycles in the same woman. Many physical and emotional factors can result in prolonged or irregular menstrual cycles. It is customary to refer to the first day of the menstrual period (menstruation) as day 1 of the menstrual cycle. *Menstruation* is the sloughing off, or shedding, of the endometrium. The usual duration of the menstrual period is three to six days, the average being four or five days.

During and after menstruation the production of FSH by the pituitary reaches its highest level. Under the influence of FSH one of the immature egg follicles (in either ovary) grows much larger, from a mere pinpoint to nearly a third of an inch in diameter. Inside the fluid-filled follicle is a maturing egg. The maturing follicle secretes much *estrogen*, which causes the endometrium of the uterus to thicken in preparation for the egg. The estrogen also feeds back to the pituitary gland, where it inhibits further secretion of FSH but stimulates production of LH. When the LH level in the blood reaches a certain critical level, the mature follicle bursts (*ovulation*), expelling the egg into the abdominal cavity, where it is picked up by the fimbria of the fallopian tube. Ovulation occurs an average of 14 days after the beginning of menstruation, although it commonly takes place from the ninth to the eighteenth day; it is known in rare cases to take place outside these limits and even during menstruation. After ovulation the egg travels slowly down the fallopian tube, carried by the cilia lining the tube. At this point the woman is fertile—capable of becoming pregnant. Although some reports differ, it is usually agreed that the egg remains viable (capable of being fertilized) for about 2 days. The total trip down the fallopian tube takes about 6 days, so if the egg is to be fertilized, the sperm must meet it in the upper portion of the fallopian tube.

If the egg is not fertilized, it continues down the fallopian tube to the uterus, where it disintegrates. The human egg is about the size of the period after this sentence and forms no significant part of the menstrual flow. After ovulation the empty follicle, under the influence of LH, recloses and becomes the *corpus luteum.* Then under the direction of LH and LTH the corpus luteum produces the hormone *progesterone,* which serves to mature the endometrium and to prevent its being sloughed off (menstruation). A reciprocal relationship exists between the levels of progesterone and LH and LTH similar to that between estrogen and FSH. As the level of progesterone in the blood increases, the production of LH and LTH is suppressed. As the level of LH and LTH in the blood drops, the corpus luteum degenerates, ceasing to produce progesterone; then menstruation occurs.

If the egg is fertilized, it continues down the fallopian tube, dividing and redividing into 2 cells, then 4, 8, 16, and so on, until by the time it reaches the uterus it consists of a hollow ball of cells resembling a tiny mulberry; see Fig. 11.11. Within 10 days after fertilization the egg (now the *embryo*) implants itself in the uterus by digesting the upper cell layers of the endometrium. Soon after implantation the embryo begins to produce a *gonadotropic hormone,* which functions much like the combination of LH and LTH in stimulating the corpus luteum to produce estrogen and progesterone. Instead of degenerating, the corpus luteum continues to grow and function for about the first 12 weeks of pregnancy. Its continued production of estrogen and progesterone causes the endometrium to continue growing, instead of de-

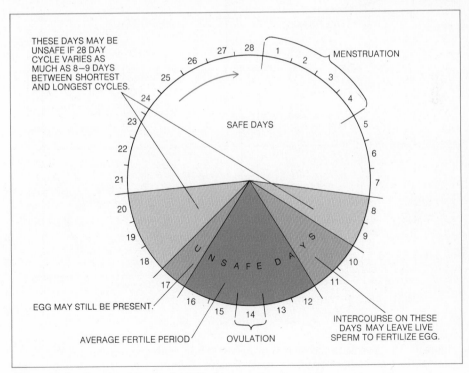

Figure 11.9   Events of the typical 28-day menstrual cycle.

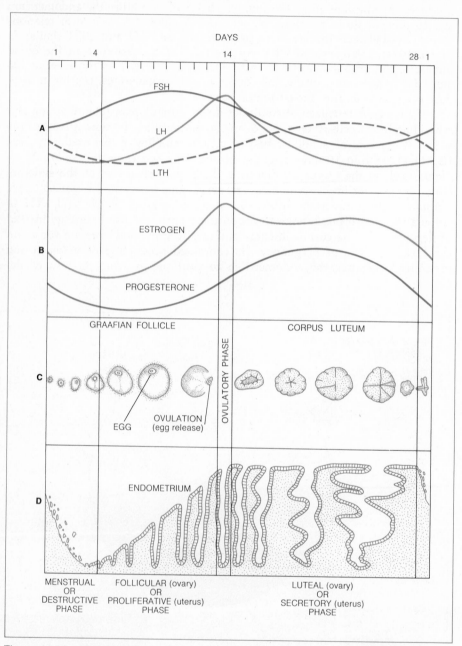

Figure 11.10   Events of the menstrual cycle: (A) pituitary gonadotropic hormones; (B) ovarian hormones; (C) development of egg (ovum); (D) changes in thickness of endometrium of uterus and development of endometrial glands.

generating, as in menstruation. The sustained high level of estrogen and progesterone also prevents further egg-follicle maturation and ovulation.

PREGNANCY

Embryology

A full-term human pregnancy usually lasts about 266 days from conception, or about 280 days after the beginning of the last menstrual period. During the first 8 weeks of pregnancy the developing child is called the *embryo*; be-

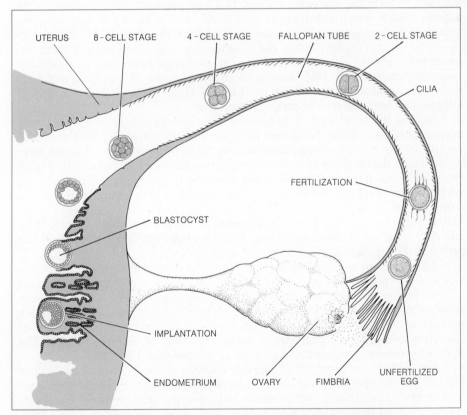

Figure 11.11 Stages of development of zygote. The egg escapes from the follicle in the ovary, is picked up by the fallopian tube, and is fertilized by a sperm cell. It moves through the tube, into the uterus, and implants (buries) into the endometrium 6–8 days after fertilization. During this time the zygote divides into 2 cells, then 4, 8, and finally into a hollow ball of cells called a blastocyst.

yond 8 weeks it is called the *fetus*. The study of the unborn child is the fascinating science of *embryology*. Today very little mystery remains regarding this aspect of human life.

The fertilized egg (*zygote*) very quickly begins cell division (*mitosis*) and becomes a multicelled *embryo* by the time it reaches the uterus. Unlike a bird egg, the human egg carries very little stored food. During the first 8 weeks of pregnancy, the embryo obtains most of its nutrition through digesting the surrounding endometrium by means of special *trophoblastic cells*, the same cells which have enabled the embryo to implant itself. The processes of *mitosis* and *meiosis* may be studied with the aid of Figs. 11.18 and 11.19. (See pp. 323 and 324.)

During the early weeks of pregnancy the embryo surrounds itself with several membranes the most important being the *amnion*, or "bag of waters," which cushions the fetus, and the *chorion*, which interlocks with the endometrium to form the placenta; see Fig. 11.13 on page 305. The *placenta* is the organ through which the fetus is nourished from 8 weeks of age until the termination of pregnancy. The fetus is attached to the placenta by the *umbilical cord*, which contains veins and arteries carrying blood to and from the placenta. It should be emphasized that no exchange or mixing of blood between the mother and child takes place in the placenta. All exchange of food and waste products between the mother and child takes place by means of diffusion through the membranes of the placenta.

During the latter part of pregnancy the placenta serves as an extremely important source of the hormones *estrogen* and *progesterone*. By the end of pregnancy the estrogen production reaches 50 to 60 times that of a nonpregnant woman, while the progesterone production increases 10 times. The higher levels of these hormones cause many changes in the body of the woman, which better adapt her for pregnancy and childbirth. For example, the uterus and external genitalia enlarge, breasts enlarge, and pelvic ligaments relax. When pregnancy is full term, the placenta is a flat disc, about 1 inch thick and 6 to 9 inches in diameter. After delivery of the child the placenta is expelled as the *afterbirth*.

The pregnant woman has a great and understandable curiosity about the size and appearance of her child at the various stages of its development. Let us then briefly describe the embryo or fetus after each month of its development. Pregnancies are customarily measured in *lunar months*, four-week periods which correspond to menstrual cycles. It is also common to speak of the *three trimesters* of pregnancy, each consisting of thirteen weeks. The month-by-month development proceeds as follows; see Fig. 11.12.

End of first lunar month (4 weeks). Embryo about ¼ inch long, including tail (all young vertebrate embryos have tails); head very large in proportion to body, mouth and jaw present, but no eyes, ears, or nose; backbone formed, curved until head almost touches tail; small buds of arms and legs; heart formed and beating.

End of second lunar month (8 weeks). Embryo now unmistakably human and from this point on is called a *fetus*; about 1 inch long; head large, face human, eyes, ears, and nose visible; arms and legs more developed, webbed hands and feet present; tail starting to be absorbed.

End of third lunar month (12 weeks). Fetus now over 3 inches long, weight 1 ounce; sex distinguishable; fingernails and toenails appear; movements occur but are too weak to be felt by mother.

End of fourth lunar month (16 weeks). Length now 6¼ inches, weight 4 ounces; fine hair appears on body; some women feel movements ("quickening"); skeleton may be visible on x-ray examination.

End of fifth lunar month (20 weeks). Length 9½ inches, weight 11 ounces; mother definitely feels movement; with a stethoscope the fetal heartbeats can now be heard through mother's abdomen.

End of sixth lunar month (24 weeks). Length 12 inches, weight 1½ pounds; skin wrinkled and red; head large in proportion to body, eyebrows and lashes formed, eyelids have opened; if born, almost no chance for survival.

End of seventh lunar month (28 weeks). Length about 14 inches, weight about 2½ pounds; if born, chance of survival about 1 in 10.

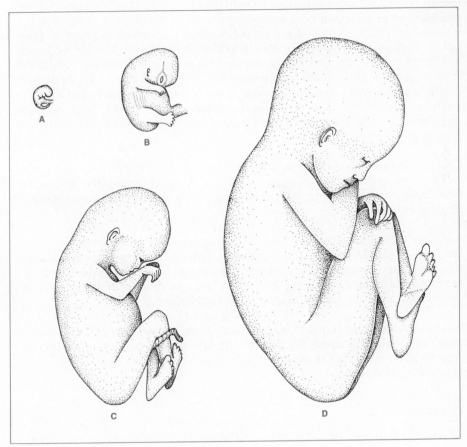

Figure 11.12   Series of human embryos: (A) at 4 weeks; (B) at 8 weeks; (C) at 12 weeks; (D) at 16 weeks.

End of eighth lunar month (32 weeks). Length about 16 inches, weight about 3½ pounds; hair on head is more abundant; if born, good chance of survival.

End of ninth lunar month (36 weeks). Length about 18 inches, weight about 6 pounds; now a fully mature infant; survival rate almost same as full term.

End of tenth lunar month (40 weeks). Full-term infant; average length about 20 inches, average weight 7 pounds if girl, 7½ if boy; see Fig. 11.13.

These weight and length figures are averages; there are considerable variations in both. Normal babies commonly vary in weight from 5 to 11 pounds. Boys tend to be slightly heavier than girls.

Labor contractions may begin about the fortieth week.

Early signs of pregnancy

Cessation of menstruation   For a healthy woman with a history of regular menstrual cycles the cessation of menstruation is often the first sign of pregnancy. Even in a woman with a very regular cycle, however, a delay of a few days in menstruation should not be automatically accepted as proof of pregnancy. Pregnancy as the cause should seldom be seriously considered before a delay of at least ten days has occurred. Absence of menstruation may result from many conditions other than pregnancy. Emotional upset very commonly delays menstruation, especially when there is fear of pregnancy. Other influencing factors are change of climate, extreme cold, anemia, and hormone imbalance. By the time the second period has been missed, the chance of pregnancy is strong.

Changes in the breasts   The swelling of the breasts, normally occurring prior to each menstrual period, is exaggerated in early pregnancy. The breasts become larger and fuller and may have a heavy feeling besides a throbbing or tingling sensation.

Frequent urination   Early in pregnancy the enlarged uterus presses against the urinary bladder, giving the impression that the bladder is always full. As the pregnancy progresses, the uterus rises away from the bladder and this symptom disappears, returning during the last two months of the pregnancy, when the head of the fetus presses against the bladder.

Nausea   About two thirds of all pregnant women experience some nausea or vomiting, beginning about the time of the first missed period and lasting for four to six weeks. This is often called "morning sickness," but it may occur at any time of the day.

Pregnancy tests

The married woman usually waits until about the time of the second missed menstrual period before she visits her physician. By that time he can usually diagnose pregnancy through visible changes in the skin, breasts, vagina, and uterus. If it is important to confirm pregnancy before this time, tests can diagnose pregnancy with a high degree of accuracy when the menstrual period has been delayed about two weeks. Several of the commonly used pregnancy tests depend upon the presence of the hormone *chorionic gonadotropin* in the urine or blood of the pregnant woman. The urine or blood is injected into a test animal (mouse, rabbit, frog, or toad); if the hormone is present, characteristic changes occur, depending on the type of animal.

In another type of test oral tablets containing estrogen and progesterone are administered for three days and then discontinued. If menstruation does not occur within fifteen days, there is a very strong possibility that pregnancy exists.

Three *positive* tests of pregnancy are fetal heartbeat, detection of active movements of the fetus, and ability to see the fetal skeleton by x-ray.

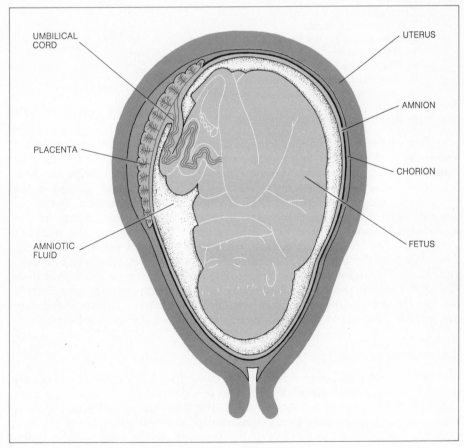

Figure 11.13   Fetus at end of tenth lunar month (full term).

Complications of pregnancy

It is impossible to overemphasize the importance of proper care of the pregnant woman. She must be under the care of a qualified physician, and she must take excellent care of herself. The quality of prenatal care can influence, not only the health and comfort of the woman, but also the future welfare of the child. The physician can detect many possible complications of pregnancy in their very early stages and can often prevent such complications from becoming a serious threat to the health of the mother or the child.

Between her routine visits to the physician there are certain possible danger signs in pregnancy to which the woman should be alert. If *any* of the following symptoms appear, she should make an immediate report to her physician:

1. Vaginal bleeding, no matter how slight
2. Regular pains or contractions in abdomen
3. Sudden escape of water from vagina
4. Chills and fever
5. Extreme shortness of breath
6. Symptoms of toxemia:
   a. Severe continuous headache
   b. Dizzy spells
   c. Dimness or blurring of vision
   d. Persistent vomiting (in later part of pregnancy)
   e. Swelling of face, hands, ankles, fingers, feet
   f. Rapid gain in weight
   g. Reduced urine output

One of the most common complications of pregnancy is the condition known as *toxemia*. This is a condition that seldom appears before the last three months of pregnancy. About 7 percent of all late pregnancies are complicated by toxemia. Although the word by derivation means "poison in the blood," no such poison has ever been isolated, and it is generally agreed today that none is involved. The causes of toxemia are not clear; it may be due to antigenic substances that have crossed from the fetus into the mother's circulation. The condition is characterized by high blood pressure, swelling, and protein in the urine. If allowed to become severe it may result in convulsions, coma, and even death. Susceptible pregnant women must limit their salt intake, which should regulate water intake. Treatment may also include plenty of rest and drugs to reduce swelling. Fortunately, early prenatal care can provide adequate detection and early management of the condition.

Diet in pregnancy

In order to safeguard her own health as well as that of her child, the pregnant woman needs to pay careful attention to her diet. The one thing she must *not* do is to "eat for two." According to the Recommended Dietary Allowances, the pregnant woman needs significantly increased quantities of protein, vitamins, and minerals but *only slightly increased* food energy (calories). She must greatly curtail her consumption of sweet, starchy, or fatty foods, concentrating on those foods which yield large amounts of proteins, vitamins, and minerals in proportion to their caloric value. She must be particularly careful to meet her daily 78-gram protein requirement. This protein requirement can be met through daily consumption of a quart of skim milk, one egg, and two average servings of lean meat. A quart of nonfat milk yields almost half the daily protein requirement, along with important calcium, yet is relatively low in calories.

One of the problems in pregnancy is maternal weight gain. Many women have concern over maintaining their prepregnant figure. Yet it is now believed that the practice of limiting pregnant women to a weight gain of only 10 to 14 pounds may be one reason for the high infant mortality rate in the United States. The higher the maternal weight gain, the higher the infant's birth weight and the better his growth and performance record during his first year of life. The National Research Council now recommends an average weight gain of 20 to 25 pounds for most women. One study showed an average pregnant gain of pounds to consist of the following:

Baby	7¼
Placenta	1
Amniotic fluid	1½
Increase in weight of uterus	2
Increase in weight of breasts	2–3
Water storage	5
Protein storage	4

Only about 11 pounds of this weight is lost with delivery. Some weight is lost within the next several weeks. Any excess weight will be likely to remain permanently. As a consequence, many women grow heavier with each child while other women—after multiple pregnancies—retain the figure of fashion models.

Terminations of pregnancy

Since most pregnancies terminate in the uncomplicated, spontaneous delivery of a full-term infant, let us first consider such a delivery. Many women look forward to their first delivery with considerable apprehension or even with fear; yet, looking back at the same event, they can find nothing to justify such emotions. Perhaps it will be a young woman's first hospitalization, in which case she may fear the unknown world of the hospital. Some women worry about not getting to the hospital in time, although such cases are so rare that they receive much newspaper attention. Other women worry about the delivery itself; yet childbirth today has been refined to the point that it presents little hazard to either the mother or the child.

The stages of labor   The word *labor* is used to describe the muscular contractions of the uterus through which the infant is expelled. Labor is divided into three rather distinct stages: the preparatory period, or *first stage*, the birth of the baby, or *second stage,* and the delivery of the placenta (afterbirth), or *third stage;* see Fig. 11.14.

· FIRST STAGE   The preparatory stage lasts from the first labor contractions until the baby is ready to be born, an average period of about 13 hours in first deliveries and about 8 hours in subsequent deliveries. Shorter or longer labors are not uncommon, nor are they abnormal. At first the contractions are weak, infrequent (every 40 or 50 minutes), and irregular. Gradually they become more frequent, more regular, and stronger. When the contractions occur at intervals of 5 to 15 minutes and last for 30 seconds or longer, the physician will probably recommend that the woman go to the hospital, following a prearranged plan. Near the end of the first stage of labor the cervix opens from a narrow slit into a wide passageway.

· SECOND STAGE   The second stage of labor begins with the dilation of the cervix and lasts until the baby is born, an average period of 50 minutes in first deliveries and about 30 minutes in subsequent ones. If the amniotic membrane has not broken late in the first stage of labor, it breaks early in the second. A small incision, *episiotomy*, is almost always made in the *peri-*

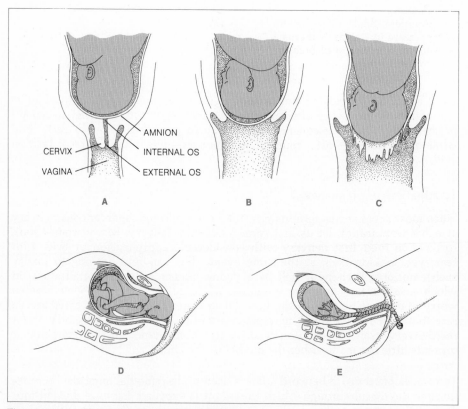

Figure 11.14   Normal delivery: (A) cervix before dilation; (B) cervix fully dilated; (C) rupture of the amnion; (D) birth of the head; (E) delivery of the placenta. Conditions A and B here correspond roughly to the first stage of labor, C and D to the second, and E to the third.

neum (floor of the pelvis), in the region extending back from the vagina toward the anus, to prevent its tearing and to make delivery easier. Once the head of the infant appears, the remainder of the delivery is usually quite rapid.

• THIRD STAGE   The final stage of labor consists of the expulsion of the afterbirth (placenta). It lasts 5 to 6 minutes and is accomplished with little or no pain. After the birth of the child the wall of the uterus greatly shrinks, causing the placenta to break loose. A few mild contractions of the uterus bring about its expulsion.

Anesthesia in childbirth   Pain is normally involved in the delivery of a child. The amount of discomfort can be reduced by preparing the mother. This preparation should include an understanding of the physical and emotional aspects of delivery. Learning controlled relaxation and breathing before delivery can reduce muscle spasms during labor. Such natural methods to reduce childbirth discomfort are referred to as *natural childbirth.*

Natural childbirth is based upon the fact that much (but not all) of the pain in childbirth is the result of fear and tension and that these are the result of lack of understanding of the birth process. Thus natural childbirth is a matter of preeducation of the pregnant woman regarding all aspects of childbirth and special exercises to strengthen the muscles that aid in delivery. Her physician may also need to coach her during labor in breathing and relaxing. Few women in the United States give birth in this manner without the benefit of any anesthesia.

Drugs are commonly used when the pain becomes too severe. Some drugs reduce the pain but allow the mother to remain conscious; others act only on selected parts of her body; some cause her to lose consciousness. Drugs may be injected into the spinal cord to deaden nerves of the uterus but not affect the woman's consciousness. The drugs used depend upon the wishes of the mother and the choice of the physician.

With mothers who are receptive to it hypnosis has been effective in allowing labor with little or no drugs. Although recognized by the American Medical Association, hypnosis has limited use. The procedure requires time and patient response.

Complications of delivery

Induced labor   Under special circumstances labor is sometimes brought about or strengthened through the use of oral or injected drugs. Such a procedure might be followed in severe cases of toxemia, diabetes, Rh incompatibility (discussed later), or prolonged and weak contractions. It must be emphasized that the drugs available for this purpose are effective only when the pregnancy is near full term; they are absolutely ineffective, and often dangerous, when used in an effort to produce abortion of an early pregnancy.

Forceps delivery   Forceps delivery, often called *instrument delivery*, is frequently used in the late stages of a difficult or prolonged labor or in presentations other than the usual head-first one. The forceps is a large, tonglike instrument with broad, flat, grasping surfaces, which fit around the head of the fetus. The physician then exerts a gentle pull and rotates the head.

Cesarean delivery   A *cesarean section* (spelled *caesarean* in Great Britain) is a major surgical procedure in which the infant is delivered through an incision in the lower abdomen and uterine wall. This type of delivery is advisable only when some condition is present that prevents normal vaginal delivery, such as too large a child for the birth canal, Rh complications, or the position of the child. As a general rule, one cesarean section limits a woman to this type of delivery for all future children, owing to the scar left on the uterus. Although many women have had more than three cesarean deliveries, the physician usually advises that the fallopian tubes be tied off at the time of the third cesarean delivery.

Extrauterine pregnancy   An extrauterine, or *ectopic*, pregnancy is one that develops outside the uterus. About 1 in 150 pregnancies is of this type. The most common site of ectopic pregnancy is the fallopian tube, although some occur within the abdominal cavity. Regardless of the place the egg lodges in the tube, the fetus usually aborts. The mother may feel severe abdominal pains and, if hemorrhaging occurs, she may show vaginal bleeding. In any event, the affected tube must be removed. This does not prevent later pregnancies, because the other fallopian tube is still available for egg transport.

Premature delivery   Premature delivery is the live birth of an infant before it is fully mature. A premature infant is one whose weight is 5½ pounds or less at delivery. The less an infant weighs at birth, the less its chances of survival. The survival chances are usually classified as follows:

1 lb 1 oz, or less	No chance of survival.
1 lb 2 oz, to 2 lb 2 oz	Extremely poor chance of survival.
2 lb 3 oz, to 5 lb 8 oz	Chances of survival range from poor to good, according to weight.
5 lb 9 oz, or more	Excellent chance of survival.

In terms of age of fetus, it may weigh 1 pound 1 ounce during the sixth lunar month (22 weeks) or 2 pounds 3 ounces at the end of 28 weeks. It is difficult to pinpoint the causes of premature delivery. Prematurity is the leading cause of infant mortality (death between birth and one year of age).

Abortion

The removal of a growing embryo or fetus from the wall of the uterus to which it is attached is defined as an *abortion*. A *natural abortion*, or "miscarriage," is the spontaneous termination of pregnancy by the body. It is believed that about 1 in 10 pregnancies ends in this manner. About 75 percent of these occur during the first 2 and 3 months of pregnancy. Common causes are an abnormally developing fetus, abnormalities of the placenta, and maternal disease. An *induced abortion* is legal or illegal, depending on state or national laws.

Legalized abortion   Early in 1973 the United States Supreme Court ruled that every woman in the United States, regardless of preexisting state laws, has the same right to an abortion during the first six months of pregnancy as she has to any other minor surgery. According to the decision, during the first three months of pregnancy the abortion decision must be left to the medical judgment of the pregnant woman's attending physician. After the first trimester, a state may regulate the abortion procedure in ways that are reasonably related to maternal health, for instance by requiring hospitalization. But it is illegal to demand that a panel of physicians approve the abortion. Only after the fetus has developed enough to have a chance of survival on its own, usually during the seventh month, may a state regulate and even proscribe abortion except where it is necessary for the preservation or health of the mother.

The court has held that a woman's right to privacy overcomes any state interest in using abortion statutes (as have some states) to regulate sexual conduct, even though indirectly. It also holds no legal right to life. Legal abortion during the first trimester is decidedly safer than childbirth. After that the dangers to the mother increase, and so the states' authority to protect the health of the mother increases also. The United States has thus joined Japan, India, the Soviet Union, and the majority of Eastern European countries in making abortion readily available.

There are several commonly used methods of aborting pregnancies. A *dilatation and curettage*, or 'D and C,' is a dilating of the cervix and a mild scraping of the inside of the uterus with a spoonlike curette; this method may be safe through the first 12 weeks of pregnancy. The most common method in early abortion is the *suction curettage*, or vacuum aspiration, a negative pressure being used to suck out the products of conception; it may be safely used through the first 12 weeks or, in conjunction with a D and C, through the first 17 weeks. Another method, called *saline injection*, is the introduction of a hypertonic solution of saline or glucose into the uterine cavity; the uterus starts to contract, and within one or two days the fetus and placenta should be expelled. It is the most common method of abortion performed after 16 weeks, and it may be used up to 24 weeks of pregnancy. The procedure usually takes one to three days. It can be difficult to use, the risk of complications being about three times higher than with the other two methods; the complications may include infection and retained placental tissue, often accompanied by fever or bleeding. A fourth method is *abdominal surgery*: a physician may either remove the fetus from the uterus by a cesareanlike section, *hysterotomy*, or remove the uterus, a procedure called *hysterectomy*. Used for pregnancies up through 26 weeks hysterotomy is about four times more likely to cause major complications than a saline solution. A most important point is that all these methods are safe *only* when handled by a qualified physician.

There is little danger to the mother when the procedure is performed at the proper time by a qualified physician in an aseptic hospital setting. According to some recent surveys, the mortality rate for legal abortions in the United States ranges from about 4.2 to 8.2 per 100,000 abortions. A rate of 4.2 represents less than one quarter the danger faced by a mother in normal childbirth. Early abortion (performed during the first 3 months) is far safer than childbirth, saline abortion is somewhat safer, while both hysterotomy and hysterectomy are riskier.

The costs of abortion vary widely. If a woman is eligible for Medicaid, it may cost her nothing. Some nonprofit clinics charge $125 to $150. The same procedure in a voluntary hospital may be about $200 for an early abortion. Late abortions usually include a hospital stay, so the price is higher. A saline abortion may cost about $350, whereas hysterotomies cost at least $800 and can cost considerably more. Insured members of certain health plans may now obtain abortions for as little as $40.00.

Few seek abortions for strictly medical reasons, such as their own health or suspected congenital abnormality of the fetus. Rape and incest account for few cases. Most requests are due to reluctance to interrupt career plans, lack of money, fear of losing personal freedom, or uncertainty about a relationship with the man involved. A few are due to psychiatric problems. Some are due to contraceptive accidents: a device improperly used, an ineffective device, or a changeover from one method of contraception to another.

Illegal abortion   Any induced abortion that is not specifically provided for by the laws of the state or country in which it is done is called an illegal (criminal) abortion. The recent Supreme Court decision has not made all abortions in the United States legal. Because it is a medical procedure, the state may require that it be performed only by a licensed physician, rather than by a dentist, chiropractor, barber, nurse, or midwife. During the second trimester the state may require that it be performed only in qualified institutions such as hospitals or clinics. The state may still regulate and even prohibit abortion after the seventh month except where it is necessary for the preservation or health of the mother (a *therapeutic abortion*). Such restriction is necessary in order to protect the health of the individual. Otherwise, permanent damage to the woman's reproductive organs, serious infections, and even death may result.

FERTILITY CONTROL

Almost every married couple has some type of fertility problem. For about 75 percent of all couples the problem is to control the excess fertility possessed by almost every species. Since almost every human born now lives to the age of sexual maturity and reproduction, it is no longer necessary to produce large numbers of offspring to ensure the survival and reproduction of a few.

Low fertility

For about 25 percent of married couples the frustrating problem of low fertility exists—difficulty in producing the desired number of children. *Sterility* is an absolute term indicating total inability to produce a child. About 10 percent of all couples in the United States face sterility in husband, wife, or both. *Fertility* is a relative term indicating the ease with which children are produced. The man who produces sperm in low numbers or the woman who ovulates very infrequently exhibits a relatively *low fertility*, but neither is sterile. About 15 percent of all couples in the United States are unable to have as many children as they wish. The probable outcome of efforts to conceive a child at various levels of fertility is summarized below:

Man and wife highly fertile	Prompt conception
Man and wife normally fertile	Conception within a few menstrual cycles
Fertility high in one, low in the other	Delay of several months likely
Fertility low in both man and wife	Conception after long delay or not at all
Either one or both sterile	Conception impossible

For every 100 cases of infertility, the wife is unable to conceive in 50, the husband is unable to induce conception in 30, and the problem is shared by both partners in 20. For a few couples the cause lies in a specific incompatibility or interaction between the individuals involved, with the possibility that each would be normally fertile with another partner. For example, the wife may produce specific antibodies that destroy the sperm of the husband. In the more common case, in which a structural problem makes conception difficult in a woman, she might be able to conceive with a highly fertile man but unable to conceive with a man having a lower sperm production.

The most common cause of low fertility among males is a low sperm count in the semen. The average volume of semen in an ejaculation is about 3 or 4 cubic centimeters, and the average sperm count is about 120 million in each cubic centimeter of semen. This means an average total of perhaps 400 million sperm per ejaculation. If the sperm count falls below about 40 or 50 million sperm per cubic centimeter, the male becomes less fertile than normal, his fertility decreasing progressively with any further diminishment in sperm count. A low sperm count is usually associated with a low level in the semen of the enzyme hyaluronidase, which is necessary for penetration of the egg. The sperm count can sometimes be raised and fertility improved through avoiding intercourse for about two weeks before ovulation is expected in the wife and then attempting to make the intercourse coincide with ovulation.

Low fertility in the female is complicated by her relatively brief periods of fertility. Sometimes the level of production of the pituitary gonadotropic hormones FSH and LH is so low that ovulation never occurs. Such cases may be treated through injection of gonadotropic hormones. Sometimes obstruction of the fallopian tubes prevents the egg from reaching the uterus or the sperm from reaching the egg. Occasionally the cervix of the uterus is so heavily plugged with mucus that the sperm cannot enter. In some cases the reason for the infertility of the female cannot be determined.

Artificial insemination

Artificial insemination, the injection of semen by syringe into the vagina or cervix, is sometimes resorted to when infertility results from a low sperm count in the husband. Occasionally the semen of the husband is collected over a period of time and preserved through refrigeration until an adequate amount is obtained for fertilization.

In other cases semen from a donor is used in artificial insemination. The identity of the donor should not be known to the couple. An effort is usually made to select a donor whose physical characteristics resemble the husband's. In addition to possible legal, moral, and religious objections to artificial insemination from a donor, there is a very great likelihood of psychological complications. The child may be distressed if told of his parentage; the parents may feel anxiety in either case. The greatest psychological risk is probably taken by the husband. Unless he is blessed with an unusual degree of maturity and self-confidence, he may see the child as a constant reminder of his inadequacy or become jealous of the biological father of the child. He may reject the child, feeling that it is more his wife's than his own. For most couples adoption is probably wiser than donor artificial insemination.

CONTRACEPTION

All normally fertile married couples must use some method of contraception or birth control if they are to space their children as they desire and limit the total number of children produced. Indeed, a very high percentage of married couples, regardless of religion, *do* make use of contraceptive methods. With the availability of today's highly effective contraceptive methods there is no medical justification for the conception of an unwanted child, with the resulting hardship and unhappiness for both the parents and child. The goal of those active in family planning is that *every* child conceived be a *wanted child*.

Mechanical contraception

Several types of device are designed mechanically to prevent the spermatozoa from reaching the ovum. Prior to the development of hormonal contraceptives, such devices were the most effective contraceptives available and were most often prescribed by physicians. Even today the popularity and use of mechanical contraception remains high.

Condom ("rubber") The condom is usually a synthetic rubber sheath worn rather tightly over the erect penis. There is a rubber ring at the open end to help hold it in place. The function of the condom is to prevent the sperm from reaching the vagina. It is almost as effective as the diaphragm in preventing pregnancy, and its effectiveness can be increased if used in conjunction with contraceptive jelly applied to the outside of the condom or foam inserted into the vagina before intercourse. The disadvantages are that it interferes with the full enjoyment of the sexual act by dulling sensation and that cheap condoms tend to be imperfect and may not be free of holes.

Diaphragm   The vaginal diaphragm is a shallow rubber or synthetic cup designed to cover the cervix of the uterus, preventing sperm from entering. A flexible metal spring or coil holds it in place. A woman must be "fitted" for the device by a physician, and it is then purchased at a drugstore. Vaginal dimensions vary among women and change after the birth of a first child. A contraceptive jelly containing a spermicide may be applied around the edge and inside of the cup before insertion. This gives further protection.

Intrauterine device   The intrauterine devices, called IUDs, are made of plastic, stainless steel, or plastic wrapped in copper. They may be shaped as a spiral, loop, bow, or ring, and they measure about an inch in diameter. When placed in the uterus they prevent pregnancy. Once in place, the device usually can remain there without any harmful effects for years. When a pregnancy is desired, the IUD is then removed, and the woman may become pregnant. The only cost comes with insertion and occasional checkups, and the devices interfere in no way with menstrual discharge. Some women may be bothered with cramps, excessive bleeding, and backache; others may expel the device spontaneously, although this possibility can be reduced by using a smaller device. Older women and those with a greater number of past pregnancies tend to tolerate an IUD better, although newer designs are proving highly successful for childless women. The copper-wrapped devices are almost as effective as the pill (pregnancy rate of 1) and have reduced the usual side effects.

Drug contraception

A variety of *spermicidal* (sperm-killing) foams, creams, and jellies are available for the prevention of conception.

Vaginal spermicides   Various chemical preparations kill or impede the movement of sperm. These vaginal spermicides are available in the form of creams, jellies, aerosol foams, and suppositories. Creams and jellies are designed for use with a diaphragm. The foams are packaged in a pressure can or in individual, measured-dose dispensers. The foam contents are placed with a plastic applicator high in the vagina. Suppositories and foaming tablets are spermicides in solid form, which melt or dissolve when placed in the vagina. They can be purchased without prescription at drugstores. Although more effective than the douches, they are somewhat less effective than the mechanical devices and the pill.

Douche   Some women believe that pregnancy can be prevented by *washing out* the semen after intercourse, emptying a large rubber bulb, or syringe, filled with water into the vagina. Sometimes it is thought that there is an added safety in the supposed spermicidal abilities of certain substances such as hot or cold water, or vinegar, lemon juice, or soap dissolved in the water, or some of the "douches" available in drugstores. However, the sperm are safely within the uterus within 30 seconds after ejaculation; a douche can wash out the vagina but not the uterus. Regardless of how soon the douching is done or what is used, after unprotected ejaculation it is too late. A douche is a *poor contraceptive method.*

Hormonal contraception   The female oral contraceptive pills are designed to prevent ovulation. Their function is based upon the hormonal control of the menstrual cycle. As already mentioned, the hormones FSH and LH from the pituitary gland are necessary for the maturation of an egg and its release from the ovary. The follicles in the ovary produce both estrogen and progesterone. The presence of both estrogen and progesterone inhibit the body's further production of FSH and LH, until the follicle deteriorates late in the month.

The pills' basic hormone is *progestin,* a synthetic progesterone. Some forms of the pill also contain estrogen. When taken daily, starting with day 5 —that is, *from the start of menstruation*—the synthetic progestin and estrogens inhibit the body's production of FSH and LH before a mature egg can be produced. Ovulation does not occur; thus there is no egg present to unite with a sperm in intercourse, and consequently there is no pregnancy.

Sold under a number of trade names, the pills preventing ovulation are commonly one of two types. The *combined* pill contains both estrogen and progestin. One type of pill is taken for 20 days from *days 5 to 25,* then stopped to allow for menstruation; the prevention of pregnancy with this pill is nearly perfect. The *sequential* pills consist of two different pills: one type, containing only estrogen, is taken *days 5 through 19,* and then a second type, containing both estrogen and progestin, is taken *days 20 through 24.* Taking the pills in sequence reduces some possible side effects found with the combined pills—such as headache, nausea, and swelling breasts. Pregnancy prevention is not quite as good as with the combined pills. Regarding other fears in the use of the pill, there is no evidence to date that it causes cancer in women. There is evidence, however, of increased blood clotting, particularly among women with blood type A.

A third type of pill does not prevent ovulation but prevents *implantation.* It is called the "morning-after pill." A woman may find herself in a situation where she engages in sexual intercourse without having access to a birth-control device. With the possibility of pregnancy the morning-after pill ensures against pregnancy *after* intercourse. Once an egg is fertilized, several days are required to move it to the uterus and several more for it to become implanted in the uterine lining. A morning-after pill taken three to five days after intercourse may prevent implantation. Consisting of a synthetic estrogen, the pill causes contraction of the uterus and the expulsion of its contents. This pill should be used only on an emergency basis and not as a regular birth-control method.

Other methods of birth control

The rhythm method   One of the least effective methods of fertility control is the *rhythm method.* Rather than a form of contraception, it is *abstinence* from intercourse during the days of each menstrual cycle when the wife is believed to be fertile. The method is based on the fact that a woman produces a mature egg once a month with some predictability. If a mature egg fails to meet a sperm within twenty-four hours, it begins to degenerate. Sperm inseminated into a woman's body and kept at normal body temperatures can remain alive from one to three days after intercourse and still fertilize an egg. Avoiding intercourse for three days each month should prevent pregnancy. This is all simple enough, but the *big* question each month is: When does ovulation occur?

Ordinarily ovulation occurs 14 days *before* the start of the next menstruation. This is no problem if the cycle lasts exactly 28 days. But in some "28-day women" ovulation actually occurs anywhere from 17 to 13 days before menstruation. Added to this, many women do not menstruate with a twenty-eight-day regularity. The average woman varies as much as 8 to 9 days between her longest and shortest menstrual cycles. Some cycles are as short as 21 days and others as long as 38 days.

Exactly how can the day of ovulation be determined? With ovulation a few women experience a low abdominal pain. With others the normal body temperature (as taken before getting out of bed in the morning) rises a few tenths of a degree after ovulation and until menstruation. This method of pregnancy control is not highly effective. In addition, affectionate couples do not enjoy regulating sexual intercourse by the calendar. The method casts undue uncertainty over a sexual relationship that should be wonderfully confident.

Withdrawal (coitus interruptus)   One of the oldest fertility control methods is the withdrawal of the penis from the vagina just before ejaculation, so that the semen is deposited outside the vagina. The disadvantages of this method are numerous. Among other things, its effectiveness is low (though better than the rhythm method or the douche), and it greatly interferes with the enjoyment of intercourse by both husband and wife.

Surgical sterilization   Though not technically considered a contraceptive method, surgical sterilization is a very positive and essentially perfectly effective method of fertility control. Increasing numbers of married couples are turning to surgical sterilization of either the man or wife after they have produced a desired number of children.

Sterilization of the male is a simple office procedure in which the vas deferens are clipped or tied off, or both, through a small incision at the base of the scrotum. This operation has no effect on either the desire or the ability to have intercourse. Ejaculation occurs as before, but the semen contains no sperm.

Sterilization of the female is more major, involving an abdominal incision, through which the fallopian tubes are tied or removed. As in the male, there is no change in the sex life. It is to be stressed that sterilization of either male or female is probably permanent. Those few specialists who do attempt to restore fertility after surgical sterilization report a maximal 50 percent rate of success.

Choice of method

The birth-control method chosen should meet the approval of both partners and also of their physician. In the method which is best for a given woman (since most contraceptives are designed for women) the most important factor is *safety*. The ideal method must neither be harmful to a woman's health nor reduce her ability to bear a child in the future, if she wants one. It should be free from harmful or unwanted side effects, both for the person using the device and for the partner. A second factor is *rate of effectiveness*. It must be effective in preventing pregnancy for the particular person. It should also have "use-effectiveness," or a high probability of continued use. The third factor is *ease of administration*. If permanently inserted, as is an intrauterine device (IUD), it is expected that a professional person will insert it; if some other mechanical device, the person using it must find it easy to apply. Ideally, the device will be one which could be applied at some time other than during actual preparation for intercourse. A fourth element is *acceptability*. Acceptance must include such factors as medical ones (medical history, absence of side effects, physical comfort), social ones (prevailing religions, cultural hesitations), and psychological ones (personal esthetics, one's own habits and attitudes). *Reversibility* is a fifth element. Whether a woman's fertility is ever utilized or not, it is important that both she and her husband know that pregnancy is possible. Sixth is *expense*. Some devices (such as the IUD) require only an initial expense, while others involve a recurring cost (pills, condoms, foams). Even in the United States economy is a factor for many couples, but in many underdeveloped countries several cents a day may be prohibitive. Last is the effect the device has on a person's *libido*, or sexual feelings. A highly sexed person will welcome the assurance that delightful feelings will not be reduced. A couple must be satisfied they have chosen the method of birth control that best suits their needs.

The reliability of birth control techniques is measured by the number of pregnancies per 100 woman-years. This means that if 100 women use a technique as directed for one year, the approximate number of pregnancies would be:

No precaution whatever	80–90
Douche	31–40
Rhythm	24–38
Withdrawal (coitus interruptus)	16–18
Condom	12–15
Foam	8–12
Diaphragm	6–10
Intrauterine devices	3–5
Sequential pills	1–3
Combined pills	0.3–1.5
Sterilization	<0.0003>

There is no single known technique that is absolutely reliable in *all* cases. The effectiveness of any contraceptive method depends upon its being used (1) as directed and (2) consistently.

For further information

The best source of family-planning information is an obstetrician or family physician. The public-health departments of many states, counties, and cities also offer aid, and certain nonprofit family-planning agencies are available. The national agencies have local offices scattered across the country; to reach them, the first thing to do is to check the telephone directory and, if no locations are given, they can be reached through their information centers in New York:

Planned Parenthood Federation of America, Inc., 515 Madison Ave., New York, New York 10022

Family Planning Information Service (FPIS), 300 Park Avenue South, New York, New York 10010

Other good sources of information are Guttmacher's *Planning Your Family*, the *Consumers Union Report on Family Planning*, and *Birth Control* (Time-Life Books, Time, Inc.), all of which may be obtained through local public libraries.

HEREDITY

The cell

To understand the mechanisms of heredity we need to consider briefly the basic structure of human cells and how cells divide. All human tissues are composed of cells, most of which are microscopic in size. By the time of birth the single cell which was the fertilized egg has divided and redivided into *billions* of cells, forming the whole human body. Although these cells are differentiated (specialized) to serve specific functions, the genetic (hereditary) material contained in each is *identical*.

Figure 11.15 represents a typical unspecialized human cell, such as might be found in the early embryo. A typical cell is surrounded by a *cell membrane;* everything inside the cell membrane is *protoplasm*. Within the cell is a *nucleus*, which contains the *chromosomes* and the *nucleolus*. All the cellular material outside the nucleus is called *cytoplasm*. Located in the cytoplasm are numerous tiny *ribosomes*, the site of protein synthesis. There are numerous other cellular structures, essential to life but not to our discussion of heredity.

Chromosomes

Within the nucleus of every cell are located the actual bearers of genetic information, the chromosomes. Every human body cell contains 23 pairs of chromosomes; every sperm or egg carries only 23 chromosomes—one member from each pair. Thus the fusion of the sperm with the egg creates a cell (the fertilized egg, or *zygote*) carrying 23 *pairs* of chromosomes, one member of each pair having come from the sperm and the other from the egg. Every one of the billions of cells which will result from the normal fertilized egg will carry the identical 46 chromosomes.

The genetic code

Every chromosome contains *thousands* of molecules of *deoxyribonucleic acid* (DNA), the chemical bearer of the information of heredity (the genetic code); see Fig. 11.16. The insight into the structure and function of DNA is one of the high points of modern science. With this knowledge has come the exciting (and to many persons, frightening) possibility of man's control over human heredity and evolution. Each DNA molecule resembles an extremely long, twisted ladder, the *thousands* of rungs of which are pairs of chemicals. The only known pairs of these chemicals are two in number: *adenine* paired with *thymine*, and *cytosine* paired with *guanine*. There are only four positional combinations of each pair possible: adenine–thymine, thymine–adenine, cytosine–guanine, and guanine–cytosine. But the thousands of sequences of these combinations in one molecule make possible an almost infinite number of different arrangements. It is the sequences in which these pairs occur that determines the characteristics of every living thing. These pairs may be thought of as *letters*, which in sequence spell out the words of the "genetic code." When we speak of "genes," we are really speaking of the *structure* of DNA.

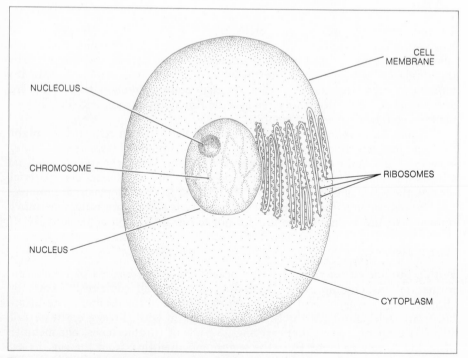

Figure 11.15　An unspecialized cell, as in the early development of an embryo.

Action of DNA

DNA has the ability, most unusual for a chemical molecule, of reproducing itself. Each time a cell divides, its DNA must first duplicate itself. It does this by "unzipping," the two sides of the ladder unwinding and the rungs breaking in the center. Each half then reconstructs the original molecule by pulling the necessary parts from other materials surrounding the molecules. Thymine attracts adenine, adenine attracts thymine, cytosine attracts guanine, and guanine attracts cytosine. When this process is complete, the cell divides, as discussed below.

The way in which DNA is believed to function as a gene is shown in Fig. 11.17. DNA controls the characteristics of a living thing by controlling the synthesis of protein within each cell. The characteristics of any living thing are determined by the types of protein it contains. The type of protein is

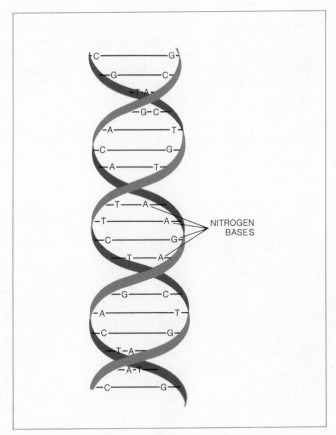

Figure 11.16   Portion of DNA molecule. Nitrogen bases consist of adenine (A), thymine (T), guanine (G), and cytosine (C).

determined by the sequence of the amino acids it contains (see Chapter 7). DNA determines the sequence of the amino acids that make up each protein, thereby determining the characteristics of the individual. It is known that the manufacture of proteins takes place in the numerous *ribosomes* in the cytoplasm of the cell. A chemical messenger carries the genetic code from the DNA in the nucleus to the ribosomes in the cytoplasm. This messenger is called *messenger* RNA (ribonucleic acid). RNA is similar to one half of a DNA molecule—as if the ladder were sawed in half lengthwise. The messenger RNA units attach themselves to the surface of the ribosomes. Other RNA units, called *transfer* RNA, transport single amino acids from other areas of the cell to the ribosome, where, with the aid of an enzyme, the messenger RNA arranges the amino acids into specific proteins. Many of these proteins are enzymes, which will in turn enable vital chemical reactions to take place within the cell.

Cell division

Only two types of cell division are known to take place in the human body, *mitosis* and *meiosis;* see Figs. 11.18 and 11.19. Of these mitosis is the commoner. All growth and replacement of cells takes place through mitosis. It is through mitosis that the fertilized egg divides into the billions of cells present at birth. The most important characteristic of mitosis is that it results in *two cells identical with the parent cell.*

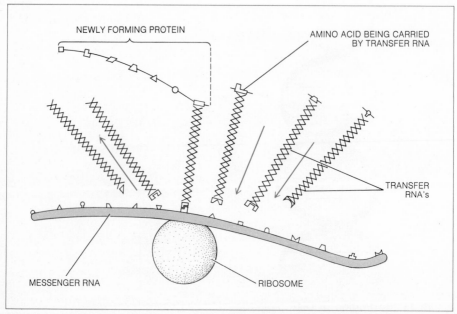

Figure 11.17 Formation of protein molecules. Note that the transfer RNA deposits amino acid according to the "blueprint" carried by the messenger RNA.

The second type of cell division, meiosis, takes place only in the ovary or testis, in the production of eggs or sperms. Through the process of meiosis, which involves 2 cell divisions and results in 4 cells, the number of chromosomes in each cell is reduced from 23 pairs to 23 single chromosomes. Each sperm or egg gets one member of each pair. The most important characteristic of meiosis is the *random assortment* of chromosomes which takes place. When a man produces a sperm, for example, that sperm gets some chromosomes that the man received from his mother (maternal) and some chromosomes that he received from his father (paternal). For each of the 23 pairs of chromosomes a random assortment takes place—a given sperm being equally likely to receive a maternal or paternal chromosome. It is this random assortment of chromosomes that leads to the independent inheritance of traits that are determined by different chromosomes. This random assortment also means that every sperm or egg a man or woman produces receives a different combina-

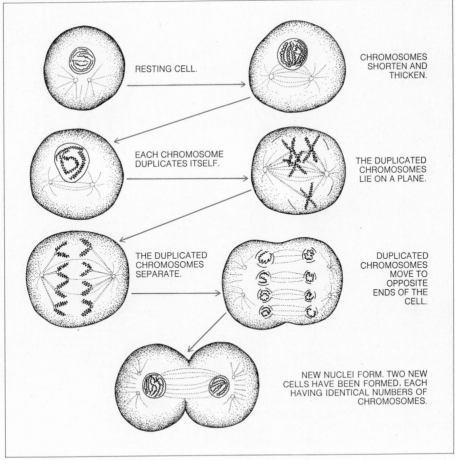

RESTING CELL.

CHROMOSOMES
SHORTEN AND
THICKEN.

EACH CHROMOSOME
DUPLICATES ITSELF.

THE DUPLICATED
CHROMOSOMES
LIE ON A PLANE.

THE DUPLICATED
CHROMOSOMES
SEPARATE.

DUPLICATED
CHROMOSOMES
MOVE TO
OPPOSITE
ENDS OF THE
CELL.

NEW NUCLEI FORM. TWO NEW
CELLS HAVE BEEN FORMED, EACH
HAVING IDENTICAL NUMBERS OF
CHROMOSOMES.

Figure 11.18   Mitosis, the production of two identical cells.

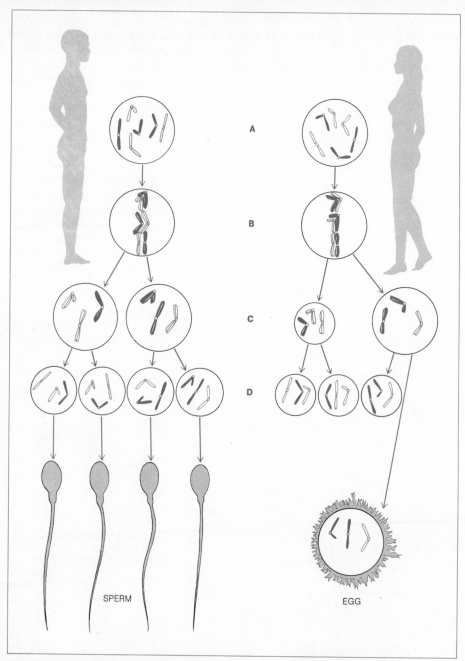

Figure 11.19   Meiosis, the production of sperms or eggs: (A) cells in the testes and ovaries contain 23 chromosomes from the mother and 23 from the father, shown in white and black, respectively (only 3 pairs are shown); (B) each chromosome *duplicates* itself, and similar pairs line up with each other; (C) first cell division, in which the number of *duplicate* chromosomes in each

tion of chromosomes. Thus a couple can produce many children, but never two with exactly the same combination of traits (except in the production of identical twins, in which case one fertilized egg divides to produce two genetically identical children).

Dominance and recessiveness

Genes (DNA patterns) are often spoken of as being either *dominant* or *recessive*. For many traits there is a contrasting pair of dominant and recessive genes. If a child receives one dominant gene from either parent, he will exhibit the dominant trait. If a child is to exhibit a recessive trait, the recessive gene must be received from each parent. Thus, when a person does exhibit a recessive trait, he is *homozygous* for that condition—meaning that he carries only the one type of gene. Every sperm or egg produced by that person will carry the recessive gene. A person showing a dominant trait may have received the dominant gene from each parent (he would be homozygous), *or* he may have received the dominant gene from one parent and the recessive gene from the other parent, a condition referred to as *heterozygous*. When dominance is complete, the appearance of the person is the same, whether he is homozygous or heterozygous. For some hereditary traits the heterozygous person presents an intermediate appearance—halfway between the homozygous dominant person and the homozygous recessive person. Such inheritance is called *incomplete dominance* or *intermediate* inheritance. For many human traits not one but *several* pairs of genes help determine the appearance of the person. In such cases (examples are skin color, hair color, and stature) there are numerous intermediate conditions between the two extremes.

Common misconceptions about heredity

It would be well at this point to clear up several common misconceptions about heredity. First of all, it is a common belief that recessive genes are always undesirable. A glance at the accompanying listing of human heredity traits in Table 11.3 will show that in many cases the recessive condition is the normal condition, the dominant being abnormal. For example, the gene producing six fingers on each hand is dominant over the gene for five fingers, yet the possession of five fingers on each hand is considered by most of us to be the preferred condition. The same example points out another common misconception: that recessive genes occur less commonly than dominant genes; obviously the recessive condition of five fingers per hand is much more common than the dominant in this case. The list of hereditary traits reveals many other similar cases.

---

new cell is reduced by one half; (D) second cell division, in which the duplicate chromosomes of each cell divide, forming a total of four new cells containing, again, single chromosomes. Four cells are formed by each meiosis; of the four male cells all are useful sperms, but only one of the four female cells is a useful egg.

Table 11.3 *Some hereditary traits in man*

	dominant	recessive
Eyes	Brown	Blue or gray
	Green or hazel	Blue or gray
	Normal color perception	Color-blindness (sex-linked)
	Nearsightedness	Normal
	Farsightedness	Normal
	Congenital cataract	Normal
	Astigmatism	Normal
Nervous system	Huntington's chorea	Normal
	Migraine headache	Normal
	Normal	Phenylketonuria (PKU)
	Hereditary tremor	Normal
	Normal	Congenital deafness
Endocrine system	Normal	Diabetes mellitus
Circulatory system	Blood groups A, B, AB	Blood group O
	Rh factor present (positive)	Rh factor absent (negative)
	High blood pressure	Normal
	Normal	Hemophilia (sex-linked)
Skin and hair	Normal pigmentation	Albinism
	Dark hair	Light hair
	Curly hair	Straight hair
	Baldness (males)	Normal (males)
	Normal (females)	Baldness (females)
Body structure	Six fingers each hand	Five fingers each hand
	Webbed fingers or toes	Normal
	Dwarfism	Normal
	Stub fingers	Normal
	Free earlobes	Attached earlobes

Genes can change

In predicting the offspring from a particular mating we assume a *stability*, or lack of change, in the genes (DNA), and 999,999 times out of 1 million we may be correct in that assumption. But about once in every million cell divisions an error is made in the self-duplication process of the DNA. If such an error is *stable* and is passed on with subsequent cell divisions, it is a *mutation*. With the change in DNA pattern a new gene has been produced. Mutations have a very important bearing upon the welfare of mankind. In the first place, mutations are the basis of *evolution*. The very small percentage of mutations that prove to be advantageous to the species is maintained through the ever-occurring *natural selection*, when mutations turn out to be selected over the original genetic composition. Man has watched such a process taking place during the past few years, as insects have become resistant to insecticides and bacteria to antibiotics. We also see mutations occurring in viruses, such as the often-changing flu viruses.

Mutations seem to occur spontaneously, but they also can be induced through exposure of cells to radiation or to certain chemicals. It is *not* possible to produce mutations through physical change in an organism; in breeds of dogs whose tails have been cut off for hundreds of years, puppies are born today with tails not one micron shorter than their ancestors of a hundred generations ago. Acquired traits in human beings, such as brain damage resulting from physical injury, are *not hereditary*. In considering the genetic desirability of a given marriage, it is important to distinguish carefully between those traits which are hereditary and those which are acquired.

Genetic counseling

The detection, prevention, and treatment of genetic diseases is a new, critical field of medicine. Its current progress is no less dramatic than what took place in medicine after Pasteur's discovery of the germ theory. Although the field is in its infancy, more than twelve hundred genetic diseases are already known, only a small number of which are so far treatable.

Detection of genetic defect is done through *amniocentesis*, a diagnosis of the chromosomes of the fetus in the uterus by extraction of both amniotic fluid and fetal cells, by *enzyme analysis* of both amniotic fluid and fetal cells, and by *skin-cell analysis* of potential parents for abnormal genes. With such information the options now open to parents are more than simply avoiding pregnancy. A number of genetic diseases can be detected early enough in pregnancy to permit therapeutic abortion of the affected fetuses. Potential parents can be informed whether or not they carry the abnormal gene for a specific condition, so that a pregnancy may be monitored. Genetic counseling is available at most major medical centers.

Genetic determination of sex

The genetic determination of the sex of an unborn child is quite a simple matter. Of the 23 pairs of human chromosomes, one pair is called *the sex chromosomes*. This is the only pair of human chromosomes in which the two members may be different in appearance. One is a fairly large chromosome called the X chromosome. The other is a very small one, the Y *chromosome*. Females carry two X chromosomes in every cell; males carry one X and one Y chromosome per cell.

During the production of eggs or sperms the sex chromosomes, like all other pairs of chromosomes, separate, each sperm or egg receiving only one member of the pair. Since a female is XX, every egg she produces carries an X chromosome. A male, being XY, produces sperm cells of which half carry an X chromosome and half carry a Y. If an egg is fertilized by an X-bearing sperm, the child will be XX and therefore female; if an egg is fertilized by a Y-bearing sperm, the child will be XY and therefore male. Once the child is conceived, nothing that the mother, doctor, or anyone else can do will have any influence on the sex of the child.

Errors during divisions of a cell lead to various kinds of abnormalities. The loss of an X chromosome during the first division of an XX fertilized egg cell can result in an XO female, an abnormal condition known as Turner's syndrome; in XO females the sex glands remain undeveloped, and the female is usually mentally defective. Or a female may produce an XX-bearing egg cell which, when fertilized by a Y-bearing sperm cell, produces an XXY male; this is known as Klinefelter's syndrome, the males having abnormal testes, being unable to produce sperm, and frequently being mentally defective.

Sex-linked heredity

Many X-linked genes are known but, except for sex factors, few Y-linked genes have been found. All other traits determined by the X chromosome are said to be X-linked. The Y chromosome carries *no* corresponding genes. X-linked recessive traits occur much more often in men than in women. The reason is that a male, with only one X chromosome, will exhibit the recessive trait if it is carried by his one X chromosome. But before a female will exhibit the X-linked recessive, she must carry the gene on *each* of her two X chromosomes. The chance of receiving the same gene twice is, naturally, the *square* of the chance of receiving it once. If the chance in a male is 1 in 20, the chance in a female will be 1 in 400. The best-known examples of X-linked traits are color blindness and hemophilia ("bleeder's disease").

Since a man transmits an X chromosome only to his daughters, an X-linked trait is passed from a man to his daughter (who probably will be an unaffected "carrier"), who in turn will pass the gene to half of her sons, who will be affected.

The Rh factor in pregnancy

One hereditary trait that occasionally complicates pregnancy is the *Rh factor*. This is a chemical substance, which is usually present within the red blood cells (erythrocytes). If a person has this factor present in his red blood cells, then he is Rh *positive,* as are about 85 percent of whites, 92 percent of blacks, and 99 percent of Orientals. If this substance is missing, then he is Rh *negative,* as are about 15 percent of whites.

The usual circumstances under which the Rh factor may complicate pregnancy comes when an Rh-negative woman, with an Rh-positive husband, bears an Rh-positive child. The Rh factor is inherited through a dominant gene, so a heterozygous positive man can father both positive and negative children. When a negative woman carries a positive child, small amounts of Rh factor diffuse across the placenta from the tissues of the child into the blood of the mother; see Fig. 11.20.

Once the Rh factor enters the body of the mother, it acts as an *antigen* (see Chapter 18). The antigen stimulates her body to produce anti-Rh factor, or *antibodies* (Chapter 18), which will *destroy* red blood cells containing the Rh factor. This process has *no effect* upon the red cells of the mother, since they contain no Rh factor. But when the level of antibodies in the mother's blood becomes high enough, these antibodies diffuse back across the placenta into the blood of the child and destroy his red blood cells. This diffusion most commonly occurs with the second or third pregnancy. The result of this destruction is a type of anemia called *erythroblastosis fetalis*, in which the blood cannot carry sufficient oxygen for the infant. In extreme cases this anemia may result in stillbirth, death following birth, or mental retardation. Such infants appear yellow (jaundiced) because of the byproducts of the breakdown of the red blood cells.

When tests indicate that a dangerous level of antibodies has been reached, labor may be induced somewhat prematurely and the infant given blood transfusions. Recently such transfusions have been performed upon infants still in the uterus—the first of intrauterine therapies. Or, if such level has been reached, a cesarean section may be performed. Or damage may be prevented in the infant by an exchange blood transfusion immediately after birth. Vaccines (such as Rho GAM) which neutralize antigens present in the mother are now available for Rh-mothers; the vaccines should be administered to the mother immediately after delivery of an Rh-positive baby. The method is

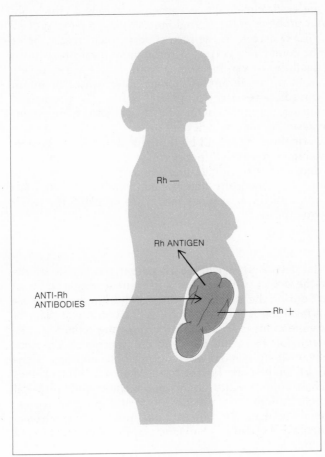

Figure 11.20   Rh incompatibility in pregnancy.

over 90 percent effective. Spacing births sufficiently is another solution; it allows the antibody level to fall low enough to cause no trouble with the next conception.

Other blood groups

In addition to his Rh blood type a person has a blood type from each of many other blood-group series. Most of these series are inherited independently of each other, for the genes are carried by different chromosomes. For a discussion of the most well-known series of blood groups, the A-B-O series, see Chapter 16. This series is inherited independently of the Rh series, so a person can have any combination of Rh and A-B-O blood types.

CONGENITAL ABNORMALITIES

Abnormal conditions that are present at the time of birth are *congenital abnormalities*. They may be environmentally *or* genetically caused. Such abnormalities remain a major problem in the United States today, 6 percent of all infants born having *significant* defects in the formation of their bodies. Some of these deformities can be completely corrected through surgical procedures; others result in lifelong debilities of varying degrees; still others are so severe that they result in the death of the infant. Although other causes of infant mortality have yielded to medical research, congenital defects have remained a major cause of death during the first year of life. In addition, many spontaneous abortions are the result of abnormal development.

Most congenital abnormalities must still be thought of as unpreventable. Although it is often possible in retrospect to determine the cause of the abnormality, little can be done today to predict and prevent these unfortunate cases. Some malformations are genetically determined, some result from adverse intrauterine environmental conditions, and some are probably the result of a combination of the two causes.

Genetic causes

Some hereditary congenital defects arise when each parent is a carrier of the same recessive gene for the defect. Other defects of genetic origin arise as the result of an "accident" during the meiotic cell division leading to the sperm or egg. The egg or sperm resulting from such faulty cell division may deviate from the normal chromosome number of 23, and the resulting offspring may show a corresponding deviation from the usual 46 chromosomes. Chromosome counts made of cells of living persons have revealed chromosome numbers ranging from 45 to 49. Individuals having other than 46 chromosomes are usually abnormal. Their abnormalities commonly include both physical deformities and mental retardation. A commonly occurring abnormality resulting from a chromosomal imbalance, and often from an extra chromosome, is *mongolism*. The mongoloid person is characterized by short stature, a broad, flat head, a large tongue, slanting eyes, and very low mentality. The incidence of mongolism increases markedly with the age of the mother. The risk of a mongoloid's being born to a woman in her twenties is about 1 in 3,000; to a woman over thirty-five it is 1 in 300; over forty, it is 1 in 70; over forty-five, it is 1 in 40. Fortunately, most women today bear their last child while still in their twenties. There is no known treatment for the child born with an abnormal chromosome number. Parents who have had one child with a chromosomal abnormality have an appreciable chance of producing more such children in future pregnancies, because one of the parents may be carrying a chromosomal abnormality in the ovary or testis. The chance of a second defective child ranges from 1 in 100 to 33 in 100, depending upon the maternal age and type of abnormality. Such parents should have genetic counsel before deciding upon another pregnancy.

Better than one half of all fetuses lost through miscarriage show abnormal chromosome numbers. In women having a history of repeated miscarriages of obviously defective fetuses there is an increased chance that a full-term infant also will be defective. Naturally, when miscarriages have been due to a maternal factor such as a low progesterone level, no such increase in defective offspring occurs.

Environmental causes

The environmental causes of congenital defects exert their greatest effect during the first 8 to 12 weeks of the life of an embryo. At this stage of development the body is undergoing rapid differentiation, the formation of most organs taking place. Among the environmental factors that may seriously affect the embryo are excessive exposure to radiation, use of certain drugs by the mother, and exposure to disease agents. Virus diseases may have an especially severe effect upon the embryo. Many normally mild virus diseases, such as German measles, have been proven to cause serious defects when an embryo is infected during the first 6 months of pregnancy.

Most defects start during the first 90 days of pregnancy. Drugs (sedatives, tranquilizers, and others) which might be safe to take under most circumstances may be dangerous in light of the rigorous demands of early pregnancy. This is especially true with the unplanned pregnancy, in which damage may be done before the woman even knows she is pregnant. Knowing that there may be other causes of a missed menstruation, a woman may take insufficient precaution in her exposure to x-rays, virus infections, or drugs. She may not see a physician for several months, by which time she has already passed the time of greatest fetal damage.

Prevention of congenital defects

Here are some simple suggestions on how prospective parents may reduce the chances of birth defects in their children.

1. Marrying a close relative increases the risk of producing a defective child. Such increased risk is the basis of state laws that prohibit close relatives from marrying each other.

2. All married couples should have a family physician, who should be made aware of any known history of family defects or sources of complication,

such as an Rh incompatibility, so he can correctly counsel the couple. They should both seek his counsel before planning a pregnancy, and then the woman should see him at regular intervals during the pregnancy. Since premature babies are more likely to be defective than full-term babies, medical care during pregnancy is essential to avert premature delivery.

3. The physician treating other conditions should be told of any suspected pregnancy. A woman who either is pregnant or apt to become pregnant should take *only* those medications prescribed by her physician.

4. The pregnant woman should avoid known possibilities of contact with diseases. If there has been known contact, she should inform her physician.

5. Except in emergency, x-ray examinations should be avoided during the first 90 days of pregnancy.

6. Smoking should be avoided during pregnancy. The more a mother smokes during pregnancy, the less her baby will weigh at birth. As already pointed out, the weight of a baby at birth can relate to its chances of survival, especially if it is exceptionally small.

7. The age of the mother must be considered. A high correlation exists between birth defects and the age of the mother and, in some cases, of the father. Mothers under 18 and over 40 produce a greater percentage of defective children than those in between.

8. Since diet affects growth, girls should learn to eat properly. Diet must be thought of both in terms of the girl's own health and the future growth and development of her children. The fetus depends entirely on the diet of its mother.

SUMMARY

   I. Human reproductive systems
     A. Male reproductive system
       1. Testis—produces both spermatozoa and testosterone.
       2. Scrotum—loose tissue covering testis.
       3. Epididymis—holds sperm cells while they mature.
       4. Vas deferens:
         a. small duct carrying sperm from the epididymis into the urethra.
         b. near the upper end is an enlargement for the storage of mature sperm until ejaculation.
       5. Fluid-producing glands:
         a. seminal vesicles—most important source of fluid for the semen.
         b. prostate gland.
         c. Cowper's glands.
       6. Penis—male organ of sexual intercourse.
       7. Nocturnal emissions—involuntary ejaculations during sleep.
     B. Female reproductive system
       1. Ovary—produces both eggs (ova) and hormones.

2. Fallopian tube (oviduct)—duct which carries eggs from the ovary to the uterus.

3. Uterus—organ specialized for the growth and protection of the unborn child.

4. Vagina:
   a. female organ of sexual intercourse.
   b. produces lubricating materials upon sexual arousal.

5. External genitalia:
   a. vulva—two pairs of labia surrounding the opening of the vagina.
   b. clitoris—sensory erectile tissue lying at the forward junction of the labia.
   c. hymen—membrane which may partially close the opening of the vagina.

6. Sexual intercourse.

II. Menstrual cycle
   A. Hormones of reproduction
      1. Menstrual cycle is under control of pituitary gland.
      2. Hormones stimulating the ovaries are:
         a. follicle-stimulating hormone (FSH).
         b. luteinizing hormone (LH).
         c. luteotropic hormone (LTH).
      3. Two types of hormones from the ovaries are important in the menstrual cycle:
         a. estrogens.
         b. progesterone.
   B. The menstrual cycle
      1. Menarche—first menstrual period; usually occurs between the ages of 11 and 15.
      2. Menopause—cessation of the menstrual cycle at about age 47.
      3. Menstrual cycle lasts an average of 28 days and includes two important events:
         a. menstruation—occurring the first 4 or 5 days of the cycle.
         b. ovulation—occurring at about the midpoint of the cycle.

III. Pregnancy
   A. Embryology—full-term pregnancy lasts about 266 days from conception.
      1. During the first 8 weeks the developing child is called the embryo.
      2. Beyond 8 weeks called fetus.
   B. Early signs of pregnancy
      1. Cessation of menstruation—result of chorion-produced gonadotropic hormone, which maintains production of progesterone by the corpus luteum.
      2. Changes in the breasts—become larger and fuller as a result of the continued high progesterone level.
      3. Frequent urination—enlarged uterus presses against the urinary bladder.
      4. Nausea—may begin at the time of the first missed period and last for 4 to 6 weeks.
   C. Pregnancy tests
      1. Most depend upon chorionic gonadotropin in the urine or blood of the pregnant woman.
      2. In other tests estrogen and progesterone are administered for a few

days in case the delay in menstruation is due to immaturity of the endometrium.

   D. Complications of pregnancy
1. Prenatal care of utmost importance for early detection of complications.
2. Pregnant woman should know and be alert to the signs of possible complications.

   E. Diet in pregnancy
1. Pregnant woman needs significantly increased quantities of protein, vitamins, and minerals, but only slightly increased calories.
2. Maternal weight gain is critical:
    a. the higher the maternal weight gain the better the child's growth and performance.
    b. a maternal weight gain of 20 to 25 pounds is now recommended by the National Research Council.

   F. Terminations of pregnancy
1. Labor occurs in three stages.
2. Anesthesia commonly given mother during delivery.

   G. Complications of delivery
1. Labor induced if life of mother or fetus in jeopardy.
2. Cesarean section is surgical delivery through abdominal wall.
3. Extrauterine (ectopic) pregnancy is one developing outside uterus.
4. Premature delivery—live birth of an infant before it is fully mature, weight being under 5.5 pounds.

   H. Abortion—any termination of pregnancy before there is any chance of survival of the infant.
1. Spontaneous—natural, often called miscarriage.
2. Induced:
    a. legal—may be done either for medical reasons (therapeutic) or on demand of the mother; dilatation and curettage (D-and-C); suction curettage; hypertonic solution, saline or glucose; abdominal surgery, hysterotomy or hysterectomy.
    b. illegal—performed outside the restrictions of the law.

IV. Fertility control
   A. Low fertility—occurs in about 25 percent of all married couples.
1. Cause may lie in either the man or the woman, or partially in each.
2. Sterility—total inability to produce a child.

   B. Artificial insemination
1. Injection of semen by syringe into the cervix.
2. Semen may be that of the husband or a donor.

   C. Contraception
1. Mechanical—several devices designed to prevent the spermatozoa from reaching the ovum:
    a. condom—sheath worn over penis.
    b. diaphragm—rubber cup worn over cervix of uterus.
    c. intrauterine device—coil inserted in uterus.
2. Drugs
    a. vaginal foams, creams, jellies, suppositories.
    b. douches—vaginal irrigants.
    c. hormonal—inhibit production of FSH and LH by means of synthetic estrogens and progesterone.

d. morning-after pill—synthetic estrogen taken after intercourse, which causes expulsion of the fertilized egg before implantation.

3. Other methods of fertility control
   a. rhythm method—periodic abstinence from sexual intercourse during the fertile period of menstrual cycle.
   b. withdrawal (coitus interruptus)—withdrawal of penis prior to ejaculation.
   c. surgical sterilization—permanent surgical interruption of passage of sex cells.

4. Choice of method—factors to consider
   a. safety.
   b. rate of effectiveness.
   c. ease of administration.
   d. acceptability.
   e. reversibility.
   f. expense.
   g. effect on libido.

V. Heredity
   A. Genetic material—identical in each cell of the body.
   B. Chromosomes contain the genetic information.
      1. Each sperm and egg contains 23 chromosomes.
      2. Each body cell contains 23 *pairs* of chromosomes.
   C. Genetic code—chemical carrier of genetic information: deoxyribonucleic acid (DNA).
   D. Action of DNA—controls the characteristics of a living thing by controlling the synthesis of protein within each cell.
   E. Cell division
      1. Mitosis results in two cells, each identical with the original.
      2. Meiosis:
         a. takes place only in production of sperms and eggs.
         b. reduces the number of chromosomes from 23 pairs to 23 single chromosomes.
   F. Dominance and recessiveness—shown in characteristics by contrasting pairs of genes.
      1. If a child receives a dominant gene from either parent, he will exhibit the dominant characteristic.
      2. The recessive gene will not produce its characteristic if the opposing dominant gene is present.
   G. Change in a DNA pattern is called a mutation.
   H. Sex of a child is determined by the sex chromosomes.
   I. Genetic counseling—concerned with the detection, prevention, and treatment of genetic diseases.
   J. Sex-linked hereditary characteristics, other than sex, carried on the X chromosome.
   K. The Rh factor in pregnancy—caused by Rh incompatibility between mother and fetus.

VI. Congenital abnormalities
   A. Abnormal conditions present at time of birth.
   B. Some of genetic origin.
   C. Prevention of congenital defects.

Glossary

If you cannot find the word you wish in this glossary, check the index for text and glossary references.

afterbirth (af'tər burth). The placenta and associated membranes, expelled from the uterus after the birth of a child.

amniocentesis (am ne o sen te' sis) (G. *amnion*, lamb; *kentesis*, puncture). Transabdominal perforation of the uterus to permit drainage of amniotic fluid.

amnion (am'nē ən) (G. *amnion*, lamb). The membrane which surrounds the embryo within the uterus, secreting amniotic fluid to form the "bag of water."

ampulla (am pul'ə) (L. *ampulla*, jug). A dilated section of a tubular structure.

cervix (sur'viks) (L. *cervix*, neck). The neck or any necklike part of an organ.

chorion (kor'ē on) (G. *chorion*, membrane). The outermost embryonic membrane, part of which unites with the endometrium to form the placenta.

chromosome (krō'mə sōm) (G. *chroma*, color; *soma*, body). Small bodies contained in the nucleus of every cell, carrying the DNA which determines the inherited characteristics of the organism.

cilia (sil'ē ə) (L. *cilium*, eyelash). Minute hairlike structures attached to the outer surface of a cell, capable of wavelike motion.

climacteric (klī mak'tər ik, klī mak ter'ik) (G. *klimakter*, rung of ladder). The physical and mental changes occurring at the termination of the reproductive years in the female.

clitoris (klit'ə-ris, klī'tə ris) (G. *kleitoris*). Small erectile sensory structure located at forward juncture of vulva of female external genitalia.

copulation (kop yə lā'shən) (L. *copulatio*). Sexual intercourse.

corpus luteum (kor'pəs loo'tē əm) (L. *corpus*, body; *luteum*, yellow). The ovarian follicle after discharge of the ovum, persisting as a yellow mass which secretes the hormone progesterone.

Cowper's glands (kou'pərz, koo'pərz) (William Cowper, English surgeon, 1666–1709). A pair of small glands located in the lower abdomen of the male, secreting a lubricating fluid into the urethra upon sexual arousal and contributing a small amount of fluid to the semen.

cytoplasm (sī'tə plazm) (G. *kytos*, cell; *plasma*, plasm). The protoplasm (living material) of a cell exclusive of that of the nucleus.

deoxyribonucleic acid (DNA) (dē ok si rī'bō nyoo klē'ik). The chemical bearer of hereditary traits, located in the chromosomes.

ectopic pregnancy (ek top'ik) (G. *ektopos*, displaced). A pregnancy outside the uterus, usually in the fallopian tube or abdominal cavity.

ejaculation (i jak yə lā'shən) (L. *ejaculatio*, expulsion). The expulsion of the semen.

embryo (em'brē ō) (G. *embryon*, unborn young). The early developing stage of any organism; in the human, during the first 8 weeks.

embryology (em brē ol'ə jē). The science which deals with the development of the embryo.

endocrine gland (en'də krin) (G. *endon*, within; *krinein*, to separate). A gland secreting into the blood a substance (hormone) that acts elsewhere in the body.

endometrium (en dō mē'trē əm) (G. *endon*, within; *metra*, uterus). The mucous membrane lining the inside of the uterus.

epididymis (ep i did'i mis) (G. *epi*, on; *didymos*, testis). An oblong body attached to each testis, in which sperm cells mature and are stored.

episiotomy (ə pē'zē ot'ə mē) (G. *epision*, vula; *tome*, cutting). Surgical cutting of the vulvar orifice to prevent tearing in childbirth.

erectile (i rek'til) (L. *erectio*, erect). Capable of erection.

erection (i rek'shən). The condition of becoming rigid and elevated.

erythroblastosis fetalis (i rith'rō blas tō'sis fi tal'is) (G. *erythro*, red; G. *blastos*, germ; L. *fetus*, unborn child). Destruction of the red blood cells of the fetus or newborn child, usually resulting from Rh incompatibility.

estrogens (es'trə jənz) (G. *oistros*, a strong desire). Female sex hormones, promoting female sexual development.

fallopian tube (fə lō'pē' ən). The paired ducts carrying the ova from the ovary to the uterus. Also called *oviducts*.

fertility (fər til'i tē) (L. *fertilis*, fruitful). Ability to produce offspring.

fetus (fē'təs). The unborn child after 8 weeks of development.

fimbria (fim'brē ə) (L. *fimbria*, fringe). The fringelike upper end of the oviduct.

follicle-stimulating hormone (FSH) (fol'i kl) (L. *follis,* bag). A gonadotropic hormone from the anterior pituitary, stimulating the maturation of the ovarian follicle and its production of estrogen.

gamete (gam'ēt) (G. *gamete*, wife). A mature egg or sperm.

gene (jēn) (G. *gennan*, to produce). A DNA pattern responsible for producing a given hereditary trait; occurs at a definite location on a particular chromosome.

gonad (gō'nad) (G. *gone*, seed). An ovary or testis.

gonadotropic hormone (gō nad ə trop'ik) (G. *tropos*, turning). A gonad-stimulating hormone.

heterozygous (het ər ə zī'gəs) (G. *heteros*, other; G. *zygotos*, yolked together). Possessing two different genes in regard to a given character.

homozygous (hō mə zī'gəs) (G. *homes*, same). Possessing two identical genes in regard to a given character.

hyaluronidase (hī'ə loo ron'i dās). An enzyme that softens cell membranes. Necessary for fertilization of human egg; also found in snake and spider venoms and produced by pathogenic bacteria.

hymen (hī'mən) (G. *hymen*, membrane). The membranous fold which may partially or wholly close the external opening of the vagina.

impotence (im'pə təns) (L. *in*, not; *potentia*, power). Lack of power; especially incapacity for sexual intercourse. May be physical or emotional in origin.

interstitial cells (in tər stish'əl) (L. *inter*, between; *sistere*, to set). In the male gonads, the cells lying between the seminiferous tubules of the testes, secreting testosterone.

labia (lā'bē ə) (L. *labia*, lips). The liplike portions of the female external genitalia.

labor (lā'bər) (L. *labor*, work). The series of processes by which the baby and other products of conception are expelled from the body of the mother.

luteinizing hormone (LH) (loo'tē ə nī zing) (L. *luteus*, yellow; G. *izein*, cause to be). A hormone from the anterior pituitary which stimulates corpus luteum formation in the ovary and the secretion of testosterone by the testis.

luteotropic hormone (LTH) (loo'tē ə trop'ik) (G. *tropikos*, turning). A hormone (also called prolactin) from the anterior pituitary which stimulates progesterone secretion by the corpus luteum and causes the breasts to produce milk.

meiosis (mī ō'sis) (G. *meiosis*, diminution). A special type of cell division occurring during the production of sperms or eggs, by which the usual double set of chromosomes is reduced to a single set.

menarche (me nahr'kē) (G. *men*, month; *arche*, beginning). The beginning of the menstrual cycle.

menopause (men'ə pawz) (G. *pausis,* cessation). Cessation of menstruation, occurring at an average of 47 years of age.

menstrual cycle (men'stroo əl sī'kl) (L. *menstruare,* to menstruate). The regularly recurring cycle of physiological events, including ovulation and menstruation.

menstruation (men stroo ā'shən). The cyclic uterine bleeding resulting from the degeneration of the endometrium.

mitosis (mī tō'sis) (G. *mitos,* thread; *osis,* process). The most common type of cell division, resulting in two cells, each genetically identical with the original.

mongolism (mong'gə lizm). A type of idiocy often resulting from the presence of one extra chromosome in each body cell. Also called *Down's syndrome.*

mutation (myoo tā'shən) (L. *mutatio,* change). A stable, transmissible change in a DNA pattern (gene).

nocturnal emission (nok tur'nəl i mish'ən) (L. *noctis,* night; *emittere,* to send out). The discharge of semen (seminal fluid) by males during sleep. Commonly first occurs shortly after puberty.

nucleus (nyoo'klē əs) (L. *nucleus,* kernel). A spheroid body within a cell, containing the chromosomes.

orgasm (or'gazm) (G. *orgasmos,* swelling). The climax of sexual excitement in the male or female.

os (os) (L. *oris,* mouth, or *ossis,* bone). (1) A mouth or orifice. (2) A bone.

ovary (ō'və rē) (L. *ovarium,* ovary). The female sex organ in which are formed ova and hormones.

oviduct (ō'vi dukt) (L. *ovi,* egg; *ductus,* duct). The tube carrying ova from the ovary to the uterus; the *fallopian tube.*

ovulation (ov yoo lā'shən) (L. *ovum,* egg). The discharge of the mature egg from the graafian follicle of the ovary.

ovum (ō'vəm). An egg.

penis (pē'nis) (L. *penis*). The male organ of copulation.

perineum (per ə ne'əm) (G. *peri* + *inein,* to empty out). The floor of the pelvis; region between the vulva and anus in a female or between the scrotum and anus in a male.

pituitary gland (pityoo'i-ter ē) (L. *pituita,* phlegm). An endocrine gland located at the base of the brain; secretes numerous hormones, many of which stimulate the function of other endocrine glands. Also called the *hypophysis.*

placenta (plə sen'tə) (L. *placenta,* a flat cake). A disc-shaped organ within the uterus through which takes place the exchange of materials between maternal and fetal blood.

progesterone (prō jes'tə rōn) (L. *pro,* before; *gestatio,* pregnancy). A hormone produced by the corpus luteum of the ovary (and by the placenta), promoting the maturity of the endometrium and the maintenance during pregnancy.

prostate gland (pros'tāt) (G. *pro,* before; *histanai,* to stand). A gland in the male surrounding the neck of the bladder and the urethra.

protoplasm (prō'tə plazm) (G. *protos,* first; *plasm,* plasma). The living material within any cell.

puberty (pyoo'bər tē) (L. *pubertas,* transition). The age at which sexual maturity is reached.

ribosome (rī'bə sōm) (ribose; G. *soma,* body). Microscopic bodies within a cell, the site of protein synthesis.

scrotum (skrō'təm) (L. *scrotum,* bag). The sac which contains the testes and related structures.

semen (sē′mən) (L. *semen*, seed). The product of the male reproductive organs, a mixture of spermatozoa and fluid secretions from the prostate and various other glands and cells.

seminal vesicle (sem′i nəl ves′i kl) (L. *vesicula*, small bladder). A gland located on each vas deferens, the primary source of the fluid portion of semen.

seminiferous tubule (sem i nif′ə əs) (L. *semen*, seed; *ferre*, to bear). The numerous small tubes in the testis, the site of sperm production.

sex-linked (seks′lingkt′). Hereditary traits transmitted by genes carried on the X chromosome.

somatotropic hormone (sō′mə tə trop′ik) (G. *soma*, body; *tropos*, a turning). A hormone from the anterior pituitary gland, having a stimulating effect on body growth.

spermatozoon (spur′mə tə zō′ən) (Plural of G. *spermatos*, seed; *zoon*, animal). The mature male germ cell; the *sperm cell*.

sterility (stə ril′i tē) (L. *sterilis*, unfruitful). The inability to produce young.

testis (tes′tis) (L. *testis*, testicle). The male gonad, producing spermatozoa and testosterone.

testosterone (tes tos′tə rōn). The male sex hormone, produced by the testes, inducing male secondary sex characteristics.

toxemia (tok sē′mē ə) (G. *toxikon*, poison; *haima*, blood). A series of conditions occurring in pregnant women, including high blood pressure, excess fluid in the tissues, and albumin in the urine.

trimester (trī mes′tər) (L. *trimestris*, of 3 months). A period of 3 months.

trophoblastic cells (trof ə blast′ik) (G. *trophe*, nutrition; *blastos*, germ). A layer of cells attaching the fertilized ovum to the uterine wall and supplying nutrition to the embryo.

umbilical cord (um bil′i kəl) (L. *umbilicus*, navel). The flexible cord connecting the fetus and the placenta, containing the umbilical arteries and veins.

urethra (yoo rē′thrə) (G. *ourethra*, urinary canal). The duct carrying urine from the bladder to the exterior of the body, and in the male also carrying semen.

uterus (yoo′tə rəs) (L. *uterus*, womb). The hollow, muscular, pear-shaped organ of the female wherein develops the fetus.

vagina (və jī′nə) (L. *vagina*, sheath). The sheathlike structure in the female for the reception of the penis in copulation.

vas deferens (vas def′ər enz) (L. *vas*, duct; *deferens*, carrying away). The duct carrying spermatozoa from the testis to the prostate.

vulva (vul′və) (L. *vulva*, cover, wrapper). The external genital organs of the female.

zygote (zī′gōt) (G. *zygotos*, yolked together). The fertilized ovum.

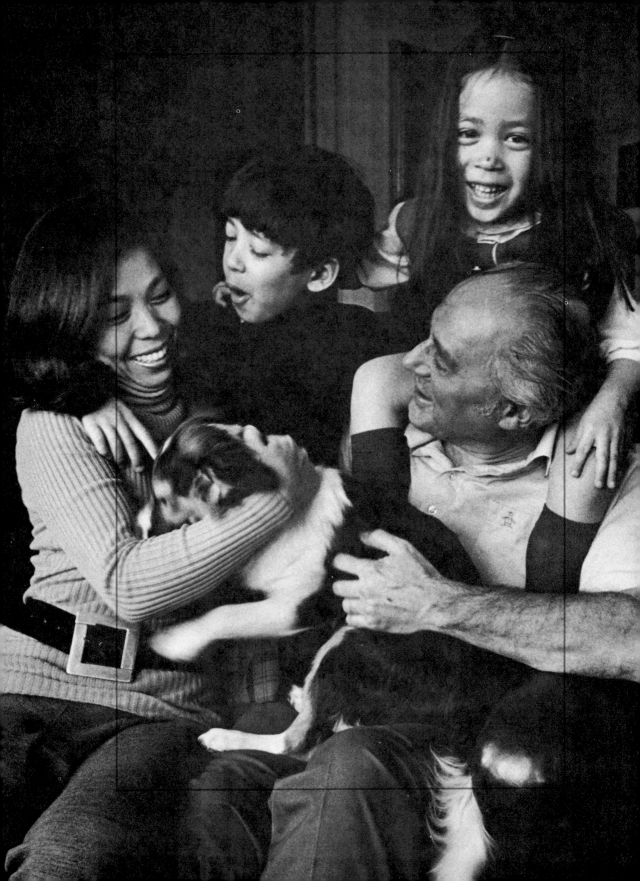

Success in marriage

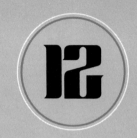

This chapter deals with the behavioral aspects of sexuality—before, within, and outside marriage. Most authorities today agree that attitudes toward standards of sexual behavior have changed and are continuing to change. While fewer young adults today are satisfied with rigid puritanical standards of sexual behavior, most young adults continue to feel a great responsibility for the consequences of their sexual behavior. Probably to an even greater extent than in the past the responsible young adult today tries to avoid sexual behavior which will result in unhappiness to either himself or another person. The emphasis has moved from dogmatic "thou-shalt-nots" to a concern for the pragmatic human values, both positive and negative, of various forms of sexual behavior. Sexuality is today recognized as a positive value in life, and sex as a potential source of great legitimate pleasure and satisfaction.

NONMARITAL SEXUAL ADJUSTMENT

The authors of this text generally prefer the term *nonmarital* to the more traditional *premarital*, because it is more inclusive, meaning not only "before marriage" but also "without marriage," as are the permanently single, the divorced, and the widowed. We shall, however, say "premarital" when it is appropriate to do so.

The sexual behavior of the unmarried person has been a source of concern throughout history. A traditional approach to nonmarital sexual adjustment was to pretend that sexual tensions, if ignored, would somehow just go away. This attitude, of course, was unrealistic because the sexual needs of the unmarried person are no different from those of the married person. Nevertheless, the traditional attitude has been to condemn any form of sexual satisfaction outside marriage.

Today American society is not unanimous in what it considers right or wrong on matters of sexual conduct. During the past fifty or sixty years there has been a definite liberalization in the general attitude toward sex. But individual codes of behavior still range from total sexual freedom to strict prohibition. Today, as always, unmarried individuals and couples must still decide on their own course of sexual conduct.

Petting

There are various degrees of sexual relationship. One is "petting," which might be defined as all relations more intimate than kissing but short of actual sexual intercourse. Petting typically includes manual or oral stimulation, or both, of the breasts and sexual organs, and it may or may not lead to orgasm in either the male or female.

Oral stimulation involves much personal preference. To some people it is extremely enjoyable; to others it is equally unpleasant. It is most important that oral sex (or any other practice) not be forced upon a partner who does not really enjoy it.

Any value judgment regarding petting should be based on such considerations as the age and emotional maturity of each individual and their individual attitudes and backgrounds. Petting is a normal step in the development of psychosexual maturity and enables one to learn his own sexual responses and those of the opposite sex.

Petting acts more as a stimulus for sexual desire than as a relief from sexual tensions. It is sexually arousing. The natural tendency of petting is to become more and more intimate, until it culminates in actual sexual intercourse. Consequently, the sexually aroused couple finds it very difficult to stop short of true intercourse. It is unplanned intercourse of this sort that most often results in nonmarital pregnancy, since adequate contraception may not be readily available. Some couples develop techniques of petting to mutual orgasm as an alternative to intercourse. If this is to be done, it is important that no semen be allowed near the vaginal opening, since pregnancy can occur even without vaginal penetration by the penis.

Nonmarital sexual intercourse

There are no universal answers to questions of whether or when to engage in nonmarital intercourse. Many individual factors must be considered. To some their religious beliefs dictate a definite "no" if the tenets of their religion are to be followed. To others, below the age of consent, state laws dictate a firm "no." But for the young adult, of legal age and holding no strong religious beliefs, it becomes a highly individual question, to be decided on the basis of personal values and philosophy, due consideration being given to all possible (positive and negative) results of such action. The following are some matters that should be given consideration in a decision about nonmarital sex.

Physical consideration

· PREGNANCY   The basic motivation behind most of the laws and religious and social regulations pertaining to marriage is to provide a stable family environment for the child and to determine who is responsible for his support. Historically our society has held contempt for the illegitimate child and his mother. The fear of pregnancy has, therefore, traditionally been the greatest deterrent to nonmarital intercourse. Even today, although attitudes toward sex have changed considerably, pregnancy out of marriage is regarded as a serious problem by many people.

Modern contraceptive methods can reduce the chance of pregnancy to a very low level if they are used properly and consistently. Anyone engaging in nonmarital sexual relations should choose a highly effective contraceptive method and be certain that it is used properly. Even though a normally foolproof method (such as pills) is chosen, there should be a definite plan and agreement on the action to be taken in case accidental pregnancy should occur. If a couple is not mature enough to discuss this problem realistically, then it is questionable whether they are mature enough to engage in sexual relations at all. Some of the paths available to the unmarried pregnant girl are given below.

· ABORTION   Abortion is now legal in the United States. Every woman now has the same right to an abortion during the first 6 months of pregnancy that she has to other minor surgery. This does not mean that every physician, hospital, or clinic will perform abortions. But the services are available. A woman wanting an abortion need only shop around until she is able to get one. However, some precautions are in order. An induced abortion temporarily interferes with the body's hormonal system, and some women may need post-abortion medical help. Repeated induced abortions may later lead to the inability to conceive or carry a child to full term. For some, religious or personal philosophical viewpoints may raise emotional or ethical questions that need to be answered. Although nearly all abortions are warranted, abortion should not be viewed as a substitute for the individual's use of a reliable contraceptive.

· SINGLE PARENTHOOD   The prospect of keeping and raising a child out of wedlock holds little appeal for many women. Yet in recent years increasing numbers of unmarried women are taking this option. It is probably preferable for both mother and child over the option of marrying just "to give the child a name" and then divorcing after a few months or years of bitter marriage.

· MARRIAGE   Although pregnancy is one of the most common reasons for getting married, it may be one of the poorest. A high percentage of forced marriages turn into disasters, leading to divorce or, perhaps even worse, to meaningless, bitter coexistence. Unless both parties truly want to marry, it is far better to take one of the other options.

· ADOPTION   In many cases adoption is the best course of action, because it should assure the child of a loving home where he is welcomed rather than resented. There is currently a strong demand for newborn infants for adoption.

Venereal disease The risk of venereal disease depends on the pattern of nonmarital sexual relationships. If the only relationship involved is between a mutually faithful couple then, of course, there is no risk of venereal disease (assuming neither is infected to start with). If a person has many casual sexual contacts or has intercourse with anyone who does have such contacts, then the risk of venereal disease is greatly increased; syphilis and gonorrhea are now epidemic.

Psychological considerations The personal motives for engaging in nonmarital sexual intercourse may be quite varied, even within an individual. They should, however, be examined, as should their effects on possible future marriage.

· MOTIVATION The individual considering nonmarital sex should consider his own motivations and the motivations of his partner. Is it to be a mutual expression of love, each being truly concerned with the welfare of the other? Or is it to be a case of exploitation, one of the two being interested only in his own sexual or ego satisfaction? Allowing oneself to be sexually exploited repeatedly may contribute to negative attitudes toward sex, which can create difficulty in future sexual adjustments.

· EFFECT ON FUTURE MARRIAGE It is difficult to isolate any one factor, such as premarital sexual activity, and then determine its exact effect on total marriage success. There are so many factors related to unhappy marriages that it is almost impossible to determine direct cause-and-effect relationships. A traditional point of view has been that premarital sex is detrimental to total marriage adjustment, but recent studies have indicated that people who enjoy full sex lives before marriage usually continue to have satisfactory sexual relationships in marriage. However, individuals with premarital sexual experience also are more likely to engage in extramarital sex. Thus there are significant qualifications to information of this type. One is that it does not establish any cause-and-effect relationship; it is quite possible that those persons with satisfactory premarital sexual lives were also psychologically or biologically predisposed toward sexual success. The person who is more sexually adventurous before marriage is likely to continue to be so after marriage. In any case, it seems that premarital sex is neither essential to nor precludes happiness in marriage.

Social considerations Different societies and different elements within one society hold varying attitudes toward nonmarital sexual intercourse, ranging from total permissiveness to total prohibition. In the United States we find an ambiguous situation, in which many people disapprove of the sexual activities of others but excuse their own similar activities. The "official" attitude here is prohibitive toward sexual activity before marriage; the "unofficial" attitude is still the highly discredited "double standard," which is much more tolerant toward the sexual activities of men than of women. This is an unfortunate carryover from the era when women were not expected to enjoy sexual intercourse.

Fear of discovery drives many couples to seek less than ideal places for their sexual relationships, often with unhappy results. The fear, anxiety, and haste may make orgasm impossible for the female, thus building a negative attitude toward sex. After several disappointing, frustrating experiences she may feel that she is sexually inadequate or that she is being exploited for the purely selfish satisfaction of the male, who may himself feel sexually inadequate because of her lack of satisfaction.

Legal considerations   In a few states any sexual intercourse between unmarried persons is illegal, but the laws are seldom, if ever, enforced. Of more importance are laws that prohibit intercourse with a woman below the "age of consent," which varies among the states from 14 to 21 years of age but is most often 18 years of age. A male having intercourse with a girl below this age can be prosecuted for statutory rape, a felonious offense. Even if a girl appears to be older and lies about her age, the male can still be convicted.

Another possible legal complication is that not uncommonly a woman will voluntarily engage in intercourse and later claim that she was forcibly raped. It can be very difficult for a man to prove otherwise.

Still another problem can arise when an unmarried girl becomes pregnant and sues for child support. Any male who has had intercourse with her during a given period of time may be named in the suit. Unfortunately, blood tests do not always identify the true father.

Masturbation

Masturbation is the production of orgasm by self-manipulation of the sex organs. In the past it was thought to lead to insanity, impotence, acne, and any number of major and minor problems. Today it is recognized as perfectly harmless and a part of normal sexuality in both the male and the female. Over 90 percent of all males masturbate at some time in their lives, as do over 60 percent of all females.

Most individuals resort to masturbation as a substitute for sexual intercourse only when the latter is unavailable. As a result, masturbation is most common among unmarried individuals, though married people also masturbate when their mates are in some way unavailable for intercourse.

The old wives' tale that masturbation leads to insanity probably originated in the fact that emotionally disturbed individuals sometimes masturbate excessively, in a retreat from reality. The fear of impotence was based on the erroneous notion that the lifetime supply of semen was limited and could be exhausted through masturbation.

Masturbation may begin at any age; the average age of first orgasm is about fourteen years. The frequency of masturbation among normal unmarried males varies considerably, from about once a month to several times daily. Females typically masturbate less frequently than males.

Parents should be careful not to lead their child to a sense of guilt over masturbation, recognizing that the practice is normal. Girls should be warned against inserting objects into the vagina for self-stimulation, because they may cause infection.

Nocturnal emissions

Nocturnal emissions, commonly called "wet dreams," are involuntary discharges of semen, often accompanied by sexual dreams. Almost all males experience these emissions at some time. They are perfectly harmless and serve to relieve the pressure of fluid in the seminal vesicles when no other sexual outlet is available.

Prostitutes

Prostitution, though it exists in all areas, plays a minor role in the sexual adjustment of the typical college student. A few college males regularly patronize prostitutes, and a few others occasionally. But the typical customer of the prostitute is older (36 to 40) and poorly educated. The obvious reasons for avoiding prostitutes are their high incidence of venereal disease, the chance of being robbed, and the chance of arrest.

HOMOSEXUALITY

A much-discussed topic today is homosexuality—sexual attraction to members of the same sex. Significant numbers of both males and females experience at least some degree of homosexual activity during their lives. Various surveys have given somewhat differing reports of the exact incidence of homosexuality, depending on survey methods and sample population. It does seem clear that the incidence of homosexuality is somewhat higher among males than among females, though female homosexuals (lesbians) are far from rare. Statistics on homosexuality have been clouded by the fact that many individuals pass through a stage of development during their adolescence or preadolescence during which they feel homosexual attractions but with further development become fully heterosexual in their attractions. Homosexuality does exist, however, among persons in all walks of life—male or female, poor or rich, ignorant or intellectual, young or old, single or married.

Among those in whom homosexuality persists into the adult life it can exist in any degree, from slight homosexual feelings in a predominantly heterosexual individual to total homosexuality with the exclusion of any heterosexual feelings. Many persons are *bisexual*, feeling attractions for both males and females.

The appearance and outward display of homosexuality is also quite variable. Despite the increased openness of homosexuality in the past few years, most male and female homosexuals still give no obvious indication by their appearance of their true sexual nature. Since the opinion of the general public is still strongly against homosexuality and the chance of arrest is still great, there are valid reasons for being guarded about it. The outward signs of homosexuality are often so subtle as to be noticed only by other homo-sexuals, if at all. The few male homosexuals who do make an obvious display of homosexuality may either adopt an effeminate mode of dress and action (the public image of the "queen") or, to attract other male homosexuals, de-velop a very masculine image, with strong muscular development, leather clothing, motorcycles, and similar symbols of masculinity. Female homo-sexuals may similarly range in appearance from masculine to very feminine.

Homosexual behavior patterns

The typical pattern of homosexual relationships differs considerably between male and female homosexuals. The female tendency is to establish long-term homosexual relationships, lasting for months, years, or even a lifetime. In these female relationships, one member sometimes assumes a more dominant, masculine role, in both dress and actions, while the other member assumes the feminine role. Since there is very little open solicitation for sexual activity by lesbians, they very seldom encounter any difficulty with the law.

The typical pattern of male homosexuality is quite different. The empha-sis among males is generally toward variety in sexual partners. Exclusive relationships are unusual and seldom last for any length of time. Instead, the male homosexual is often engaged in a constant, seemingly desperate, search for new sexual encounters. He may spend much of his time haunting "gay" bars and similar homosexual gathering places. Since there is much open solici-tation for homosexual activity, the chance of arrest of male homosexuals is great. Though it is illegal to do so, some police departments still use "baiting" and entrapment techniques in arresting homosexuals. It has been estimated (Gebhard *et al.*, 1965) that the average number of different sexual partners of the aggressive homosexual male is about two hundred per year. Individual male homosexuals have reported sexual contact with as many as a thousand different partners per year. This constant search for new sexual partners ex-poses the male homosexual, not only to the possibility of arrest, but also to the veneral diseases. The VD rate among male homosexuals is extremely high. The behavior of the male homosexual seems to indicate that his life is not as satisfactory as that of the female homosexual.

Among the practices used by male homosexuals to achieve orgasm are mutual hand manipulation of the penis, oral-genital contacts, and anal-genital contacts. Techniques used in female homosexual contacts include kissing, manual and oral manipulation of the breasts, and manual or oral stimulation of the genitalia.

Some homosexuals enter into heterosexual marriages. There are several possible motivations behind such marriages. Sometimes the individual is truly bisexual and enjoys relationships with both sexes. More often, the marriage is an attempt by the homosexual to live a "straight" life, thinking the mar-riage may solve the problem of homosexuality (it seldom does). Or marriage can be a "front" for homosexual activity, an attempt to appear socially ac-ceptable while secretly engaging in homosexual activities. The mates in these marriages are often relatively "sexless" individuals who will make few hetero-sexual demands on the homosexual.

Causes of homosexuality

Homosexuality is the result of emotional, rather than biological, causes. Homosexuals are physically no different from heterosexuals; their hormone levels are no different, and they do not respond to hormone treatments. Homosexuality is an emotional phenomenon, an indication of fixation or regression in emotional development. Most homosexual people do not know why they are homosexual; in fact, it is often difficult for even the trained psychiatrist to know the definite cause. What may cause one person to become homosexual may not hold true of another. It is generally agreed that the influences leading to homosexuality take place during childhood. In fact, whether an individual is going to be homosexual or heterosexual is so strongly determined by the time he or she is twenty years old that the chance of a change in sexual attraction after that time is remote.

The relationship between the child and his parents is often implicated as a contributing factor in the development of homosexuality. Failure to identify with a parent of the same sex is a common finding in homosexuals. The homosexual male is often found to have had an unusually strong attachment to his mother or sister. Psychoanalytically oriented psychologists sometimes relate fear of incest to homosexuality; that is, a male may identify all females with his mother and so be reluctant to engage in sexual activity with them. An important determining influence in the development of homosexuality can be the realization by a child that his sex was a disappointment to one or both of his parents, especially if their disappointment leads them to treat the child as if he were of the opposite sex. Occasionally a mother is found to have used a boy as a husband-substitute, showering love on him and preventing him from developing a normal attraction to girls by sheltering him from contact with them and by her derogatory remarks about girls and normal heterosexual relationships.

Some authorities stress masochism (sexual pleasure in being abused) as an underlying cause of homosexuality. The entire personality structure of the homosexual is seen as filled with an unconscious wish to suffer. Through homosexual activity this wish is often fulfilled through arrest, imprisonment, venereal diseases, beatings, and other problems that homosexuals encounter.

Isolated incidents of homosexual behavior usually result from temporary needs and drives rather than from any deeply rooted homosexual attitudes. Sexual play between children of the same sex is common and does not usually lead to any adult homosexuality. Occasional episodes of homosexual experimentation in adolescence similarly do not necessarily mean that the individuals will become homosexual adults. Even adults, when isolated from the opposite sex, such as in prison, may engage in homosexual activities without being regarded as true homosexuals. The same may be true of isolated cases of homosexual behavior under the influence of alcohol or drugs.

Treatment of homosexuality

As was previously mentioned, homosexuality has emotional rather than physical causes. Its treatment, therefore, revolves around psychotherapy. Unfortunately, the rate of success in treating homosexuality has not been as great as that for many other types of emotional problems. There are two essential requirements for success. The first is that the homosexual must really want to change. The second is a therapist who understands homosexuality and has experience in its treatment. The success rate is about one third.

Much has been said and written regarding the attitude that society and the law should assume toward homosexuality. Opinions range from those favoring strict enforcement of strict laws against all forms of homosexuality to total permissiveness toward homosexual behavior. It is generally agreed today that punishment of the homosexual by jailing him does not change his homosexuality or result in any subsequent change in his behavior. In fact, those who support the masochistic theory of homosexuality would say the threat of jail reinforces homosexual behavior. The authors of this book believe that there must be continued legal restrictions to discourage adult homosexuals from soliciting homosexual acts from children and adolescents. Many youths spend several years wavering between homosexual and heterosexual feelings. Anything that would push them toward the homosexual side should be discouraged. We base this statement, not on any moral or religious grounds, but on the fact that the homosexual life is seldom as happy or rewarding as the heterosexual life. Most of the arguments given by homosexuals in favor of their mode of living are merely a series of rationalizations to justify their unhappy lives. In all fairness, though, we should point out that many homosexuals live useful, well-adjusted lives and that many of the problems of the homosexual arise from the social stigma attached to homosexuality and from the homosexual's resulting alienation from the mainstream of heterosexual society.

FACTORS TO CONSIDER BEFORE MARRIAGE

At no time in recent history has traditional marriage been the subject of such skepticism and criticism as it is today. To many young people contemporary marriage is just a mockery of everything of value in life. They have watched their parents' marriages end in divorce or exist in a grindingly destructive combination of emotional estrangement, anxiety, and hostility. They have seen the beautiful romances of their friends turn into dull marriages, in which lovers gradually become bitter adversaries. Not surprisingly, increasing numbers of people are deciding that marriage is just not for them. Yet the majority of young people still hold hopes for a successful marriage, and the majority of people still do marry. The success of their marriages depends largely upon their reasons for marrying, their own personal readiness for marriage, and their selection of a marital partner.

Some poor reasons for marriage

Many marriages fail because they were motivated by the wrong reasons. Some of the wrong reasons for marriage are given below.

Pressure from parents   Parents often exert upon their offspring obvious or subtle pressures to get married. This may reflect the social goals of the parents, their desire for grandchildren, or the projection of their values onto their children.

Social pressures   Some people marry because "everyone is getting married" and they fear rejection if they do not follow suit. Friends may keep asking "When are you going to get married?" There is also the very unfortunate existence of economic biases against unmarried people. For example, some employers favor married people in their hiring practices, and often single people (especially single women) experience difficulty in obtaining credit or loans.

Fear of being "left out"   Some people marry sooner than they really want to because they fear that all of the desirable marriage partners will be gone if they delay. This, of course, is just not true—there are always desirable mates available.

Transfer of dependency   Many people never develop an adequate degree of emotional independence and self-determination because they live with their parents until marriage and then transfer all their dependencies directly to their marriage partners. Not only does this thwart their own emotional growth and self-actualization, but it often contributes to later marital problems. Few people today can remain satisfied with a "clinging vine" who has few interests and little identity outside the marriage. A man may not remain satisfied with a woman whose only identity is as his wife; a woman seldom remains satisfied with a man to whom she must play the role of "mother." To help avoid such problems it is important to live independently, away from one's parents, for a period before marriage. Anyone who is not mature or secure enough to do so is certainly not ready for marriage.

Pregnancy   As previously mentioned, one of the worst reasons for getting married is pregnancy. The chances of lasting happiness are very slight, and often everyone is hurt by the marriage, including the child for whose supposed benefit the marriage took place.

Are you ready for marriage?

Success in marriage demands considerable emotional strength and maturity. Many marriage failures can be traced to inadequate emotional development of one or both of the partners.

Age at marriage   The age at which a person marries is influenced greatly by such individual factors as educational goals, military duty, and social and cultural background. The national average age at the first marriage is just under 23 years for men and between 20 and 21 years for women. Many people, girls in particular, feel pushed to marry at a fairly young age to avoid getting "left out" and becoming "old maids." Such fear is not warranted, because at any age numerous individuals eligible for marriage will be found. In fact, some of the best marriage prospects delay marriage for several years in order to reach educational or career goals.

Many studies have shown that the average happiness level in marriage increases with the age of the couple at the time of marriage. Emotional conflict, sexual maladjustment, money problems, in-law trouble, and divorce are all much more common among those couples who marry in their teens. Marriages in which the husband was in his teens are particularly unhappy.

One of the sources of problems with young marriages is that many people greatly change their value systems somewhere between the ages of 16 and 22; during this period one's interests, tastes, ideals, standards, and goals usually undergo a complete change. If people marry before this change, there is a strong possibility that they will no longer meet each other's tastes and emotional needs.

A related problem is that early marriage often interferes with the development of a mature philosophy. There is a tendency of intellectual growth to stop with marriage. This can be prevented, of course, but many young married people fall into a deep philosophical and intellectual rut from which they never escape.

Emotional maturity   The emotional demands of marriage are much greater than those a couple experience during dating. Thus an important requirement for marriage is emotional maturity. This generally increases with age, but some individuals remain emotionally adolescent even though they have legally become adults.

Before marriage a person should be as free as possible of emotional maladjustments, such as moodiness, jealousy, anxiety, depression, and insecurity. Their presence in a marriage can be disastrous. A person who is subject to such maladjustment should seek qualified professional counsel.

The truly mature person has skill in establishing and maintaining good interpersonal relationships. He recognizes the needs of others and is willing to assume some responsibility for meeting these needs. Each partner in a marriage must have such a concern for the other if happiness is to result.

Social maturity   Social maturity develops through social interaction. Before marriage social maturity should be built through dating many different individuals. This gives a better basis for the selection of a marriage mate and helps satisfy social curiosity. The person whose dating is more restricted may later, after marriage, feel he has missed something and try to compensate through extramarital affairs.

We have discussed the need for a period of single, independent life before marriage, a time of freedom between the bondage of childhood and the bondage of marriage. Most people appreciate this freedom to a point, after which they feel ready for marriage. A few find this freedom permanently satisfying and prefer not to marry. There is no reason why these people should feel any obligation to themselves or to society to marry.

Financial resources   Although less important than the preceding personal factors, financial factors must be considered before marriage. The minimal amount of money a couple needs to live on is highly variable. Most young couples enter marriage without great amounts of money. But if the husband is to be a student, there must be a careful evaluation of the marriage plans, to avoid the unfortunate situation of an education terminated for financial reasons.

Often the parents of student couples offer some financial help. But the couple should evaluate this possibility with respect to their sense of independence. If such help is going to be a source of conflict, then some other financial arrangement must be developed. If the couple is to rely on the earnings of the wife, then obviously it is important that a highly reliable method of contraception be used. A pregnancy in this situation could be a serious financial and emotional burden.

Selecting for happiness

The chances of a happy marriage are determined by one's own personal traits, those of one's chosen partner, and how those traits act upon each other. Let us consider, then, some of the traits to look for in a potential mate. Right away let us dispel the notion of the "one and only" or the "marriage made in heaven." For every person there are thousands of potentially good mates. If the person you might be considering for marriage seems to have a serious deficiency in some respect, just keep looking. On the other hand, if no one seems to fit your ideal for marriage, you might well be overcritical or just not ready for marriage.

Positive personality traits   By far the most important characteristic to evaluate in a potential marriage partner is his or her personality. Some people have positive personality traits which enable them to enjoy life to its fullest and to bring joy to anyone in contact with them. Others are so burdened with negative reactions that their own happiness is impossible, as is that of anyone who must live with them. Traits which help produce happiness in marriage include the ability to adjust easily to changes in conditions, optimism, a sense of humor, an honest concern for the needs of others, a sense of ethics, and the freedom from such negative traits as anxiety, depression, insecurity, and jealousy.

Mutual-need satisfaction   The marriage that is happy and lasting is one in which the needs of each individual are adequately satisfied. While the idea may not appeal to romanticists, the basic reason why people marry is to satisfy their needs. A good marriage satisfies many needs—sex, love, companionship, security, and subtle psychological needs. Since everyone is unique in his psychological needs, the characterization of the "ideal" partner for each person is a highly individual matter. Only through knowing each other very well, over a long period of time and in a variety of situations (both pleasant and unpleasant), can two people learn how well they are able to fulfill each other's needs.

Genuine mutual love   The distinction between genuine love and infatuation is not always clear. Infatuation is frequently associated with immaturity, a "puppy love." It is a kind of substitute for love until a person has the capacity to love someone fully and deeply. It tends to involve sexual attraction more than personality attraction. Infatuation is unrealistic, a fantasy. The object of the infatuation is seen as a "dream mate," lacking any undesirable traits. Infatuation is often immediate, whereas love develops with time. Infatuation often wears off quickly, yet it may, with time, develop into mature love.

A person truly in love is concerned with his loved one's happiness and well-being. He is tender, considerate, and constant. He is willing to sacrifice some of his own pleasures in order to bring pleasure to his loved one. There is a desire to share ideas, emotions, goals, and experiences. Love continues to grow indefinitely with the passage of time.

There should definitely be a strong sexual attraction between any persons considering marriage. It would be an unusual couple who would want to marry in the absence of sexual attraction. However, many people mistake sexual attraction for love, when it is actually just part of love. A couple can have a very good sexual relationship without loving each other, but such a relationship would make a weak basis for a happy marriage.

Agreement on parenthood   Any couple considering marriage should reveal their true feelings about having children. Ideally, they should agree on whether they want children and, if so, how many. It is always unfortunate when a person who wants children chooses a partner who would rather remain childless. Automatically, one or the other of them is destined to be unhappy. If there is serious disagreement on this matter, it would be well for each individual to look for another mate.

Incidentally, if neither person wants children, there is *no* reason to feel guilty about a decision to remain childless. Studies have shown that children are not essential to happiness in marriage. In fact, they have been found to place additional strain on an already unhappy marriage. A couple need feel no obligation to themselves or to society to produce children.

Hereditary traits   Some individuals carry obvious hereditary defects. Others seem perfectly normal but come from families in which such defects are known to occur. The latter individuals may or may not be carrying undesirable hidden genes. If there is any question regarding the possibility of transmitting defective genes, it is wise to seek genetic counseling, either from a physician or a specially trained genetic counselor whom a physician may recommend. Any decision to marry and have children, marry and not have children, or not to marry at all should be based upon such advice and not on the advice of uninformed friends and relatives.

Similarities in background   It is important for any couple considering marriage to take a critical, objective look at their differences in general background. These differences may be minor and insignificant or major and have a great bearing on the marriage. Many studies have shown that the more similarities between two individuals, the greater their chances of marital success. Significant differences may involve age, nationality or ethnic background, economic status, education, intelligence, religion, or previous marital status. Most marriages can be successful, despite these differences, if the couple is willing to work out the special problems involved.

• AGE   When there is a wide difference in age, the individual must examine why he wants to marry a person considerably older or younger than himself. Is it the desire for immediate economic security? Is it the inability to find a partner close to one's own age? Is it a feeling of flattery at commanding the attention of a more mature or more youthful person? Is the older person seen as a "father" or "mother" image? Does the older person need to dominate or the younger to be dominated? Is it just an infatuation? On the average, marriages are happiest when the man and wife are within a few years of each other in age. However, if the marriage with a wide age difference fulfills the needs of each person, then such a marriage may be quite happy.

• ETHNIC ORIGIN   Marriages between members of different races or nationalities may face the most difficult problems of any type of mixed marriage. Not only can there be problems within the marriage, but the couple may experience resentment and prejudice from family members and unenlightened members of society.

The internal problems in these marriages may revolve around customs, standards, and points of view. For example, the attitudes toward women and their rights, duties, and status may be quite different. Family patterns of authority and the role expected of each member may conflict. Attitudes on raising children and care of elderly relatives may be another area of disagreement. These are not always problems in mixed marriages, but such topics should be discussed objectively before any marriage between different races or nationalities takes place.

The problems caused by prejudices of family members and society are particularly frustrating, because they should not exist in an enlightened society. The source of many of these problems is the ethnocentric attitude of groups which guard the ethnic heritage to excess and often sincerely believe in the supremacy of their group over all others. The elders of some of these groups encourage their youth to maintain a distance from outsiders, to continue to respect the traditions and customs of the group, and to marry within the group. The young man or woman who marries outside the group may experience total rejection by even immediate family members.

Other problems may arise in finding housing and employment, especially in black-white marriages. There may even be problems in finding friends that will fully accept both partners. The amount of social prejudice felt by the interracial couple will vary from city to city and with the part of the country. Interracial couples may find their best acceptance today in college towns, where the general attitude is usually more enlightened and liberal than in many other places.

It is likely that the number of interracial marriages will continue to increase, if the trends of the past few years can be projected into the future. The breakdown of social prejudices is painfully slow, but it can be hoped that the need for a discussion such as this will eventually be a thing of the past.

• ECONOMIC STATUS   Even though our society has always claimed that one of its goals is social equality regardless of economic status, patterns of behavior do vary greatly with economic level. Behavior that is "correct" at one economic level may meet with disapproval at another level. Attitudes toward authority, freedom, ethics, education, and other values may differ. Marriage of individuals of different economic backgrounds may require some adjustment of these attitudes.

A problem area in marriages involving different economic backgrounds may be "in-law" relationships. The wealthier set of in-laws may not entirely accept the son-in-law or daughter-in-law who comes from a less affluent background.

Other problems can arise when a woman who has been raised in affluence marries a young man of limited income. This couple has two choices. One is to accept financial aid from the girl's family (if it is offered), which may be psychologically damaging to the young man. The other is live within their income, which may require a difficult adjustment for the girl, if her values are materialistic. There may be no problem at all, but this is another area which should be discussed and agreed upon before marriage.

• EDUCATION   Even with the increasing educational opportunities available today it is not unusual for two young persons to have wide differences in level of education. A change in reading tastes, personal goals, and social sophistication usually accompany a greater extent of education. A better educated partner may be interested in entirely different recreational activities. Compatibility in marriage is largely a matter of common interests, and differently educated persons are likely to have few common interests. There is a tendency for boredom to develop and for each to go increasingly his own way.

Yet there are individuals who, though short on formal education, have horizons that are wider than many college graduates who have confined their interests to a specialized major field of study.

• INTELLIGENCE   Perhaps a similarity in level of intelligence is even more important than similarity in level of education. In marriages in which there is a wide contrast in basic intelligence, there is a tendency of the partners to drift apart. Not only may the more intelligent partner long for stimulating exchanges of ideas with someone else, but also the less intelligent person may develop feelings of inferiority. Each may grow lonely. These marriages can be successful if each partner recognizes the other's strong points and allows each to excel in his own way. Common interests discovered *before* marriage can be cultivated after it.

• RELIGION   Religious differences can be one of the most disruptive influences in a marriage. The important factor is not simply the fact of difference in religious affiliation, but the significance the individuals attach to their religious beliefs. To some religion means nothing. To others it is the unifying force in their lives. A religion shared in marriage can form a powerful bond between man and wife. Religious conflict can act as a powerful wedge, forcing man and wife far apart.

Most of the differences we have thus far discussed *can* be worked out satisfactorily. However, in certain combinations of religious beliefs, if each person remains faithful to his religion, there may be constant conflict throughout the marriage. Such marriages should be entered into only after mutually acceptable answers to all possible questions and problems of mixed-marriage life have been reached. Nothing should be left to chance or to resolution after marriage. Having made these decisions, the couple should go together to discuss them with the parents and the clergy of each faith. Their decisions should be clearly in mind and well stated (in writing, if possible), so there can be no possibility of a misunderstanding. If after such discussions with parents and clergy there still seem to be conflicts, it probably would be better for each to look for someone else whose religious beliefs are more similar to his own. This may seem to be a pessimistic view of the problem, but it *does* seem the best way to avoid the problems of a religiously incompatible marriage.

Previous marital status   One out of every four or five marriages today involves a person who has been married before. The chances of falling in love with a divorced or widowed person are not remote. Marrying a person who has been divorced or widowed is not the same as marrying one who has never been married before. A past marital experience affects the attitudes a person brings to a second marriage. These attitudes may be the product of memories of a happy marriage or the bitter aftertaste of marital disappointment.

Second marriages can turn out to be very desirable and happy, or the problems that were causes of trouble in the first marriage may reappear. Before marrying a previously married individual one must have definite answers to several questions. Has the divorced or widowed person recovered sufficiently from the feeling of loss to make a wise choice, or is he desperate? If the former mate is still living, what are his attitudes toward that person? What are the chances of the former mate's coming between the new partners? Can the new mate be content to live in a home previously occupied by the former partner? Are the real causes of the divorce, not simply the legal grounds, known to the new mate? (Remember that you have heard just one side of the story.) Is there any assurance that the same problems will not recur? Has the person been divorced more than once? (Third and subsequent marriages are *very* poor risks.)

If the divorced or widowed person has custody of children from a prior marriage, a prospective mate should want to be assured of acceptance by them. Also, one's own attitude toward these potential stepchildren should be honestly appraised. In the event there are children born into the second marriage in addition to children present from the first one, the parents must make every effort to avoid any showing of partiality toward one set of children.

Danger signals in a relationship

Many people are married only a short time before they realize that their marriages are mistakes. As a result, the divorce rate is very high during the first few years of marriage. It is obvious that many divorces are the result of the wrong people's getting married in the first place. Much misery could be prevented if such incompatible couples could be identified before they made the commitment of marriage. Actually, many unfortunate marriages can be predicted by the following danger signals in the premarital relationship.

Quarreling Quarreling is a very serious danger signal in any relationship that is moving toward marriage. Such quarreling is almost certain to continue after marriage, probably at an escalated frequency and intensity. Quarreling almost always means that the needs of one or both partners are not being fulfilled in their relationship. As long as needs are mutually met, there is no need to quarrel, and a relationship runs smoothly. Couples must *not* rely on the folk belief, so often reinforced by movies, television, novels, and other media, that true love seldom runs smoothly and that they should not be concerned over their "lovers' quarrels." The theme of lovers fighting, breaking up, making up, marrying, and living "happily ever after" occurs frequently in the entertainment media but very rarely in real life. Constant quarreling calls for serious evaluation, in which the real reasons for the quarrels are determined through open and honest communication of feelings. If an area of conflict cannot be clearly resolved, it would seem foolish for a couple to marry.

Lack of communication If either partner cannot openly and freely express his feelings on any subject to the other, this casts considerable doubt upon their chances of a happy marriage. Not only is lack of communication a problem in itself, but it can also be an outward symptom of a personality problem in one of the individuals or a basic incompatibility of the two. It is important that any couple considering marriage thoroughly discuss their feelings about sex (role, frequency, techniques, etc.), parenthood, contraception, family finances, role of each partner in a marriage, in-law relationships, and general life style. Any inability to communicate or any open disagreement in one of these areas can only be interpreted as a danger sign and portent of an unhappy marriage.

Lack of confidence that the marriage will be good Another prime indicator of unhappy marriage is when either person has serious doubts about the possibilities of the success of the marriage. Retrospective surveys of married couples have shown that the happiest married couples are those who had the least doubts before marriage that they would be happy. By contrast, a large percentage of unhappily married couples recall serious premarital doubts about the ultimate success of their marriages.

Off-again on-again relationships A history of temporary breakups in a relationship is strongly predictive of failure in marriage. Such breakups indicate that one or both partners may lack a strong commitment to the relationship, that needs are not being well fulfilled, or that other serious problems exist. The same problems that cause temporary breakups are likely to remain after marriage, leading to continued trouble. Couples with a history of breakups should carefully consider the underlying causes before entering into marriage.

MARRIAGE LAWS

Every state has laws regulating marriage. Although the laws vary somewhat from state to state and are changed periodically, there are certain similarities among them.

Minimal age for marriage

Every state has a minimal-age requirement for marriage. The age ranges from 14 to 17 for girls and from 15 to 18 for boys. The most common age requirements are 16 for girls and 18 for boys. Two thirds of the states allow exceptions when the girl is pregnant or has an illegitimate child or in certain other special circumstances.

All states require parental consent for marriage if either partner is below a given age. Most commonly such consent is required if the age of the boy is below 21 or the girl below 18.

Physical examination and blood test

All but a few states now require a medical examination of some kind which generally includes a blood test. In most states this is for venereal disease only. A few states also examine for one or more of the following: feeblemindedness, uncontrolled epileptic seizures, infectious tuberculosis, chronic alcoholism, mental illness, and drug addiction. About two thirds of the states require that the examination be given not longer than 30 days before the issuance of the marriage license. In some cases the blood test must be within 10 days of the issuance of the license.

Waiting period

Most states have legislated a "cooling off" period either between the application for a marriage license and its issuance or after the license is issued but before it can be used. The purpose of these laws is to prevent marriage on a sudden impulse with its often unhappy results. Typical waiting periods are from 3 to 7 days. Thousands of unhappy marriages are believed to have been prevented by these waiting periods. Those states with no waiting periods are common marriage sites for eloping couples.

Prohibited marriages

Every state prohibits marriage between close relatives such as brothers, sisters, fathers, or mothers. More than half the states prohibit the marriage of first cousins and a few even of second cousins. All states prohibit the marriage of a person who is already married to one living spouse (bigamy). Marriage of a person who is legally judged to be mentally ill is prohibited in all states. Other prohibitions in some states include feeblemindedness, epilepsy, and the "biologically unfit." No state considers a marriage valid which involves force or willful misrepresentation. To represent oneself falsely is usually grounds for the annulment of the marriage.

Common-law marriages

A common-law marriage is one in which both parties agree to live together as husband and wife without benefit of license or ceremony. Such marriages are now officially recognized by only a few states. Since there are no records of these marriages, they have no status in most states.

ENGAGEMENT

Engagement today means the private agreement between a man and woman to marry each other. The engagement may or may not be made "formal" by public announcement. If such a formal announcement is made, it is usually after a period of informal testing of the arrangement. There is, however, no obligation for the couple to announce their engagement formally at all, any couple is free not to announce their engagement if they so choose. If there is no formal announcement, then it is easier to break off the engagement if the couple later desires to do so.

Purposes of engagement

One of the main purposes of engagement, whether formal or informal, is to let each partner feel how he reacts to a prolonged, intensive relationship with the other. During this time they can test their reactions to the new relationship in a more intense and exclusive manner. Since most people still feel that marriage should involve exclusive sexual fidelity between the couple, it is important that a similar fidelity exist in engagement. It is very unlikely that the individual who is unfaithful during engagement will be faithful in marriage. Yet during engagement the two people need not seal themselves off from society. If, for example, one of them is away in school or military service, the other should be allowed the liberty to date. Such dating should be limited to pleasure and convenience, without serious interest or sexual activity and should not be limited to one person. Such dating can relieve some of the loneliness of separation and can be a good test of a couple's devotion. If their love can withstand a minor test like this, the chances are better that it can withstand the tests of marriage. If the relationship cannot stand such a trial, and either jealousy or a new love interest develops, then it is good to discover this before marriage, since the same thing is likely to happen in the marriage. It is always far easier to break an engagement than a marriage.

Other purposes of engagement are to allow time to answer the many questions essential to a successful marriage. Often the attempts to answer these questions will indicate that no marriage should take place. Some of these questions are the following. When and where will the wedding be held? Who will be invited to attend? Where should the honeymoon be, and how much money should be spent on it? Do the partners adequately understand sexual intercourse, reproduction, and contraception? Are they going to want children and, if so, when and how many? What are their attitudes on the use of contraceptives? Where is the couple going to derive their income, and how much will it be? How will their money be spent? Does the wife plan to work? Where do they plan to live? Will either be continuing with college? These questions and many more require definite answers before marriage.

Sexual relations during engagement

The extent of intimacy during engagement is a matter for each couple to decide. Some couples feel that sexual intercourse during engagement is desirable and engage in it without any apparent problems. Other couples question the advisability of intercourse at this time, agree on definite limits to their love-making, and then respect these limits. The training of still other couples places them in a dilemma—they want to have intercourse but do not think they should. If intercourse is going to result in guilt feelings, then it is probably better to wait for marriage.

Some people approaching marriage worry about the effect that past sexual experiences may have on their marriage. They may wonder whether their own sexual adjustment will be difficult or whether they will experience rejection by their partners. The best way to avoid any such problem is to minimize the past and build on the future. What is done is done; the past should not be allowed to interfere with the present and the future.

There may be a question of how much should be told about past sexual experiences. There certainly is no need to confess everything to the partner. Uncalled-for confessions may only arouse basic suspicions and create doubts. Minute details regarding the past are better left untold. However, anything that could affect the marriage should be told before, not after, the wedding.

Some things that should be told because they can affect the marriage and would probably be revealed with time anyway are previous marriages and how they terminated, any serious health defects, particularly if they relate to childbearing, any record of felony convictions, and any financial debts or obligations. Again, these should be revealed before marriage, not after.

Length of engagement

There is no definite length for an engagement. It should, of course, last long enough for all of its functions, as we have discussed, to be carried out. It is well documented that the divorce rate is very high among couples who know each other for only a short time before marriage. As a general rule, it is good to have at least one year of close relationship before marriage. Countless poor marriages would be prevented if all couples were to know each other well for a year before marriage.

Breaking the engagement

Although broken engagements can be unpleasant, they are certainly preferable to broken marriages; if a partnership is incompatible, it is far better to admit it before marriage than after. If, at any time, either partner wants to break an engagement, it should be broken. Once a person makes up his mind to break an engagement, he should act promptly and kindly. He should not allow the opinions of family or friends, the fact that the wedding plans are under way, or embarrassment or pride to prevent him from carrying out his decision. He should disregard any pleas, promises, or threats the other person might make. The wishes of the other party should not be "given in to" out of pity or fear. In time both parties will get over the experience, and an unhappy marriage will have been avoided. No person should ever assume a "this one or nobody" attitude. There are thousands of good marriage partners available to anyone who will seek them out. To the "jilted" party, this advice: please do not act "on the rebound" and hastily start another serious relationship, either for spite or to salvage your own hurt feelings. Such swift actions can lead to an even worse marriage than was avoided.

PREMARITAL COUNSELING

Increasing emphasis is being placed on premarital counseling to assist couples in making an adequate marital adjustment. It has been found that the probability of happiness in marriage can be predicted by examining certain background factors, personality traits, engagement relations, engagement adjustment, and other anticipated factors.

The counselor may be a professional marriage counselor, a clergyman, or a physician. Some marriage counselors use personality tests to indicate a person's suitability for marriage or the likely compatibility of a couple. If either member of the couple has inadequate knowledge of sexual intercourse and reproduction, he or she may be counseled by books or discussions. The couple should be prepared to discuss with the counselor any fears or inhibitions they may have regarding normal sex life. The counselor should question them regarding financial plans, housing, budgets, and any other phase of marriage that may be a subject of adjustment.

Even though a state law may require only a blood test for syphilis, each prospective partner should have a thorough physical examination, to detect any condition that might interfere with sexual relations, childbearing, or earning a living. There should be a consultation with a gynecologist regarding the preferred method of contraception for the couple. A genetic counselor should be consulted if there is any history of hereditary disorders in the family of either partner.

BEGINNING A MARRIAGE

Starting a marriage should be one of the most pleasurable and memorable stages in life. There is the excitement of setting the date, looking at apartments, making wedding plans, the actual ceremony, and the honeymoon.

The wedding ceremony

The particulars of the wedding ceremony are usually determined by the marriage partners and their families. The role of the parents of the couple can be small or large. Although many couples want their weddings to be something they and their friends will remember, no wedding should place a heavy financial burden on either the couple or their families. The central idea in planning a wedding and honeymoon should be to minimize the stress-producing factors, and financial burden is one of the greatest stress producers.

A wedding is merely the beginning of a new relationship and is not an end in itself. It does not need to be a "big production." Plans should be made carefully so that, in the effort to carry out an impressive ceremony, the couple does not become so nervous, confused, and fatigued that the setting for a good honeymoon adjustment is lost. The wedding should fit the desires of the couple, not the social aims of their parents.

The wedding rite may be a brief statement before a judge or justice of the peace or a modest or elaborate church ceremony. The wishes of the couple should be respected. Many religious groups have typical ceremonial forms that are followed, some being more symbolic than others. Regardless of the form chosen, the ceremony should fit the social and emotional needs of the couple, affirming their goals and pledging their commitment in terms that are meaningful to them.

Elopement and secret marriage

An elopement is a kind of "runaway" wedding in which the fact of the marriage is made known after the wedding. In a secret marriage the fact of both the wedding and the marriage are kept secret for an extended period. There may be valid reasons for elopement. Parents may have an unjustified opposition to the marriage, in spite of the reasonable age and maturity of the couple. Family factors such as illness, recent death, or parental disharmony may make elopement more desirable. Many couples elope to save the high cost of the typical wedding ceremony and reception.

There are also arguments against elopement and secret marriage, especially the latter. The couple may be acting too hastily because of fear of pregnancy. They may be bypassing some of the important functions of engagement (the divorce rate is much higher after elopements and secret marriages). Parents, friends, and relatives, whose support is needed during married life, are sometimes hurt and alienated. If the marriage is to be kept secret for a period of time, the couple faces frustration in keeping it quiet and yet fulfilling their marriage. If the wife becomes pregnant, the explanations become rather awkward and unconvincing.

The honeymoon

A honeymoon is a special period during which, in privacy and isolation, a couple takes the first steps in adjustment to shared living. Although not every couple can or does have a honeymoon, it can help smooth the transition from single to married life. A honeymoon should be well planned, to make the adjustment as easy as possible. Ideally it should allow the partners to concentrate on each other, sexually and socially, rather than on business, extended travel, or crowded activity schedules. The place chosen for the honeymoon should be one both can enjoy. The cost should not create an undue burden. The honeymoon should last long enough to allow for adjustment yet not so long that it leads to boredom.

MARITAL SEXUAL ADJUSTMENT

A sexually inexperienced bride and groom may be very likely to have some anxieties about their wedding night. Each partner hopes for a mutually satisfactory sexual experience, but each may have many doubts. Much of the anxiety may be reduced with proper preparation. The bride's premarital consultation with a gynecologist can help considerably. At that time a contraceptive method should be prescribed that will minimize the fear of pregnancy and not interfere with total abandon in sexual expression. The gynecologist should also check a virginal bride-to-be for the presence of an unusually tough hymen. Such a hymen can make her sexual initiation painful and unpleasant. It is a simple matter for the gynecologist to dilate or cut such a hymen, eliminating the possibility of an unpleasant introduction to marital sex.

Even with these precautions, a virginal couple should not expect their first efforts at sexual intercourse to be entirely satisfactory. The inexperienced man may seldom have adequate sexual control, and on the first attempts at intercourse may ejaculate and lose erection almost immediately after vaginal penetration, or even before. But after a few minutes he should be able to attain erection once again and, with seminal pressure reduced, delay ejaculation for some time.

An inexperienced bride may be disappointed in her failure to achieve orgasm on her wedding night. But many studies have shown that the virgin bride often does not reach orgasm through intercourse for a matter of several days, weeks, or even months. In fact, some women achieve orgasm only after a year or more. Marital adjustments take time. Time is required to break down fears and inhibitions and to learn sexual techniques. The sexual happiness of the wife depends greatly upon her husband. His attitudes toward sex and toward her will considerably influence her sexual responses. The sexual adjustment of the wife is made easier when her husband is free in his expressions of love and tenderness toward her. His attitude of patience with her is also critical.

Sexual satisfaction is not the only aim of marriage. Placing too high an expectation on sex can be disappointing. The success of a marriage cannot be measured by the number of orgasms per month, as some of the "marriage manuals" seem to indicate. Sex must be viewed as only a part of marriage. On the other hand, a couple should not neglect working toward a satisfying sexual adjustment.

COMMON SEXUAL PROBLEMS

Sexual problems are important in the lives of millions of people. A sex problem can be a problem in itself, a symptom of a problem in emotional adjustment, or the result of some difficulty in the complex interaction between a woman and a man.

Increasing numbers of people are now seeking professional help for their sexual problems. In the past, when women were not really expected to enjoy sex, conditions such as female sexual dysfunction and premature ejaculation would not have been recognized as serious problems, but in an age when a woman expects to achieve orgasms in a majority of her sexual experiences and is expected by her sexual partner to take an active, enthusiastic role in sexual relationships any sexual problem assumes great importance.

Since sexual adequacy is an important part of a positive self-concept, it is often difficult or impossible to admit to others that a sexual problem exists. If people realized how common sexual problems really are, it might be easier for them to seek help for their own.

Female sexual dysfunction

Within the general category of female sexual dysfunction (*dys* means "difficult" or "painful") may be grouped a variety of female sexual problems. Although the symptoms are diverse, the underlying causes are often quite similar. Common forms of female sexual dysfunction include hyporesponsiveness, or "lack of interest," difficulty in attaining orgasm, painful coitus, and so-called "nymphomania."

The word *frigid* has been applied to the hyporesponsive woman, but many authorities, such as Masters and Johnson (1966 and 1970), reject any use of the word because of its vagueness, its negative tone, and its history of misuse. For example, the word has too often been used by a male as an expression of hostility toward a woman when, for any reason, their sexual relationship has been unsatisfactory to either of them. Calling a woman "frigid" is a nice ego-protective device for a man, since it relieves him of any responsibility for their sexual problems. The careless use of the word may do much psychological harm to a woman, adding anxiety, shame, and low self-esteem to whatever psychological problems she may already have.

Owing to the variety of definitions given to female dysfunction there are a corresponding variety of published figures on its incidence. Most of the studies on sexual response have concentrated on married women, ignoring any women who might have remained single as a result of their hyporesponsiveness. Another variable is the basis of the survey. Some have been based on how often coitus is desired, some on how often it actually occurs, and some on how often orgasm is reached in coitus or on the total orgasmic achievement from all types of stimulation. In any case, it seems that sexual hyporesponsiveness is a perennial problem for many women (perhaps 15 or 20 percent) while transient or situational dysfunction in response to temporary conditions would occur at some time during the life of almost every woman.

Sexual dysfunction can have many obvious and subtle effects on a woman and her relationships with men. It may, in its more severe forms, influence even her nonsexual relationships with men, especially if her problem is associated with a fear or resentment of men. The effects on a marriage are usually obvious and predictable. The husband will feel angry, unloved, rejected, and sexually inadequate and will often, as an ego defense, become involved in extramarital affairs in order to confirm his own sexual adequacy. The effects on the woman herself are difficult to separate from the psychological characteristics which are likely to underlie her dysfunction. In other words, the dysfunction is usually the cause, as well as the effect, of emotional problems. Traits often associated with sexual dysfunction, either as cause or effect, include anxiety, depression, tension, frustration, general unhappiness, and a multitude of psychosomatic complaints. Any direct physical effects would occur mainly in a woman who is sexually responsive and becomes highly aroused for long periods of time but without the relief of orgasm. In such cases the pelvic blood vessels remain dilated and a painful pelvic congestion may result.

Causes of female dysfunction   Problems in female sexual response are almost universally accepted as usually having psychological rather than physical causes. The basic biological drive and capacity for sexual satisfaction usually is seen as being present but blocked by psychological factors. Some cases, however, are in fact caused by biological factors, such as hormone imbalance, so a first step for any woman concerned with her sexual responses should be a complete physical examination to find or rule out any possible biological causes of her problem.

Many psychological factors are implicated in female dysfunction. Fear is often the cause of inadequate female response. There may be a fear of men, fear of the penis, fear of pregnancy, fear of venereal disease, fear of being physically or emotionally hurt, fear of loss of identity, or fear of being physically or emotionally close to someone. Hostility is another obstacle to female response; it may be hostility toward men in general or toward a specific man. Many women who are not "turned on" by their husbands are highly responsive to their lovers.

Many daughters of strictly moralistic parents are left with a persistent feeling that sex is wrong or evil and therefore punishable. Although they may rationally know otherwise, it may be difficult to overcome the inhibiting effect of this feeling.

A previously responsive woman may become unresponsive after being emotionally hurt a few times in her relationships with men. As an ego defense she learns to avoid full emotional commitment for fear that she might once again be disappointed and hurt. Similarly, a woman who was emotionally deprived as a child, raised perhaps by cold and unloving parents, may as an adult find herself unable to take the risk of disappointment that is inherent in any close interpersonal relationship. In either case the woman consciously or unconsciously decides that, rather than love a man and take the chance of his rejecting her, she will reject him first. Such a woman may be very independent in all aspects of her life, driven to perform in school, in a career, and perhaps in sports. She may be successful by most objective measures of success but in many cases seem never really very happy.

The role of the male in causing female dysfunction deserves further emphasis. Many men are really directly responsible for their partner's unresponsiveness. Some men never display any trace of love or attention to the woman and then cannot understand why she is not instantly aroused when they want sex. Other men are so sexually inhibited that they in turn make a woman feel that sex is something dirty. Their inhibition may prevent them from adequately arousing the woman with precoital sex play and may also lead to their premature ejaculation. After enough instances of premature ejaculation, a woman often finds that she would rather not bother to risk further disappointment and becomes unresponsive.

Dyspareunia (painful coitus) A few women find coitus to be physically painful, perhaps so much that they cannot attain orgasm or even avoid coitus entirely. Female dyspareunia can result from either physical or psychological factors. A woman suffering from dyspareunia should have a gynecological examination for any possible physical causes of her problem. Among the possible physical causes are vaginitis (inflammation of the vagina), presence of an unusually tough hymen, childbirth injuries, and other anatomical abnormalities. Any of these physical problems are correctable, either with medications or minor surgery.

Penis size would seldom, if ever, be a factor in dyspareunia. First, there is not a great variation in size among erect penises. Second, the vagina is flexible enough for a woman sexually aroused to be able easily to accommodate even the largest penis.

When painful coitus is associated with emotional factors, it should be thought of as part of the total picture of female dysfunction. The problem in such cases is either that the acting emotional factors cause the muscles of the vaginal opening to contract tightly (*vaginismus*) or that there is so little sexual arousal that the production of vaginal lubricant is inadequate to prevent coital pain. The underlying causes of dyspareunia and its treatment are usually of the same general nature as in other forms of sexual dysfunction.

"Nymphomania" In general use the word *nymphomania* is usually applied to a woman who is thought to have an extremely strong sex drive, expressed in a multitude of sexual adventures with a variety of partners. In reality, the "nymphomaniac" is typically a woman of normal sex drive who has great difficulty in achieving satisfying orgasms and is desperately searching for sexual satisfaction. She often fakes orgasms in coitus to hide her condition from her partners. She pivots from man to man, always hoping that the next one will provide the satisfaction she needs. Of course, she will never find such a man, because the problem is her own.

The psychological bases of "nymphomania" include most of those of the other forms of dysfunction, plus a few more. There may be personality traits, such as a low self-esteem or guilt feelings, that make a woman feel inadequate, inferior, or unworthy of the "reward" of orgasm, so she may unconsciously deny herself this pleasure as a form of "punishment." Like other forms of dysfunction, "nymphomania" can often be successfully treated by a qualified therapist.

Treatment of female dysfunction Since female sexual problems are most often caused by psychological factors, their treatment usually involves psychotherapy, counseling, or behavior therapy. Of course, physical causes should be ruled out before such treatment begins.

A traditional form of treatment was psychoanalysis (an extensive probing of the unconscious mind), but this process is often slow and expensive and the results may be disappointing. The needs of the majority of patients are probably better met through nonpsychoanalytic methods. There are many approaches. One is to attempt to correct a woman's faulty attitudes about sexuality with more positive feelings about sex and her own sexuality. Since the problem often involves the interaction between a woman and her mate, the husband or lover is often brought into the therapeutic situation. If he refuses to cooperate, that in itself is strong evidence that he is a major contributor to the problem.

Behavior therapy, based on the idea that behavior is determined by modifiable stimulus-response patterns, centers around the reconditioning of responses to given stimuli, with the goal of developing more appropriate responses. It is often quite successful. The treatment of sexual problems ideally combines both educational and psychological aspects, aimed at the woman's accepting her need for and right to sexual pleasure and the demolition of her old sexual inhibitions.

Male sexual dysfunction

Impotence   Impotence is defined in many ways. Typical definitions are "the inability to achieve or maintain an erection of quality sufficient to accomplish coital connection," "a persistent inability to maintain an erection sufficient to allow orgasm and ejaculation to be accomplished during coitus," and "the inability sexually to satisfy a normally responsive female in coitus." Some authorities thus include premature ejaculation as a form of impotence, while others consider it a separate problem. The authors of this text prefer to follow the lead of Masters and Johnson in defining *impotence* in terms of erectile incompetence and considering premature ejaculation a separate problem, though in many men the two problems coexist and result from the same causes.

· CAUSES OF IMPOTENCE   Impotence may be caused by physical (biological) or psychological factors or a combination of the two. The great majority of cases (more than 90 percent) are mainly psychological in their origin, but before automatically treating impotence as a psychological problem it is important to rule out any possible physical cause.

Many physical factors may cause impotence. Fatigue and heavy use of alcohol or other drugs rank high among these causes. Also many prescribed drugs, such as tranquilizers, may cause impotence as a side effect. The possibility of hormonal problems must also be considered. Diabetes is a common hormonal cause of impotence. Insufficient hormone secretion from the pituitary gland (gonadotropic hormones) or the testes (testosterone) will also cause impotence. There may be abnormalities in the sex chromosomes. Certain surgical procedures, such as those necessary in cancers of the prostate or colon, are followed by a high incidence of impotence. The normal aging process is usually associated with some decline in potency, though there is a great variation among men in this respect. In this, as well as in most of the other causes of impotence, a man is likely to develop a great concern over his declining potency, which tends to compound the problem, for the fear of impotence ironically is one of the most important psychological causes of impotence.

A multitude of psychological factors can act, either singly or in various combinations, to produce impotence. There is no one underlying psychological conflict present in all cases of impotence nor any impotence-causing conflict that is not also present in many normally potent men. In fact, the same case of impotence might be interpreted quite differently by several different therapists, depending on their type of training. The Freudian psychoanalyst and the behavior therapist, for example, would probably come to entirely different conclusions.

As previously mentioned, the fear of impotence is almost universally recognized as a major cause of impotence. There is in the minds of many men much exaggeration regarding the "inevitable" loss of sexual potency with aging. Millions of men secretly fear that any day their potency will suddenly fail them. The first instance of impotence for a man often occurs when he has been drinking or using other drugs, is under some great temporary emotional stress, or is fatigued. Perhaps he attains an erection but loses it halfway through coitus or during the preliminary sex play. You may be sure that the next time he attempts coitus he is going to be worried about his potency. Erection of the penis is controlled through the parasympathetic branch of the autonomic nervous system. The autonomic nervous system is not under direct conscious control, but its actions are determined by the emotional state of the individual. The parasympathetic branch is stimulated by a feeling of well-being and inhibited by emotions such as fear, anxiety, or anger. It is quite impossible to attain an erection by conscious will, no matter how much one is desired, if the basic emotional state is such that the parasympathetic nervous system is being inhibited. Thus the fear of failure can set up a cycle in which failure is assured.

Other sources of impotence-causing anxiety include fear of being detected in an extramarital affair (may cause impotence with either woman or with both), fear of premature ejaculation, fear of being judged sexually inferior, fear of causing pregnancy, and fear of venereal disease.

Other psychological causes are resentment toward the sexual partner, as in the case of a passive man who is dominated by an aggressive wife or of a man who feels a woman is overly dependent upon him. Impotence is sometimes seen as an unconscious means of "punishing" a woman by denying the fulfillment of her sexual needs. There may be a hostility toward women in general, conscious or unconscious negative feelings or disgust about sex, or a variety of neurotic personality disturbances.

· TREATMENT OF IMPOTENCE   The treatment of psychogenic impotence follows the same general patterns as the treatment of dysfunction in women. The approach varies considerably from therapist to therapist, depending largely upon the school of thought. As in female problems, it is often useful to treat both the man and his sexual partner as a unit, since the impotence often revolves around the complex network of interactions between the two.

And now a word to the women: If ever a man has trouble attaining or keeping an erection (which is common enough), be aware that the man's sexual future could be in jeopardy. The woman's reaction to his impotency will greatly influence his success in that attempt and future attempts at coitus. The female's immediate feelings may be those of hurt and rejection, and the natural impulse may be to hurt in return, perhaps through ridicule, by comparing him with other men or by accusing him of being unfaithful. Such a reaction will produce enough anxiety practically to ensure that his next attempt at lovemaking will also fail. On the other hand, a *reassuring* female response, perhaps including gentle manual or oral stimulation of his male organs, may result in immediate potency or in any case will not interfere with his future attempts at intercourse.

Premature ejaculation   When is ejaculation premature? Anyone would agree that ejaculation prior to or immediately after vaginal penetration is premature. But what about ejaculation after two minutes? After five minutes? What about ejaculation after the partner has had one orgasm but would like to have several more? What about a man who can last for 30 minutes but whose partner needs an hour of intensive coitus to reach her orgasm? Obviously, there can be no clear-cut definition of premature ejaculation. Masters and Johnson (1970) consider a man to have a problem of premature ejaculation if he cannot delay ejaculation long enough to satisfy his *normally responsive* partner in at least 50 percent of their coital experiences. Perhaps ejaculation is best considered premature if it seems so to either sexual partner.

Indeed, premature ejaculation has not always been recognized as a problem. In fact, there was a time when a man might have been proud of how quickly he ejaculated, as a supposed sign of great virility. As long as women were not really expected to enjoy coitus, it made little difference how long coitus was sustained.

Very few men are likely to get through life without at least a few instances of "premature" ejaculation. In fact, under certain conditions premature ejaculation must be considered an entirely normal and predictable physiological event. For example, it is unrealistic to expect a young man who has been without any sexual release for many days to withhold his ejaculation while his partner thrusts vigorously and incessantly in her effort to achieve her own orgasm. Similarly, the first act of coitus with a new and highly exciting woman may be normally expected to result in a "premature" ejaculation.

How then do you distinguish "normal" premature ejaculation from the "problem" variety? The distinction here is that, if a man has regular and frequent intercourse with the same woman, and it often ends in premature ejaculation, it is a problem. In such case there may be underlying psychological causes that may be quite similar to those causing impotence. Examples are hostility toward the woman, when premature ejaculation is used to deny her sexual satisfaction, guilt about sex, in which premature ejaculation is used to "get it over with," feelings of sexual inadequacy, in which there is a rush to prove that the penis is still "working," fears, and love conflicts.

Ejaculation, like erection, is controlled through the autonomic (involuntary) branch of the nervous system. Thus, ejaculation cannot be controlled by direct conscious effort ("willpower"). As in impotence, the reaction of a man's sexual partner greatly influences his chances of overcoming premature ejaculation. If she ridicules or chastises him, he is in trouble. If she *reassures* him and minimizes the problem, then he has a very good chance of overcoming it.

There is no shortage of "advice" for the man who is bothered by premature ejaculation. For persistent premature ejaculation there should be, first of all, a physical examination for such physical causes as urethritis, prostatitis, cystitis (bladder infection), and diabetes. If no physical cause can be found, then psychotherapy is often recommended. As in impotence, if there is a regular sexual partner, it is important that she be included in the therapeutic process. Masters and Johnson in *Human Sexual Inadequacy* take a more directly physical approach, recommending an "exercise" for premature ejaculation, in which the woman's hand stimulates the man's penis almost to the point of orgasm and then with the thumb and fingers tightly squeezes the base of the glans of the penis. Done repeatedly, as detailed in their book, this technique often solves long-term problems of premature ejaculation.

If premature ejaculation occurs in one of the "normal" situations, as described above, then the male is likely to be highly enough aroused for a second erection to be attained in a few minutes and, with seminal pressure reduced, prolonged intercourse should be possible. If premature ejaculation occurs repeatedly in second and subsequent erections, then the premature ejaculation is of the "problem" type and professional counsel should be sought. In many cases reerection after premature ejaculation is impossible, even in a young man who should be capable of a second erection, illustrating the close relationship between premature ejaculation and impotence.

Many other suggestions are offered for the prevention of premature ejaculation. These would be of value only when there is no serious underlying psychological cause. Some physicians prescribe mild tranquilizers for their patients who complain of premature ejaculation. Some doctors recommend that a topical ointment containing a local anesthetic be applied over the glans of the penis to reduce the sensory stimulus. A similar effect can sometimes be obtained by wearing a condom (rubber) over the penis. Regular sex partners can learn to prolong coitus by their both holding very still for a few seconds whenever ejaculation seems imminent. Some men learn to fantasize about nonsexual objects when ejaculation threatens. Premature ejaculation is sometimes associated with inadequate foreplay and with penetration of the vagina while it is still poorly lubricated and tight; the increased friction makes control difficult. Through experimenting with different coital positions a couple may find one or more in which ejaculatory control is improved. Positions with the woman lying, sitting, or kneeling over the man are sometimes helpful. There are really very few men who cannot be successfully prevented from premature ejaculation in some way, though professional help may be necessary.

HAVING CHILDREN

Children play an important role in most marriages. For many couples children are an important source of satisfaction and fulfillment. Yet the attitudes and values of a growing minority of couples lead them to a decision to remain childless. Fortunately, the highly effective contraceptives available today allow couples to make definite plans and decisions regarding children and in most cases to carry out their wishes successfully.

An important decision

Few decisions in life have as far-reaching effects as the decision to have a child. Such a decision carries many responsibilities. One obvious responsibility is financial: children are expensive. Although it will vary somewhat with a family's income and level of living, the cost of supporting a child to college age is estimated to be in excess of $25,000 today. A couple should plan the size of its family in terms of the income and desired standard of living of both. The child will have a need to love and be loved. He will need to acquire a sense of security from his parents and their family relations within the home. Since children have many kinds of needs, parents must be committed to supplying them for the many years of childhood and adolescence—and in some cases even longer.

There is only one good reason for having a child—namely, a genuine desire of both parents to have that child. On the other hand, there are many poor reasons for having a child. The worst possible reason is to try to bring happiness to an already unhappy or unstable marriage. Studies have shown that bringing a child into an already troubled marriage does not solve any problems, and quite commonly it leads to a further deterioration of the marriage. It is certainly unfair to the child to bring him into such a situation.

Another poor reason for having a child is to try to satisfy the desires of the parents of the couple for grandchildren. A young couple has absolutely no responsibility to their parents in this respect; nor are they responsible to the urging of their friends to have children. Similarly, there is no responsibility to society for the production of children. The population of the world is already increasing quite well!

Even with the use of modern contraceptives there is still some chance of an unplanned pregnancy. Aside from accepting the child, two other options remain open to the parents: abortion of the embryo or carrying the fetus to term and giving the child up for adoption. To react against the situation by keeping the child and then resenting or abandoning it, or by one of the parents either deserting the marriage or seeking a divorce is surely a demonstration of immaturity. The child has no choice either of the situation or of his parents. Parents should overlook any disappointment and give the child the type of home he deserves.

Timing

If possible, the first pregnancy should come only after the couple has had sufficient time to make a reasonable marital adjustment. It may be wise for pregnancy to come before the couple becomes too attached to material possessions and set schedules. The optimal biological time for childbearing is between the maternal ages of twenty and thirty years.

A teenage mother frequently is still faced with problems of emotional and social immaturity that distract from her effectiveness as a well-balanced mother. On the other hand, if the mother is too old, the physical dangers of childbirth to both herself and the baby are increased.

Spacing of children

The raising of children places great demands upon parents, particularly mothers. Today, through the intelligent use of contraceptives, a couple can space and plan the birth of children to match their desires and resources. There are many reasons for doing so. The couple should be ready financially for each child, the previous child should be old enough for the mother not to need to carry him around during the second pregnancy, and sufficient time should be allowed for the mother to regain her vitality. The amount of spacing will depend upon the wishes of the couple. Many consider a two- or three-year spacing most convenient. One should not forget that children spaced too far apart can be a problem in that too wide an age spread between children makes it difficult for them to share common interests. A degree of companionship between children not only assists in their development but also often makes it easier for the mother, since the children tend to entertain each other and thus require less directed entertainment from the parents.

The total number of children desired is a personal matter. Hopefully, the number should reflect the planned desires of the couple in terms of their financial and emotional capabilities, their social settings, and the world populations.

Involuntary childlessness

Approximately 10 percent of all marriages are childless in spite of repeated attempts at pregnancy. A couple approaching marriage should not take for granted that it will be possible to have children. For some people childlessness is difficult to accept.

A number of physical factors may be responsible for sterility; some can be changed with medical attention, others cannot. Sterility may be due to improperly formed reproductive organs, cervical obstructions, defective sperm, glandular deficiencies, or other conditions. It may result from developmental disease or emotional difficulties. If the condition is known before marriage, it is the responsibility of the sterile partner to inform the other one. It is important that, if such a couple wants children, both partners seek the aid of a physician, a fertility clinic, or the Planned Parenthood Federation. If after proper deliberation and consultation a pregnancy is not forthcoming, and if the partners still desire children, they may consider either artificial insemination or adoption.

Adoption

There are well over a hundred thousand adoptions in this country each year. In most localities the demand for adoptions is greater than the supply of children. The first step is filing with an adoption agency an application to adopt a child. The processing of the application requires time, sometimes months.

Some state laws even require a one-year waiting period, during which the home is thoroughly checked by a local welfare agency.

Although some adoptions are independently handled directly between natural and adoptive parents or their representatives, many states prohibit such independent adoptions. Such prohibition is based on cases in which children have been given away without sufficient cause, or adoptive home life was not suitable, or babies were not properly matched to their adoptive parents, or the adoptive parents were not legally protected either in terminating an unacceptable adoption or in maintaining an exclusive guardianship that was questioned by the natural parents.

It is preferable in all cases to work through either a private state-licensed agency or a public welfare department. Such agencies collect all available facts regarding the child's background, race, intelligence, education, and health. They collect the same regarding the prospective adoptive parents, plus information regarding their social and economic position, their emotional acceptability as parents, and their reputation among their friends. The agency often checks out their homes. After the application for adoption has been approved, the child is matched as closely to his adoptive parents as possible. After the child is left with the agency, he is often held for medical observation for a few days. If healthy, he is placed in an adoptive home on probation for several months or a year, during which time the legal adoption papers are drawn up. During this time most abnormalities are noticed, so that there is a slim chance of an undesirable abnormality's cropping up afterwards. Actually, there is little more chance of having an imperfect adoptive child this way than there would be of having an imperfect child of one's own.

Unique problems are faced in adoptions, none of which is unsolvable. The adoptive child fills an important emotional place in his adoptive parents' lives and they in his. If relations are well handled, the child-parent relationship should be just as satisfying as a natural one.

EXTRAMARITAL SEXUAL RELATIONS

Within American culture sexual exclusiveness in marriage is still considered important by a majority of people. At the time of marriage most people plan to remain faithful and expect their new mates to do the same. Yet recent surveys show that infidelity occurs at some time in more than half of all marriages. Thus there seems to be a definite gap between what we believe (or say we believe) and what we actually practice. It is interesting to examine some of the causes of infidelity.

Often it is difficult to pinpoint the real causes of infidelity, because most people try to justify their behavior with elaborate rationalizations. Although infidelity is often attributed to an unsatisfactory sexual relationship within a marriage, it also occurs when the marital sexual adjustment is entirely satisfactory. In fact, the real motivations for infidelity are probably more often nonsexual than sexual. Among the more common reasons given for infidelity are boredom with the marital partner or the home situation in general, lack of sexual interest by or in the marital partner, and lack of warmth, love, or affection in or for the marital partner. Some people even rationalize their extra-marital affairs as evidence of their true love for their partner: their affairs enable them to remain married and to tolerate both the marriage and the spouse. Some people explain their infidelity on the simple basis of a healthy heterosexual interest in a variety of partners. This is, of course, part of the philosophy of the "swinger."

The amount of guilt associated with infidelity varies greatly. Those most bothered by guilt would be people whose behavior contradicts their own values and standards. But guilt presents little or no problem for many people, sometimes because there are no conflicting values to produce guilt. Others so thoroughly rationalize their infidelity that guilt is escaped. For many people the worst psychological problem associated with infidelity is some degree of anxiety related to a fear of getting "caught" by either their own or their paramour's spouse, an unpleasant situation at best.

When the rationalizations are stripped away, there emerge three principle causes of infidelity. All are interrelated, and all reveal an underlying inability to be fully committed to a relationship of love and mutual regard and respect. It is a mistake always to assign the "blame" to the partner who is unfaithful, for the problem may involve characteristics in the "innocent" partner that almost force the infidelity of the other as a matter of ego preservation. Thus, the problem may lie in either partner or in both. Any lasting relationship requires commitments and compromises, which one or both partners may be unable or unwilling to make. The three basic problems are as follows.[1]

1. *Lack of commitment.* Some people marry even though their degree of love and commitment are uncertain. Such marriages may be motivated by financial, social, religious, or psychological factors. An often expressed attitude is, "Well, if it doesn't work out, I can always get a divorce." Any expectation of fidelity in such a case is totally unjustified. Obviously, anyone so weakly committed should avoid marriage.

2. *Failure in adjustment.* Marriages in this category begin in love, loyalty, and commitment, but the partners gradually drift apart, until one or both must go outside the marriage in order to fulfill emotional needs. A cause of such problems may be the unrealistic expectations that so many people hold for marriage. Almost from birth we are conditioned by various media and the national folklore to expect to marry and "live happily ever after." The ideal marriage is portrayed as a state of perpetual euphoria in which problems just don't exist. Sex is supposed to be supremely enjoyable, with both partners always in the mood for sex at the same times and each sexual act ending in simultaneous, earthshaking orgasms, each bigger and better than ever before. *Nonsense.* In every marriage there are going to be problems. Money problems, in-law problems, sexual problems, illnesses, child-raising problems, role and identity problems, conflicting interests, conflicting careers, and, if the marriage lasts that long, problems of aging and retirement. When the realities of married life are compared with the unrealistic expectations that most of us hold, then even a very good marriage can look like a dismal failure. In our

---

[1] After Leon Salzman, "Female Infidelity," in *Medical Aspects of Human Sexuality*, February 1972.

disappointment we feel entirely justified in going outside marriage to satisfy our various needs. Into this category fall the millions of people who excuse their infidelity on the basis that it sustains their marriage.

3. *Personality disorders.* In this category are a variety of personality structures that make fidelity impossible. Included are the sociopath, the paranoid, the jealous, the immature, and the egocentric types. A very common trait associated with infidelity is insecurity about one's sexual attractiveness or adequacy. The person who has numerous short-term affairs is often motivated by a need for reassurance that he or she can attract lovers and perform well sexually. In the male this is called the "Don Juan" personality.

In conclusion, it seems that, although infidelity is occasionally part of a neurotic or psychotic personality development, it more often represents an understandable form of behavior. It may occur with people who are basically loyal and faithful, in response to compelling emotional needs. It may occur as a single brief affair, as a series of occasional brief affairs, or as a chronic situation.

The incidence of infidelity has traditionally been higher in men than among women, but this is believed to have been the result of social pressures rather than any basic biological or psychological differences. Such factors as fear of pregnancy and the "double standard," by which society has winked at male infidelity while frowning at the same behavior in women, have tended to create the different behavior patterns. Improved contraception, readily available abortion, and the general liberation of women are acting to remove these restraints on the expression of female sexuality. As a result infidelity is becoming equally common among both sexes.

The infidelity of either partner is certainly no reason to terminate an otherwise satisfactory marriage. It may, however, be taken as evidence that the needs of the unfaithful partner are not being adequately met within the marriage. If the marriage partners can calmly and rationally discuss their needs and feelings, then the resulting mutual understanding often results in each partner's being better able to satisfy the needs of the other, so that the need for infidelity ceases to exist. A realignment of unrealistic expectations for marriage is often necessary. If a couple cannot work out their own problems, they should not hesitate to seek the help of a qualified marriage counselor. If both partners are willing to "forgive and forget" and work to correct their shortcomings, then even a very shaky marriage may be returned to a state of relative happiness.

DIVORCE

In some marriages it becomes evident that because of unresolved conflicts there is no longer a basis for trying to continue the relationship. The relationship of marriage can be broken either formally or informally. It may be broken informally by desertion, in which one partner simply disappears, or by separation, in which the couple agrees to live separately. Neither desertion nor separation constitutes a legal divorce nor terminates the marriage. A marriage can be legally terminated by annulment if it can be established that some legal requirement for marriage was never met (due to fraud, deception, illegal age, bigamy, or some other violation). Or divorce can be obtained if it can be established that one partner violated the marriage rights of the other partner. Technically, divorce must be based on such grounds rather than just a mutual agreement.

The grounds for divorce among the various states include irreconcilable differences, adultery, cruelty (physical or mental), desertion, nonsupport, alcoholism, drug addiction, impotence, insanity, pregnancy at time of marriage, bigamy, fraud, force or duress, felony conviction, and imprisonment. A particular state might recognize many or few of these grounds. Persons seeking divorce often go to extremes to establish complaints within these categories, even though the actual cause of failure was something entirely different. This practice is so common that the number of decrees awarded in certain categories tells very little of the true nature of the marital conflicts among the couples involved.

The majority of divorce decrees are awarded to women. There are several reasons for this. Generally, women have access to more grounds for divorce than men. The courts tend to be more sympathetic to the divorce suits of women and tend to award alimony more readily to them. It is also more common for the woman to be awarded custody of the children, if any, than the man. The man typically makes child-support payments to his ex-wife until the children reach a given age.

Incidence of divorce

The divorce rate in the United States, as shown in Fig. 12.1, is near its all-time high. The high point occurred during the readjustment period following World War II, with a peak rate of 4.3 divorces per 1,000 population in 1946. The trend in recent years has been a gradual rise in the divorce rate. In 1972

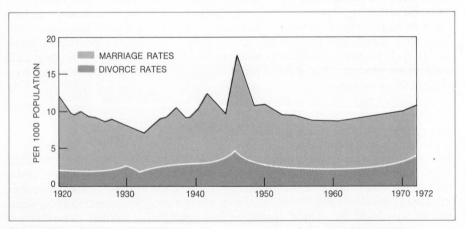

Figure 12.1   Marriage and divorce rates in the United States, 1920 to 1972. (From the Public Health Service, U.S. Department of Health, Education and Welfare.)

the rate was about 4.0, in 1968 it was 2.9, and in 1957 it was 2.2. The current divorce rate represents 1 divorce for every 2.7 marriages. The incidence of divorce probably will continue to rise in response to more liberal attitudes toward divorce as well as to the liberalization of laws in many states. It should be noted that this rise does not necessarily indicate greater unhappiness in marriage; it may indicate a decreasing willingness to tolerate the continuance of unhappiness in marriage.

The incidence of divorce can be correlated with several characteristics of marriage. Divorce occurs more frequently in cities than in rural areas and more often among those of lower income than those of higher income. It is more common during the first five years of marriage than later. Marriages in which one or both parties were less than age twenty at the time of marriage are more likely to end in divorce.

It must be remembered that divorce rates are only a partial indication of marriage failure. There are many additional couples whose marriage has failed but who have not obtained a divorce for economic or religious reasons, fear of loss of social or professional standing, the presence of children in the home, or fear of admitting failure. The increase in divorce rates is due to many factors, which may or may not include increasing unhappiness in marriages. The evolving criteria for success in marriage place a greater importance on love and companionship, without which a marriage today is more often considered to be a failure. Public opinion toward divorce is increasingly liberal. More and more people are deciding that the temporary pain of divorce is better than living in the continuing turmoil of an unhappy marriage. The increasing independence and the freedom of women to be self-supporting have probably been influential too.

Effects of divorce upon partners

The emotional effects of divorce are greater than the average person, who has never been through it, realizes. Both parties involved usually find it to be a painful experience—emotionally, socially, and financially. It usually does not solve the basic human problems that were its true cause. New problems are created for both the divorced couple and any children they might have. There is often a mixture of guilt and resentment. For some the readjustment demanded is severe enough to call for the help of friends, clergymen, and psychiatrists.

Effects of divorce upon children

Divorce is particularly bewildering to children. They are in a no-man's land, being pulled in two directions. The best affection the divided parents can bestow is not comparable to the security a child should feel in a warm home relationship. He is helpless in resolving his position with each of his parents, since he feels loyalty to both of them. Any court battle over custody only aggravates the damage. Some children become so emotionally disturbed that their attitudes toward their school work and friends are noticeably affected. Their world has collapsed. The child often feels that somehow he was responsible for the divorce. As the child matures, it becomes necessary for him to achieve an outlook on the matter that does not warp his own chances for a successful marriage. He must be convinced that his parents' problems do not reflect upon him. Most of all, he must learn from his parents' experience, so that he does not make similar mistakes.

Divorce prevention

The most effective divorce prevention takes place before marriage. This means the development of desirable attitudes toward marriage and the selection of the right marriage mate. It also means that the partners in an unhappy marriage should not hesitate to try the services of a qualified marriage counselor. Under the direction of a counselor, and within the "safe" environment of his office, points of conflict often can be brought to the surface and rationally discussed and, surprisingly often, resolved.

Care should be taken in the selection of a marriage counselor; there are many "quacks" in this area. Preferably, a referral should be obtained from a family physician, a family service agency, or a clergyman. Furthermore, adequate time should be allowed for the results of counseling to become apparent. The improvement is rarely of the "overnight" nature and frequently takes the form of a gradual improvement in a relationship over a period of several months.

Remarriage

The remarriage rate among divorcees is high, indicating that few of them are completely soured on the idea of marriage. According to the U.S. Bureau of Census, a divorced man or woman of any age is more likely to remarry than is the never-married person of the same age to get married. The bureau reports, for example, that at age 30 a single woman has a 50 percent chance of marrying, while a divorcee of that age has a 94 percent chance of remarriage.

The divorce rate among second marriages is somewhat higher than among first marriages, and it soars in third and subsequent marriages. On the other hand, a remarriage often results in much greater happiness than the original marriage. Remarriages can turn out well if the new partners earnestly try to avoid the problems that destroyed the first marriage.

SUMMARY

    I. Nonmarital sexual adjustment
      A. Petting
        1. A normal step in development of psychosexual maturity.
        2. Arouses, rather than relieves, sexual tensions.
        3. Many couples pet to mutual orgasm.
      B. Nonmarital sexual intercourse
        1. Material considerations:
          a. Pregnancy, resulting in choice of
            abortion.

            single parenthood.
            marriage.
            adoption.
      b. Venereal disease.
    2. Psychological considerations:
      a. motivation.
      b. effect on future marriage.
    3. Social considerations.
    4. Legal considerations.
  C. Masturbation
    1. Perfectly harmless.
    2. Part of normal sexuality.
  D. Nocturnal emissions
    1. Perfectly harmless.
    2. Relieve seminal pressure.
  E. Prostitutes.
II. Homosexuality
  A. Homosexual behavior patterns
    1. Females tend to form stable relationships.
    2. Males tend toward variety in homosexual partners.
  B. Causes of homosexuality
    1. Emotional rather than biological.
    2. Parent-child relationships.
  C. Treatment of homosexuality
    1. Rate of success in treatment has not been great.
    2. Jail does not cure the homosexual.
III. Factors to consider before marriage
  A. Poor reasons for marriage
    1. Pressure from parents.
    2. Social pressures.
    3. Fear of being "left out."
    4. Transfer of dependency.
    5. Pregnancy.
  B. Readiness for marriage
    1. Age at marriage:
      a. average 23 for men and 21 for women.
      b. high divorce rate in teenage marriages.
    2. Emotional maturity.
    3. Social maturity.
    4. Financial resources.
  C. Selecting for happiness
    1. Positive personality traits.
    2. Mutual need satisfaction.
    3. Genuine mutual love.
    4. Agreement on parenthood.
    5. Hereditary traits.
    6. Similarities:
      a. age.
      b. ethnic origin.
      c. economic status.
      d. education.
      e. intelligence.

       f. religion.

      7. Previous marital status.

  D. Danger signs in a relationship

    1. Quarreling.

    2. Lack of communication.

    3. Lack of confidence that the marriage will be good.

    4. Off-again on-again relationships.

IV. Marriage laws

  A. Minimal age

    1. 14 to 17 for girls.

    2. 15 to 18 for boys.

  B. Physical examination and blood test

  C. Waiting period

  D. Prohibited marriages

  E. Common-law marriages

V. Engagement

  A. Purposes of engagement

    1. To test reactions to a prolonged, intensive relationship.

    2. To allow for preparations for marriage.

  B. Sexual relations during engagement

    1. The extent of intimacy during engagement is a matter for each couple to decide.

    2. There is no need to confess all past sexual experiences during engagement.

  C. Length of engagement

    1. There is no definite length.

    2. It is desirable to have at least one year of close relationship before marriage.

  D. Breaking engagement

    1. A broken engagement is better than a broken marriage.

    2. If either partner wants to break an engagement, he should do so promptly.

VI. Premarital counseling

  A. The probability of marital happiness can be predicted.

  B. Counselor may be a professional marriage counselor, a clergyman, or a physician.

  C. There should be a consultation with a gynecologist to determine the preferred method of contraception for the couple.

VII. Beginning a marriage

  A. The wedding ceremony

    1. Should not create a financial burden.

    2. Should fit the desires of the couple, not the social aims of their parents.

    3. Should be planned to minimize stress-producing factors.

    4. There may be valid reasons for elopement.

    5. Secret marriages should be avoided.

  B. The honeymoon

    1. Can help smooth the transition to married life.

    2. Should be well planned.

VIII. Marital sexual adjustment

  A. A sexuality inexperienced couple should not expect their first efforts at sexual intercourse to be entirely satisfactory.

B. Complete sexual adjustment may take some time.
IX. Common sexual problems
    A. Problems in female sexuality
        1. Dysfunction:
            a. many definitions—may include low level of sexual interest, difficulty in achieving orgasm, or both.
            b. usually caused by psychological factors, including fear, hostility, and inhibition.
        2. Dyspareunia:
            a. may have physical or psychological cause.
            b. if psychological, would have same causes as female sexual dysfunction.
        3. "Nymphomania":
            a. actually a variety of sexual dysfunction.
            b. a desperate search for sexual satisfaction.
        4. Treatment usually psychotherapy.
    B. Problems in male sexuality
        1. Impotence:
            a. inability to achieve or maintain erection.
            b. usually psychological, occasionally biological.
            c. biological causes include fatigue, alcohol and other drugs, hormonal problems, surgical procedures.
            d. Psychological causes include fear (especially of impotence), anxiety and worry, and hostility.
            e. treatment usually psychotherapy.
        2. Premature ejaculation:
            a. no clear-cut definition.
            b. to be expected at times.
            c. cause usually psychological.
            d. treatment usually psychotherapy.
X. Having children
    A. Modern contraceptives allow definite plans and decisions regarding children.
    B. Parenthood carries many responsibilities.
    C. There are many poor reasons for having a child.
        1. To try to bring happiness to an unhappy marriage.
        2. To supply the parents of a couple with grandchildren.
        3. To satisfy friends.
    D. Even though a pregnancy is unplanned, the parents should still accept the child.
    E. Timing—couple should allow for reasonable marital adjustment before having children.
    F. Spacing—should allow for physical and emotional health of the mother.
    G. Involuntary childlessness
        1. affects about 10 percent of marriages.
        2. can often be corrected.
    H. Adoption
        1. Over 100,000 in United States each year.
        2. Should be handled through an agency.
XI. Extramarital sexual relations
    A. Occur at some time in over half of all marriages.

     B. Usually result of unfulfillment in marriage, often nonsexual.
     C. Possible causes
        1. Lack of commitment.
        2. Failure in adjustment.
        3. Personality disorders, especially sexual insecurity.
     D. Symptom of a problem, not a reason to end marriage.
     E. Qualified professional marital counseling can often return a rocky marriage to happiness.
  XII. Divorce
     A. Grounds vary from state to state.
     B. Currently 1 divorce for every 2.7 marriages.
     C. Occurs more frequently in
        1. cities than rural areas.
        2. low-income families than in high-income ones.
        3. first 5 years of marriage.
        4. marriages of under-20 partners.
     D. Emotional effects greater than many realize.
     E. Particularly hard on children of divorced couple.
     F. Remarriage rate of divorcees high.
     G. Remarriages can be very successful.
     H. Divorce prevention
        1. Development of desirable attitudes.
        2. Selection of right mate.
        3. Qualified marital counseling.

Glossary

If you cannot find the word you wish in this glossary, check the index for text and glossary references.

abortion (ə bor'shən) (L. *abortio*, miscarriage). The expulsion of the human fetus from the womb before the fifth or sixth month.

age of consent. The minimum legal age a person must have reached in order legally to give consent to sexual intercourse. See *statutory rape.*

annulment (ə nul'mənt) (L. *annullare*, to bring to nothing). A legal dissolving of the marriage relation on grounds the marriage was not valid according to the laws of the state.

artificial insemination (ahr ti fish'əl in sem i nā'shən) (L. *inseminatus*, sown, from *in*, into and *semen*, seed). The deposit of semen into a female by artificial means.

bigamy (big'ə mē) (L. *bi*, two; G. *gamos*, marriage). Criminal offense of entering into a second marriage while a previous one is still legally in effect.

coitus (kō'i təs) (L. *coitio*, going together). Sexual intercourse.

common-law marriage. A marriage not solemnized by religious or civil ceremony but effected by agreement to live together as husband and wife.

contraceptive (kon trə sep'tiv) (L. *contra*, against; *conceptus*, from *concipere*, to conceive). A device for the prevention of the fertilization of the human ovum.

desertion (di zur'shən) (L. *desertus*, solitary, desert). Act of abandoning a marriage partner.

divorce (di vors') (L. *dis*, apart; *vertere*, to turn). A legal dissolving of the marriage relation.

dyspareunia (dis pah roo′nē ah) (Gr. *dyspareunos,* badly mated). Painful or difficult coitus in a female.

frigidity (fri jid′i tē) (L. *frigidus,* cold). Low level of sexual interest or difficulty in attaining orgasm in a female; preferably called female dysfunction.

heterosexual (het′ər ō sek′shoo əl) (G. *hetero,* other; L. *sexualis,* sexual). Sexual attraction or relationship between members of the opposite sex.

homosexual (hō′mō sek′shoo əl) (G. *homos,* same; L. *sexualis,* sexual). Sexual attraction or relationship between members of the same sex.

illegitimate (il lə jit′i mit) (L. *in,* not; *legitimare,* to make lawful). Born to parents not married to each other.

impotence (im′ pə təns) (L. *in,* not; *potentia,* power). The inability to attain or to maintain erection of the penis.

lesbian (les′ be an). A female homosexual.

masturbation (mas tər bā′shən) (L. *manus,* hand; *stuprare,* to rape). Self-excitation of one's genitals.

nymphomania (nim fo mā′nē ah) (L. *nympha,* the labium minus; Gr. *mania,* madness). Popularly, exaggerated sexual desire in a female; usually a search for sexual satisfaction by a woman having normal sexual drive but difficulty in achieving satisfying orgasms.

premature ejaculation (i jak yə lā′shən). Inability of male to delay ejaculation long enough to satisfy a normally responsive woman.

rape (rāp) (L. *rapere,* to seize). The crime of having sexual intercourse with a woman by force and without her consent.

separation (sep ə rā′shən). An arrangement by which a husband and wife live apart and separately by agreement.

statutory rape (stach′yoo tor ē rāp) (L. *statuere,* to set or ordain). Sexual intercourse, either voluntarily or forcibly, with an individual below the age of consent. See *age of consent.*

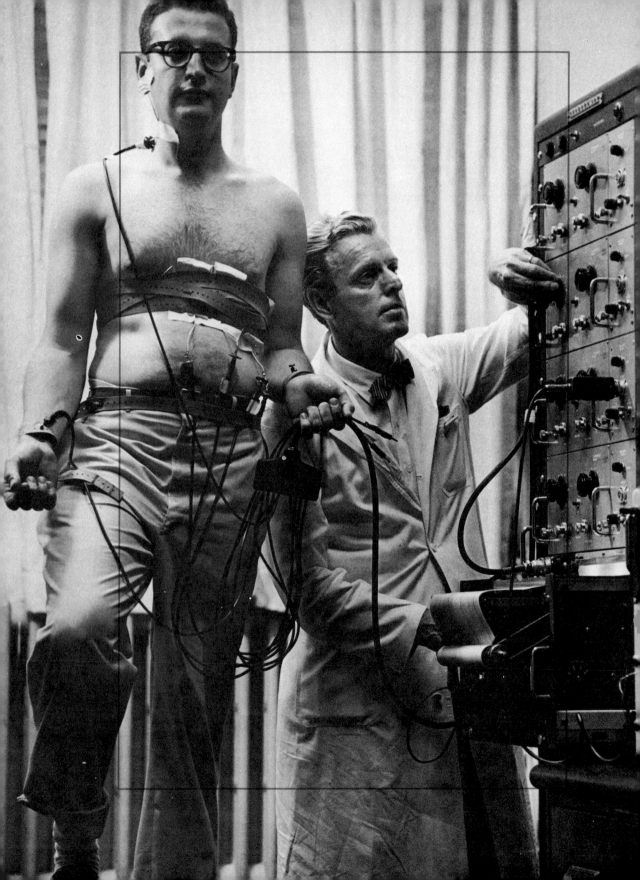

Choosing and financing health services

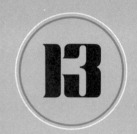

13

During the past century medicine has made unbelievable strides. Maladies that carried the fear of death for our grandparents—diphtheria, scarlet fever, poliomyelitis, whooping cough, and typhoid fever—are now controlled to such a point that few of us give little, if any, thought to them today. A child born today can look forward to a life half again as long as his ancestors could have fifty years ago. More exciting yet, medical men believe that life expectancy may well be further increased. Health problems that have so far gone unsolved now seem to be within reach of cure or prevention through the greatest research efforts that have ever been mounted. Medical advances do not come to us automatically. They come through proper medical counsel and care, availability of hospital services, and use of appropriate drugs.

Finding the answers to all diseases is not the only goal of modern medicine. Of equal concern is getting good medical care to the public. The finding of a cure for a dreaded disease will mean little to the average citizen unless he can find a satisfactory answer to the question "How do I get the best in modern health care for my family and myself?"

MODERN MEDICINE

Aims of modern medicine

The hopes of medicine today may be expressed in four major objectives:

1. Good medical care must be available to *all* people. Economically depressed communities, both in this country and elsewhere, have the right to expect cures for their diseases and infirmities.

2. The *prevention* of disease must be given top attention. As much as possible the physician must replace concern over how to remedy an already existing condition with interest in an effective way to prevent its initial occurrence.

3. The needs of the whole man must be administered to. Areas of medical specialization tend to treat parts of a man. Important as specialization is, man is still an integrated individual of interrelated systems. When one part becomes ill, the whole man to a degree is ill and therefore needs attention.

4. Research into unconquered diseases and better methods of treatment must be pursued. Medicine can never stand still in terms of research if the best of medical care is ever to be attained.

These objectives have not yet been attained. The medical profession must remain alert to better ways of solving the problems standing in their way.

Problems faced by today's physician

A major problem facing the medical profession today is the increasing shortage of physicians. In spite of the fact that there are more medical schools today, the ratio of physicians to patients is slimmer than it was fifty years ago. In 1909 there was a physician for every 568 persons; in 1970 there was one for every 603 persons (statistics for the United States; in some countries the ratio is far more startling). Worse yet, the available physicians are not always distributed evenly in the population. The physician-patient ratio is often somewhat better in urban centers and somewhat poorer in rural areas. Many physicians prefer to practice in urban locations close to modern medical facilities, where they can render the highest type of health care. However, the urban concentration reduces the number of physicians available for rural practices, sometimes depriving scattered, rural populations of adequate medical personnel. Another problem is that not all physicians are available for general health care. Actually, at present there is only one *general practitioner* available for every 3,700 persons and only one *internist* (specialist in internal medicine) available for every 5,000 persons. Compounding this dilemma is the greater demand the American public is making on the physician. Today the average American sees a physician five times a year, twice as often as he did in 1930.

Perplexed by the flood of new medical findings, more and more physicians have felt the need to restrict their practice to specialized areas of medicine, changing the traditional reliance upon a "family physician" for all health services; see Fig. 13.1. Patients have been confused about "what kind" of physician to consult.

The image the public has of the medical profession has changed. Rapid changes in medical practice have occurred, and the public has accepted certain new trends but is skeptical of others. As therapy has become more mechanized and organized, the busy physician has not always communicated sufficiently with his patient. People have become somewhat wary when they have not properly understood the techniques being used.

Some patients who have not been referred to specialists by their family physician or a general practitioner have been disappointed with their own choices of specialists. Since the "miracle drugs" have been found useful in treating many diseases, others feel these drugs have tended to reduce the important relationship a person in distress needs with his physician. Medical practitioners today make greater use of the office, clinic, and hospital, and less use of the patient's home, than they did in the past. They believe that

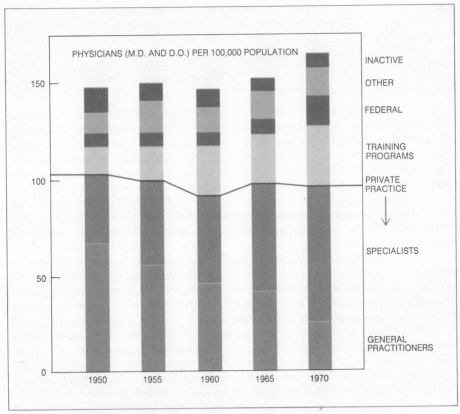

Figure 13.1 Types of physician (M.D. and D.O.) in relation to population (in hundred thousands) from 1950 to 1970. (From Health Resources Statistics, 1971, National Center for Health Statistics, *DHEW Publication No. (HSM) 72-1509*.)

treatment can be more effective when administered at some centralized location where better therapeutic tools are available. Some of the tasks formerly handled by the physician can now be safely delegated to the hospital's highly trained staff. This has made it possible for the physician to carry a heavier case load. On the other hand, these practices have tended to give the physician less contact with home conditions and thus have deprived him of background information that would enable him to know the whole patient.

Physicians are expected to keep abreast of the mounting mass of medical data. The physician is faced with increasingly informed patients who want to know the nature of their ailments. Thus, even though a physician has been professionally trained to communicate in concise technical terms, he must successfully bridge the communication gap between the forefront of research and the understanding of his patients, in order to warrant their confidence.

Medical costs have risen sharply during the past two decades and will continue to rise. Although hospital costs have risen faster than other medical costs, the lay public tends to place the blame for these higher costs on the physicians. It is understandable that these higher costs are the price to be paid for improved but costlier diagnosis and therapy. However, it is important that rising costs of medical care not get out of reach of the public and prevent some people from receiving adequate medical care.

Changes in the medical profession

As a result of rapid social changes during the past two decades there have been certain changes in the traditional methods of medical practice. The medical profession has been increasingly conscious of the problem of preparing professional people who are sufficiently broad in their training to treat the whole man yet who have adequate depth in the specialties to utilize and apply the latest information. There is increasing concern for giving emerging specialists more experience in general practice and in giving more specialized information to the general practitioner both before and after graduation. This change amounts to less emphasis on narrow specialties and more emphasis on general medicine.

There is a general feeling in the profession that health insurance must be extended. This extension is necessary if low-income families are to be sufficiently covered against mounting medical costs. The federal government has taken the responsibility to provide health insurance when, in its eyes, private methods have not kept abreast of the need.

The patterns of medical practice have been changing. More group practices combining varying specialties are being established, providing a kind of unified medical service. There is increasing use of clinics and outpatient departments of general hospitals. In the past, as better medical tools became available in city or general hospitals, physicians tended to move their practices closer to urban areas. This centralization has, in some cases, left large territories in which few, if any, medical services were readily available. But now more demand is being made for physicians to return to suburban and rural areas.

CHOOSING A PHYSICIAN

The informed person knows that good health requires good medical counsel. But he still needs an answer to the question "What kind of physician makes the ideal medical adviser, and where do I find him?" Before this question can be adequately answered, it is necessary to become acquainted with the training necessary for each type of medical practitioner.

Requirements for practice

Before a man is licensed to practice medicine, he must have met certain professional and ethical requirements. Although standards vary somewhat from state to state, training as a physician usually takes a minimum of seven years after graduation from high school. Three years of college work is the usual minimal requirement for entry into schools of medicine and osteopathy, but four years is preferable. This is followed by four years of study, leading to the M.D. or D.O. degree (doctor of medicine or doctor of osteopathy). Some medical schools recently have so revised their curricula as to enable medical students to get their M.D. degree in three years. After graduation almost all physicians serve a twelve-month internship in an approved hospital, to gain hospital experience. Then, before a physician is allowed to practice in a given state, he must be licensed by a board of medical examiners. The license is granted only after he has passed either a state or a national board examination, depending upon the particular state. Those who wish to become certified specialists must have two to four years of advanced hospital training (residency) and then two or more years of supervised practice in the specialty.

The standards for training physicians and the ethics of medical practice are set by the medical profession itself. As far as possible the profession attempts to regulate the ethics of its members. Much of this regulation is handled through the local and county medical societies. Most of them have adopted standards for their members on such things as prohibiting advertising, refraining from guaranteeing cures, adhering to all legalities regarding the taking of a human life and the administration of drugs, cooperating with legal authorities, and giving evidence (through all public and private contacts) of their trustworthiness. Admittedly, some physicians fail to meet all of these standards. In choosing a physician we have both the right and the obligation to be satisfied with the reputation, private and public, of the man to whom we entrust our lives.

A family physician

Everyone should have a physician whom he can regard as a personal or family physician. This physician should know his patients well and provide their basic medical care. In addition he should advise the services of specialists when required. General family care usually can be provided by either the general practitioner or the general internist.

General practitioner   Customarily Americans have looked to a single physician to diagnose and treat all the family's illnesses, and the physician practiced general medicine and attempted to handle the full range of health conditions. Twenty years ago general practitioners (GPs) outnumbered specialists three to one. Today it is just the opposite: specialists outnumber general practitioners three to one (Fig. 13.2). General practitioners are more commonly found in rural, semirural, and suburban areas.

A physician may practice general medicine after he has completed his basic training and has served his internship. Although not required, more of these physicians today are taking additional, or postgraduate, training of some kind. Many of them have completed at least two years of residency training and are members of the American Academy of General Practice. Some of them direct this postgraduate study to a given area of medicine and confine their practice more or less to a type of specialty.

Some unique problems face the general practitioner today. First, in order to have a high-quality practice he must keep abreast of the mass of new scientific information and developments. Second, he must face a demanding load of work. The average GP puts in a ten-hour workday, many seeing as many as 135 patients a week. Third, he is called upon to treat most of his patients' illnesses, since he is in the best position medically to minister to the whole person.

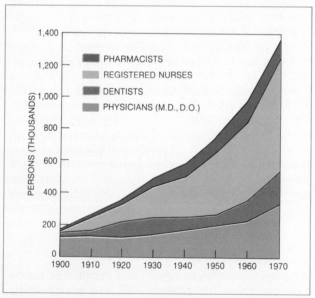

Figure 13.2   Growth of various health professions in relation to population from 1900 to 1970. (From Health Resources Statistics, 1971, National Center for Health Statistics, *DHEW Publication No. (HSM) 72-1509.*)

General internist   The specialist in internal medicine may or may not fill the role of family physician. He is generally better qualified to serve as a personal physician to adults than to children. To become an internist he must have completed six years of training in an approved hospital after medical school and have successfully passed the examination given by the American Board of Internal Medicine. Since his training is primarily in diagnosis, he is particularly suited for preventive medicine as well as for coordinating the work of specialists needed to treat the specific problems the patient faces. Not all internists desire to practice general medicine; some confine their work to subspecialties such as allergies, heart diseases, digestive-tract problems, or lung ailments. Generally, internists do not deliver babies, practice surgery, deal with troubles of the eye, or treat children.

The specialties

The more a physician concentrates his attention on a given system of the body, the less time he has for the whole person and the less proficient he may be in general practice. To know one area of medicine in depth he must confine himself to it to the exclusion of other areas. Such concentration has enabled medicine to make its great strides in heart surgery, cancer therapy, psychiatry, and other areas. Usually, a certified specialist has completed the hospital residency and passed the examination required of his particular specialty and is therefore recognized as a *board diplomate* by that particular specialty.

Internal medicine   Although internal medicine often deals with the total person, the practice of internal medicine is recognized as one of the specialties. The characteristics of that specialty have been described.

Obstetrics and gynecology   Obstetrics, the care of the woman in pregnancy and childbirth, is frequently combined with gynecology, the care of women's diseases. Stressing preventive medicine, the obstetrician sees the mother early in pregnancy, supervises her health, and handles the delivery. Such attention has reduced infant mortality to a low rate in this country.

Pediatrics   Pediatricians specialize in the care of infants and children. They advise parents, give checkups, diagnose congenital deformities, administer immunizations, treat childhood diseases, and so on. Some pediatricians confine themselves to certain types of children's illness, such as heart disease and children's allergies (cardiology and pediatric allergies).

Surgery   The surgeon is concerned with operating upon the patient to correct an unwanted condition. Surgery may involve removing a cancerous growth, repairing a damaged heart, stopping a brain hemorrhage, or setting a broken bone. This specialty commonly tends to be subdivided into specific areas—neurosurgery, thoracic surgery, orthopedic surgery, and so on.

Psychiatry   The psychiatrist deals with emotional illnesses and disturbances. He generally treats his patients through psychotherapy, shock therapy, drugs, or combinations of these. Some psychiatrists are also neurologists. To be a psychiatrist a person must first earn an M.D. degree and then study psychiatry.

Other   Among many other specialties are the following, which we list rather than describe in detail.

>   Anesthesiology—the administering of general and local anesthetics
>   Dermatology—the treatment of diseases of the skin
>   Neurology—the treatment of physical diseases of the brain and nervous system
>   Ophthalmology—the treatment of the eye and its diseases
>   Otorhinolaryngology—the treatment of diseases of the ear, nose, and throat
>   Pathology—the study of the structural changes that cause or are caused by
> disease
>   Radiology—the diagnosis and treatment of disease by means of x-rays, radium,
> and other radioactive sources
>   Urology—the treatment of diseases and abnormalities of the urinary tract in
> the female and the urinary and genital (urogenital) tract in the male.

In all there are thirty-four recognized fields of medical specialization. Each is governed by its respective American Board for purposes of examination and certification.

Osteopathy

Recent development in the relationship between osteopathy and medicine in certain states requires that something be said here about this field. Originally osteopathy was based on a theory proposed in 1870 by Dr. Andrew Still. This theory held that disease could be based on disturbed nerve function resulting from a pinching of the nerves as they leave the spinal column. This theory considered a disease or condition in any particular organ of the body to be due to a malcondition in the nerve supplying that organ.

The medical profession has considered this theory unfounded and contradictory to its knowledge of human anatomy and pathology. Over the course of years, however, osteopathic physicians have been quietly abandoning many of the tenets originally held in osteopathy and have increasingly emphasized the practice of sound medicine. This change has progressed to the point where their training and practice is similar to that of traditional medicine. However, osteopaths are often barred from practicing in medical hospitals. As a consequence, osteopathic physicians often open their own hospitals or clinics as they are able to finance them. Some individuals prefer the services of an osteopath. Today's osteopathic physician utilizes both drugs and physical manipulation in the treatment of patients. A qualified osteopathic physician may satisfactorily serve as a family physician.

Osteopaths constitute about 4 percent of all the physicians in the country (M.D. and D.O.). Students are trained in six four-year osteopathic schools. They are licensed in all the states. In California the state osteopathic board does not grant new licenses but does renew existing ones.

Types of practice

In recent years there has been another significant change in the nature of medical practice. Physicians have increasingly favored banding together in various kinds of groups to provide better care than they could give when located in isolated, single-man offices. Although the clinic idea has been commonly used for years in larger medical centers, such as the Mayo Clinic in Rochester, Minnesota, the average local physician practiced independently prior to World War II. Since 1946 the number of medical groups and the number of physicians in the groups have tripled. Various types of group practices can now be found in any community.

The tendency is for group practices to represent something more than simple office-sharing. More commonly, it is an organization of full-time physicians with centralized bookkeeping and laboratory facilities. In the main, medical groups consist of physicians from different specialties banding together with the idea of giving complete medical care to their patients. The majority of them are composed of fewer than six physicians. Since the physicians work to some extent as a team, this arrangement allows for more frequent consultation and for less inconvenience to the patient in making and keeping appointments.

Selecting the right physician

In seeking medical care an individual will have to determine what his family's needs are and then settle on what is available. If he is seeking general medical care, he may prefer either a physician in general practice or several specialists in selected branches of medicine. Since some general practitioners further restrict themselves to a narrow branch of practice, the family will need to know the nature of a physician's practice. If there are young children in the family, the physician chosen should be one who enjoys working with children. Elderly people may prefer choosing a physician who is involved in geriatrics. If a family cannot find the single ideal physician, it may be desirable to settle for several specialists, such as a pediatrician for the children and an internist for the adults.

In choosing a physician a family may find it useful to follow some or all of the following suggestions:

1. Select the names of a number of family physicians in the general area. A physician's office should be located close enough to make medical care readily accessible. It is a good idea to choose one whose office is located either in the patient's home town or in his part of the city. Compose a list of names from suggestions given by friends, a local hospital, or the local medical society.

2. Look into the credentials of each physician on the list by contacting the local or county medical society or by going to your public library and asking for the *AMA Directory* or *The Directory of Medical Specialists*. Find out whether he is licensed to practice in your state. Determine whether he has

taken additional training beyond basic medical training and, if so, where and when. Check on how long he has been practicing. If he is a general practitioner, find out whether he is a member of the American Academy of General Practice; if he is an internist, see whether he has been accepted as a fellow in the American College of Physicians. Although these memberships do not guarantee a good medical man, they are some indication of a physician's interest in improving himself. Membership in the local medical society is important: not all physicians who are licensed to practice are accepted for membership in these societies. Acceptance is based upon a physician's adherence to the ethical standards of the society.

3. Find out whether a physician is a staff member of, or practices in, an accredited hospital. A phone call or visit to the hospital administrator can supply a person with this answer. Good hospitals select their members with care. Remember, if a person must go to a hospital, he will be permitted the services of his family physician only if the physician is allowed to practice there.

4. Evaluate the physicians on the list with friends and neighbors who have gone to them. Look for reasons why individuals like or dislike their physicians. If a person detects any pattern of repetition of complaint, it could well be a problem with the physician and not just the grievances of a patient. The person should likewise overlook excessive praise if he suspects it is unrealistic rather than objective.

5. The patient should make an appointment to see the physician he would most like to have. He should find out whether the physician is accepting new patients and whether his office is neat and clean and well run. The patient should discuss his family needs with the physician, determine whether the physician could supply most of them, and discuss the specialists he consults with. He should find out whether the physician can be expected to make house calls, whether he is usually available for emergencies and, if not, whether another physician fills in for him and who that other physician is. The patient should be frank in discussing with the physician his fee schedule in relation to those of other physicians in the same community.

6. When the patient has left the physician's office, he should review his visit. Is he pleased with the physician's personality? Does he seem to be the sort of physician he would want to confide in? Was he businesslike and thorough? If he can answer these questions affirmatively, he has found his family physician.

The patient-physician relationship

The patient will, in all probability, expect a satisfying relationship with his physician. However, neither the patient nor the physician should be exposed to unreasonable expectations about human relationships. As a patient one is entitled to receive careful, effective service, including the use of necessary laboratory tests and consultations with appropriate specialists in order to provide himself with adequate treatment. Although it is not always within the physician's power to cure—and sometimes not even to provide relief—the patient should always be able to feel that his physician is doing his best.

The physician should administer inoculations or have them administered. He should advise the family, particularly when it includes children, when inoculations should be given. A careful physician will notify adults when certain kinds of periodic examination should be made. Then his suggestions should be acted upon. In the practice of preventive medicine it is sometimes hard for patients to grasp the full benefit of medical care and to justify the cost of it. A good physician will not suggest treatment or prescribe medicines he does not think the patient needs. Remember, a physician would much rather keep a person from getting ill than attempt to bring a patient back to health once he is ailing. Prevention of illness is not only easier but also less painful—and cheaper.

If a patient is not completely satisfied with a physician's diagnosis and treatment, he ought to ask for further consultation with his or another physician. If the patient is convinced that he can no longer trust the medical care provided by his physician, he may seek out a new doctor. However, before this step is taken, the patient should be sure that the new physician will be able to offer him better treatment. There are often various ways to treat a given malady. Every physician will have his weak spots, his moments of fatigue, his failings. There is value to be gained in building up a personal health history with one physician. In the event the patient seeks a new physician he should first be sure a basic improvement in medical care will be gained rather than mere relief from petty grievances.

If he is to expect medical care, the patient should be acquainted with a physician who will be able to provide it when it is needed. Some individuals moving into a new community fail to contact a new physician until they need him in an emergency or late at night. Then, if they encounter any difficulty in obtaining care, they make complaints against the medical profession. It is legitimate for a physician to question what responsibility he has toward a nonpatient who has made no attempt to acquire a family physician but who expects care in the middle of the night.

If a patient is not satisfied with a physician's fee schedule, it is the patient's obligation to discuss it frankly with the physician. If the cost of medical care is imposing a hardship on the patient or his family, the physician wants to know about it. Often low-cost medical care is provided where conditions warrant it. The patient should be open and fair in discussing costs with his physician, and the physician should be expected to be understanding and fair in return.

In relations with his physician the patient should treat him the way the patient would want to be treated and expect that the physician will behave similarly. A physician can give his best service when he feels his patients appreciate his efforts. Much as he would enjoy being able to cure every physical ailment, medical research has not provided him with all the necessary answers to accomplish this aim. But a good physician will go just as far in diagnosis and treatment as his ability, training, available facilities, and patients allow him to go.

ALLIED HEALTH PROFESSIONS

Complete health service requires the services of a number of professions. These workers are employed in many places—hospitals, pharmacies, nursing homes, laboratories, and private offices. Below is a limited discussion of a few significant allied health fields.

Dentistry

Dentistry treats ailments or abnormalities of the gums and teeth and attempts to prevent their recurrence. The dentist does this by locating and filling cavities, extracting teeth, if such procedure is warranted, straightening crooked teeth, treating gum and mouth diseases, and replacing missing teeth with artificial dentures (prostheses) constructed to give each patient chewing comfort and efficiency. As in preventive medicine, there has been increasing emphasis on prevention of tooth diseases by routine cleaning of teeth, fluoridation of water supplies, and adequate periodic brushing. Most dentists are general practitioners who provide many types of dental care, although the small number of specialists is increasing. The specialties of dentistry deal with *orthodontia*, or straightening of teeth, *oral surgery*, or the extraction of teeth and surgical procedures, *pedodontics*, or dentistry for children, *periodontics*, or treatment of gums and underlying bone, *prosthodontics*, or providing artificial replacements for missing teeth, *endodontics*, or root-canal therapy, *oral pathology*, or treating diseases of the mouth, and *public-health dentistry*.

Dental training consists of four years of professional training following two to four years of required college work. The dental specialties usually require two or three years of additional professional training.

Nursing

More people are engaged in the nursing services than in any other health occupation; see Fig. 13.2. The nursing team is led by the *registered nurse* (R.N.) but also includes the vocational (practical) nurses, nursing aides, orderlies, and attendants.

Registered nurses handle the largest share of nursing services. They administer medications and treatments prescribed by physicians, observe, evaluate, and record symptoms and the progress of patients, assist in patient education and rehabilitation, improve the surroundings of the patients, and instruct other medical personnel and students. Although the majority of them work in hospitals, they also perform in private duty, offices, public health, industrial plants, and nursing schools.

There are three types of training program for registered nurses. *Diploma* programs are conducted by hospital schools and usually require three years of training, *associate degree* programs are usually located in community colleges and are approximately two years in length, and *baccalaureate* programs usually require four years of study in a college or university, although some require five years. Additional training can be taken to qualify for a nursing specialty in obstetrics, pediatrics, psychiatry, or surgical nursing.

Medical technology

As the physician works to detect, diagnose, and treat diseases, he will frequently call for laboratory tests to confirm the presence or absence of a condition. Much of the laboratory work can be time-consuming. Therefore *medical technologists* are trained to assist the physician. Generally working directly under the supervision of a pathologist, the technologist makes blood counts, urinalyses, and skin tests, examines body fluids and tissue samples microscopically, runs cultures of microorganisms to determine their identity and reaction to drugs, types and cross-matches blood samples, measures basal metabolism, and analyzes food, water, or other materials for bacteria.

The great majority of medical technologists work in hospitals and conduct tests in connection with the examination and treatment of patients. The *medical technologist* is not to be confused with the *medical technician* or *laboratory assistant*. The technologist is required to take four years of college, including twelve months in a medical-technology educational program. The college work is based heavily on the basic biological and physical sciences. The training program must be affiliated with a degree-granting college or university.

Pharmacy

Pharmacists help in health care through making drugs and medicine available and providing information on their use. They dispense prescriptions ordered by medical practitioners and sell general drugs and medical supplies. They are trained to understand the composition of drugs and to be responsible for the drug's purity and strength. Only a registered pharmacist may fill a prescription. A registered pharmacist must be a graduate of an accredited college of pharmacy and have passed a rigorous examination in the state in which he practices. The training of five years of professional study and one year of internship includes the compounding of drugs. However, many drug products today are manufactured in the form in which the patient purchases them, not requiring compounding by the retail druggist. But this fact does not diminish the importance and responsibility of the pharmacist. He is responsible for all drugs dispensed and has the prerogative to question any prescription as being dangerous in either quantity or kind. If not fully satisfied, he can validly refuse to fill a prescription.

Physical therapy

This branch of the healing arts serves in the rehabilitation of people with injuries or diseases affecting muscles, joints, nerves, and bones. The *physical therapist* works under the direction of a physician, to administer therapy through the use of therapeutic exercise and massage and various types of treatment with heat, water, light, and electricity. Physical therapy has been invaluable in the treating of victims of poliomyelitis, cerebral palsy, arthritis, and muscular dystrophy. Preparation for this type of work usually calls for either a bachelor degree in physical therapy or a one- or two-year graduate program.

Optometry

The *optometrist* is especially trained and licensed to examine eyes and test their refractive abilities, determine the deviation from normal, and prescribe lenses and visual training that does not require drugs or surgery. He should not be confused with *ophthalmologists* or *oculists* (medical specialists dealing with the medical and surgical care of the eyes and their refractive corrections) or *opticians* (those who interpret the prescription of the ophthalmologist or optometrist and select the frames to hold the lenses). The usual training consists of two years of preoptometry education and four years of professional education. Most graduate optometrists are in private practice.

Podiatry

Sometimes called a *chiropodist*, the *podiatrist* diagnoses and treats diseases and deformities of the feet or tries to prevent their occurrence in his patients. His work is important, since more than half of the people in the United States have foot troubles ranging from simple corns to difficulties requiring special shoes or foot appliances and even to problems requiring the attention of a medical specialist. The field of podiatry is far from overcrowded. Most podiatrists, when they have completed their four years of professional training after the required two years preprofessional training, engage in private practice.

Chiropractic

Chiropractic, or "drugless healing," is based on the belief that the nervous system largely determines a person's state of health and that any interference with this system impairs normal functions and lowers the body's resistance to disease. Patients are treated by manipulation. In the forty-eight states licensing the practice, four years of training in a school of chiropractic following high school or, in most states, one or two years of college work are required. Chiropractors are licensed in all states except Louisiana and Mississippi.

Most chiropractors are better trained in therapeutics, such as body manipulation and adjustment, than they are in adequate understanding and diagnosis of the underlying disease. Consequently, although the chiropractor may bring relief to conditions in which the spinal column is maladjusted, there are many common medical conditions he is not prepared to care for. Accordingly, a chiropractor should not be sought out as a family physician.

FACILITIES FOR PATIENT CARE

As modern medicine has progressed, the providing of improved medical care has become more involved. Not many years ago most patients were seen in their homes by the family physician. The diagnosis and treatment were limited either to what was on hand or to what the physician could bring with him.

The home served as a kind of "hospital" for the delivery of babies and the treatment of pneumonia and tuberculosis and as a nursing home for those suffering from chronic diseases. Only patients with the most complicated conditions were admitted to the town hospital.

Today only minor illnesses are cared for at home. Improved standards of diagnosis and treatment require facilities that are available only in physicians' offices, clinics, nursing homes, and hospitals.

Clinics and nursing homes

The services of hospitals are frequently supplemented by the services of clinics and nursing homes. Clinics are often set up in conjunction with a hospital to provide various types of specialized service for patients with venereal disease, tuberculosis, cancer, and communicable diseases and for patients needing maternal care and child dental care. Their services are for patients who are not severely ill enough to require hospitalization yet who need medical care. Although they deal in diagnosis and treatment, they direct their effort toward instructing expectant mothers, providing social services, and giving advice on matters of nutrition and other public health problems. Patients who can afford the service are charged; however, many patients pay little or nothing.

Nursing homes provide services for convalescing patients or for those with chronic illnesses, but not on as large a scale as a hospital supplying qualified services. They help to free needed hospital beds for patients with more acute illnesses. The quality of their care should be no different from that of a hospital.

Hospitals

Hospitals provide complete medical facilities for the acutely ill, including expensive, centralized equipment and services not available in the local physician's office. The centralized hospital enables the busy physician to see his patients as a group. It also serves to protect the public from individuals with easily communicated diseases. The greater use of hospitals today, compared with that of a few years ago, along with the natural increase in population, has substantially increased the demand for available hospital facilities.

Generally, hospitals have been constructed with funds from communities, private philanthropists, local or state tax dollars, and grants of federal monies. During the past two decades the number of available hospital beds in the United States has doubled. In addition, costly hospital facilities have been increased. Although many communities have been able to keep up with the demand in providing up-to-date hospital facilities, some parts of the country today either lack hospital facilities or have substandard ones. Yet in spite of the continuing need for more and better hospital facilities, considerable thought must precede the locating of new hospitals and the enlarging of existing ones. Preliminary questions that need to be answered are the following: Will the hospital be large enough to provide necessary equipment and facilities? Are there enough physicians in the vicinity to staff it adequately? Are enough nurses, trained technicians, and other qualified personnel available to man it? Can it be large enough to make the operation of the hospital plant self-supporting? Is the surrounding population large enough to warrant the cost of operating it? If there is already an existing hospital in the area, would it be cheaper to add more beds to it than to build an entirely new hopsital and duplicate expensive equipment?

Hospitals often are established to provide certain kinds of medical service to certain groups of people. Generally, they may be grouped according to their type of ownership and method of operation: government hospitals, voluntary hospitals, and proprietary hospitals.

Government hospitals The federal government has established institutions for personnel in the military services and the Public Health Service and their dependents, for American Indians, for merchant seamen, for veterans, for patients of leprosy, and for narcotics addicts. Individual states have established either *specialized* hospitals for individuals—such as for the emotionally disturbed patients or the tubercular—or *general* hospitals, which are usually associated with a state-supported medical school. City and county hospitals are commonly general hospitals, providing general medical care but frequently giving special attention to communicable-disease control and the care of the indigent. In many cases the government hospital is set up for the long-term patient.

Voluntary hospitals Voluntary hospitals are public hospitals set up on a nonprofit basis. They have been established by churches, philanthropic individuals, charitable organizations, or the local community. They are run by governing boards, selected from the community, which are responsible for all phases of operation, financing, and construction. Mostly short-term institutions, these hospitals provide for more than two thirds of all hospital admissions. Although they attempt to meet their own expenses, they frequently are underwritten financially by local organizations. Since the end of World War II the federal government has aided somewhat in the construction of voluntary hospitals by making monies available under the Hill-Burton Act.

Proprietary hospitals Owned and administered by individuals or corporations, proprietary hospitals are set up as profit-seeking investments. They are often established by real-estate promoters and then leased to groups of physicians at no cost to the community. Although this arrangement frequently appeals at first to the community, the operations of proprietary hospitals in many places have raised some degree of controversy and question. They are primarily short-term hospitals catering to the most profitable type of hospital business. They hesitate to admit patients who are unable to pay their way. The majority of them are small and unaccredited (only about one third of them are accredited). Although not all are poorly administered, they generally have gained questionable reputations.

Accreditation of hospitals

Concern over standards of hospital care resulted in the establishment in 1952 of the Joint Commission on Accreditation of Hospitals (JCAH). A voluntary, nonprofit organization, it is sponsored by the American College of Physicians, the American College of Surgeons, the American Hospital Association, and the American Medical Association. Its functions have been to set up national standards of hospital care, to accredit hospitals meeting these standards, and to see that these standards are maintained in accredited hospitals. In order to become accredited, a hospital must have twenty-five or more beds, have been in operation at least one year, be listed with the American Hospital Association, and have passed a rigid inspection by JCAH physicians. Upon application a hospital is thoroughly evaluated in all respects, including cleanliness, laboratories, food handling, records and, in particular, the practice of its staff physicians. A full accreditation is good for two years, after which the hospital must be reexamined.

Increasing value is being given to JCAH accreditation. A nonaccredited hospital may not train interns, residents, or nurses, all of whom contribute to making a better hospital. Nonaccreditation also threatens the cutoff of Medicare income. Under law, any hospital accredited by the JCAH is automatically certified for Medicare; unaccredited hospitals must be separately inspected and approved for Medicare by state health officials. The Blue Cross insurance organizations have in some cases refused to make payments of insurance monies to nonaccredited hospitals. Since many of the larger hospitals in the country are accredited, hospitals representing over 89 percent of the total bed space are accredited. More than 75 percent of all voluntary hospitals are accredited, but less than 50 percent of all proprietary ones are.

How to choose a hospital

Although many individuals today live in communities in which there is but a single hospital, an increasing majority of people live within easy commuting distance of two or more hospitals. Some of these individuals at some time or another have the choice of selecting a hospital. The choice of a physician may be based in part on which hospital he practices in. In our larger cities a physician may have access to more than one hospital; in such case the patient may select the one he prefers. Even though he may never have the choice of a hospital, any individual concerned with the quality of health care he is getting should want to be informed on his local hospital. For these reasons he should have some basis for judging a hospital. In so doing there are three basic questions that should be asked.

1. *Is the hospital accredited?* Accreditation by JCAH will not guarantee a first-rate hospital, but it will mean that it has met certain minimal standards, both in facilities and in staff practice.

2. *Is it a teaching hospital?* A hospital that has a program for training personnel is equipped to provide better medical service. The higher the level of this teaching, the better. The best situation is one in which a hospital is

associated with a medical school. Here one can expect to find well-qualified specialists as instructors and qualified resident physicians training in the specialties. Although there are rather few medical-school hospitals in the country, many more hospitals have some type of resident training program. If this type is not available, one should look for a hospital that at least trains interns or nurses.

3. *Who owns the hospital?* In other words, is it a voluntary, nonprofit community hospital or a privately owned, proprietary hospital? Generally, a voluntary hospital is to be preferred over a proprietary one. Ultimate responsibility for the conduct in a voluntary hospital rests with its board of trustees chosen from the community, whereas in the proprietary hospital responsibility rests only with its *owners*, and its quality will rise and fall with the owners' dedication, sense of ethics, or desire to make a profit.

Decisions before hospitalization

Even after a person is satisfied that his hospital is a good one, it is advisable, when it is suggested that he or a member of his family enter the hospital, to learn whether the hospital is the best place to obtain the needed services. For instance, could the suggested treatment be taken care of just as well in a clinic providing infant or child care or in a nursing home for older individuals? Elderly people sometimes develop serious psychological problems over entering a hospital. Cost, also, is not to be overlooked, even by those holding some form of hospitalization insurance. Even if one has such insurance, the more it is utilized, the higher will be the premium rates among its subscribers. Accordingly, hospitalization for convenience only cannot be sanctioned. Generally speaking, if a person is fortunate in having a reliable physician, he should be able to rely upon that physician's recommendation on matters of hospital admission. A good physician will always be concerned with his patient's best interests.

Upon entering a hospital a person may have the choice of a ward or a semiprivate or private room. Although a ward location costs less, the patient will also have less privacy. The room selection should depend upon the need for privacy and other personal requirements as well as on financial ability.

Patients admitted to teaching hospitals and those who are not under the care of a specific physician are often assigned to intern or resident physicians. Since such students are being trained in diagnosis and treatment, patients attended by them will also be under the observation of teaching specialists. Such patients, therefore, often receive the best of professional care.

FINANCING HEALTH CARE

There remains, however, the problem of paying for this care. Adequate health care today can be quite expensive. In the minds of many people there arises the question why it must be as expensive as it is. Is health care overpriced? Is a greater share of the average wage-earners' paycheck going for medical and dental expenses than it has in past years? Have the costs of all health services risen uniformly? Are people more interested in using their dollars for other personal needs and less interested in effective (and expensive) health care?

Any comparisons of an individual's costs of health care one year with his costs of some past date are futile, because there is no standard of comparison. Health care has become more complex, and the quality of treatment expected today far exceeds that expected in the past. Although we would be happy to return to the "old-fashioned" costs, we would not wish to return to methods of care that reduced our chances of survival.

Why health care is so costly

The cost of health care has been increasing faster than the *Consumer Price Index*, which is the U.S. Department of Labor index that shows us what it costs us to live; see Fig. 13.3. Yet not all kinds of health care costs have risen equally, as Fig. 13.4 shows. Overall health care has gone up 28 percent

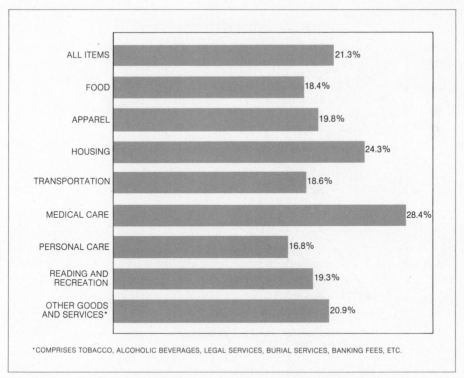

Figure 13.3   Percentage increases in medical-care costs and other major living expenses over the Consumer Price Index in the United States for the period of 1967 to 1971, costs in 1967 being base 100.

since 1967, hospital room rates have increased 160 percent, and drugs have increased 5 percent (by comparison, they cost less than they did in 1967).

Why the great increase in hospital rates? One reason is that the number of hospital admissions is twice what it was twenty years ago. Physicians make greater use of hospitals than they used to, both saving them time and providing a higher quality of care. Another reason is the greater hospital operating costs due to the continued rise in wages paid hospital personnel, as their wages have been moving to parity with other professions. Yet another reason is more and more hospital construction. While in some places this is needed, because all existing facilities are full, in other places there are many bed vacancies. Some communities or private groups build new hospitals too close to adequate existing hospitals; unnecessary duplication of hospital facilities too close to existing hospitals significantly raises hospital costs for *all* patients within the area.

Not only is hospital construction very costly, but so is a hospital's equipment. The major scientific equipment used in hospitals is being improved so rapidly that a new piece of major equipment is obsolete long before it is

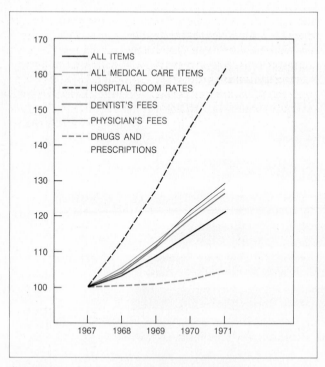

Figure 13.4 Increases in kinds of health-care costs over increase in the Consumer Price Index in the United States for 1967 to 1971, costs in 1967 being base 100.

Table 13.1 *Cost of hospitalization for coronary occlusion, per patient, compared with number of fatalities*

year	no. of patients	fatalities	cost per patient
1920	100	40	$200
1940	100	30	$400–600
1970	100	16	$3500

worn out. Yet such increasingly expensive equipment is helping save the lives of more patients. A study from Massachusetts General Hospital is a case in point. In a comparison of patients coming to the hospital with coronary occlusions (heart attacks), in terms of cost per patient to fatalities for the years 1920, 1940, and 1970, the results were as shown in Table 13.1. In addition, such expensive equipment must be available every moment of the day and every day of the year—and qualified technicians must be available to operate these devices. All of these factors have increased the cost of hospital confinement.

Health insurance

It is the boast of the health-insurance field that more than 90 percent of our population holds some form of health insurance; see Fig. 13.5. However, health insurance benefits cover only about one third of the health expenses of the average family. Consequently, the typical family looks with some suspicion on the rising costs of health insurance. Insurance companies are facing the predicament of balancing higher benefit costs against premium rates. They have the choice of either increasing the rates or reducing the benefits. Still, as

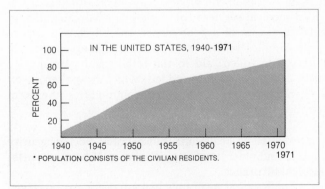

Figure 13.5   Percentage of civilian population with some form of health insurance protection for period 1940 to 1971. (From Health Insurance Institute; Health Insurance Council; U.S. Department of Commerce, Bureau of the Census.)

far as policyholders are concerned, their health care tends to be a little cheaper in the form of a prepaid plan. They are protected somewhat against sudden large medical costs by being forced systematically to lay away funds.

The traditional method of financing health costs has been for each family to pay medical and dental bills as they arise, hoping to have sufficient savings for the major episodes. This individual financing has been a "pay-as-you-go" matter for some and a matter of budgeting for others. Were health expenses "average" and predictable from month to month, much like rent, food, or other recurring expenses, a family could budget a certain amount of money for this purpose. But because of the unpredictable nature of health problems, such budgeting is impossible. Health expenses are usually erratic, with periods of heavy expense separated by periods of little or no expense. And some families are repeatedly hit by heavy expenses which go far beyond the average.

As a result of these problems there has been an increasing trend toward collective financing of health costs. This is not a new concept, but one that dates back to ancient times. The current methods of collective financing fall into one or two basic approaches—public (tax-supported) health services and private (voluntary) health insurance.

Public health care (tax-supported)

Public health care has been made available to some extent to a great number of Americans through a number of programs. These include federal, state, county and, sometimes, city facilities and services. These many programs may be categorized in several main groups.

Care of the indigent   The oldest of the public programs for specific groups are the organized health programs for the poor, or indigent. In 1935 the federal Social Security Act, a milestone in the organization of health services in the United States, provided medical services for three principal categories of indigent persons: the aged (65 years of age or older), the blind, and dependent children (minors from families unable to provide adequate support). In the 1950s a fourth category was added: aid to the totally and permanently disabled. Since then a fifth category has been added, which is spoken of by the welfare people as "general welfare." In some communities the term "home relief" has been applied to these general-welfare cases.

Medicare   Medicare is a program of health insurance under Social Security that helps Americans 65 years and older pay for medical care. It has two parts: hospital insurance and medical insurance.

· HOSPITAL INSURANCE   The hospital insurance helps pay for care received as a hospital inpatient and for certain follow-up services. It does not pay physicians' bills. At the present time it covers the following:

1. Up to 90 days of inpatient care in any participating hospital in each

benefit period (a new benefit period begins after a person has not been an inpatient for 60 days).

2. A "lifetime reserve" of 60 additional hospital days.

3. Up to 100 days of care in each benefit period in a participating extended-care facility after one leaves the hospital. A participating extended-care facility must be staffed to furnish skilled nursing care and other related health services.

4. Up to 100 medically necessary home health "visits" by nurses, physical therapists, home health aides, or other health workers.

There are certain minimal charges for some of these services. The covered services in a hospital or extended-care facility include the cost of room and meals in semiprivate accommodations (two to four beds) and regular nursing services, and the cost of drugs, supplies, appliances, and equipment furnished for use in the hospital or facility.

Hospital insurance does not cover physicians' bills, private-duty nurses, items furnished for one's convenience, and the cost of the first three pints of blood needed as an inpatient.

· MEDICAL INSURANCE   The medical insurance helps pay physicians' bills and a number of other medical items and services not covered under hospital insurance.

Medical insurance is voluntary, and people must sign up for it. The monthly premiums are shared equally by these people and by the federal government. Almost anyone can apply for it at age 65, whether they are under Medicare or not. A person may register only during specified periods. Benefits include payment for the following:

1. Physicians' services.

2. Up to 100 home health visits each year furnished by a home health agency taking part in Medicare, if a physician arranges the treatment and certifies the patient's need for such services.

3. Other medical or health services prescribed by a physician—such as x-ray, radiation, surgical dressings, splints, artificial limbs, and rental or purchase of medical equipment.

4. Office medical supplies, outpatient physical-therapy services, certain ambulance services, clinical laboratory, x-ray and other radiological services supplied by a pathologist or radiologist while one is a hospital inpatient.

A subscriber pays the first $50 of his medical expenses each year and then 20 percent of the balance. Insurance benefits are usually paid directly to the physician. The physician or supplier agrees to make only reasonable charges.

Health insurance does not cover routine physical checkups, prescription drugs and patent medicines, eyeglasses or eyeglass examinations, hearing aids, immunizations, dentures and routine dental care, or orthopedic shoes. A person can drop out of this health insurance plan any time he wishes by filing written notice.

Aid to veterans   The veterans' program is divided into two principal parts: care of service-connected disabilities and care of nonservice-connected disabilities. Any condition that was inflicted or activated during service, if noted on the individual's medical-service record, will be taken care of at government expense through the Veterans Administration. For treatment of nonservice-inflicted disabilities or conditions the individual must be able to prove inability to pay for treatment before the Veterans Administration will accept the patient for treatment. Nonservice disabilities do not qualify for treatment if the ex-serviceman received a bad-conduct, dishonorable, or "undesirable" discharge.

A great network of hospitals and clinics provides this care. There is also a so-called "home town" program for veterans, which makes provision for local care of service-connected disabilities for a veteran who lives in a place distant from a Veterans Administration hospital.

Aid to military dependents   A program of importance in recent years is that for military dependents. The wives and children of military personnel who are on active or inactive duty or who are retired from the service are the objects of this program. Children are covered until they are 18 years of age.

Started during World War II, this program was meant to serve as a small token of appreciation to the men overseas. Service wives having babies were provided with care. Dropped at the end of the war, the program was later reintroduced as it became harder to recruit military personnel and have them stay on beyond their six-month to four-year tours of duty. The government promised to see that the dependents of military personnel received adequate health care. The program extends such care to several million people either at military posts or at freely chosen places.

Special groups (general government health care)   Several other groups of citizens are of interest to the government for various reasons.

· MILITARY PERSONNEL   Military persons receive all health care while on active duty or upon retirement from the military service. Many of the young people in our country have had their best experiences with first-class medicine during the time they were in the service.

· AMERICAN INDIANS   Over half a million Americans who are Indians are entitled to health care through a network of hospitals and clinics operated by the United States Public Health Service.

· UNITED STATES MERCHANT MARINE   The Merchant Marine members' government-financed health care goes back to 1798 and represents the first public tax-supported medical-care program.

Special diseases   There are tax-supported programs for special diseases. The most important is for emotional disorders. For about eighty-five years care of the emotionally ill has predominantly been a public function and often provided for in a state hospital. The whole approach to care of the emotionally ill is being revitalized, and the financial support for local, state, and federal agencies is in the process of revision. In addition, more private hospitals are providing coverage for emotional illnesses. As indicated in an earlier chapter, clinics for alcoholism and drug abuse are maintained by local, state, and federal agencies. These clinics are the major treatment centers for these conditions in the United States.

Communicable diseases   Venereal-disease diagnosis and treatment are of high public concern. Programs for control of venereal diseases have changed as the nature of the treatment has changed. During the early 1940s the treatment of venereal disease was a long process. Most of the venereal-disease therapy was administered through public clinics. When penicillin became available in the 'forties the picture changed. The treatment of venereal disease became relatively rapid and, therefore, inexpensive. Therapy shifted largely to private offices. The veneral-disease programs in most health departments are now largely concerned with public education and the epidemiological conditions of the diseases. Then there are rare diseases such as leprosy, for which there is a public hospital in Carville, Louisiana. In some of the larger cities there are special hospitals for other infectious diseases.

Crippled children   There are special provisions for health care of crippled children, administered usually by the state health departments and to some extent by welfare departments. Crippled children receive both medical and educational care. The Crippled Children's Program is one of the best examples of a service in which the leadership has been very insistent on high standards. A child who gets health care under the Crippled Children's Program must be treated by a specialist certified in his field—such as orthopedics, physical medicine, or surgery.

Crippled adults   There are two principal kinds of organized health-care programs for crippled adults. The oldest are those growing out of litigation over industrial injuries—workmen's compensation insurance. Although the cost of this program is not tax supported, the program in each state is the result of legislation. The health care is financed under law through the insurance carried by the employer.

Other kinds of disabilities affecting adults (amputation, blindness, crippling arthritis, and others), which may or may not be related to employment, are also covered by health care programs. A federal-state program of vocational rehabilitation is usually administered by the State Department of Education, because an important feature of the plan is job retraining.

General hospital care   General public hospitals are tax supported to provide general hospital care for people with any condition. They are usually operated under city or county government. In most cities throughout the country the special publicly operated hospitals are strongly oriented to the care of indigent persons and those with chronic illnesses.

Local or county health departments   Finally, under the tax-supported services is the local health department, which provides various special services. Although these services vary in kind and extent from county to county, the following services are often provided, particularly in the better organized counties:

Communicable disease control	Maternal health consultations
Area health offices	Public health dentistry
Tuberculosis control	Sanitation inspection and supervision
Venereal disease control	Vital records (births and deaths)
Public health nursing service	Industrial health services
Public health social services	Public health education
Public health nutrition services	Air pollution control
Child health consultations	School health services

Private health-insurance programs

The several widespread forms of private health insurance currently available are based upon the idea that individuals cannot successfully budget against the potential costs of illness. The best hope for protection, then, lies in large numbers of persons' pooling the risks through health plans so as to spread both the chances and the costs. Insurance companies sell these health plans through employee groups, professional organizations, and individual subscriptions.

Kinds of subscription The most reasonable premium rates have been gained through the formation of groups of subscribers. Group plans are available only through an employer. Typically, only one type of plan is available, with a set, group-wide premium charge for each subscriber with the same contract (with some differences, depending upon the size of the family of the subscriber). An individual, nongroup subscription frequently will cost more than a comparable group policy or will provide fewer benefits. More than 75 percent of the people covered by health insurance today belong to group plans, according to the Health Insurance Institute.

Types of benefit In terms of benefits, there are three general types of plan: service benefits (full payment), cash-indemnity benefits, and a combination of the two. The majority of subscribers are enrolled in combination plans.

The service plans are generally in the form of contracts between the policyholder and the hospital or physician. The hospital agrees to provide certain services upon presentation by the policyholder of his policy identification card. The hospital or physician then agrees to accept fee allowances under that plan as full or near-full payment for care rendered. After the service is rendered, a claim form is filled out and sent to the insurance company by the hospital or physician. Reimbursement is then made directly to the hospital or physician, according to the provisions of the policy.

The cash-indemnity plans pay benefits in the form of cash to the policyholder. He is reimbursed for the medical costs he has incurred or paid. The patient is usually required to present either a physician's or hospital statement showing the exact amount due or a receipt for payment already made.

Types of insurer   There are many types of health insurance available today. Several main examples will be discussed here.

· BLUE CROSS   Blue Cross is a nonprofit operation with more than 75 million members. This is more than 36 percent of the population, or one out of every three. Of Blue Cross members, 88 percent are served through group subscriptions. Through seventy-five plans in the United States the organization insures members against costs of hospital care, physicians' services, drugs, and laboratory tests. Each plan is independently governed by a local board made up of community, hospital, and medical leaders. Blue Cross is officially endorsed by the American Hospital Association.

Owing to the number of Blue Cross plans across the country, it is difficult to describe a typical plan. Each plan is a separate, regional, autonomous organization under the national name of Blue Cross. Each plan sets its own policies, rates, and benefits, and makes its own contracts with hospitals in its territory. Each Blue Cross organization reserves the right to contract only with those hospitals meeting its standards of acceptability. Consequently, not all hospitals are eligible to receive Blue Cross payments.

Types of coverage range from several weeks to a full year of hospital service. The most widely sold policies cover the partial or complete cost of 30 days of hospital care. Other plans also cover services of physicians, anesthetists, x-ray diagnosis and therapy, drugs, and laboratory tests. Most plans offer *extended benefits*, which may include dental care and nursing, and coverage in the event of a long siege of illness. Hospital claims under the Blue Cross plans are paid directly to the contracting hospital; physicians' claims may be paid first to the subscriber, who then pays the physician.

· BLUE SHIELD   Set up along the same general lines as Blue Cross, these nonprofit physicians' plans today have more than 66 million subscribers through 71 different plans. Organized in 1946 and endorsed by the American Hospital Association, Blue Shield plans are designed to provide prepaid coverage for physicians' services and at the same time help to assure physicians the collection of their fees. Payment of claims is based either on a *set amount* for the service or on what is a *usual* fee for that locality. The Blue Shield schedule of rates is completely covered according to the payment schedule. If the family income is over this set level, the plan covers only a percentage of the physicians' charges.

Blue Shield is available in most states. Certain other physicians' insurance plans are available in individual states, such as the California Physicians' Service plan in California.

· COMMERCIAL   Today the majority of the hospital and surgical policies are being written by commercial insurance companies; see Fig. 13.6. Although their coverage is similar to that of Blue Cross and Blue Shield, the approach of the insurance companies is often different. Their plans are of the cash-indemnity type or a combination of the service benefits and cash-indemnity benefits. The commercial insurance company in no way engages in contracts with hospitals or physicians and, consequently, does not seek to control the quality of medical services rendered to their policyholders. These plans sometimes involve deductibles and coinsurance features and often offer a wide variety of plans that can be tailor-made to the wishes of the individual applicant.

Commercial companies have led the way into other forms of health insurance:

Major medical. These plans are designed to give large amounts of coverage for major expenses. They are not designed to pay for the expenses the insured can easily pay out of his own pocket or which can be covered by the regular type of hospital, surgical, and medical contract. Consequently, major-medical plans usually contain a deductible of $100 to $500. The policyholder is expected to pay this amount himself or with a regular type of policy. In addition, a coinsurance feature provides that the insured himself must bear the cost of 20 to 25 percent of the expenses above the deductible amount, and the insurance company pays the other 75 to 80 percent. Major-medical plans cover expenses resulting from both accidents and sickness.

Comprehensive plans. Comprehensive contracts are newer than major-medical plans. Contracts of this type are designed to provide regular (basic) medical care plus major-medical coverage. In other words, they are a basic and a major-medical plan combined into a single policy. Available on either an individual or a group basis, they are designed to combine the best features of the other two types of policy.

• INDEPENDENTS   The "independent" insurance plans are, generally, the three hundred smaller local plans that do not fit any of the previous categories. They have been organized by labor unions, corporate managements, physicians, and laymen. Most of them have their own staffs of salaried physicians,

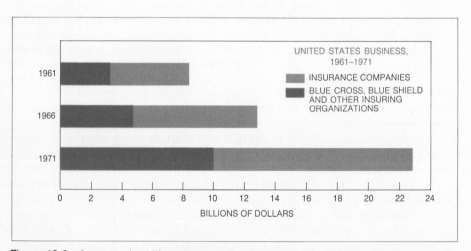

Figure 13.6   Increase in dollars spent on health insurance premiums according to type of insurer for the period 1961 to 1971. (From Health Insurance Institute; U.S. Department of Health, Education and Welfare; and *Health Insurance Review.*)

some their own hospitals, and many their own clinics. Their main emphasis is placed on diagnostic services and on care outside the hospitals. Examples are the Health Insurance Plan of Greater New York, Group Health Insurance of New York, Kaiser Foundation Health Plan, and the Community Health Association of Detroit. Not uncommonly, the patients must use a staff physician under these plans and may not bring a nonstaff physician in from the outside. Plans lacking their own hospitals have agreements with existing hospitals for service to their members. Although the independents are generally local, many are large organizations. New York State and California have a number of such plans. Nevertheless, their growth has been relatively slow in relation to the growth of other health-insurance plans.

· DENTAL PLANS   A fairly recent development in health insurance is that of plans providing benefits for dental care. In the past ordinary dental care has usually been excluded from health-care plans except as a necessary provision in accident insurance. The rates depend upon the type of coverage provided and the makeup of the particular group. Most coverage provides a limited amount of care, the patient paying a portion of the cost. These plans are set up to cover necessary procedures for a sound, healthy mouth. Usually excluded are dental services not deemed necessary for normal chewing.

A complete listing of plans can be found in the *Directory of Prepaid Dental Care Plans,* U.S. Department of Health, Education, and Welfare, Public Health Service, Bethesda, Maryland 20014.

PURCHASING AND REVIEWING HEALTH INSURANCE

The sale of hospital, health, and accident insurance is too serious a matter to become a battle of wits between buyer and seller. Buyers can be misled as much by the omission of facts as by the deliberate distortion of facts; they also may be presented with so many facts that truths become lost. Quite often the buyer can unwittingly put himself in a position where he has only limited legal action if his claim is disputed.

Provisions to look for when purchasing health insurance

Overall, a person should determine, first, the type of health-care expenses he desires to be protected against and, second, the extent (proportion) to which he wishes these expenses insured.

Types of health-care expenses   There are three general types of health-care expense: *hospital expenses, professional services* (those performed by physicians licensed to practice medicine), and *paramedical services* (laboratory, x-ray, nursing, and so forth). The first two lend themselves more readily to the principles of insurance.

Extent of coverage Purchasers should consider the extent or proportion of medical expenses they want to have insured:

1. Total probable costs.
2. The portion of the total costs.
3. The category of these costs.

A person should have some idea of what health-care expenses amount to. It is wise to look into and determine the following:

1. The prevailing hospitalization costs in the community.
2. The kinds of hospital service preferred (private, semiprivate, or ward).
3. Professional costs—information on a physician's charges can be obtained by discussing the matter with the physician himself or with a local medical society office.

Underwriting organization (insuring company) Some questions to find answers for are these:

1. Is the company or prepayment plan licensed to do business in your state?
2. What is the general reputation of the organization in fulfilling its obligations to its policyholders?
3. Is there a claims-paying office located either in your state or otherwise reasonably near?
4. Does this company or its agent, or both, have a good reputation in your community?

Contract provisions Contracts involve both privileges (benefits) and obligations. It is one's responsibility to read and understand a contract *before signing it*. In particular look for the following items:

· INSURING CLAUSE Know the scope of coverage (be sure it contains types of benefit you desire).

· EXCLUSIONS, OR CONDITIONS NOT COVERED Most policies have some exclusions (the amount of the premium is determined largely by the number and nature of the exclusions). Most insurance companies will exclude some of the following:

1. Plastic or cosmetic surgery.
2. Elective surgery (that which can be done at the patient's convenience). In some policies this is covered 6 months or so from the date of the purchase of the policy.
3. Occupational illnesses and accidents covered by workmen's compensation.
4. Conditions resulting from acts of war or riot (including injuries and illnesses sustained in the armed forces).
5. Preexisting illnesses.
6. Dental care and operations.

· WAITING PERIODS This involves the time interval between issuance of a contract and the date certain benefits are payable. Examples would be maternity benefits, elective surgery, or preexisting illnesses. These provisions are included because an insurance company usually agrees to cover only those conditions that commence after the insurance is written.

· BENEFIT REDUCTIONS   This means reducing benefits below the amount otherwise payable (for example, if the hospital has no contract with this company, or if a physician is nonparticipating).

· WHO IS COVERED   This usually includes spouse and unmarried dependent children and usually *only the names specified in the policy*.

· AGE LIMITS   Some policies specify minimal and maximal age limits (most policies will cover a dependent child for only so many years).

· CANCELLATION AND RENEWAL PROVISIONS   Many policies are cancellable by the insuring company; some policies state that the company can elect not to renew the policy at any premium due date; some policies are *both* noncancellable and guaranteed renewable to a specified age (these commonly are more expensive, but they are a better type of insurance).

· IS CHOICE OF A PHYSICIAN OR HOSPITAL LIMITED?   This should be clearly understood. For example, what happens in case of travel or employment out of a home area, when a medical emergency makes it impossible to get to a designated physician or hospital?

By keeping these points in mind one should be able to make a wise selection of health coverages that best suit family needs. Further questions should be addressed to one's insurance counselor, the local Blue Cross or Blue Shield representative, the union office, or another source in which confidence can be placed.

Clarification of terms used in policy

The buyer should go over the entire contract word by word whenever he purchases any form of health insurance or income-protection insurance. He must rely mainly upon the reputation of the individual agent and the company issuing the policy.

If there are statements or definitions that are not completely clear to the buyer, he may ask the insurance company for a letter of clarification; the buyer may write out all terms that are not completely clear to him, mail this to the main office of the insuring company, and request them to return to him the official definitions of these terms. Upon receipt of the reply, he should study it very carefully, and if the definitions are acceptable, then—and only then—sign the contract for the insurance. When he receives his copy of the insurance policy, he should clip his letter of clarification onto the policy. Whenever presented with a claim, the insurance company is legally bound to the definitions they have set down.

Advice from a physician or hospital

It is also advisable to ask a personal physician his reactions to a specific medical plan. It is a good idea to contact the hospital in the area to see whether the amounts payable for specific hospital care are adequate to pay for at least 80 percent of their charges.

Periodic review of a prepayment plan

At certain times a person should take time out to review his health-insurance coverage. (1) During a three-year period changes may occur in income, the relative needs of a family, and possibly even the number in a family. For this reason it is wise to review every three years. (2) Every time a person changes his employment he should review his insurance coverage, because he may lose certain types of coverage with one employer and receive new coverage with another employer. (3) Whenever there is a change in residence, he should review his insurance to bring his address up to date. Many policies are issued in a specific area and are not in force when the individual leaves this specific area. (4) Whenever a family's situation changes—as by divorce, death, or birth—the insured should review his insurance policy to be sure of exact coverage.

During these periods the insured should write down the following information as a guide to the information he is looking for: any facts that will help determine the coverage he needs (auto coverage, life insurance, health, and so on); how large a premium he can afford with his current income (for example, can he afford coverage against catastrophic illness and events?). With this information, he must also take into account facilities and services available through the state and federal agencies. He should also determine whether he would qualify for such aid if it were needed. Next, what demands income protection—car, home, school, food, clothing, and so on. Then he should write out the coverage that he has through sick leave, disability benefits, workmen's compensation, and any insurance provided through his employer. He should note any discrepancies that can be eliminated and take action.

Regardless of *how* a family provides for its health care, there can be no question that such care must be available. The human life has a clear value which, to some extent, can be guaranteed through a reliable insurance program. Since the great majority of people depend upon their ability to work and thereby to earn money, the protection of their lives from physical disability will be one of their most important assets. A family *must* be protected in its ability to earn money as well as against unnecessary loss of money owing to medical and hospital costs.

SUMMARY

    I. Modern medicine
      A. Aims
        1. Good health care must be available to all people.
        2. Prevention of disease must be given top attention.
        3. The needs of the whole man must be ministered to.
        4. Research into unconquered diseases and better methods of treatment must continue to be pursued.

B. Problems
   1. Shortage of physicians.
   2. Rapidity of change in medical knowledge and technology.
   3. Rise in medical costs.
C. Changes in the medical profession
   1. Deemphasis of narrow specialties and reemphasis of general medicine.
   2. The belief that more people must be covered by health insurance.
   3. Increased use of group practices, clinics, and outpatient departments of general hospitals.
II. Choosing a physician—involves choosing a satisfactory medical adviser and knowing the facts regarding his training and background.
   A. Has he obtained the requirements to practice?
   B. Family physician
      1. General practitioner, or GP—practices general medicine, either by choice or because he lacks training in one of the specialties.
      2. General internist—a specialist who confines himself primarily to diagnosis and will, if necessary, refer a patient to other specialists.
   C. The specialties
      1. Internal medicine—diagnosing internal ailments and treating them with medicine if advisable.
      2. Obstetrics and gynecology—care of women in pregnancy and child-birth and care of women's ailments.
      3. Pediatrics—care of infants and children.
      4. Surgery—operating for unwanted conditions.
      5. Psychiatry—treating emotional illnesses and disturbances.
      6. Anesthesiology—administering general and local anesthesia.
      7. Neurology—treating brain and nervous-system diseases.
      8. Ophthalmology—treating the eye and its diseases.
      9. Pathology—identifying structural changes and diseases.
      10. Urology—dealing with diseases of the urogenital tracts.
   D. Osteopathy
      1. Originally considered diseases due to nerve malconditions.
      2. Present training and practice generally based on sound medical principles.
      3. Serves satisfactorily as a family physician.
   E. Types of practice
      1. The past favored the independent, single-man office.
      2. Has moved toward group or clinical practice.
   F. Selecting the right physician—depends upon one's personal needs and preferences.
   G. The patient-physician relationship should:
      1. Be reasonable for both.
      2. Respect a physician's professional advice.
      3. Begin with a patient contact before an emergency arises.
      4. Include satisfaction with fees charged and payments made.
III. Allied health professions—include medical services which help the physician to provide complete medical care; they include the following professions.
   A. Dentistry
      1. Treats abnormalities of the gums and teeth and attempts to prevent their recurrence.

    2. Includes the following branches of practice:
      a. general practice—general dental care.
      b. orthodontia—straightening of teeth.
      c. oral surgery—extracting of teeth and surgical procedures.
      d. pedodontia—children's dentistry.
      e. periodontia—treatment of tissues that support the teeth.
      f. prosthodontics—art of making artificial teeth and dentures.
      g. oral pathology—treatment of diseases of the mouth.

B. Nursing—done by a team led by the professional or registered nurse (R.N.).
    1. Vocational nurse.
    2. Nursing aide.
    3. Orderly.
    4. Attendant.

C. Medical technology—involves performing laboratory tests under the supervision of a pathologist.

D. Pharmacy—involves making general drugs and medical supplies available for sale and dispensing prescriptions ordered by a medical practitioner.

E. Physical therapy—aids the rehabilitation of people with injuries or diseases affecting muscles, joints, and bones.

F. Optometry—involves testing the refractive ability of the eyes, determining any deviation from normal, and prescribing lenses to provide correction without use of drugs or surgery.

G. Podiatry (chiropody)—treats diseases and deformities of the feet and correction and prevention of foot problems.

H. Chiropractic—a system of treatment based on the belief that the nervous system determines a person's state of health and that physical impairments are basically related to the nervous system.

IV. Facilities for patient care

A. Clinics and nursing homes supplement the services of hospitals.

B. Hospitals provide complete medical facilities for the acutely ill patient.
    1. Kinds of hospitals grouped according to their type of ownership and administration:
      a. government hospitals—may be federal, state, city or county.
      b. voluntary hospitals—public hospitals operating on a nonprofit basis, governed by a board of community leaders.
      c. proprietary hospitals—owned and administered by individuals or corporations and are set up as profit-seeking investments.

C. Accreditation of hospitals determined by the hospital's meeting the standards of excellence set by the Joint Commission on Accreditation of Hospitals (JCAH).

D. Choice of hospital
    1. Is the hospital accredited (by the JCAH)?
    2. Is it a teaching hospital?
    3. Who owns the hospital?

E. Decisions before hospitalization
    1. Whether hospital admission is required.
    2. Whether the needed care could be provided just as well in a clinic or nursing home.

      3. Whether a private or semiprivate room is required or desired.

      4. How the cost of services provided is to be paid.

V. Financing health care—people expect far better health care today than in the past; more complex health care has boosted health costs.

  A. Health care costly

  B. Health insurance

    1. Public (tax-supported) health services.

    2. Private (voluntary, prepaid) health insurance.

  C. Public health care

    1. Care of the poor (indigent).

    2. Medicare:

      a. basic benefits—covering primarily hospital care.

      b. supplemental benefits—covering primarily the physician's care.

    3. Aid to veterans.

    4. Aid to military dependents.

    5. Special groups (general government medical care).

    6. Special diseases.

    7. Communicable diseases.

    8. Crippled children.

    9. Crippled adults.

    10. General hospital care.

    11. Local or county health departments.

  D. Private health-insurance programs

    1. Kinds of subscriptions:

      a. group plans—set up by employer in a given firm.

      b. individual (nongroup) plans—set up for each person or family.

    2. Types of benefits

      a. service (full payments)—contract between policyholder and hospital or physician.

      b. cash indemnity—pay cash benefits to the policyholder.

      c. combination of service and cash-indemnity policies.

    3. Types of insurer:

      a. Blue Cross—nonprofit policy for hospitalization.

      b. Blue Shield—nonprofit policy for physician's services.

      c. commercial—usually provides cash-indemnity benefits, engages in no service contracts with hospitals or physicians; common coverage includes major medical and comprehensive plans.

      d. independents—set up by special groups to provide for prepaid medical service from hospitals, clinics, nurses, and physicians.

      e. dental—provides a limited amount of care, patients paying portion of the costs.

VI. Purchasing health insurance

  A. Provisions to look for

    1. Types of health care expenses—hospital, physician, paramedical.

    2. Extent of coverage.

    3. Underwriting organization (insuring company).

    4. Contract provisions:

      a. insuring clause.

      b. exclusions.

      c. waiting periods.

      d. benefit reductions.

      e. who is covered.

      f. age limits.

      g. cancellation and renewal provisions.

      h. limits on choice of physician or hospital.

  B. Clarification of terms used in policy—should be obtained in writing from the insuring company before the contract is signed.

  C. Advice from a physician or hospital should be sought before the contract is signed.

  D. Periodic review of a prepayment plan

    1. Changing needs of a family insurance program should be reviewed:

      a. every three years.

      b. with every change in employment.

      c. with every change in residence.

      d. with every change in family situation.

    2. Guideline for future purchases should include:

      a. what facilities and services are already provided through public facilities and workmen's compensation.

      b. amount of coverage needed.

      c. extent of a person's present commitment for essential items.

      d. how large a periodic premium can be afforded.

Glossary

If you cannot find the word you wish in this glossary, check the index for text and glossary references.

anesthesiology (an əs thē zē ol'ə jē) (G. *an,* without; *aisthesis,* sensation). The science of anesthesia (the partial or complete loss of sensation with or without loss of consciousness resulting from the administration of drugs).

cash-indemnity benefit. A cash benefit paid by a health insurance policy to a policyholder for an insured loss.

chiropodist (kī rop'ə dist) (G. *cheir,* hand; *pous,* foot). A person who specializes in the minor disorders and care of the human foot; see *podiatry.*

chiropractic (kī'rə prak'tik) (G. *cheir,* hand; *pratein,* to do). A system of therapy based upon the claim that disease is caused by abnormal function of the nervous system.

coinsurance. A policy provision, often found in major-medical insurance, by which the insured person and the insurance company in a specific ratio share the hospital and medical expenses resulting from an illness or injury.

collective financing. The financing of medical expenses through the prepayment of fees, either through public taxes or through a private insurance plan.

deductible. That portion of covered hospital and medical charges which an insured person must pay before his policy's benefits begin.

dentistry (den'tis trē) (L. *dens,* tooth). That branch of health services dealing with the care of the teeth and related structures, as practiced by the dentist.

dermatology (dur mə tol'ə jē) (G. *derma,* skin; *logos,* understanding). The branch of medicine dealing with diagnosis and treatment of diseases of the skin.

diplomate (dip'lə māt) (G. *diploos,* double; L. *atus,* to become). A holder of a certificate of the National Board of Medical Examiners or of one of the American Boards in the specialties.

disability. A physical condition that makes an insured person incapable of doing one or more duties of his occupation.

exclusion. A specific hazard for which a policy will not provide benefit payments.

extended benefit. Coverage providing benefits for extended medical care due to severe injury or prolonged sickness, usually in addition to basic coverage for short-term medical care.

general practitioner (prak tish′ə nər) (G. *praktike*, business). One who practices the general, usually unrestricted, profession of medicine.

government hospital (hos′pi təl) (L. *hospitalis*, pertaining to a guest). A hospital which is owned and operated by some level of government: federal, state, or city.

guaranteed renewable. A policy which the insured has a right to continue in force by the timely payment of premiums to a specified age, during which period the insured has no right, on his own, to make any change in any provision of the policy while it is in force.

gynecology (gī′nə kol′ə jē) (G. *gyne*, women). The study of the diseases of the female, particularly of the genital, urinary, and rectal organs.

indigent (in′di jənt) (L. *indu*, in; *egere*, to need). Poor or needy.

individual financing. The financing of medical expenses without the benefit of any prepayment or insurance plan, either on a pay-as-you-go basis or by budgeting for expected expenses.

internal medicine (in tur′nəl med′i sin) (L. *internus*, within). That department of medicine which deals with diseases that cannot be treated surgically.

internist (in′tur nist, in tur′nist) (L. *internus*, within). One who treats internal organs and diseases (not a surgeon) and who frequently confines his practice to adults.

medical technology (med′i kəl tek nol′ə jē) (L. *medicus*, physician; G. *techne*, art). The practice of medical laboratory procedures.

National Board Examination. A national examination in the medical, dental, or paramedical professions given by Board of Examiners from that particular profession which, if passed, qualifies a person to practice in that profession. Certain states require a state examination to be passed in the profession before one is entitled to practice in that state.

neurology (nyoo rol′ə jē) (G. *neuron*, nerve). That branch of medicine dealing with the nervous system and its diseases.

obstetrics (əb stet′riks) (L. *obstetrix*, midwife). That branch of medicine which deals with the care and treatment of women during pregnancy, childbirth, and the period immediately after.

oculist (ok′yə list) (L. *oculus*, eye). A physician specializing in the treatment of diseases of the eye; also called an *ophthalmologist*.

ophthalmology (of thal mol′ə jē) (G. *ophthalmos*, eye; *logos*, study). The branch of medicine dealing with the eye and its diseases.

optician (op tish′ ən) (G. *optikos*, pertaining to the eye). A person who makes or sells eyeglasses and other optical instruments.

optometry (op tom′ə trē) (G. *optos*, seen; *metron*, measure). The profession of testing the refractive powers of the eye and fitting lenses to correct eye defects.

oral pathology (or′əl pa thol′ə jē) (L. *os, or*, mouth; G. *pathos*, disease). The branch of dentistry treating the nature of diseases of the teeth. Also known as *dental pathology*.

oral surgery (or′əl sur′jə rē) (ME. *surgerie* from G. *cheirourgia*, handwork). The branch of dentistry which treats conditions of the mouth and associated structures, especially the teeth and jaws, by surgical methods.

osteopathy (os tē op'ə thē) (G. *osteon*, bone; *pathos*, disease). A system of treating ailments originally based on the belief that they generally result from the pressure of displaced bones on nerves and are cured by manipulation.

otorhinolaryngology (ō'tō rī'nō lar ing gol'ə jē) (G. *otos*, ear; *rhis*, nose; *larynx*, larynx). The branch of medicine dealing with the ear, nose, and larynx and their functions and diseases.

paramedical (par ə med'i kal) (G. *para*, beyond; L. *medicari*, to heal). Having a medical aspect or a secondary relation to medicine.

pathology (pa thol'ə jē). That branch of medicine dealing with the nature of disease, especially the structural and functional changes caused by disease.

pediatrics (pē dē at'riks) (G. *paidos*, child; *iatreia*, cure). The branch of medicine concerned with the development and care of children and the diseases of children and their treatment.

pedodontia (pē də don'shə) (G. *paidos*, child; *odous*, tooth). The branch of dentistry which deals with the teeth and mouth conditions of children.

periodontia (per'ē ə don'shə) (G. *peri*, around; *odous*, tooth). The branch of dentistry dealing with the study and treatment of diseases occurring around the tooth.

pharmacy (fahr'mə sē) (G. *pharmakon*, medicine). The profession which prepares and dispenses drugs and medicines.

physical therapy (fiz'i kəl ther'əpē) (G. *physikos*, natural; *therapein*, treatment). The treatment of disease by physical means (nonmedical).

physician (fi zish'ən) (Fr. *physicien* from G. *physikos*, natural). A person authorized by law to practice medicine.

podiatry (pō dī'ə trē) (G. *pous*, foot; *iatreia*, cure). The diagnosis and treatment of disorders of the foot. See *chiropodist*.

preexisting condition. A physical condition of an insured person which existed prior to the issuance of his policy.

proprietary hospital (prō prī'ə ta rē) (L. *proprietarius*, pertaining to property). A hospital owned and operated by private individuals or corporations as profit-seeking investments.

prosthodontics (pros tho don'tiks) (G. *prosthesis*, "a putting to"; *odous*, tooth). The branch of dentistry dealing with the mechanics of making and fitting dental appliances and substitutes.

psychiatry (sī kī'ə trē) (G. *psyche*, soul; *iatreia*, healing). That branch of medicine which deals with the diagnosis, treatment, and prevention of emotional illness.

radiology (rā dē ol'ə jē) (L. *radius*, ray). The branch of medicine which deals with roentgen rays and other radiant energy in the diagnosis and treatment of disease.

registered nurse (rej'īs tard nurs) (L. *regere*, to record; *nutrix*, a nurse). A graduate nurse who has been registered and licensed to practice by a State Board of Nursing Examiners or other state authority.

service benefits. A contract benefit which is paid directly to the provider of hospital or medical care for services rendered.

specialist (spesh'ə list) (L. *specialist*, special). A practitioner who restricts himself to a special type of disease.

State Board Examination. A state examination in the medical, dental, or paramedical professions given by a State Board of Examiners from that particular profession, which, if passed, qualifies a person to practice that profession in that particular state. See *National Board Examination*.

surgery (sur'jə rē) (ME. *surgerie*, from G. *cheirourgia*, handwork). The branch of medicine which treats diseases, partially or completely, by manual and operative procedures.

urinalysis (yoo ri nal'i sis) (L. *urina,* urine; G. *ana,* apart; *lysis,* a loosening). Chemical or microscopic analysis of the urine.

urology (yoo rol'ǝ jē). That branch of medicine dealing with the urine and urinary tract; includes the genitourinary tract in males.

voluntary hospital (L. *voluntas,* will; *hospitalis,* pertaining to a guest). A public hospital owned and operated on a nonprofit basis.

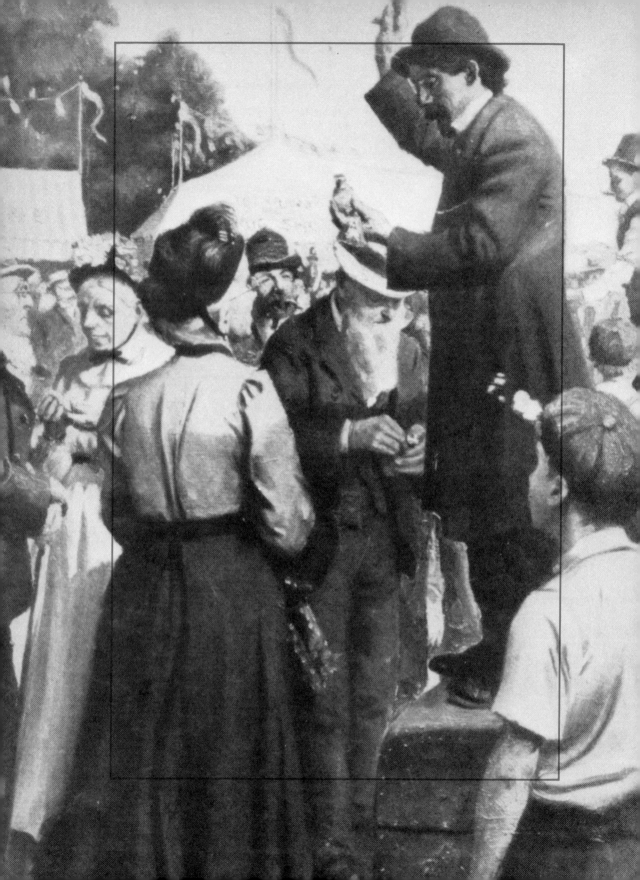

Quackery

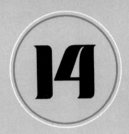

Although the colorful "snake oil" salesman with his medicine show is a thing of the past, his counterpart is still very much on the scene. Today's quack is much more sophisticated than his predecessor, but his goal remains the same—to separate the unsuspecting from their money. Regardless of how sincere his interest in a person's health may seem, his real interest is financial. Today over two billion dollars a year are spent in the United States for worthless or fraudulent remedies. Although much of today's quackery involves a direct "doctor"-patient relationship, a still larger field is promotion through the mail and in drug and "health food" stores of various patent medicines and remedies of questionable value.

WHO IS A QUACK?

A *quack* may be defined as a boastful pretender to medical skill or one who promises health benefits that he cannot deliver. He may attempt to go beyond the limits of medical science or to exceed the limits of his own training. The quack often sells or treats patients with a *nostrum*, a cure-all drug or machine (any drug, machine, or treatment for which broad, sweeping claims are made may be called a nostrum).

A common stereotype of a quack is probably that of an odd or sinister-looking individual. On the contrary, the real quack usually inspires confidence. Quacks possess varying types of educational background. A few licensed physicians enter into quackery, sometimes authoring books which have great sales success. More commonly a quack may have chiropractic or naturopathic training or no professional training. There also exists today a certain amount of "corporate quackery," where proprietary compounds ("patent medicines") are sometimes overzealously promoted by advertising departments. Any individual may enter into quackery if he attempts to diagnose and treat a serious illness by himself, for *self-treatment is quackery.*

WHY PEOPLE TURN TO QUACKERY

Fear, ignorance, and gullibility

Much quackery preys upon fear. There are those who have a constant fear of imminent ill health. As preventives they use special diets, exercise routines, gadgetry, or even subscribe to mystical philosophies or alleged religions. Others are actually threatened with death. Such a person, told by his physician that he has an incurable disease, lives in fear—fear of death, fear of pain, fear of the unknown. He may always have followed good health practices yet, in the moment of desperation grasps at any hope offered, regardless of how unscientific or expensive it may be. Sometimes fear keeps a person from seeing an ethical physician in the first place.

The quack need not confess that his treatment may not work—to him integrity is not essential. Stock in trade for him is to oversimplify. More important, he pays more attention to the person than to the ailment. Since he can't provide a cure, if disease is present, he's generous in promises, sympathy, and compassion. Oddly enough, patients often remain loyal to the quack even though his promises have failed.

Quackery is the legitimate offspring of ignorance. Gullibility, especially in combination with ignorance, is the chief ally of the quack. A segment of the American public is almost unbelievably gullible. When ill, a person may either seek help or depend upon self-treatment. If he chooses self-treatment, he probably will use some folk remedy, such as garlic, or some recent innovation, such as huge doses of vitamin C. He judges all results in the same way: Did it work? Did his nerves calm down? Did his head clear up? Did his indigestion disappear? If so, quackery has another new convert. He fails to realize two common observations in medicine: symptoms often disappear by themselves (treatment or no), and the taking of *anything* (even a placebo, the useless "sugar pill") is a great psychological force toward improvement. A definition of effectiveness may cover not only physical but also psychological factors. The U.S. Food and Drug Administration says of sedatives, "they are easily open to exploitation, since 30 to 70 percent of any group of persons tested will experience relief of anxiety when given a placebo and told it will be effective."

Teenager to senior citizen

Although no age group is immune to the quack, the teenager and the senior citizen contribute significantly to his support. The teenager is particularly receptive to mail-order quackery. He finds in some of the magazines many deceptive advertisements that appeal to his age group and may receive many direct-mail advertisements, since his name is often sold for "sucker lists." Since the teenager is often very self-conscious about his appearance, most of the products offered promise good looks, sex appeal, and popularity. Some of the current offerings include products to add weight, take off weight, build muscles, and add to the bust line. Other popular products offer more attractive skin or hair.

The senior citizen finds appeal in products that promise to renew lost youth and vigor. He is often duped in schemes to relieve arthritis, impotence, prostate conditions, colitis, and "tired blood." The nutrition quack finds a ready market in elderly people who are eager to believe that all their aches and pains can disappear through the use of a food supplement. In addition, the elderly are attracted to so-called "clinics," "health ranches," and "hospitals" which claim cures for all types of chronic disease through chiropractic, diet, and other limited measures. Such places offer the hope of a quick, easy, painless treatment, usually provided by practitioners who are not licensed physicians.

SOME MAJOR TYPES OF HEALTH QUACKERY TODAY

Cancer quackery

Cancer quacks are estimated to make about $50 million a year for worthless treatments. Although some of their methods have repeatedly been exposed as quackery by agencies of the United States Government, these charlatans continue to prosper. Cancer quackery can be one of the most tragic of rackets when a person having an early cancer spends vital time waiting for a worthless remedy to cure his cancer. In too many such cases the cancers reach an incurable stage before the victims seek ethical treatment, although early treatment by an ethical physician using standard methods might have resulted in a complete cure.

The strongest ally of the cancer quack is many people's fear of surgery. The quack always offers treatment without surgery, but the ethical physician knows that surgery is the most positive treatment for most types of cancer.

The quack is very successful in treating cancers that never existed and thereby gains some of his most solid supporters. The patient who believes he may have cancer, not having seen an ethical physician, will almost always have his suspicions confirmed by the quack. After a series of expensive treatments the quack will pronounce the nonexistent cancer cured. The patient is then forever grateful to the quack for having saved his life and is eager to write letters of testimonial, picket the state capitol, testify in court, or do whatever will aid the quack in his running battle with the authorities.

Arthritis quackery

The word *arthritis* is a general term used to indicate an inflammation of the joints. About twelve million Americans suffer from this painful, crippling condition. The ethical physician can offer a complete cure for very few of the many types of arthritis. Thus the door is wide open for one of the most lucrative fields of quackery. An estimated ten thousand arthritis quacks sell about a quarter of a billion dollars worth of useless drugs, devices, and treatments each year. Half of all arthritis sufferers try some of these worthless remedies.

The least offensive (though often extremely highly priced) of the arthritis remedies are the glorified aspirin products. At the other extreme are the dangerous drugs and the treatments that may actually be harmful. Since by their nature some types of arthritis tend to come and go, a worthless treatment is often given credit for curing arthritis, when actually the symptoms would have disappeared even if nothing had been done. As with every other disease, the ethical physician can still be relied upon to offer the most effective, up-to-date treatment.

Reducing without dieting

There is always a ready market for any treatment that promises weight loss without unpleasant diets. Since one out of every four Americans attempts to lose weight each year, any device offered is sure to find acceptance among some of these fifty million people. Some of the most common schemes are as follows:

Reducing pills are sold by mail or over the counter without prescription. Such pills, if strong enough to be effective, should be used only under medical supervision.

Dietless reducing plans are of every description. Many plans, although advertised as dietless, actually do involve a strict diet, which must be followed if any weight is to be lost.

Vibrators are supposed to remove fat mechanically. It is impossible to vibrate weight away.

Massaging devices are like the vibrators: weight cannot be massaged off.

Spot reducing claims to remove fat only from certain parts of the body, as the person wishes. It is absolutely impossible to control from which part of the body fat is lost.

Reducing creams obviously are worthless, yet their sales are brisk.

This is but a sampling of the many approaches available to the person who is looking for an "easy" way to lose weight. Some of the plans promoted are worthless but harmless; other can be actually dangerous.

Food fads

Today *fifteen million Americans* are living in the shadow of confusion cast by the food faddists and "health food" quacks. These unfortunate people find themselves following expensive, complicated, and often unpleasant diets; instead of being better fed, they are actually more likely to be suffering a nutritional deficiency than those who eat ordinary diets following simple rules of basic nutrition.

In addition to their sale in health food stores, health food products and food supplements are commonly promoted in two other ways. One method is door-to-door selling, in which the salesman takes advantage of the privacy of the home to prescribe his expensive food supplement as a remedy for any disease or condition the resident may mention. The other widespread approach is "health food" or "nutrition" lectures. The lecturer, posing as a highly qualified scientist, gives an emotionally appealing presentation of a mixture of scientific fact and superstition concerning nutrition, never failing to mention repeatedly whatever product he happens to be pushing. What appears to be science is in reality *pseudoscience*, with lectures and slick-paper brochures emphasizing half-truths, quarter-truths, and false implications.

Regardless of the sales approach used, the food quack makes use of scare tactics, basing his presentation on certain modern myths used by almost all operators in his field. Although each idea contains an element of truth, the conclusions drawn are not supported by scientific evidence. Some of the common misrepresentations are described below:

Myth that all diseases are due to faulty diet. There is absolutely no basis in such a claim.

Myth of the indispensable food product. Promoters often represent their products as being the *only* source of a vital food substance. Every substance known to be important in nutrition is available from a variety of common grocery-store foods. The promoter often counters this fact with the implication that his product contains a substance not yet known to science. Of course, there is absolutely no basis in such a claim.

Myth that soil depletion causes malnutrition. A common story is that repeated cropping of the land has removed some substance, which is therefore lacking from the foods produced. The only substance of which a deficiency in the soil is reflected in the crop produced is iodine. Since people today obtain adequate iodine through diet and the use of iodized salt, iodine deficiency is rare. If any other mineral is lacking from the soil, this deficiency is reflected in a lowered *quantity* of produce, but the nutritional *quality* is not affected.

Myth of "organic" or "natural" foods. Two key words in the health food business today are "organic" and "natural." According to biological or chemical definition of the word *organic* (see a dictionary), all foods are organic. As to the word *natural*, the claim is often made that foods grown with commercial fertilizers are inferior to those grown with "natural" fertilizer (manure). The fallacy of this claim lies in the fact that a plant can absorb from the soil only certain simple inorganic nutrients and, if manure is used as fertilizer, before any absorption into the roots of the plant can take place, the compounds present must be broken down by bacteria into the same simple compounds present in commercial fertilizers.

A related claim is that the synthetically produced vitamins are inferior to naturally occurring vitamins. This statement usually is made by salesmen of high-priced food-supplement products to indicate the superiority of their products over lower priced ones. Actually, the man-made vitamins are chemically identical with the naturally occurring vitamins, are absorbed in the same manner, and function in the body in exactly the same way.

The very word *chemical* is often used in a derogatory manner by the salesman, who apparently does not know or chooses to ignore the fact that all food is nothing but a mixture of chemicals. He deplores the use of chemical food additives such as antioxidants, coloring agents, mold inhibitors, and numerous other additives important to modern food processing. Since the 1958 amendment to the Federal Food and Drug Law such chemicals are thoroughly screened by their manufacturers for any possible harmful effect, before the Federal Food and Drug Administration permits their use in foods. Although some are dangerous in large dosages, in the amounts used, today's additives are perfectly safe. The food quack is apt to decry even the use of pasteurization, a process of indisputable value and importance for milk and certain other food products.

Myth of overprocessing. The food quack exaggerates the loss of food value through modern food-processing methods. Although some loss definitely does occur, the public today is much better fed than at any time in the past as a direct result of modern food technology. Highly nutritious processed fruits, vegetables, and meats are available throughout the year, not just during limited seasons. Today's processing methods are often less destructive to vitamins than were those of the past.

Beauty aids and baldness remedies

Human vanity provides a steady income for numerous beauty and baldness quacks and companies preparing "miracle" cosmetics. There is always something new in the beauty-cream business, often featuring such exotic ingredients as mink oil, orchid pollen, royal jelly, vitamins, and turtle oil. Excessively dry skin is definitely benefited by the use of a simple oil, lotion, or cream, but any effort to "nourish" the skin through the external application of vitamins or other substances is futile. Skin is nourished from within, and beautiful skin is usually the result of good diet, cleanliness, and general good health. Hormones *are* absorbed through the skin, but because of their possible side effects a person should consult a physician before using hormone skin creams.

Expensive baldness treatments are sold by mail through magazine and newspaper ads, and traveling baldness "clinics" often temporarily operate in hotels and motels. Although the baldness quacks sometimes include in their ads a brief statement that they cannot cure hereditary baldness, the implication is always left that they can cure *your* case of baldness. The person who is losing hair excessively should see a qualified dermatologist (M.D.), who can determine whether the baldness is of a type that can be treated. Baldness of an irregular, blotchy nature may be the result of some disease or local infection and may be treatable by the dermatologist. Certainly, the ethical dermatologist is able to offer every method of treatment available from the quack, along with many effective types of therapy the quack cannot use. If the baldness is of an incurable type, the dematologist will not hesitate to say so and will not administer a useless series of expensive treatments, as the quack often does. When progress is made in the prevention of hereditary baldness, the dermatologist will have the latest, most effective treatments.

Breast development

In our national obsession with female breasts some girls have come to feel sexually inadequate, unattractive, or self-conscious because of their small breasts. The size of the breasts is influenced by hormone levels and hereditary factors. The "girlie" magazines, movies, and other entertainment forms have contributed to an exaggerated concept of ideal breast size, since they feature those few girls with unusually large breast development.

Many schemes for breast development are offered to the "flat" girl. Unfortunately, most of them are ineffective and some are actually harmful. They are as follows:

Special exercises. Of all the plans offered, special exercises offer the most hope of a larger *appearing* bust line without danger. Exercises will *not* increase the size of the breast. Breasts consist of fatty tissue with the slightest bit of muscle beneath the nipple. The only hope for the most modest of breast enlargement would be to exercise the chest muscles underlying the breast, giving the appearance of greater breast development and improved posture. Regardless of the ads, breast massagers—manual or machine—will not increase the bra size "from 32A to 36D."

Special diets. Nothing beyond a normal, well-balanced diet can be eaten that will contribute to breast development.

Breast-development creams. No cream applied to the breasts could safely increase their size. If a product contains hormones, its use could be dangerous, unless one is under adequate medical supervision.

Silicone implants and injections. National magazines have given much publicity to silicones as a means of increasing breast size. Most medical authorities and the Food and Drug Administration strongly condemn this method of enlarging the breasts. The dangers inherent in these procedures are great and far outweigh any possible benefits.

The "flat" girl should realize that there is no relationship between breast size and sexual adequacy or femininity. Large breasts might be of value to a "topless" dancer, but they are of no particular value in everyday life. In fact, breast size does not even relate to the ability of a mother to nurse her baby. Thus a girl should accept her figure as it is and save her anxieties for more important problems.

Patent medicines

In a typical drugstore one is confronted with literally hundreds of highly advertised remedies for the common ailments of man. Although the products are commonly called *patent medicines,* a more correct name is *proprietary* compounds, since the formulas are seldom patentable. Most patent medicines are of little value and usually do not cause any direct harm. However, some do have potentially harmful effects if used to excess or by a physiologically sensitive person. Certain medicines that are normally harmless become very dangerous when used in combination with a particular physical condition. For example, usually harmless laxatives may be quite hazardous when taken by a person with appendicitis. Other products may produce so much drowsiness that driving a motor vehicle becomes hazardous.

A major problem with proprietary medicines occurs when their use replaces or delays a qualified physician's diagnosis and prompt treatment of a serious disease. The user then may suffer from *self-diagnosis* and treatment unsupported with adequate knowledge. It is all too familiar in many drug and health food stores to observe customers prescribing medicines for each other, often with the aid of "helpful," but medically untrained, clerks, when the symptoms they describe could easily indicate a very serious disease.

It is important that proprietary medicines be used only for minor symptoms and that their use be discontinued and a physician consulted if those symptoms do not disappear in a very few days.

Probably the most effective substance sold without a prescription is aspirin (acetylsalicylic acid), which today forms the basis for a myriad of proprietary compounds. The beneficial properties of aspirin, in addition to relief of pain, are that it reduces fever and inflammation. The "glorified aspirin" products—which usually contain aspirin, phenacetin, and caffeine, or just aspirin and caffeine—along with the buffered aspirin products, have been shown to be no more effective for most individuals than plain aspirin. Several products that originally contained phenacetin no longer do, since (in large doses) this agent has been shown to cause permanent kidney damage. Aspirin should be purchased in small quantities (about a three-month supply), because it breaks down in storage. The breakdown is indicated by a vinegary odor in the bottle, owing to the presence of acetic acid.

Of the more than $1 billion spent in the United States each year on nonprescription remedies about $350 million goes for aspirin and its products and another $350 million goes for cold remedies. Every year new "miracle" cold remedies are offered to the public with great fanfare from their manufacturers, only to drop quietly out of the picture a few years later, when the producer releases a newer "miracle." The fact remains that, despite the many advances in other areas of medicine, there is still no way to prevent or cure the common cold. Some of the products offered do provide some symptomatic relief, such as opening a stuffed nose, drying up nasal drip, and reducing fever, but the best advice for the early cold sufferer still is that he go to bed for twenty-four hours. This rest helps him avoid secondary infections and complications. The actual cold will last no longer than a week, but these secondary problems may last considerably longer. Antibiotics have no effect upon the actual cold, since antibiotics are not effective against viruses. Antibiotics should be reserved only for those cases in which secondary bacterial infections occur. The cold sufferer should not press his physician into prescribing antibiotics.

SOME SPECIFIC EXAMPLES OF QUACKERY

The following specific examples of quackery have been selected from recent issues of *FDA Papers*, an official publication of the Food and Drug Administration. They should serve to illustrate the types of fraud and deception to which the public is being subjected today.

Mail fraud

Given below are a few examples of mail fraud that were reported by the U.S. Post Office Department in the last few years (with dates of reports).

Advertising and sale by mail of "The Original Waist-Away Belt" to remove and eliminate fat deposits from the midsection of the wearer. (February 1972)

Solicitations of orders and sales through the mails of "Formula LDX-33," designated to nourish the sex organs and restore lost sexual interest, potency, or fertility. (March 1972)

Advertising and sale of products called "Frenchie's Make Them Hot Pills," "Frenchie's Whisky Pills," and "Frenchie's Spanish Fly Chewing Gum," represented to be effective as sex stimulants. (March 1972)

Firm advertised that "newest Grapefruit Super-C diet" enables subscribers to eat all they want while losing and retaining a substantial weight loss year after year. (September 1971)

Advertising and sale by mail of "Excit-X" liquid capsules, guaranteed in writing to induce sexual desire and represented as a true, safe aphrodisiac. (April 1971)

Advertising and sale by mail of "La Vive Body Creme," an alleged bust developer, purported to increase the size of, and give shapelier contours to, the breasts of female users. (November 1970)

Advertising and sale by mail of the "Paradise Grapefruit Diet," represented as enabling subscribers to stuff themselves with "forbidden foods" while losing 10 pounds in 10 days. (August 1971)

Products

Given below are some examples of products that were seized by the U.S. Food and Drug Administration in the last few years (with dates of seizure).

Estrogen tablets: False and misleading claims to be effective for menopause, senile vaginitis, and prostatic carcinoma; inadequate directions for use. (11 April 1969)

Piosan (niacin and vitamin C): Misbranded while held for sale; false and misleading claims for strengthening of teeth and pyorrhea prevention; false and misleading claims for relieving kidney aches and correcting inflammation of the urinary tract. (14 May 1970)

Scalp and hair conditioner: False and misleading claims for treatment of itchy scalp, loose dandruff, all hair and scalp miseries; no warnings to discontinue use and consult a physician if undue skin irritation develops or increases. (8 August 1969)

Protein hair spray with mink oil: False and misleading claims to prevent evaporation of skin and hair moisture, prevent and treat contact eczema, dermatitis, dandruff, promote rapid healing of burns, and have remarkable curative powers. (14 August 1969)

Skin cream: New drug not approved for safety and efficacy; inadequate directions for use in contracting breast muscles to make sagging breasts firm and round; implied claims for enlarging underdeveloped breasts. (7 January 1970)

Vitamined sunburn cream: False and misleading claims to kill pain of sunburn and to prevent dry skin and scaling, "may even prevent skin cancer"; inadequate directions for use. (5 September 1968)

Vitic Circuit electronic device: False and misleading claims to maintain healthy functioning of the body, retard aging, beneficially affect the nervous system through a magnetic current. (24 September 1970)

Electronic air cleaner: False and misleading claims to filter the air in 14 to 18 minutes, remove bacteria and viruses from the air, make breathing easier, and reduce discomfort of asthma. (31 December 1970)

Pollen-extract tablets: False and misleading claims of revitalizing old people and aiding patients suffering from a wide range of physical ailments. (2 October 1970)

Replacement for natural oils: False and misleading claims to be effective for replenishing of natural oils in dry or aging skin, hair, and fingernails; inadequate directions for diagnosis and treatment by laymen; not in conformity with the Fair Packaging and Labeling Act. (10 September 1970)

Vacuum cleaning device: False and misleading claims for preventing family epidemics, internal poisoning, skin infections, and respiratory disorders. (6 January 1971)

PROTECTION AGAINST QUACKERY

Personal protection

Although governmental agencies are actively and fairly successfully combating quackery, it is still everyone's responsibility to be able to recognize deception and avoid its snare. Some of the signs useful for recognizing quackery are given below. The first five pertain to mail-order quackery and proprietary medicines. The last ten pertain to the more direct practices of quackery—those given in offices, clinics, and such. Several of the signs apply equally to both types of quackery.

Diagnosis by mail This is *pure* quackery. Not even the most skilled physician could accurately diagnose all disease by a mailed-in description of symptoms or sample of blood or urine. Yet such a diagnosis is the basis of much mail-order medicine.

Free trial package Many mail-order health or beauty aids offer a free or low-cost trial package. Others send a free book which promotes their product. The generous provider of the "free 30-day trial supply" knows that since man is a creature of habit, after thirty days the user will probably continue with the product, which he will then purchase at a high price. People often believe that a product is physically benefiting them, when the only actual effect may be imaginary. Another practice of the mail-order house is to sell names of customers for "sucker lists," often for promotion of products even more shoddy than the original.

"Limited supply—act at once"   "Don't miss this once-in-a-lifetime opportunity." This sales approach, so commonly used in all lines of business, is intended to stampede the customer into acting without taking time to think about the offer and check its validity. The salesman who successfully applies this high-pressure tactic is referred to as a "closer," because he closes a sale before the customer realizes what is happening to him. Usually an ample supply of any product can be promoted in this way.

"Recommended by doctors and nurses" The advertisement seldom states *which* doctors and nurses or even what type of doctor.

"Approved by independent research laboratories" It is not difficult for the patent-medicine producer to find some chemist who is willing to set up an "independent research laboratory," perhaps in his garage and, for a fee, to approve almost any product. He may test its safety without checking its effectiveness, or, conversely, he may find it to be effective without checking its safety.

Offer of free or low-cost diagnosis The practitioner who gives a free diagnosis must make his living from the treatment he renders, so he is naturally inclined to make a diagnosis that is going to lead to some of his treatments. In ethical practice an accurate diagnosis is often much more costly than the resulting treatments, since the treatment of an accurately diagnosed condition may be very efficient.

Boastful advertising The code of ethics of most medical, dental, and similar professional societies prohibits or restricts the advertising of services by members.

Location The ethical practitioner usually chooses a professional environment for his office rather than a rented space in a department or discount store. Medical offices often are centered around a large hospital.

Claim to cure disease that others cannot cure The quack often claims that he can cure a condition that the physician cannot, such as cancer, arthritis, or the common cold.

Guarantee of cure or satisfaction The ethical doctor never guarantees a cure; medical science has not progressed to the point where treatment is that certain. Even though the quack may guarantee his treatments, it is doubtful that he often refunds money.

Testimonial letters The testimonial letter is a common device of the quack. His letters are often from several sources:
   The paid testimonial: some people, including celebrities, will say anything if they are paid enough.
   Person cured of a nonexistent disease: such cases are discussed under cancer quackery.
   Author of letter is dead: often, during the legal investigations of quacks that follow their arrests, it is discovered that persons who wrote letters of

testimonial died a short while later of the same disease of which they claimed to have been cured.

Claims of secret machines or formulas Claims for wonder-working machines and magic formulas are meaningless, because the ethical physician will have knowledge of and access to any effective therapy.

Use of seemingly impressive degrees The quack often lists several high-sounding degrees after his name and plasters his walls with the corresponding diplomas. Such degrees can be easily obtained through nonaccredited "diploma mills" or can be made up to order in print shops.

Belittling the use of surgery and drugs The quack is quite naturally against the use of valuable treatment methods such as surgery and drugs, since the physician can use them and the quack cannot. He therefore noisily claims the superiority of his own nonsurgical and nondrug (and worthless) methods of therapy.

Claims of persecution The quack often takes a very defensive stance, crying that the government and the medical associations are out to get him. And for once he is right. The government agencies and ethical medical societies are determined to make life miserable for the quack and eventually to eliminate quackery from the United States.

Public protection

Governmental agencies At every level of government efforts are being made to control fraudulent health practices. The Federal Trade Commission is active in cases involving fraudulent or deceptive advertising. The Post Office Department may move rapidly in cases of mail-order fraud. The Food and Drug Administration regulates the purity, safety, and proper labeling of drugs and food products moved across state lines. Certain state, county, and city governments also are active in suppressing quackery. In 1967 the state of California became a leader in the fight against quackery by enacting laws making fraudulent practice a felony.

Nongovernmental organizations Several privately financed groups actively participate in the restraint of health frauds. Among these are the Bureau of Investigation of the American Medical Association, Better Business Bureaus, and Chambers of Commerce. Although these organizations have no legal regulatory powers, they can bring cases of fraud to the attention of the public and the proper legal regulatory authorities.

When one is in doubt about the merit of a particular product or treatment, it is often worthwhile to check with a local Chamber of Commerce, Better Business Bureau, local medical society, or a licensed and registered physician.

THE PERSISTENCE OF QUACKERY

Why does quackery persist in spite of the intensive efforts by government and individuals to suppress it? The reason is that, although the quack is not very skilled in treating disease, he is very adept in other areas. He often operates at the very borderline of legality, perhaps obeying the letter but not the spirit of the law. When he is convicted, he usually serves a short jail sentence, pays a stiff fine (which he can well afford), then immediately changes his location and perhaps his name and is back in business again.

Often even getting a conviction proves to be very difficult. Juries may be swayed by the emotional testimonies of former patients of the quack. Large corporations engaged in sales of proprietary compounds retain excellent lawyers to fight their battles with the authorities, and the corporations often win. It took the federal government, for example, sixteen years to get the word *liver* removed from Carter's Little Liver Pills on the basis that they had nothing to do with the liver.

The private citizen can aid the campaign against quackery through reporting incidents of suspected quackery to his local district attorney's office or the local medical society. It is often only through such complaints that authorities are alerted to a fraudulent operation. It is apparent, then, that today, as always, it is the responsibility of the individual to be alert to health fraud and quackery and to avoid falling into its trap.

SUMMARY

Quackery today includes fraudulent treatments, "health" foods, patent medicines, and remedies of questionable value.

  I. Who is a quack?
     A. One who promises medical benefits he cannot deliver.
     B. One who promotes cure-all drugs, machines, and treatments.
     C. One who practices self-treatment.
 II. Why people turn to quackery
     A. Fear of death, pain, and surgery; ignorance; gullibility.
     B. Desire by teenagers and senior citizens to achieve attractiveness or regain youthful vigor.
III. Some major types of quackery today
     A. Cancer quackery
        1. Cure promised without surgery.
        2. Diagnosis and treatment of cancer when none exists.
     B. Arthritis quackery
        1. Ethical physician can cure only a few of the many types of arthritis.
        2. Half of all arthritis patients try quack remedies.
     C. Reducing without dieting
        1. One out of four Americans tries to lose weight each year.
        2. Some common "easy" but ineffective schemes are:
           a. nonprescription reducing pills.
           b. dietless reducing plans of many types.

       c. vibrators.

       d. massaging devices.

       e. spot reducing.

       f. reducing creams.

D. Food fads

  1. "Health foods" and "food supplements"—often sold by:

     a. "health food" stores.

     b. door-to-door salesmen.

     c. "health" lecturers.

  2. Commonly used misrepresentations include the following *myths:*

     a. that all diseases are due to faulty diet.

     b. that some food products are indispensable.

     c. that soil depletion causes malnutrition.

     d. of "organic" or "natural" foods.

     e. of overprocessing.

E. Beauty aids and baldness remedies

  1. Skin creams often feature exotic ingredients:

     a. most of these ingredients are of no value.

     b. physician should be consulted before one uses hormone skin creams.

     c. beautiful skin is usually the result of good diet and general good health.

  2. Expensive baldness treatments are sold through baldness "clinics" and by mail, whereas the dermatologist is the one best qualified to treat baldness.

F. Female breast development

  1. Schemes offered may be either ineffective or harmful:

     a. special exercises—can increase development of chest muscles, but not of breast tissue.

     b. special diets—of no value.

     c. breast-development creams—hormone products should not be used without medical supervision.

     d. silicone implants and injections—dangers outweigh benefits.

  2. No relationship between breast size and sexual adequacy or femininity.

G. Patent medicines

  1. Most are of little or no value.

  2. Probably the most effective substance sold without a prescription is aspirin:

     a. aspirin is the basis for many proprietary compounds.

     b. aspirin should be purchased in small quantities, because it breaks down in storage.

  3. None will prevent or cure the common cold:

     a. bed rest remains best treatment.

     b. antibiotics should be reserved only for secondary bacterial infections.

IV. Some specific examples of quackery

V. Protection against quackery

A. Personal protection

  1. Personal responsibility is to recognize and avoid quackery.

  2. Signs of mail-order or patent medicine quackery are:

     a. diagnosis by mail.

b. free trial package.
c. "limited supply—act at once."
d. "recommended by doctors and nurses."
e. "approved by independent research laboratories."
3. Signs of direct quackery are:
a. offer of free or low-cost diagnosis.
b. boastful advertising.
c. location.
d. claim to cure disease that others cannot cure.
e. guarantee of cure or satisfaction.
f. testimonial letters.
g. claims of secret machines or formulas.
h. use of seemingly impressive degrees.
i. belittling the use of surgery and drugs.
j. claims of persecution.
B. Public protection
1. Governmental:
a. active federal agencies—Federal Trade Commission, Post Office Department, Food and Drug Administration.
b. state, county, and city governments.
2. Nongovernmental:
a. Bureau of Investigation of the American Medical Association.
b. Better Business Bureaus.
c. Chambers of Commerce.
VI. The persistence of quackery
A. Operates at the borderline of legality.
B. Getting conviction is very difficult.
C. The quack convicted
1. Pays a stiff fine.
2. Serves a short jail term.
3. Is soon back in business.
D. Private citizens should be alert to health fraud and report incidents to the local district attorney's office or medical society.

Glossary

If you cannot find the word you wish in this glossary, check the index for text and glossary references.

nostrum (nos'trəm) (L. *noster*, our). A medicine recommended by its preparer; a quack remedy; a cure-all.

patent medicine. A nonprescription medicine advertised to the public; often of secret composition. See *proprietary compound*.

proprietary compound (prō pri'ə te rē). A preparation for the treatment of disease, protected against free competition as to name, composition, or manufacturing process by secrecy, patent, copyright, trademark, or other means.

pseudoscience (soo'dō si'əns) (Gr. *pseudes*, false). False science.

quack (kwak). A boastful pretender to medical skill.

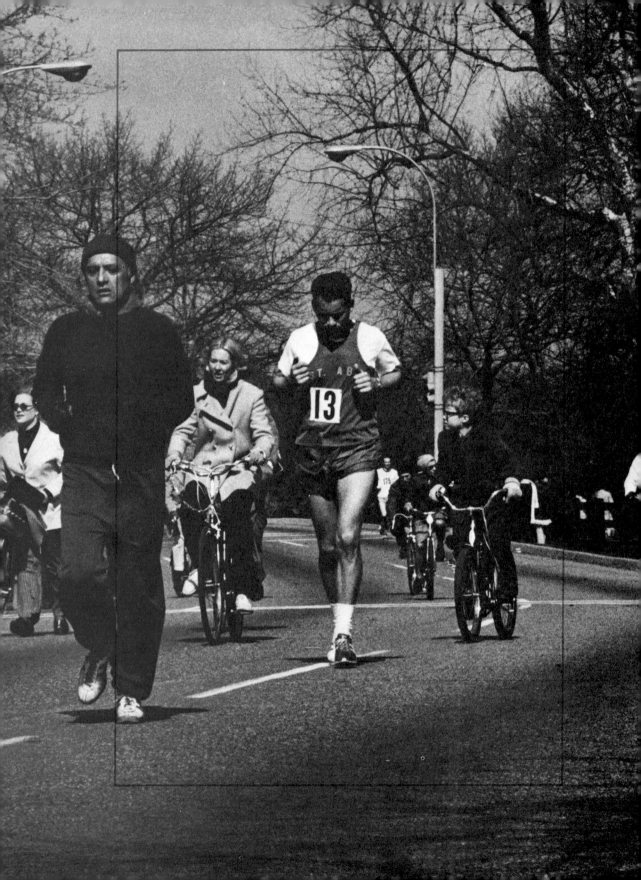

The meaning of physical fitness

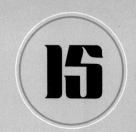

Fitness, according to Dr. Roger Bannister (the first person to run the mile in four minutes), is one of the most misused words in the English language. It can mean anything from "that feeling of pleasure which a person experiences when he stands by an open window early in the morning to—for those with vested interests—some recommendation that we ought to drink more milk or beer." True fitness implies the ability to function at an optimal level of efficiency in all daily activities. Such fitness is beyond *physical fitness;* it actually means *total fitness,* which means *the strength, speed, agility, endurance, and emotional adjustment appropriate to a person's age.* To even begin functioning at this level a person must have a physically fit body. In this chapter are guidelines to help you work toward establishing a level of total fitness that you will be able to maintain throughout your life.

TOTAL FITNESS

All body activities require energy. How the body acquires and uses energy is explained in Chapter 7. But, very simply, this energy is produced by breaking down foods (carbohydrates, fats, and proteins) in the presence of oxygen. The body can store food, but it cannot store oxygen. If more food is eaten each day than is needed by the body, the body uses what it requires and stores the rest for later. Not so with oxygen. We cannot store oxygen, so we breathe in and out every moment of our lives to keep the supply coming in. If the oxygen supply were suddenly cut off, the oxygen stored in the body would not last more than a few minutes. The brain, the heart, and all body tissue would cease to function, and we would die.

The oxygen in the air is readily available; as we need it, we breathe it in. The problem is one of getting enough oxygen to all parts of the body where food is burned. Food and oxygen combine chemically to produce energy.

Most of us produce enough energy to perform ordinary daily activities—that is, walk, talk, think, or study. However, as the activities become more vigorous, we sooner or later reach our maximal performance capacity. This spread—the difference between our minimal energy requirements and our maximal capacity—is the measure of our fitness. The most totally fit persons have the greatest spread; the least fit, the least spread. In some, the minimal energy requirements and maximal capacity are almost identical.

A standard definition of fitness and also a standard way of measuring how fit a person is have eluded both physical educators and exercise physiologists for years. Overall fitness of the body systems would seem to be an accurate means of measuring how fit a person is. As explained above, we need a constant supply of oxygen to all parts of the body, and a valid trend in physiology is to consider *aerobic capacity* (the maximal oxygen intake of a person) the indicator of overall fitness. This means that a person should have the ability to engage in prolonged physical activity, such as tennis, swimming, and golf, without undue fatigue.

This definition of fitness implies that a person must be "in condition" to be classed as totally fit. Such overall fitness, endurance fitness, or working capacity (the ability to do prolonged work without undue fatigue) has very much to do with the body's overall health—the health of the lungs, the heart, the entire cardiovascular system, other body organs, as well as the muscles.

Many individuals may be classified into one of three fitness categories, which are discussed below.

Passive fitness

The nonexerciser belongs to the category of passive fitness. This individual makes no effort to keep his body fit. He does only what he has to do during his daily routine. There is nothing physically wrong with him—not yet—nor is there anything really right with him. If he is lucky, he may remain in this condition for years. However, his body is essentially deteriorating. It will continue to deteriorate unless he increases his physical activity.

Muscular fitness

Individuals who overemphasize *isometrics* or *isotonics* represent muscular fitness. These people have the right motives but the wrong approach. Such individuals subscribe to the myth that muscular strength is equivalent to overall fitness. The skeletal muscles make up only one system in the body; it is by no means the most important system.

Isometrics and isotonic exercises affect primarily the muscular system; although they have some effect on other body systems, their effects on total fitness are limited. Individuals who have only muscular strength may not have the endurance and agility necessary for total fitness.

Total fitness

This condition exists when someone engages in balanced activities, strengthening all body systems—particularly the cardiovascular system, the respiratory system, the nervous system, and the muscular system. But it is very important to realize that total fitness is produced by *optimal* intensity and duration of physical activity. Overworking the systems of the body not only fails to produce the desired effects but might actually result in decreased fitness and damage. The amount and duration of physical activity required is different for every person. The physical activities chosen should match one's likes and needs.

PRINCIPLES OF EXERCISE PROGRAMS

An individual, while he is in school or college, should develop skills in several different activities to participate in throughout life. Four major factors should be considered as one plans his fitness activities for later life. He should develop *strength, endurance, flexibility,* and *skill.* Knowledge should be gained in activities and sports that develop and maintain these factors.

Activity programs

Individuals differ greatly in the amount of exercise they need and can take, and certain precautions should be observed. A desirable fitness level is best achieved through activity that is regular and vigorous. Consequently, someone who has a history of health problems or anyone over thirty-five years of age who has truly been a "nonexerciser" for the major portion of his life should never engage in vigorous physical activity without a complete physical examination and consultation with a physician as to what activities he is best suited for.

A physically active person may need little, if any, additional exercise to maintain fitness, while an inactive individual must add exercise to prevent becoming less fit. Also, advancing age is not a reason to discontinue exercise; actually, it is an indication for exercise. A healthy person of any age will do himself no harm by suitable physical activity.

At least five principles should be applied by the individual as he plans for an activity program for later life. The individual planning for the future should adopt them while in school or college.

1. Take courses in which *individual* or *dual* sports are taught.
2. Learn activities that will remain interesting and challenging.
3. Become proficient in activities through which a vigorous workout can be obtained in a relatively short period of time.

4. Learn activities through which a moderate workout can be obtained when it is indicated.

5. Learn activities that can offset the conditions of a chosen profession or job.

Motivation is the key to total fitness. If a person is to maintain a regular activity program throughout life, he must start early and form the necessary habits. Today there are too many "weekend athletes" who die of heart attacks because they have not participated in regular programs throughout the week.

Total fitness is valuable for both males and females. Thus all of the discussions in this chapter are directed toward both sexes. Contrary to some common thought, women who participate in exercise programs and sports do not develop large muscles. Programs that overdevelop specific muscles are unhealthy for both men and women.

Exercise improves the figure by "normalizing" it, or causing it to become better proportioned. If the arms or legs are too heavy, exercise slims them; if they are too thin, exercise develops them. American female Olympic athletes, such as skiers, track participants, gymnasts, and skaters have feminine body builds.

Although women are usually neither as strong nor as powerful as men, they have better flexibility, poise, and grace. They enjoy participating in sports aimed at developing a beautiful, womanly figure—one that is slender, graceful, and has curves in the right places. Most beautiful women participate in daily exercise programs and in sports.

Muscular strength and muscular endurance

Muscular strength is the maximal amount of force, or tension, a muscle can exert in a single contraction. Muscles develop strength when they are subjected to tension in progressively increasing amounts. Muscular endurance is the ability of the muscles either to maintain a maximal contraction or to respond repetitively for a relatively long time. Before a person undertakes any total fitness activities, he must possess sufficient strength to support his body weight easily throughout the activity. Two types of muscular contraction, isometric contractions and isotonic contractions, may be used to develop muscular strength and endurance.

Isometric contractions are produced by pushing or pulling against an immovable object. When held for a long period of time, they produce tension, or static contractions. Such exercise programs began to gain popularity in the late 1930s because of a vigorous advertising campaign, which appealed to young men interested in developing muscular physiques. The person who designed the isometric program called "Dynamic Tension" was Charles Atlas.

The systematic isometric contraction of the muscles of the body will, within days, improve muscular strength, provided the program is of sufficient time duration. Best results appear to be obtained by means of maximal contraction strength, held for 5 to 8 seconds and repeated 5 to 10 times daily. Care must be taken to exercise opposing muscle groups at equal strength, or unequal strength patterns will develop. Isometric exercises do not develop muscular endurance or flexibility. These exercises develop large muscles which can produce great muscle tension during isometric contractions. Sustained for longer periods of time (over 8 seconds), such contractions produce a rapid rise in blood pressure; in 1 minute the mean blood pressure can rise to 140.

Isometric contractions are also produced when people move or lift extremely heavy loads—when, for example, they open a window which is stuck or shovel snow (a common cause of heart attacks). Isometric contractions occur, too, when overweight individuals try to do pushups or pullups. A reasonably fit person may use 30 percent of his muscle power to do a pushup while someone 20 pounds overweight uses 40 percent of his muscle power to do the same thing. Blood pressure rises in response to the intensity of the tension and the length of time it is held. Therefore, untrained, older, or overweight persons should not use isometrics, move heavy objects, or become overly tense. The high blood pressures produced may be very dangerous to them. The size of the muscle group in use seems to have nothing to do with increases in blood pressure. Small muscles in the back of the neck which become overly tense because of nerves or fatigue produce a rise in blood pressure equivalent to that produced by large leg muscles pushing against a stationary object.

Isotonic contractions are produced when an individual continues to raise, lower, or move a moderate load. Within isotonic-exercise programs it is possible to do many combinations of *repetitions*[1] (the total number of executions), *resistance* (weight to be lifted), and *sets* (the number of groups of repetitions done consecutively without resting).

Muscular strength is best developed when the resistance is relatively high and the number of repetitions is low. Muscular endurance is best developed when the resistance is relatively low and the number of repetitions is high. For example, in weight training muscular strength is most successfully developed by lifting a selected weight only six times; muscular endurance, flexibility, and coordination are better served by selecting a lighter weight and lifting it fifteen to twenty times.

Resistance may be applied in different ways. Because body weight is considered to be resistance, isotonic contractions are produced whenever someone moves. Calisthenics and weight training are good ways to apply resistance, especially for people who start a total-fitness program after a period of sedentary living. Isotonic programs are most successful in developing strength and endurance if they are performed prior to and during an organized fitness training program.

Isotonic programs have several advantages. First, the exercises may be systematically planned to cover all muscle groups of the body and to emphasize areas of greatest need. Next, it is easy to adjust the degree of exercise from very mild forms to vigorous efforts. Finally, the exercises may be performed easily in the home. Many activities producing isotonic contractions will occur to the person seeking variety and interest in activities designed to develop adequate muscular strength and endurance.

---

[1] In many exercise programs the word *repetition* is used incorrectly. *Execution maximum* (EM) or *repetition maximum* (RM) should be used to indicate repetitions. Both terms indicate the maximal weight that can be lifted for an indicated number of repetitions. For example, 10 EM (RM) is the greatest weight that can be lifted ten times.

Circulatory endurance

Exercises for circulatory endurance stimulate an increase in cardiorespiratory functioning, producing results known as *conditioning, training effect*, and *aerobic capacity*. Essentially, such exercises involve isotonic activities which are continued over a period of time (a minimum of 15 minutes) and at a pace necessary to increase the pulse rate to between 130 and 132 beats per minute during the exercise. In addition to circulatory endurance, these activities produce flexibility and coordination.

During long periods of sustained activity, heavy demands are made on the lungs and the circulatory system, including the heart. Improved circulatory endurance results in increases in the oxygen-carrying ability of the blood, the number of the capillaries, and cardiac efficiency and output.

Isometric exercises develop strength but usually do not improve circulatory endurance. However, if the repetitions of weight training are done rapidly and are continued until a person is perspiring and breathing heavily (pulse rate is nearing 132), they may be helpful to circulatory endurance. Furthermore, isometric exercises may be performed in conjunction with jogging, hopping, or running in place.

Individual sports such as hiking, brisk walking, jogging, skipping, skating, running, cross-country skiing, bicycling, and swimming are particularly good for circulatory endurance. Distance, speed, and duration may be regulated to the capability of the individual. Progression in the amount of exercise may be planned from day to day. Other sports have a potentially good effect on circulatory endurance. Among these are the dual sports handball, squash, and tennis and the team sports soccer, basketball, and ice hockey.

Exercise tolerance

Exercise tolerance is the level at which the body responds favorably to exercise. An individual's exercise tolerance is his ability to perform a series of exercises, participate in a sport, or enjoy a walk without undue fatigue. All exercises should be adapted to an individual's tolerance level. Activities that are too easy for someone fall short of his tolerance, while exercises that are too difficult or are impossible should not be attempted.

One indication of exercise tolerance is pulse rate. Exercise physiologists have found that if a person works at 60 percent of his capacity, his body undergoes favorable circulatory changes, which lead to a trained, or fit, condition. People under 30 years of age work at 60 percent of their capacity when their pulse rate is 151 beats per minute; people over 30 work at 60 percent of their capacity when their pulse reaches 131 beats per minute. The decreased work capacity of people over thirty is caused partly by the decrease in heart rate which comes with advancing age and partly by the reduced elasticity of the blood vessels.

A person who performs calisthenics, lifts weights, or participates in an individual or dual sport can monitor his own pulse rate. To do this he should take his pulse rate for 10 seconds immediately after he stops exercising. He may then multiply the ten-second rate by 6 to obtain his rate per minute. If he is over thirty and his pulse rate is 22 × 6, or 132 beats per minute, he has worked adequately but has not overexercised.

If a person engages in 4 periods of exercise each week and in each period works at 60 percent of his work-load capacity for 15 minutes, he can maintain his body in a trained condition. Of course, not all people should work at 60 percent of their capacity; people with cardiovascular conditions, for example, should not elevate their pulse rates to 131 beats per minute. Before beginning any exercise program, a person should consult his physician; once in a program, he should continue to have periodic physical examinations. He should also consult a competent physical educator for instruction in individual and dual sports and for advice on the best exericse program for him.

Overloading and progression

The body has great ability to adapt to stress. Therefore, people who wish to improve their performance and their general condition should continually increase the duration and intensity of their exercises. The process of extending oneself beyond usual physical effort is called *overloading*, or, more recently, *interval training*. Harder work with less energy output may be accomplished by overloading. Overloading involves gradually increasing stress, in terms of the following factors:

1. Gradually and progressively increasing the speed of performance.
2. Gradually increasing the total load (resistance).
3. Progressively increasing the total time that a given position can be held.
4. Maintaining a constant resistance and progressively increasing the total number of repetitions.

In exercises designed to develop strength or circulatory endurance the intervals of overloading should be of extremely short duration (15 or 20 seconds) and should be kept within one's tolerance level. Fatigue may be delayed by reducing the work load, by slowing the rhythm, and by breathing regularly and deeply. In using interval training a person may alternately run and walk to give himself periods to recover from stress.

The principles of overloading should help you increase your efficiency and performance. As you master an exercise program, you should progress to more strenuous exercises.

Progression is accomplished when increments of work, or sets, are added at appropriate steps. All exercise plans should provide for progression. Generally, increasing the intensity, or the tempo, of an exercise is more important than increasing its duration. Through progression people begin with easy exercises and work toward more and more difficult ones.

Warming up

In the way that an athlete must train to reach the level of total fitness at which he can perform safely, a nonathlete must also take time to develop the strength, coordination, and endurance demanded by any sport. When individuals have not exercised on a regular basis for a number of years, they should recondition themselves on a warm-up basis. Too often, sedentary people who exercise become sore or injured because their muscles and joints are not ready for activity. A warm-up program of 15 to 20 minutes followed by slow walking and jogging will help prevent soreness and muscle injury. Such a program should be followed until the body is reconditioned enough to withstand more vigorous exercise. An individual should allow a minimum of one month of reconditioning for each year he has been out of condition.

Also, each time a person exercises or participates in a sport, he should first warm up. A proper warm-up prepares a person for exercise by increasing body temperature, stretching ligaments, and slightly increasing cardiovascular activity. The amount of warm-up necessary varies among individuals and generally increases with age.

You should begin at a very slow pace with light, rhythmical exercises, accompanied by stretching and deep breathing. Deep breathing before exercising temporarily increases your oxygen supply and will help you to take deeper breaths while exercising. The next activity should be a series of exercises to stretch and loosen the muscles and raise the heartbeat and body temperature enough to promote sweating.

Easing off

Just as the body needs warming up, it also needs easing off after exercise. This helps return the blood to the heart and the body temperature back to normal. You should keep moving for several minutes after vigorous activity, until your breathing has returned to normal, the stress of the exercise has subsided, and the body has cooled.

TOTAL-FITNESS CONDITIONING

The three principles of physical fitness (muscular strength, muscular endurance, and circulatory endurance) should be incorporated into any total-fitness program. Exercise alone, however, does not guarantee fitness. The American Medical Association has stated that sufficient rest and sleep, an adequate diet, and regular exercise are all necessary for total body fitness.

The minimal exercise recommendations are from 30 to 60 minutes every 2 days. For a total-fitness program to be effective, exercise should be regular. However, the value of exercise depends more on how it is done than on how often it is done. Exercise must be vigorous enough to raise the pulse beat to 131 beats per minute for people over thirty and 151 for people under thirty; increased pulse beat should be sustained for at least 15 minutes. A five-hour game of golf over eighteen holes won't do this for anyone. This is the reason why such popular sports as golf and bowling should be supplemented by an exercise program.

To follow a daily exercise program, use a combination of programs consisting of interval training and change of pace. Change of pace includes one or both of the following: (1) the shifting from one activity to another that involves a different set of muscles and a different kind of exercise, and (2) the changing of the intensity of exercise.

The time of day that you exercise depends on your schedule and your preferences. Some people enjoy an early-morning workout; others like to exercise after a day's work. Individual exercise programs must subject stress to the body within the limits of a person's exercise tolerance. The body will develop to meet the demands placed on it, and overloading and progression should be employed as tolerance extends. Each exercise program session should be started by warming up and ended by easing off.

TOTAL-FITNESS PROGRAMS

It is important to consult a professional physical educator, because he can design a balanced total-fitness program that does not overemphasize one aspect of physical development. Isometric exercises have limited benefits, because their value is restricted largely to the development and maintenance of muscular strength. Calisthenic exercises and weight training exercises improve both muscular endurance and muscular strength. However, these exercises have minimal value for circulatory fitness.

Brisk walking, jogging, and running are excellent circulatory exercises, but they do little for the abdominal, back, shoulder, and arm muscles. Therefore, they should be accompanied by exercises that strengthen these parts. There are few sports in which all parts of the body are exercised equally well. People who have been inactive and have a low exercise tolerance should pace themselves carefully when participating in vigorous sports. In fact, such people may want to avoid vigorous sports until they are in condition. Conditioning requires a minimum of *six weeks* of warming up, calisthenics, or weight training.

Women should take special care to select exercises that provide a balanced program—one that develops muscular strength, muscular endurance, and circulatory endurance. They should emphasize exercises that strengthen abdominal and back muscles and participate in sports that improve posture and balance, such as tennis and volleyball.

Pregnant women should consult their obstetricians about exercise programs. If such programs are not too strenuous, the doctor will approve of them. Even when doctors decide that exercise is not advisable during pregnancy, women are usually able to resume exercising very shortly after they give birth.

If a pregnant woman has been participating in a regular daily exercise program that includes activities to strengthen abdominal and back muscles, she should be able to carry her child easily, deliver easily and swiftly, and rapidly regain her figure after the delivery. Normally such a woman should be able to continue her regular exercise program up to the sixth month of the pregnancy. During the last three months she may engage only in a simple walking program.

Calisthenics

Calisthenics provide the opportunity to exercise specific groups of muscles. A great variety of calisthenic programs have been developed to exercise every group of muscles in the body. Some of these are "spot" exercises, which change body contours in specific places. No exercise affects only one part of the body, but some emphasize development of one area or one muscle group. Others are series of calisthenics that exercise the whole body. You should begin performing calisthenic exercises early, so that you can do them correctly and effortlessly when you reach your thirties.

There are many basic calisthenic programs designed for the whole body. In the early 1960s the Royal Canadian Air Force originated two programs which have proved to be very successful. The *5BX* [Five Basic Exercises] *Plan for Physical Fitness* for men and the *XBX* [Ten Basic Exercises] *Plan* for women are two series of relatively simple calisthenic exercises that can be done in 11 minutes each day. You should either follow an organized program like this one or have a physical educator design a program especially for you.

Weight training

If you are interested in weight training, remember that hard work is required to obtain results, and they appear very slowly. You should remain at a program for three months to determine whether there is an improvement in strength. A weight training program can be designed for you by a physical educator. Weight training classes and workouts are often part of a college or university curriculum, a men's club, the YMCA, or a gym.

In weight training programs *repetition* refers to the number of times a specific weight is to be lifted; *resistance* is the amount of weight to be lifted; a *set* is the period during which a given number of repetitions are performed without the weights' or barbells' being set down.

It is impossible to select a standard starting weight that is appropriate for everyone. If you begin a weight training program, start with an amount of weight that feels comfortable when you start repetitions. If you are going to work out three times a week, you should increase the original weight by 5 or 10 pounds each week. Use the same weight for at least 1 week or for 3 workouts. Often individuals starting their second workouts find themselves stiff, sore, and tired, and the weights feel heavier than they did during the first workout. If this happens to you, reduce the weights by 5 pounds for 1 week or by 10 pounds for 2 weeks; continue the reduction until the weights feel comfortable. Then progress to the point at which you began, and continue on ahead, gradually increasing the weights. This principle should also be used when you return to your weight training program after a short layoff.

Work out three times a week on alternate days, giving yourself a two-day rest at the end of the week. You may, for example, work out on Monday, Wednesday, and Friday, or on Tuesday, Thursday, and Saturday. An exercise session should last from 1½ to 2 hours. You should perform about 8 or 10 different exercises and 3 sets of each exercise. Rest about 1 minute between sets and approximately 2 to 3 minutes between exercises. At each set increase the weight you are lifting by 5 to 10 pounds.

Weight training does not develop circulatory endurance. It does increase muscular strength and endurance through application of the principle of *progressive resistance exercise*. In other words, as strength increases, resistance is increased. Progressive resistance occurs when a person moves a given resistance (barbells or weights) a definite number of times (repetitions).

Weight training combines weight lifting with calisthenics. Weight training programs may be as extensive or as simple as the individual desires, but they should not deviate from the principle of resistance progression. A person who simply wants to see how much he can lift may sprain muscles and joints. Weights should be increased only as strength increases. Weight training takes time; a person reaches his maximal strength only after three to five years of continuous progression.

Plan your program in writing. Make out a program card on which you list your exercises, your starting poundage, the number of repetitions, and the number of sets. As you increase the weights in each exercise, mark the changes on your card. The program card may be referred to before and during the workout. You may also use it to make changes in your program.

Every month or six weeks change your exercises. Substitute different exercises for the ones you have been doing, until you have done all the exercises in your program. Then return to the ones you started with. Such program changes help you to maintain your interest, and they vary the pressure and resistance on each muscle.

Exercises for circulatory endurance

As you have learned, circulatory endurance, or stamina, is the ability of the body to perform under stress without undue fatigue. Circulatory endurance is attained through physical activity in which the circulatory and respiratory systems are stimulated for relatively long periods of time. The normal, healthy heart cannot be injured by such exercise and will respond beneficially to the demands placed on it. However, individuals engaging in a planned circulatory-endurance program should progress in graduated increments and should avoid placing drastic demands on their hearts. An individual may determine whether or not he is exercising safely by taking his pulse rate periodically during endurance exercises. The pulse rate should never rise above 151 beats per minute for people under thirty years of age or above 131 beats per minute for people over thirty. If individuals will engage in activities that increase their pulse rates to these maximums, and if they sustain such activities for 15 minutes four times a week, they will improve their circulatory endurance to an adequate level.

Walking, jogging, and running Each year many deaths from cardiac failure occur because of jogging and running. These deaths occur because people with heart defects place excessive demand on their hearts. Anyone with a known or suspected heart or lung disability should exercise only under the direction of a physician. All "apparently" well individuals over thirty years of age should be considered to have a suspected heart or lung disability until a physician proves otherwise.

Graduated increments of walking, jogging, and running, done after a physical examination and with medical approval, improve appearance and endurance. Such a program can provide energy for the enjoyment of life and help to prevent fatigue.

Walking is the most natural of all forms of exercise. A person may walk at any time with almost no medical risk. Brisk walking accelerates the pulse and strengthens the heart, lungs, and legs. Extremely inactive people may obtain some endurance effects by walking; later, however, they must increase their rate of speed to obtain further benefits. Inactive, sedentary men (more than women) over fifty years of age should walk for exercise; they should not try jogging or running because of the increased chance of heart attack after fifty.

Jogging, the next step up from walking, is steady, slow running. Jogging may be alternated with breath-catching periods of walking. Jogging became popular in the late nineteen-sixties with the publication of *Jogging* by William J. Bowerman, track coach at the University of Oregon, and W. E. Harris, M.D., a heart specialist. This book presents a detailed, complete program for anyone interested in jogging as part of his exercise program. Jogging is pleasant, free, easy, relaxing, and fun. It can be done alone or in groups. Jogging is especially good for maintaining circulatory endurance. To achieve this purpose, however, it must be alternated with intervals of hard running after the first month or two of progression.

Jogging may be satisfactory to an individual during the initial phase of conditioning. The progression of jogging and walking outlined previously may be used to progress toward the goal of running 1 mile. Before you try to run a mile, be sure that you can jog comfortably for this distance. Don't worry about your time at first. When you can jog for a mile, start pacing yourself and reducing your time. You should pace yourself so that you are running at a constant rate. Avoid any bursts of speed, because they greatly reduce your efficiency and cause fatigue. Reduce your time by 10 seconds a week until you can run a mile in 6 minutes. This is considered excellent time for maintenance of circulatory endurance.

When space or weather restricts your ability to run, running in place can be a very effective means of maintaining circulatory endurance. The important factors in running in place are the cadence of the step and the duration of the activity. The most comfortable time length seems to be 5 minutes. To reach a five-minute goal, begin by running in place for 1 minute; then increase your time by 30-second intervals. Run for five sessions at each time level before progressing to the next interval. See Table 15.1. When you can run in place for 5 minutes, you may begin to increase your step cadence.

Aerobics Aerobics is a total-fitness program first published in 1968. The originator of the program was Major Kenneth H. Cooper, M.D., of the U.S. Air Force Medical Corps. The key concept in this program is oxygen consump-

Table 15.1 *Program for running in place*

number of sessions	running time (minutes)
1 to 5	1
6 to 10	1½
11 to 15	2
16 to 20	2½
21 to 25	3
26 to 30	3½
31 to 35	4
36 to 40	4½
41 to 45	5

tion. Because oxygen cannot be stored in the body, it must be continually replenished. Consequently, the fatigue level of an individual is controlled by the ability of his respiratory and circulatory systems to supply oxygen to the muscles.

Dr. Cooper's aerobics system consists of a point count assigned to different physical activities that increase circulatory endurance. In his physical activities an individual progresses to the point where he can perform activities worth thirty points each week. The number of points represents the amount of the physical activity necessary for maintenance of the cardiorespiratory system.

Points are obtained by performing specific circulatory endurance activities in a specific amount of time. Such activities include running, swimming, bicycling, walking, running in place, and participating in strenuous games of squash, handball, and basketball. Dr. Cooper's book *The New Aerobics* (a revised version of the program published in 1968) provides standards against which a person may gauge his aerobic fitness. For beginners to the program the test of aerobic fitness is the distance that can be covered in 12 minutes of running. See Table 15.2. After you have determined your fitness category, refer to *The New Aerobics* and choose the schedule you should follow to obtain thirty aerobic points per week.

Table 15.2 *Distances covered in twelve minutes by running for age groups*

fitness categories	distance (miles)			
	Under 30	30 to 39	40 to 49	Over 50
Very poor	under 1.0	under 0.95	under 0.85	under 0.80
Poor	1.0 to 1.24	0.95 to 1.14	0.85 to 1.04	0.80 to 0.99
Fair	1.25 to 1.49	1.15 to 1.39	1.05 to 1.29	1.00 to 1.24
Good	1.50 to 1.74	1.40 to 1.64	1.30 to 1.54	1.25 to 1.49
Excellent	1.75 and over	1.65 and over	1.55 and over	1.50 and over

Circuit training In circuit training *circuit* refers to a number of carefully selected exercises which are arranged and numbered consecutively; the person runs between exercises over a given area. Each numbered exercise within the circuit is called a *station*. An individual moves at his own speed from one station to another until he completes the entire circuit. In most cases he repeats the total circuit more than once (usually three times) and records the total time of performance. This is a convenient and different approach to exercising—one that is physically, physiologically, and psychologically sound.

Circuit training involves two valuable activities. The best physical activity for development of muscular strength and muscular endurance is weight training. The most effective method for developing and maintaining circulatory and respiratory endurance is running. (Also effective are swimming, bicycling, and rope skipping). Some people are able to participate quite regularly in either weight training or running, but very seldom are they able to participate in both. A well-planned circuit involves both weight training and running. Thus circuit training increases muscular strength, muscular endurance, and cardiovascular endurance.

The value of circuit training lies in its extreme adaptability to a great variety of situations. A circuit can be designed to fit any individual, group, area, or condition; it is even adaptable to medical rehabilitation. Circuit training enables an individual or a group of people to progress through a series of exercises and check the progress against a clock. When circuit training is used in schools, the student knows in advance exactly what he will be required to do. Furthermore, circuits may be tailored to fit each individual in the class. Consequently, students can work alone or in groups without direction from the instructor. During classroom instruction an individual should be taught how to plan and construct his own circuit for use outside class.

Circuit training utilizes three variables: load, repetitions, and time. Weight training exercises provide the load, and sets provide the repetitions. Interval running, engaged in between stations, provides repetitions and time.

On a circuit the progression is produced by decreasing the time required to complete one circuit, increasing the work load (weight or sets), or a combination of both. Progression is assured because an individual works at his current capacity and can progress as his capacity increases. Circuit training provides a series of progressive time goals, which are achieved step by step. This time factor provides built-in motivation; it encourages a person to push himself to do better. The circuit layout in which a person moves from one station to another offers variety; this is appealing to most people.

The progressions used in weight training may be used in circuit training if loads can be increased by progressively increasing the size of the weights to be lifted. In circuit training it is not necessary to change weights as frequently as it is in weight training, because weight training is only one of the variables involved in the program.

Calisthenic exercises may be used in a circuit. When this is done, the load is a person's own body weight. The load is increased by modifying the exercise. For example, the following changes will increase the work load in a push-up: standard push-up; push-up, pushing hands off the floor; push-up, pushing off the floor and clapping hands; pushing up, pushing off the floor and slapping the chest. Such modifications make calisthenic exercises very useful in circuit training. Load can also be increased by increasing the number of repetitions, or sets, at each station or by increasing the number of times the circuit is run. Laps may be added; in that case, a person runs the length of the circuit without performing at the stations. Another way to increase the load is to decrease the time needed to perform a circut. In maintaining good progression the most important factor is to increase the workload gradually and at a rate that can be handled with ease and safety.

Rope skipping   Rope skipping is an excellent cardiovascular exercise. A person who jumps steadily for 5 minutes is getting a good workout. A 10-minute daily program of rope skipping improves and maintains cardiovascular endurance as well as a 30-minute program of jogging. Rope skipping may be either a program in itself or a bad-weather substitute for a jogging, running program.

Rope is inexpensive. Cut a piece which is anywhere from 6 to 9 feet long; the correct length is the one most comfortable for you. Tape the ends so they will not fray.

Variations within a rope-skipping program can add interest and incentive. They may also provide progression. (Progression may also be achieved by performing a specific number of jumps in a certain amount of time.) The normal skipping style may be modified by jumping on one foot, alternating feet, or jumping with both feet together. Running while skipping increases timing and coordination. Jumping backward is a simple maneuver in which various foot styles can be used. Make some forward-to-backward changes and then some backward-to-forward changes. This is difficult, because you must jump an extra time as the turn is completed.

A double jump is challenging. This is done by spinning the rope faster and jumping a little higher. When you have increased your skill, shorten the rope slightly by winding it within the hand, and stay in the air longer by bending the knees and keeping them high. You may achieve a triple jump. Double and triple jumps have an effect similar to that caused by sprints in running; they rapidly increase the heart rate.

A front cross may be achieved by crossing the arms when the rope starts downward. This makes a loop through which you may jump. On completion of the jump the arms are uncrossed, and the next jump is made in the normal manner. If you have difficulty performing a front cross, lengthen the rope slightly and either lower the hands as the arms cross or cross the arms far enough to bring the elbows together. These changes will give you a wider loop to jump through. A back cross may be done by performing a regular back jump with arms crossed in front of the body (cross your arms so your elbows touch each other).

Make your own modifications. Try jumps such as a double jump with a front cross, or try to run while you change jumping forms. Again, make some forward-to-backward changes and then some backward-to-forward changes.

SPORTS—USE OF LEISURE TIME

Sports and other recreational activities may serve as conditioning programs. However, some individual and dual sports require such small amounts of physical activity that they are not adequate for a fitness program. Golf is such a sport. It has many psychological and social values but little physical value. The main energy expenditure in golf comes from walking. This walking is usually not vigorous enough to elevate the pulse significantly.

If a sport is to supply the requirements of a total-fitness program, it must be vigorous. Moreover, a person should participate in it for at least three sessions a week. Each session should last for a minimum of 30 minutes. Ideally, a person who is using a sport as the basis of a fitness program should participate in the sport for 60 minutes every day.

When you participate in a sport, you should remember that your expenditure of energy depends on several factors:

1. *The number of participants.* In calisthenics, weight training, and running you control the expenditure of energy. In dual sports, however, you must consider the number of participants. Handball may be least demanding in a game of doubles, more demanding in a game of singles, and most demanding in a game involving three people ("cutthroat").

2. *The skill of the participants.* Generally, a high level of skill is reflected in greater efficiency. Thus, a skilled person can participate at a lower energy cost. As your skill develops, you should either increase the amount of time you devote to a sport or pit yourself against people who are more skillful than you are.

3. *The duration.* The longer the duration of an activity, the greater the energy expenditure. Each participant should be vigorously active for 30 to 40 minutes. In a 60-minute game, then, you should be moving one half to two thirds of the time.

4. *The speed of the necessary physical movements.* Sports which require occasional bursts of speed are more demanding and require a greater expenditure of energy than are sports in which the participants can establish a steady pace. You should participate in such sports only after you feel your physical condition is adequate.

In choosing sports remember the value of developing and maintaining circulatory endurance. Sports that improve circulatory endurance include individual activities such as swimming, scuba diving, snorkeling, hiking, running, and bicycling, dual activities such as wrestling and judo, and court games such as badminton, handball, squash, tennis, and volleyball.

Dual sports and court games require at least two participants. Court games further require a court. These requirements may limit your opportunities to engage in exercise. Individual activities usually offer more opportunities for participation.

Some sports are much more beneficial to fitness than are others. Golf is the least beneficial. It is followed, in increasing benefit, by court games, dual sports, individual sports, weight training, jogging, and running. Remember, whenever you exercise, begin with warm-up exercises, then proceed to your basic routine, whether it is an exercise activity (weight training, jogging, running, for example) or a sport (swimming, handball, tennis, and so forth). Always finish with an easing-off period.

SUMMARY

I. Total fitness
   A. The concept—persons should have the strength, speed, agility, endurance, and emotional adjustment appropriate to their ages.
   B. All body activities require energy.
      1. Energy is produced by breaking down foods in the presence of oxygen:
         a. eating three times a day provides more than enough food for most of us; the body uses what it needs and saves the rest for later.
         b. oxygen cannot be stored; we breathe in and out every moment of our lives to keep the supply coming in.
      2. Most of us produce enough energy to perform ordinary daily tasks; this is not true as activities become more vigorous.
   C. The spread between our minimal energy requirements (to perform daily tasks) and our maximal capacity (point of fatigue) is the measure of our physical fitness.
      1. The most fit persons have the greatest spread.
      2. The least fit, the least spread.
   D. *Aerobic capacity* (maximal oxygen intake of a person) is an indicator of degree of fitness.
      1. Overall fitness of the body systems seems to be an accurate measurement of a person's fitness.
      2. This means that a person should have the ability to engage in prolonged physical activity without undue fatigue.
   E. Three categories of fitness
      1. Passive fitness—the person makes no effort to keep his body fit.
      2. Muscular fitness—individuals emphasize isometrics or calisthenics.
      3. Total fitness—persons engage in balanced activities that strengthen all body systems.
II. Principles of exercise programs
   A. Activity programs
      1. While in school or college an individual should develop skills in several different activities to participate in throughout life.
      2. Total-fitness programs are valuable for both males and females.
   B. Muscular strength and muscular endurance
      1. Muscular strength is the maximal force, or tension, a muscle can exert in a single contraction.
      2. Muscular endurance is the ability of the muscles either to maintain maximal contraction or to respond repetitively for a relatively long time.
      3. Isometric contractions produce muscle strength.
      4. Isotonic contractions produce both muscle strength and endurance.
   C. Circulatory endurance—cardiorespiratory functioning which produces results called conditioning, training effect, and aerobic capacity.

D. Exercise tolerance—the level at which the body responds to exercise favorably.
    1. Pulse rate of 151 for individuals under thirty years of age.
    2. Pulse rate of 131 for individuals over thirty years of age.
E. Overloading and progression
    1. Overloading is the process of extending oneself beyond his usual physical effort.
    2. Progression is a gradual increase in complexity of exercises.
F. Warming up—has two interpretations.
    1. Each time one exercises or participates in a sport, he should first warm up.
    2. Individuals who have not exercised regularly for a number of years should recondition themselves on a warm-up basis over a period of weeks or months before participating in a regular exercise or sports program.
G. Easing off—gradually returning the body to normal after exercising.

III. Total-fitness conditioning
A. Should always include the three principles of fitness.
    1. Muscular strength.
    2. Muscular endurance.
    3. Circulatory endurance.
B. Should be performed regularly.

IV. Total-fitness programs
A. Important to consult a physical educator to design a balanced program.
    1. Women should take special care to select balanced programs.
    2. Exercises during pregnancy should be upon consultation with an obstetrician.
B. Calisthenics—value is that you can exercise specific groups of muscles.
C. Weight training—a combination of weight lifting and calisthenics.
D. Exercises for circulatory endurance
    1. Walking, jogging, and running, done in graduated increments, improve appearance and endurance:
        a. walking is the most natural of all forms of exercise.
        b. jogging is a steady, easy-paced running.
        c. running can be very effective in maintaining circulatory endurance.
    2. Aerobics—a total-fitness program designed to improve cardiovascular endurance.
    3. Circuit training:
        a. carefully selected exercises arranged and numbered consecutively and ranging over a given area, or circuit.
        b. increased muscular strength, muscular endurance, and cardiovascular endurance.
    4. Rope skipping:
        a. excellent cardiovascular exercise.
        b. for cardiovascular endurance, 10 minutes as good as 30 minutes jogging.

V. Sports—use of leisure time
A. A sport may serve as a conditioning program.
B. If a sport is to supply the requirements of a total-fitness program, it must be vigorous; should be participated in at least three times a week; and should produce at least a 60-minute workout.

Glossary

If you cannot find the word you wish in this glossary, check the index for text and glossary references.

aerobic capacity. The maximal oxygen intake of a person.

agility (a jil'ə ti). The ability to move quickly and easily.

calisthenics (kal'əs then'iks) (G. *kallos*, beauty; *sthenos*, strength). Athletic exercises; simple gymnastics.

circulatory endurance. The ability of the body to perform under stress without undue fatigue.

dual sports. Sports that require two participants, such as tennis and badminton.

exercise tolerance. The level at which the body responds favorably to exercise.

individual sports. Sports that require only one participant, such as golf, running, jogging, and swimming.

interval training. Alternate periods of vigorous activity and walking or reduced activity.

isometrics (isə met'riks) (G. *isometro*, equal; *metron*, measure). A method of physical exercise in which one set of muscles is briefly tensed in opposition to another set of muscles or in opposition to a solid surface.

isotonic (ī'sə ton'ik) (G. *isotonos*, equal; *tonos*, a stretching). Any exercise in which muscles are put through their full range of movement while a moderate weight or load is sustained.

resistance. In exercise, the weight to be lifted, or work load.

repetitions (rep'ə tish'ənz) (L. *repetere*, to repeat). In exercise, the total number of times a weight is to be lifted within a set.

set. In exercise, the number of groups of *repetitions* done consecutively without resting.

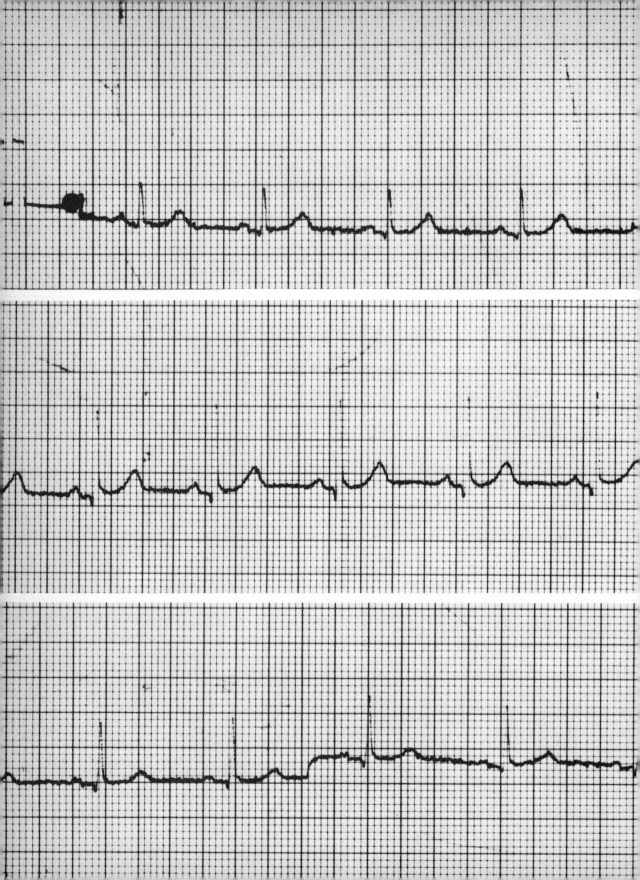

The heart and circulation

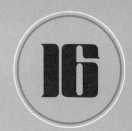

Seventy-five years ago in the United States acute infectious diseases were the most pressing health problem. Dr. Paul Dudley White, the famous Boston heart specialist, recalls that when he was a young physician, hospital staffs had difficulty making hospital beds available fast enough to take care of the many cases of typhoid fever. Today all of this has changed.

Today we can look forward to a longer life than our grandparents. The average life expectancy of 49 years in 1900 has risen to over 70 today. Medicine and public health have successfully overcome the great historic killers—acute infectious diseases. But dimming this bright picture is the high death toll of chronic diseases. Among these the *cardiovascular* ailments are by far the chief producers of illness, disability, and death among both middle-aged and elderly people. One in particular, *atherosclerotic* heart disease, accounts for almost one third of all deaths. Researchers, public and private, have mounted a massive campaign against this number-one villain—in terms not only of treating those already afflicted, but also of identifying the factors causing cardiovascular diseases and preventing their complications. Although there are encouraging omens, the task is far from complete. This chapter describes the structure and functions of the circulatory organs and their disorders and surveys the present state of heart research.

CIRCULATORY SYSTEM

The billions of cells of the human body must have, not only a sure source of food and oxygen, but also protection against the waste materials that are produced in them as food is turned into energy. The *circulatory system* is responsible for the continuous and rapid movement of materials to and from the cells. It carries its materials in a fluid medium, blood. It directs blood to the lungs, where oxygen is obtained, and then carries it to the cells and tissues (groups of cells). By the blood wastes are picked up from the cells and carried to the kidneys and other excretory organs, from which they are excreted, digested foods are picked up from the digestive tract and carried to tissues for storage or use, and hormones are carried around the body to regulate and coordinate activities. The blood also regulates body temperature and protects the body against disease. The blood is kept circulating by two muscular pumps contained in a single organ, the *heart*; see Fig. 16.1.

Vessels called *arteries* carry the blood away from the heart; other vessels called *veins* return it to the heart. The arteries are large as they leave the heart, but divide into smaller and smaller vessels, *arterioles,* the farther they go from it. These arterioles lead into microscopic vessels called *capillaries.* The capillaries, whose total length is more than fifty thousand miles in man, form profuse networks through the various body tissues. Through their very thin walls the exchange of materials between the blood and the tissues occurs. Each cell is bathed in this *tissue fluid* from the blood. The tissue fluid coming from the blood to the cell is rich in food and oxygen, but it is rich in waste products as it returns to the blood. As the tissue fluid from the cells collects in the capillaries, it passes to small veins, called *venules,* which combine into larger veins, the largest of which open into the heart.

The heart

Structure of the heart Approximately the size of a person's fist, the heart is an amazing bundle of muscle fibers richly interwoven with blood vessels. Nerves connecting the brain to the heart transmit information that "tells" the heart the amount of work required of it. For its size (about three fourths of a pound) this little pump turns out an astonishing amount of work. It is centrally located between the lungs, a bit to the left of the midline of the body; see Fig. 16.2. The heart is shaped like a cone; its tip (*apex*) is directed downward and to the left.

· HEART CHAMBERS   The heart is divided into four chambers, two on each side; see Fig. 16.3. The two upper chambers are called the *atria;* the two lower ones, the *ventricles.* The ventricles, the pumping chambers, are larger and have thicker muscular walls than the atria, which are the receiving chambers. The two halves of the heart are separated by a partition called the *septum;* the upper portion separating the atria is called the *interatrial septum;* the lower portion separating the ventricles, the *interventricular septum.*

· WALLS OF THE HEART   The walls of the heart are composed of three different layers. The interior is lined by a thin, smooth, shiny membrane called the *endocardium* (Fig. 16.3). This lining is continuous with the lining of the blood vessels and of the *valves* inside the heart. Inflammation of this lining is referred to as *endocarditis*. The middle and thickest layer is composed of muscular tissue; it is called the *myocardium*. The muscular tissue of the myocardium is somewhat layered, with thicker layers in the ventricles than in the atria. Externally the heart is covered by a membrane, the *epicardium*. The wall of the heart is supplied with blood from the *coronary arteries*, which lie on its surface; see Fig. 16.4.

· HEART VALVES The right atrium receives deoxygenated blood from the heart muscle and from all other body areas by way of a network of veins.

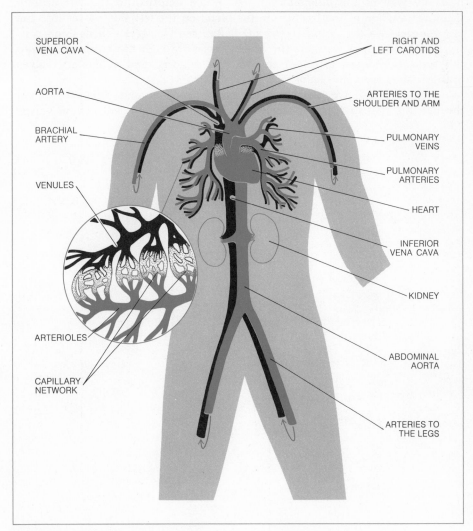

Figure 16.1   Human circulatory system showing principal arteries and veins.

These veins terminate as the *superior vena cava,* which collects blood from the upper portions of the body, and the *inferior vena cava,* which collects blood from the lower portions of the body. It transmits this blood into the right ventricle through the *tricuspid valve,* which allows blood to pass from the atrium into the ventricle but prevents its movement in a backward direction. Blood passes through this valve when the right atrium contracts, after which the right ventricle contracts. When the ventricle contracts, blood cannot pass backward through the now closed tricuspid valve but, instead, must pass on through the *pulmonary valve* into the *pulmonary artery* and on to the lungs for oxygenation. After oxygenation the blood returns to the left side of the heart by way of the *pulmonary veins,* which empty into the left atrium. Upon contraction of the left atrium the blood on the left side passes into the left ventricle via the *mitral (bicuspid) valve;* see Fig. 16.5. Then, upon contraction of the right ventricle the blood passes through the *aortic valve* into the *aorta,* the largest artery of the body. The aortic and pulmonary valves are also called *semilunar valves.*

Actually, the two atria contract simultaneously and drive the blood through the tricuspid and mitral valves at the same moment. These valves

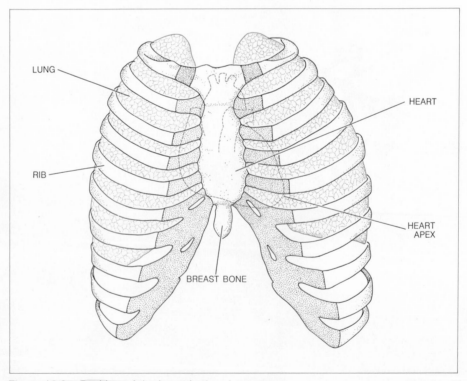

LUNG

HEART

RIB

HEART APEX

BREAST BONE

Figure 16.2   Position of the heart in the chest cage.

both close when the ventricles contract. Then both the right and left ventricles contract at the same moment and drive the blood through these two semilunar valves into the respective arteries, after which the valves close.

To prevent the tricuspid and bicuspid valves from collapsing when the ventricles contract, strong cords, the *chordae tendineae*, which are attached to the valves at one end and to the papillary muscles in the ventricle wall on the other end, contract and shorten (Fig. 16.3).

Physiology of the heart   When the body is at rest, more than 10 pints of blood are passed through each of the heart's chambers every minute. During strenuous activity the capacity of the heart increases 5 to 10 times. This organ begins its activities months before birth and never ceases until the moment of death. To give the muscle some measure of rest there is a rhythmic alternation of the contraction phase (*systole*) with a resting phase (*diastole*). The time needed for contraction and relaxation varies. At the usual rate of 70 beats per minute the diastole is twice as long as the systole. The systole phase begins in the atria, then passes into the ventricles. The systole phase results in the familiar "lub-dub" sounds of the heart. The "lub" sounds are caused

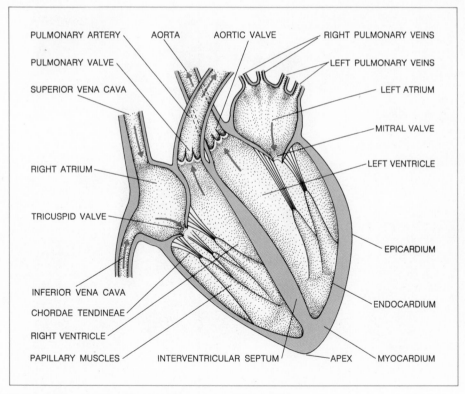

Figure 16.3   Heart, with chambers and major vessels.

mostly by the closure of the atrioventricular valves, the tricuspid and mitral, and the "dub" sound, by the closure of the semilunar valves (Fig. 16.5). If a valve fails to close properly, blood moves back through the valve, causing a swishing sound, called a *murmur*. (Other abnormalities of the heart will be discussed later.)

The heart muscle operates in a manner completely different from that of any other muscle of the body. Although the heart is under the control of the central nervous system, its beat originates independently inside the heart. The beat starts in the right atrium at a spot called the *sinoatrial node (SA node)*, also called the "pacemaker"; see Fig. 16.6. From the right atrium the impulse travels over the entire atrial muscle, causing the atria to contract. The wave action is passed to a second specialized area, the *atrioventricular node (AV node)*, located in the septum between the right atrium and ventricle. From this spot the wave action is transmitted to the *bundle of His,* a band of specialized cells which pass down the interventricular septum and divide into two main branches, called the *Purkinje fibers.* These fibers spread throughout the ventricular walls, causing the ventricles to contract.

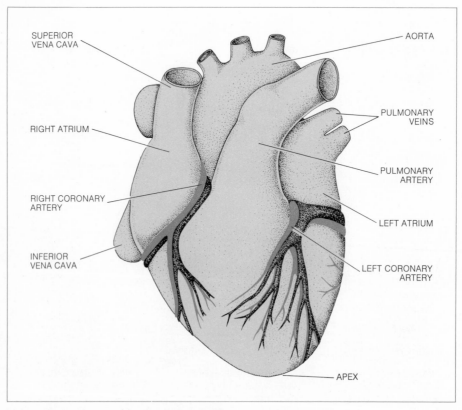

Figure 16.4   Heart, with coronary vessels.

Blood vessels

The *pulmonary circulation* carries the blood from the right ventricle toward the lungs; the *systemic circulation,* from the left ventricle to all parts of the body. Blood traveling to the heart muscle leaves the aorta through the *coronary circulation* (Fig. 16.4). Blood vessels may be divided into three groups: *arteries, capillaries,* and *veins;* see Fig. 16.7.

Arteries   Arteries carry blood away from the pumping chambers of the heart to other parts of the body. The arterial system begins with the main artery of the body, the aorta, from which lesser arteries branch off until the entire body is supplied with blood (Fig. 16.1).

Arterial walls are relatively thick, since they must sustain the pressure created on the blood by the heartbeat. The walls are composed of three layers. The elastic quality of the arteries allows them to stretch but prevents them from collapsing upon themselves. The walls contain muscle tissues that contract when the nerves supplying them are stimulated. Such contraction narrows, or constricts, the internal diameter of the arteries (*vasoconstriction*).

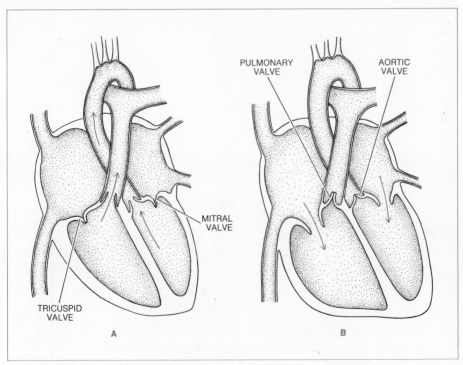

Figure 16.5   Ventricular and atrial contraction (systole): (A) contraction of the ventricles; (B) contraction of the atria. The pulmonary and aortic valves are also called the pulmonary and aortic *semilunar* valves.

When the nerves are not stimulated, the muscles relax and dilate, giving a larger internal diameter (*vasodilation*). Through branching the arteries eventually become very small. The smallest subdivisions, the arterioles, lead into the capillaries.

Capillaries The capillaries are minute, thin-walled tubes connecting the arterioles with the *venules* (Fig. 16.1). Because the capillaries have thin walls, materials carried by the blood move through them very slowly, allowing for an interchange of materials. The capillaries are exceedingly numerous. No living cell of the body is more than a few cells away from a capillary.

Veins Veins drain the tissues and the organs and return the blood to the heart. Their walls are much thinner than those of arteries, have much less muscle and elastic tissues and are easily collapsed. Consequently, they are less extensible and elastic. Since the blood pressure is reduced as it moves through the capillaries, the veins cannot depend solely upon heart pressure to move

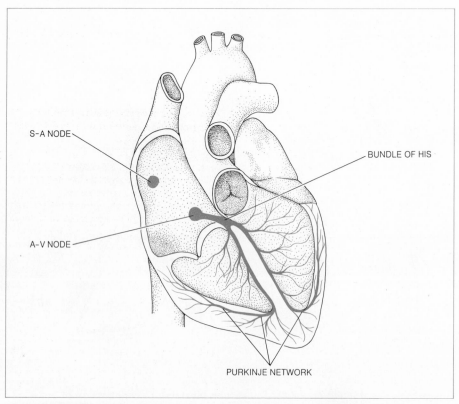

Figure 16.6   The sinoatrial node, atrioventricular node, and Purkinje system of the heart.

the blood through them. They are thus provided with one-way *valves* that prevent the blood from flowing back into the capillaries; see Fig. 16.8. Many veins are located in the skeletal muscles. As one exercises and stretches, he assists the movement of the blood through the veins.

Lymphatics

The food and oxygen leave the blood in the capillaries and enter the tissue fluid. This tissue fluid, which bathes all cells of the body and acts as a connecting link between the blood and the cells, is known as *lymph*. It is made up of certain fluid portions of the blood. Lymph accumulates faster than it is

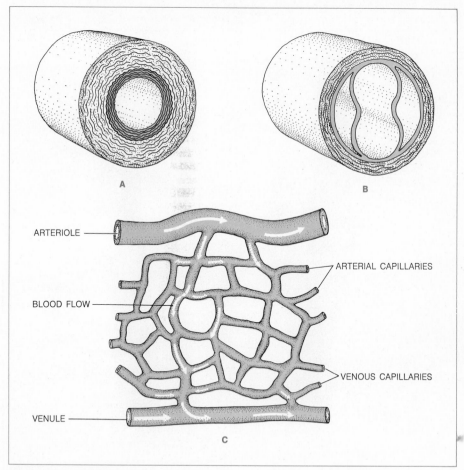

Figure 16.7   Cross sections of (A) an artery and (B) a vein; (C) diagram of a capillary bed showing arteriole and venule. Arrows indicate direction of blood flow.

able to move back into the blood capillaries. It is continually drained from the tissue spaces through a system of tubules called the *lymphatic system*. Completely separate and apart from the blood capillaries, these lymph, or collecting, capillaries begin as microscopic, blind (closed) ducts. As they become larger, they finally converge into veins near the neck. In the intestinal wall the lymphatic capillaries are called *lacteals*.

The lymphatic vessels are thin-walled and are provided with valves, like the valves of the veins, to prevent backflow. Exercise and changes in body position help to maintain the flow of lymph. The lymphatic system has no pump, or heart, to push the lymph along.

As the lymph is returned to the veins, it passes through a series of filters

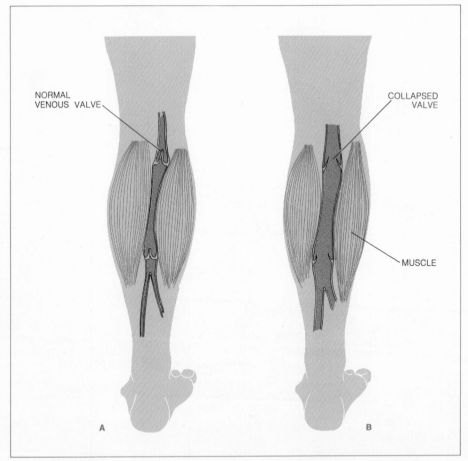

NORMAL
VENOUS VALVE

COLLAPSED
VALVE

MUSCLE

A   B

Figure 16.8   Veins of leg: (A) with closed one-way valves; (B) with collapsed valves in varicose veins.

called *lymph nodes*. Here certain undesirable particles are taken out of circulation. Made of specialized tissue, called *lymphoid tissue,* the nodes remove and to some extent destroy impurities such as carbon particles, cancer cells, dead blood cells, and pathogenic organisms. These foreign proteins and bacteria are ingested and partly destroyed by certain white blood cells normally present. The nodes manufacture *lymphocytes,* which make up about one fifth of all white blood cells and produce antibodies (Chapter 17).

Lymph nodes are quite variable in size and tend to occur in groups. They are located in chains of several nodes up to several hundred, the greatest masses being found along the side of the head and neck, in the nose-throat area, under the armpits, and in the groin. Lymph nodes close to cancer sites tend to collect wandering cancer cells; thus nodes near known cancer sites are commonly surgically removed along with the cancerous tissue. An example would be the removal of lymph nodes in the armpit of a woman at the same time that her cancerous breast is removed.

Fetal circulation

During fetal life the blood of the unborn child travels through the umbilical arteries (in the umbilical cord) to the mother to be oxygenated. It returns to the child from the mother by way of the umbilical vein, is passed to the liver, and thence into the right atrium; see Fig. 16.9. Accordingly, the blood in the right atrium is rather well oxygenated. Since the child's lungs are not yet functioning, and since much of the blood entering the right side of the heart is already oxygenated, the unborn child is normally provided with two short circuits that allow much of the blood to bypass the lungs. An opening in the interatrial septum, the *foramen ovale,* provides for some of this short-circuiting, and a connection between the pulmonary artery and the aorta, the *ductus arteriosus,* provides for the rest. The main volume of blood passes through the foramen ovale.

At birth the child's lungs become functional, and the placental circulation is broken. Normally, during the first year a septum closes over the foramen ovale. This closure is incomplete in about 20 percent of all individuals. The ductus arteriosus normally closes during the first month of life.

Blood

Blood is the fluid that circulates through the closed circulatory system to all tissues of the body. Under normal conditions it consists of a straw-colored fluid, or *plasma,* in which are suspended the *corpuscles,* which are the red blood cells, or *erythrocytes,* the white blood cells, or *leukocytes,* and the *platelets;* see Fig. 16.10. The fluid portion makes up about 55 percent of the whole blood; the cells, or solid portion, about 45 percent. Since blood is continuously exchanging materials with tissues it services, its composition is constantly changing.

Plasma   The plasma, the liquid portion of the blood, is about 90 percent water; the remaining 10 percent contains many different substances, including proteins, carbohydrates (principally in the form of glucose), lipids (fats), and mineral salts (including compounds of calcium and sodium).

Red blood cells (RBCs) The red blood cells are tiny, disc-shaped bodies. They are normally formed in the bone marrow and usually live no longer than 120 days. Their main purpose is to carry oxygen from the lungs to the tissues. This function is made possible by the pigment *hemoglobin*, which is also responsible for the red color of these cells. The more oxygen present, the brighter the red; the less oxygen, the darker the red.

White blood cells (WBCs) The white blood cells consist of various types of colorless cells. Although generally spherical, they have the ability to change

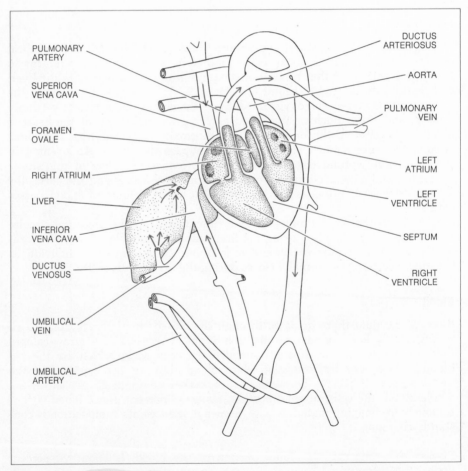

Figure 16.9 Fetal circulation.

shape. Their flexibility allows some of them to leave the capillaries, which the red blood cells cannot do. Monocytes and neutrophils play an active role in protecting the body against infection and in destroying bacteria and dead tissue by a process called *phagocytosis*. In this process the white blood cells surround and engulf, then kill and digest, the bacteria with enzymes. Sometimes they are affected by the poisons given off by the pathogens and die. They then become a part of the accumulation of material we know as *pus* or an *abscess*. The white blood cells that return to the bloodstream generally do so by the way of the lymph.

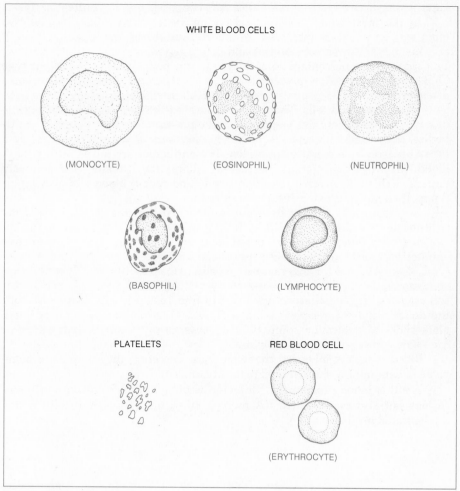

Figure 16.10   Blood cells.

Platelets Derived from large bone-marrow cells which fragment, *platelets* or *thrombocytes* are essential to blood clotting, or *coagulation*. When they come in contact with a blood-vessel injury, they adhere to the damaged area. They then disintegrate and release a chemical, which reacts with the protein in the plasma. *Fibrinogen,* a soluble plasma protein, with the aid of certain other blood constituents, changes into a solid mass called *fibrin*, which forms the clot.

Blood types and transfusions

If, for any of a number of reasons, the amount of blood in the body is too severely reduced, a person may need additional blood in the form of a *transfusion.* Before the twentieth century transfusions often had disastrous results. Later it was discovered that *red blood cells* contained specific protein *antigens.*

In the most widely used blood-typing system, the *ABO System,* two main antigen types are identified, A and B. Type A persons inherit A, type B persons B, type AB persons both A and B, and type O persons neither A nor B. The approximate percentage of each type in our population is 47 percent type O, 41 percent type A, 9 percent type B, and 3 percent type AB. A person's *plasma* contains other proteins, called *antibodies,* which complement the antigens in the red blood cells. There are two such antibodies, *a* and *b*. The plasma of a type B person contains *a* antibodies, the plasma of a type A person *b* antibodies, the plasma of a type AB person neither antibody, and the plasma of a type O person both *a* and *b* antibodies. If *a* antibodies are mixed with type A blood, the RBCs will gather together in clumps (agglutinate) and seriously impede circulation. A mixture of *b* antibody and type B blood will also agglutinate. If clumping is extensive, death follows.

In transfusions it must be firmly established that the *recipient's plasma* will not destroy the *donor's RBCs.* It is always best to give blood of the recipient's own type. It may be possible in an emergency, however, to give another type of blood. Type O persons can give blood to a recipient of type O, A, B, or AB, and for this reason are called *universal donors.* Type AB persons can receive blood from donors of type O, A, B, and AB, and for this reason are called *universal acceptors.* Prior to transfusion small volumes of both the donor's and the recipient's blood should be *cross-matched* (mixed on a glass slide) to determine compatibility. Absence of clumping indicates that the two blood specimens are compatible.

Blood types are inherited characteristics. Therefore they may be of some value in determining the disputed paternity of a child.

Another blood protein, the Rh factor, is of significance not only in transfusions but also in childbirth. (A more detailed discussion of the Rh factor can be found in Chapter 11.)

Blood count

The normal RBC count is 4.5 to 5.5 million per cubic millimeter of blood; the normal WBC count is 6,000 to 8,000 per cubic millimeter. This is a ratio of

RBCs to WBCs of 700 or 800 to 1. An apparatus for counting the number of blood cells, the *hemocytometer*, is generally used. Since the numbers of red and white cells vary rather quickly in response to certain physical conditions, a count can be used for diagnostic purposes.

Blood disorders

There are many abnormalities involving the blood. A brief discussion of several of the more common forms follows.

Anemias Anemia means a deficiency of red blood cells. Some anemias are *functional*—due to physical problems in the body; others are *hereditary*, and they tend to result in very fragile red blood cells.

· FUNCTIONAL ANEMIAS Functional anemias may be caused either by a reduction in the number of red blood cells or by the amount of hemoglobin in the cells. A reduction in the number of cells may be due to a hemorrhage (loss of blood), to destruction of red cells by organisms such as malarial parasites or by coal-tar products, or to abnormalities in the RBC-forming mechanism as a result of overexposure to x-rays, radioactive substances, or organic poisoning. Since hemoglobin contains iron, an iron deficiency may reduce the hemoglobin concentration and cause an iron-deficiency type of anemia, a type that responds well to treatment. Anemia may also result from a dietary deficiency of protein or certain vitamins.

· HEREDITARY ANEMIAS The hereditary anemias constitute one of the most serious kinds of blood disease. The two most prevalent types are concentrated in specific "races."

Sickle-cell anemia. Affecting chiefly blacks (about 8 percent in the United States), the condition results in a twisted, sickle-shaped red blood cell. Inheritance of the gene from one parent causes a mild condition with scattered sickle-shaped cells. Inheritance from both parents causes extensive cell sickling; death occurs in about 50 percent of the population of such persons before the age of 20. Overexertion or oxygen shortage can bring on a crisis in which cells become sickle shaped, bunch up in tiny capillaries, impede blood flow, and clot, often causing death. The cells are also very fragile, leading to serious anemias.

Cooley's (Mediterranean) anemia. In this hereditary anemia the red blood cells are small, have fragile membranes, and are easily ruptured upon passing through the tissues. A gene from one parent produces a mild blood abnormality, but genes from both parents produce, not only severe anemia, but skeletal abnormalities, mongoloid features, and death, usually in early life. The disease is preponderant among persons of Italian, Greek, and Armenian descent.

Leukocytosis An elevation of the WBC count to 10,000 to 25,000 cells per cubic millimeter, or higher, is *leukocytosis*. It is a natural response to infection and fever. *Leukemia* is an extreme leukocytosis due to an enormous, uncontrolled increase of one or more kinds of white blood cells, a form of cancer. Leukemia is further discussed in Chapter 17.

Leukopenias   *Leukopenias* are diseases or conditions that reduce the number of white blood cells below a satisfactory level. They may result from infections (such as typhoid fever and malaria), side effects of various drugs and treatments, radiation injury, and certain poisonings. Individuals with this condition run great risk of infection. The condition usually disappears after the agent responsible for the leukopenia has been withdrawn.

Hemophilia   In *hemophila* the normal coagulation process is delayed, leading to abnormal bleeding. It is an inherited trait, in which the blood clots very slowly and the clot is quite fragile. It is associated with a genetic deficiency in one of several blood components. A hemophiliac is in danger of excessive bleeding. At this time all known treatment is either ineffectual or temporary. There is no effective oral medication. The best known treatment is the administration of the blood factor that is deficient, but even this is a temporary measure. Many persons with this condition die early in life.

Pulse and blood pressure

With each beat of the heart, which averages about 70 per minute in humans, blood is forced out of each ventricle. It flows into the aorta from the left ventricle with great force, and from the right ventricle into the pulmonary artery with moderate force. The rapid contraction of the heart makes this discharge of blood rapid, spurtlike, and intermittent. During the interval of each beat the heart collects as much blood from the body as it discharges. With each beat of the left ventricle (Fig. 16.3) a wave of pressure starts at the heart and travels along the arteries. This wave is called the *pulse*. The pulse can be felt on any arteries that are close to the surface of the body, such as on the wrist, the sides of the throat, or the temple. The pulse is the result of the pressure of the blood on the walls of the arteries—the *blood pressure*. This pressure is highest in the aorta; it gradually decreases as it travels through the arteries, capillaries, veins, and into the right atrium. Although the blood pressure is greater after the left ventricle contracts, there is always some pressure in the arteries. The blood pressure at the moment of contraction is the *systolic pressure*; it should normally be sufficient to displace about 120 millimeters of mercury (mm Hg) in a glass tube. The blood pressure at the moment of relaxation of the heart is the *diastolic pressure*; it should normally displace about 80 mm Hg. The average blood pressure of a normal young person is about this, which is customarily written 120/80 and spoken of as "one-twenty over eighty."

The usual instrument for determining arterial blood pressure is called a *sphygmomanometer*; see Fig. 16.11. It consists of a rubber cuff wrapped around the arm and connected by a tube to either an aneroid indicator or a scaled mercury column. The cuff is inflated so that it collapses the brachial artery in the arm. By listening to the flow of blood through the artery with a *stethoscope* as the air in the cuff is let out, a physician can determine systolic and diastolic blood pressure.

Factors influencing pulse rate   A number of things can influence pulse rate. It tends to be faster in smaller people and in women. It tends to be faster in a newborn infant than in an adult. It increases proportionately with increases in bodily activity, and it decreases during sleep. It is also faster when a person has not been getting sufficient physical exercise. It increases under emotional

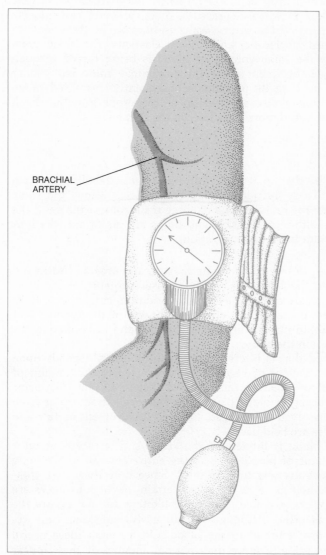

BRACHIAL
ARTERY

Figure 16.11   Sphygmomanometer for measuring blood pressure.

excitement, even when no muscular activity is involved. Many infections will increase the pulse rate as the temperature increases.

Factors influencing abnormal blood pressure   The nature of the blood pressure may indicate any number of factors of importance in a person's circulation. It can indicate the strength of the heart action. It can reflect the volume of blood in circulation. A decrease in circulation or volume, as through shock or hemorrhage, will cause a drop in blood pressure. An increase in volume will cause a corresponding increase in pressure. Blood pressure can indicate whether the elastic quality of the artery walls is normal. In the event an artery becomes "hardened" (sclerotic) and loses it elasticity, the blood pressure will increase, since the same volume of blood is being forced through a smaller opening. Any impediment along the circulatory route will hinder the flow of blood and increase its pressure. Consequently, increased blood pressure may indicate kidney disease, uremia, or cancerous growths. High blood pressure will be discussed more fully later in the chapter.

Elimination of blood waste

After the food brought by the blood to the cell has been metabolized, certain waste products remain. These include urea, carbon dioxide, water, and salts. They are eliminated from the body by one of three main routes: the skin, the lungs, and the kidneys. Although the skin and lungs are important, the kidneys are the most important in blood purification.

The kidneys   The kidneys serve to eliminate most of the urea and salts and much of the water from the body. As the body uses proteins, it produces nitrogenous wastes, which are excreted as urea. In addition, certain salts from the blood plasma also are excreted. Excretion is only one of the functions of the kidneys: they also aid in maintaining water balance and in regulating the balance of acids and bases in the body.

The amount of blood that is filtered through the kidneys depends upon the blood pressure. This amount of blood flow is reflected in the amount of urine produced. If the blood pressure falls too low (below 40 mm Hg), urine ceases to flow. In the filtering of blood plasma the kidneys extract water from the blood along with dissolved substances. Blood cells, droplets of fat, and other very large molecules are held back.

A large volume of blood is filtered by the kidneys. The rate is about 1 quart per minute. A volume of blood equal to the entire amount in the body flows through the kidneys every 4 to 5 minutes. Since only the larger components of the blood are held back in filtration, certain useful substances are filtered along with the waste products; these the kidneys reclaim before the wastes are passed out as urine. Although not all useful substances are reclaimed, most of them are returned to the blood. On occasion these useful substances appear in the urine in more than normal amounts if they appear in the blood in higher than normal concentrations, such as excess glucose in diabetics.

The general body blood pressure tends to increase if the *renal* (kidney) arteries are obstructed or narrowed. Occasionally such rise is due to tumors of the kidneys. Either of these can be a cause of persistent hypertension.

The role of exercise With a daily exercise routine the lungs begin processing more air with less effort, the heart grows stronger, more blood is pumped with fewer strokes, the blood supply to the muscles improves, and the total blood volume increases. The body's capacity to deliver oxygen to tissue cells is improved, and more energy is produced. In short, a person increases his endurance capacity or total fitness.

During muscular activity the amount of carbon dioxide is increased. The body can maintain sufficient oxygen supply and elimination of carbon dioxide during light or moderate exercise. During severe exercise, however, the carbon dioxide concentration begins to increase faster than the supply of oxygen, and it takes the body some time after the exertion has ceased to catch up on the necessary elimination of the oversupply of carbon dioxide. For a further discussion of exercise see Chapter 15.

CARDIOVASCULAR DISORDERS

Like any other tissues of the body, those of the heart and circulatory system are subject to disease and infection. Diseases in tissues of an arm or leg may cripple a person, but diseases of the heart muscle frequently lead to early death. Cardiovascular diseases are the leading causes of death among adults all over the world. Some conditions arise during fetal development or near the time of birth and are said to be *congenital;* others occur later to a normally developed heart and are said to be *degenerative.*

Congenital heart disease

Abnormalities in the development of the heart may occur during the first three months of fetal life. Although the specific causes of congenital malformations of the heart are generally unknown, the known causes include certain maternal illnesses or metabolic upsets during the first three months of pregnancy, such as German measles, mumps, or influenza. Ionizing radiations (such as x-rays) and certain drugs may have similar effects. According to the President's Commission on Heart Disease, Cancer and Stroke, more than twenty thousand babies with heart deformities are born each year in this country. These malformations are common to all parts of the world and all races, and most of them present a severe handicap to the child. Such inborn heart defects are thought not to be inherited. A mother with a congenital heart defect has about a 2 percent chance of passing such a malformation on to her children.

Congenital heart defects Heart malformations may take many forms. They may affect any part of the heart. The extent of the malformation may be slight or extensive. Because some of them cause reduction in the normal supply of oxygenated blood, the skin takes on a bluish hue; thus they are generally called "blue baby" conditions.

· SEPTAL DEFECTS   An abnormal opening in the septum may occur between the two atria (*atrioseptal defect*). The most common is the persistence of the foramen ovale, a normal fetal opening between the two atria (Fig. 16.9). Incomplete closure (*patent foramen ovale*) occurs in about one out of every four individuals. This foramen allows the deoxygenated blood from the right side to move to the left atrium, which should be transmitting oxygenated blood. In a small number of cases the presence of sufficient impure blood passing into the aorta may give a bluish hue to the skin, hence the term "blue baby."

A ventricular septal defect has a different effect. Since the blood in the left ventricle is under more pressure than that in the right ventricle, the defect, which is an opening in the septum, allows some of the blood to move from the left ventricle into the right ventricle rather than into the aorta. Thus less blood is available for the aortic flow. To compensate, the heart usually works harder, placing an extra load on it and causing it to fail at an earlier age.

· PATENT DUCTUS ARTERIOSUS   Earlier it was noted that in the fetal circulatory system a duct, the ductus arteriosus, exists between the pulmonary artery and the aorta and that this duct normally closes during the first month of life (see Fig. 16.9). If it fails to close, it is a *patent ductus arteriosus*. Since aortic blood is under greater pressure than pulmonary blood, some of the pure aortic blood passes into the pulmonary artery. The systemic (body) circulation is thus deprived of some blood. To compensate, the heart works harder. This condition allows the person less reserve for strenuous activities and high altitudes and also reduces the life span of his heart. Usually, if this condition is not corrected by surgery, the patient dies between the ages of 20 and 40. Corrective surgery is quite effective.

· STENOSIS   A stenosis is a fusing of the leaflets of either of the semilunar valves, pulmonary or aortic. Such fusion (narrowing) hampers the flow of blood and increases the work the heart must do. Surgery can be performed on selected patients. A severe, uncorrected case can place such a work load on the heart that the heart is likely to fail earlier than it normally would.

· TETRALOGY OF FALLOT   Caused by a combination of defects, the tetralogy of Fallot results in poor oxygenation of the blood. It includes (1) a hole in the septum between the ventricles, (2) displacement of the aorta to the right, so that it receives blood from both ventricles, (3) stenosis of the pulmonary valve, restricting blood flow to the lungs, and (4) enlargement of the right ventricle. It is the most common cause of "blue babies." The condition usually is treated relatively successfully by surgery.

Future for congenital deformities   Until thirty-five years ago about one out of every three congenital heart patients survived to the age of ten. Today the development of the *heart-lung machine*, a device which takes over the functions of the heart and lungs while they are bypassed for surgical repair, has made *open-heart surgery* possible. Such surgery involves operating on the heart directly. The heart-lung machine is also used when repair is called for in a major artery or vein. Although new improvements are being made in congenital heart surgery, the ultimate goal of cardiology is to discover what causes congenital heart defects and to find ways of preventing them.

Degenerative heart disease

Although the heart is very resistant to disorders, many things can impair its efficiency. Heart disease may result from infections, toxins, injuries, insufficient nutrition, or other disturbances that weaken an otherwise healthy organ. The following kinds of degenerative heart disorders are common.

Rheumatic heart disease   As explained in Chapter 19, about 3 percent of persons suffering from certain streptococcal infections develop, two or three weeks later, the symptoms of *rheumatic fever;* these symptoms are swelling and pain in the joints, accompanied by fever. The original infection may be in any part of the body, but it is commonly a "strep throat" or tonsillitis. Rheumatic fever is an allergic response to such streptococcal infection. Often the heart is inflamed and may be permanently damaged.

Although other layers of the heart may be affected, the most common damage is to the endocardium, the inner lining of the heart. This *endocarditis* (inflammation of the endocardium) causes the heart valves, particularly the mitral valve, to become scarred, since the valves consist mostly of endocardium. Material from the blood deposits on the scarred valves; they thicken and tend to stick together and thus are prevented from opening properly. Or the scarring may prevent the valve from closing tightly, so that blood leaks back through the valve, forcing the heart to pump harder in order to circulate an adequate supply of blood. Open-heart surgery has been increasingly effective in relieving such damage. The scar tissue may be removed, or the damaged valves may even be replaced with artificial valves.

Antibiotic therapy has lowered the incidence of and death rate from rheumatic fever. As a preventive measure, all streptococcal infections should be treated promptly. The person with a history of rheumatic fever must be particularly prompt in seeking treatment for infections, since one attack of rheumatic fever leaves a person highly susceptible to repeated attacks for the rest of his life.

Coronary heart disease   The blood vessels surrounding the heart, the coronary arteries and veins, derive their name from the fact that they encircle the heart like a crown, or *corona.* They transport almost 0.5 pint of blood every minute over the heart muscle. Any sudden obstruction of one of the coronary arteries will deprive that respective part of the heart of its blood supply and will cause the muscle to cease to function; see Fig. 16.12. This deadening of an area of heart muscle is called a *myocardial infarction;* it is manifested by a typical pain in the chest and sometimes by an arrest of the heart. If a coronary artery is completely obstructed, whatever the cause, the condition is called a *coronary occlusion* or *heart attack.* Sudden death usually occurs if the occlusion occurs in a main coronary artery. If the obstruction is only partial or is in a smaller coronary tributary, sufficient nutrition and rest may lead to the patient's recovery. The agonizing pain caused when such an area of dead tissue is formed may be felt in the region of the heart and in the left arm and shoulder. Severe heart pain is called *angina pectoris*. Angina pectoris may be accompanied by a sensation of suffocation and a feeling of impending doom.

Fortunately, the great majority of heart-disease patients recover and are able to lead active, useful lives—provided they get proper treatment under good medical supervision. Better than one third of all deaths in the United States, however, result from coronary artery disease. Almost all elderly persons have at least some impairment of coronary artery circulation.

In all cases, the best medical care is essential. Great care is necessary, particularly during the critical time of the second and third days after an attack, when the rhythm of the heart may be disturbed. After the infarction, the dead portion of the heart is replaced in a few weeks by fibrous tissue.

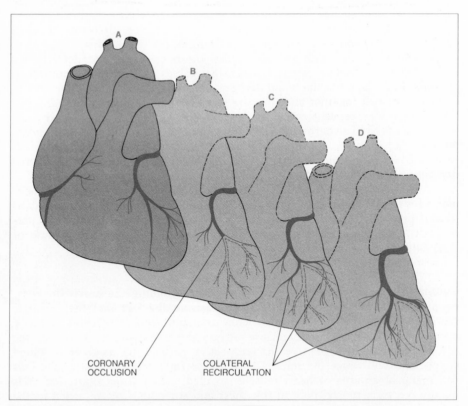

CORONARY OCCLUSION

COLATERAL RECIRCULATION

Figure 16.12   Development of heart obstruction and repair: (A) coronary arteries of heart; (B) coronary occlusion; (C) collateral circulation; (D) restoration of coronary circulation.

At the same time new blood vessels begin taking the place of the occluded artery. Eventually, if full recovery is made, all that will remain on the heart will be a scar.

It is important to distinguish between a coronary *attack* and a coronary *failure*. An attack may be mild or severe and may or may not lead to death. A coronary failure is the stoppage of the heart and, in most cases, will lead to the death of the patient unless emergency treatment is successful in reviving the victim.

Heart block   As a result of degeneration or disease in the nerve cells of the heart the rhythmic transmission of nerve impulses regulating the heartbeat may be disturbed. The exact type of heart block produced will depend upon the location of the destruction, although in all cases some degree of impulse interference, or blockage, occurs. A *sinoatrial block* affects the nerve transmission through the atria. The ventricles pick up a new rhythm and perform normally. An *atrioventricular block* prevents the transmission of the impulse from the AV node to the ventricles. Although a complete stoppage of the ventricular beat would mean death, this type of blockage often only reduces the number of ventricular contractions to the atrial contractions. For every two atrial beats the ventricles may beat only once, creating a 2:1 rhythm, or perhaps a 3:2 or a 3:1 rhythm, instead of the normal 1:1 rhythm.

Atherosclerosis   Atherosclerosis is a disease principally of the large arteries. Platelike lipid (fat) deposits, called *plaques*, appear at one or more points in the inner walls (*tunica intima*) of the arteries. As these plaques enlarge, they commonly protrude into the channel (*lumen*) of the artery. The roughness of this inner surface may cause blood clots (*thrombi*) to develop at these sites. A thrombus may cause the partial or complete obstruction (*occlusion*) of the vessel at this spot and shut off blood flow. On occasion a thrombus may break loose into the bloodstream. Such a moving clot, or *embolus*, may be carried to a point where it completely blocks the flow of blood. Although other substances, such as air, fat plaques, or tumorous material also may cause emboli, clots are the most common cause. Owing to the absence of calcium in atherosclerotic arteries, x-rays do not show a clear picture of them unless some dye is injected into the artery before the x-ray.

Although atherosclerotic damage may occur in any vessel, it is most severe in certain places. If it occurs in the heart muscle, the patient has a heart attack; if in the brain, a stroke; if in the foot, gangrene; if in the kidney, high blood pressure. The patient may be fortunate and be able to develop *collateral circulation* (enlargement of other vessels in the same area to make up for the lost circulation). Although the consequences of atherosclerosis usually appear during old age, there is evidence of it in some young adults. The full-blown disease in older people probably is the result of a lifetime of lipid deposition within the arteries.

Although some medical scientists believe that cholesterol in the diet is the chief contributor to atherosclerosis, it appears that there are other contributing factors. Some now strongly suspect refined sugar (sucrose, table sugar) as a primary cause of deaths from heart disease. While saturated-fat consumption in the United States has gone down slightly since 1900, sugar consumption has doubled. Some researchers consider sugar consumption more closely related to heart disease than saturated-fat intake.

Hypertension Hypertension simply means high arterial blood pressure. Sometimes it can be traced to a known disease, and that disease can be cured. Most commonly, however, it is a hereditary factor, called *essential hypertension*, that tends to run in families. Whatever the cause, the increase in blood pressure puts added strain on the left ventricle, sometimes causing it to enlarge and thus reducing its ability to respond to the demands made on it.

The causes of essential hypertension are known in a minority of cases. Among them are chronic inflammation of the kidneys and certain diseases of the endocrine glands. Fortunately, a number of effective drugs are available, including sedatives, which can satisfactorily reduce the blood pressure if prescribed in time. Some sufferers from hypertension have been successfully treated by a drastic reduction of the quantity of sodium in their diets, but the resulting reduction in blood pressure brought about by this treatment involves an incompletely understood mechanism which probably has something to do with the kidneys.

Cerebrovascular accidents The brain demands more than one fifth of all the blood pumped by the heart. As with the heart, any interruption in the normal flow of blood to the brain can have serious consequences. Such interruptions, commonly called *strokes,* or *apoplexy,* may come about in any of several ways: blockage of an artery by the formation of a clot (*thrombus*), blockage due to an *embolus* carried from some other place in the body, rupture of a blood vessel in the brain as a result of high blood pressure or of an *aneurysm* (ballooning of a vessel at a weakened spot), and a cutting off of the flow of blood by a tumor that places pressure on a blood vessel; see Fig. 16.13.

Depending upon its size and location, the stroke may be severe enough to cause rapid death or be too slight to be noticed. The common symptoms of moderately severe strokes include speech impediments, loss of memory or mental activity, and often partial paralysis. Since nerve cells on one side of the brain control the muscles on the opposite side of the body, a cerebrovascular accident in one side of the brain usually causes paralysis on only the other side of the body, a condition called *hemiplegia.*

Great progress has been made both in the treatment of stroke patients and in their rehabilitation. Most patients who survive the acute phase are able to lead a life which, although restricted to some extent, is nevertheless satisfying.

Vascular disorders In addition to the abnormal conditions of the blood vessels already discussed, there are several others.

· ANEURYSMS As mentioned, an aneurysm is a saclike or ballooned section of the wall of an artery or vein resulting from a localized weakness in that part of the vessel. Most commonly the aorta is the vessel affected. Such damage may result from lesions caused by syphilis or from the effects of atherosclerosis. Regardless of the cause, aneurysms tend to enlarge and thus weaken the walls affected. Under excess pressure, the aneurysm may suddenly burst; if it bursts in a critical location, as in the aorta, immediate death results. In some cases modern surgery can replace weakened aortic sections with synthetic materials.

· HEMORRHAGE   Hemorrhage is the profuse escape of blood from the vessels. It may occur from any vessels, external or internal, regardless of size or location. If only a small vessel is involved, normal clotting mechanisms will usually stop the flow. Loss of blood from a larger vessel, particularly an artery, may often be rapid and fatal. Immediate first aid through the use of direct pressure on the wound or the manual compression of the artery at a critical pressure point where the artery crosses a bone may successfully halt the loss of blood.

· SHOCK   Shock is a general, highly dangerous condition in which circulation is suddenly reduced. A state of shock may be brought on by a number of conditions—severe hemorrhage, a sudden nervous disturbance, burns,

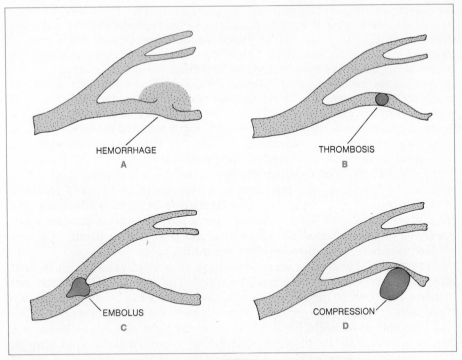

Figure 16.13   Causes of stroke: (A) hemorrhage, or bleeding; (B) thrombosis, or clot formation; (C) embolism, or traveling clot; (D) compression. Tumor or swollen tissue may stop the flow of blood. Cause may vary, but the effect of reduced circulation is the same in each case.

prolonged surgery, certain drugs, cold or exhaustion, or anything that causes a lack of oxygen in the blood. One or more of these factors may cause the small vessels to expand, with the result that blood drains from the large vessels into the small vessels of the tissues and stops circulating. Thus the blood volume is in effect markedly reduced, and essential organs that need constant circulation are deprived of the contents of the blood and soon begin to die. The victim may die quickly unless steps are taken to restore adequate circulation. A transfusion of whole blood is the best therapy, although plasma and plasma substitutes (such as glucose solutions) may also be used. These increase blood volume and help restore the circulation to normal.

A person in shock usually has cold, clammy skin, lowered body temperature, very low blood pressure, and shallow breathing. Temporary relief, such as keeping the patient warm and adjusting his body so that it is either horizontal or in a tilted position with feet up, is desirable until better measures can be taken.

· VARICOSE VEINS   Since blood in the veins is under less pressure than that in the arteries, the veins are equipped with internal valves arranged so that the movement of the blood through them can only be toward the heart (Fig. 16.8). These valves, along with any muscular movement, "squeeze" the nearby veins, helping to "pump" the blood back to the heart. Unfortunately, the valves are frequently destroyed. This destruction occurs when the veins have been overstretched (undue pressure placed on them) for an extended period of time, as in pregnancy or prolonged standing; this condition is more frequent in women than in men. The veins stretch so that the valves can no longer block the backflow of blood, and eventually the valves are destroyed. As a result the person develops *varicose veins*—large swollen veins either beneath the skin or deep in the tissues. Although these disfiguring veins may occur in various places on the body, they commonly are found along the lower leg. The resulting accumulation of venous blood in these damaged vessels creates pain and weakness in the affected muscles. (Varicose veins in the rectum are commonly referred to as hemorrhoids.)

Treatment includes elevation of the patient's legs, the wearing of elastic stockings or bandages, and the injection of sclerosing (hardening) solutions to restrict the swelling. Surgery may be resorted to in cases in which the vein lies just under the skin. Called *stripping* the veins, the process involves ligating (tying off) the affected section of vein and then pulling it out. The flow of blood is then rerouted through other connecting veins.

· PHLEBITIS   Phlebitis is an inflammation of a vein, resulting in distinct pain and much swelling at the point involved. The general inflammation and irritation may lead to the formation of a blood clot, a condition called *thrombophlebitis*. The same danger exists with this clot as with any other clot in the body. An embolism might break loose, enter the right side of the heart, and then be circulated to the lungs (*pulmonary embolism*), where it could form an obstruction and cause sudden death. Phlebitis has been reduced in recent years through greater use of anticoagulants, earlier exercise after surgery to ensure proper circulation, and prevention of infections.

Incidence of cardiovascular diseases

Approximately 25 percent of American adults have definite or suspected heart disease. Cardiovascular deaths account for more than 50 percent of all deaths among all ages. The causes of cardiovascular deaths in decreasing order are coronary heart disease, stroke, and hypertension. These three are responsible for more than 80 percent of all cardiovascular deaths.

Blacks in the United States are generally less prone to coronary heart disease than whites. The incidence among whites was approximately three and a half times that among blacks in some recent studies. More exactly, the studies showed that to avoid coronary heart disease it helps to be lean, black, poor, nonsmoking, and physically active. Although both genetics and environment appear to figure in the picture, physical activity rather than race may be the main protection against coronary heart disease.

The incidence of death from the major cardiovascular diseases increases markedly with age (for both sexes and among all races in this country). The only pronounced decline in deaths during the past three or four decades has been among those under 35 years of age. The greatest decline has been for those under 25 years of age. For those between 25 and 34 the mortality decline has been less for males than for females. Beyond age 35 the death rate from cardiovascular disease has been either leveling off or increasing since 1930. The most evident increase in death rates is among those over 65 years of age. Cardiovascular death rates in terms of geography show a higher mortality in the East and Far West and a lower rate in the Central and Mountain areas. The rates are higher in metropolitan than in nonmetropolitan areas. It must be noted once more that this general decline in cardiovascular deaths, although encouraging, has not been substantial and for the most part reflects a reduction in death rates from rheumatic and syphilitic heart disease. Furthermore, deaths from coronary heart disease have increased during the past decade.

ENVIRONMENTAL EFFECTS ON THE CIRCULATORY SYSTEM

According to the World Health Organization, cardiovascular disease is common to all races; it is not, as is sometimes claimed, a disease confined mainly to people of Europe and North America. Any differences in frequency and distribution of the major cardiovascular diseases can be explained by differences in environment, in nutrition, and in the general way of life. These diseases are particularly prevalent among middle-aged men.

Heart research has been unable either to place these factors in order of importance or to show that any one of them might be decisive. Nevertheless, evidence is accumulating that some factors tend to increase the risk of cardiovascular disease. Studies have made it possible to pick out individuals who are high risks for the development of atherosclerotic heart disease. Some of the risk factors that are clearly important will be discussed here.

Serum cholesterol levels

Coronary heart victims show a higher level of serum (blood) cholesterol than does the population as a whole. A man with a serum cholesterol of more than 240 milligrams (per 100 milliliters of whole blood) has more than three times the possibility of acquiring heart disease than does a man with a serum cholesterol of less than 200.

Hypertension

High blood pressure, or *hypertension*, occurs in about one out of every five persons. It can cause rupture of blood vessels in the brain, kidney, or other vital organs. Persons with systolic blood pressure greater than 160 are four times more likely to acquire heart disease than are those with pressures of less than 120. This risk has been shown to be particularly true when the higher blood pressure of the patient has caused his left ventricle to enlarge.

Smoking

Various studies have been conducted on the relationship between cigarette smoking and coronary heart disease. Present research has shown the cigarette smoker to be nearly twice the risk for developing heart disease as the non-smoker, his chances varying somewhat according to the number of cigarettes smoked. Those who have stopped smoking cigarettes have lower rates than those who have continued. Pipe and cigar smoking do not appear to be associated with an excessive risk of developing coronary heart disease.

Obesity

Heart researchers have not completely agreed with the insurance companies in finding obesity a cause of heart disease. Insurance companies have maintained for years that all overweight persons show a higher mortality. Other recent research, however, has shown that there is increased likelihood of development only among the grossly obese.

Sugar intake

Certain researchers now feel that the dramatic increase in coronary heart disease during the past 50 years is more closely related to high sugar (sucrose) consumption than to any other dietary factor. Consumption of refined sugar in the United States has doubled in the past 70 years, whereas the proportion of saturated fat in the United States diet has actually gone down slightly. It is suspected that the high sugar consumption leads to atherosclerosis through an impairment of glucose tolerance.

Social factors

Men from rural areas appear to have a lower incidence of coronary heart disease than men from urban areas and, as rural areas become urbanized, men living in these areas show an increasing rate of heart disease. Men of European background tend to show a lower incidence than American-born men. Men with frequent changes of residence or occupation seem to have a higher frequency than other men.

Other factors

Patients with diabetes mellitus and hypothyroidism show higher risk factors for cardiovascular disease. One study demonstrated that the incidence of coronary heart disease rises progressively as risk factors are combined. The absence of risk factors accompanies a distinctly lower incidence of coronary heart disease. Although some factors not mentioned appear to be involved, further study is needed to confirm their relevance.

Reducing cardiovascular diseases

In general terms the incidence of cardiovascular diseases can be reduced by (1) eating the proper foods in reasonable amounts, (2) avoiding infections and securing adequate treatment when infections do exist, (3) avoiding excessive emotional upsets, (4) getting adequate and regular rest, (5) exercising regularly, and (6) having regular periodic physical examinations.

SYMPTOMS AND TREATMENT OF HEART ATTACKS

Symptoms

The presence of cardiovascular disease may become evident in several ways. It may be revealed by a routine physical examination, electrocardiogram, or chest x-ray in a patient who may have had asymptomatic (without symptoms) heart disease for many years. It may manifest itself by affecting other organs, so that the true diagnosis becomes clear only after detailed diagnostic studies. The physician must be alert to the identification of the cardiac basis for symptoms that appear to be those of other diseases, such as allergy, pulmonary disease, or disease of the gastrointestinal tract.

Most patients with heart disease, however, come to the physician complaining of common indications of heart disease. The following are some important symptoms that should be looked for.

Breathlessness   Breathlessness is both the most common and most important of all symptoms. It signals a marked oxygen shortage at some place in the body. It tends to be more intense when there is pulmonary congestion along with a heart disorder. If, for instance, a person is out of breath after climbing one flight of stairs, he should see his physician.

Pain (angina pectoris)   Cardiac pain is due to oxygen deficiency. Brought on by exercise or stress, the pain is often located in the center of the chest, and it may last 1 to 5 minutes. It may radiate to the neck, left shoulder, and inner part of the left arm. It is described as very pressing, heavy, squeezing, bursting, or burning. If it occurs after exertion, it forces the patient to stop or slow down. Rest brings relief in many cases. *It is recommended that a person with chest pain see a physician immediately.*

Edema   If the heart fails to pump with usual vigor, blood flow slows down and fluid may gather in the tissues. Such swelling is called *edema*. This may be first noticed in the feet and ankles. It may also occur from other causes.

Persistent fatigue   Frequent feelings of extreme tiredness (even when a person is not unusually active) may be a sign of heart difficulty or hypertension. Heart patients may complain of a heavy feeling in their limbs, feelings of weakness, or a lack of vigor during or following exertion.

Other symptoms   Some symptoms that may occur in some cardiac patients are *cyanosis* (blueness of the skin due to insufficient oxygen in the blood), loss of consciousness, recurrent bronchitis, and heart palpitations.

Treatment

The kinds of treatment selected for the heart patient will depend upon the nature of the disease and how critical the case is. A chronic illness that affects the patient slowly should allow for planned diagnosis and treatment. Surgery for the repair of congenital conditions may often be planned well in advance. In critical, sudden cardiovascular illness, however, the story is far different. Of most common concern is the kind of treatment used for heart seizures.

Emergency care   The heart-attack patient is in need of emergency care; his life is at stake. In most cases he should be taken to a hospital immediately. The first medical care will depend upon his general condition. It may include the use of oxygen, drugs to dilate obstructed blood vessels, electric or drug stimulators to revive his faltering heart, measurements for pulse and blood pressure, electrocardiograms to record the electric impulses of his heart, or x-ray and fluoroscopic examinations to measure the size and outline of his heart. All efforts must be made to reduce the load placed on his heart. He should be physically and mentally relaxed and given absolute rest to preserve his strength. The degree of his heart cell death will depend upon the severity of the coronary obstruction and the care he receives after the attack. Dead cells cannot be revived. However, heart cells alive but starving for adequate oxygen-food supply may be saved, if the load on the heart can be reduced.

The first week is the most critical. Most deaths occur during the first forty-eight hours after the attack. The danger lessens from the second week on. Gradually new blood vessels form around the obstructed vessels, setting up a new circulation and adequate oxygen-food supply to the deprived cells. Fibrous scar tissue forms over the affected area. Blood cells work to remove the dead cells. Slowly, as the heart returns to normal, the patient can resume normal activities.

Long-term care   The cardinal rule of all treatment for heart patients is to prevent anginal discomfort (pain brought on by inadequate oxygen supply). Drug routines are often established—digitalis to cause a fuller heartbeat, nitrates, such as nitroglycerine, to dilate coronary blood vessels, anticoagulants to reduce the possibility of clotting, sedative drugs to quiet the patient, and drugs to cause specific actions to take place in the kidneys. A selective diet must be set up, including do's and don'ts. The patient must learn the need for rest and for limitation of activity. Schedules of moderate exercise must be established.

Through careful control the patient may be enabled to resume much or all of his previous routine. As a rule, the patient lives a good many years after the first attack of angina pectoris. This longevity will depend, however, upon his properly understanding his condition, faithfully using all medicine prescribed, and preventing situations that tend to precipitate other attacks.

ADVANCES IN CARDIOVASCULAR RESEARCH

The ultimate aim of heart research is to find ways of preventing heart disease entirely. As noted above, great strides have been made in this quest, but much remains to be done. In the meantime, with increased knowledge of the complexities of the human heart new types of surgery and new drugs are being developed.

Surgery

Today heart operations are being performed almost as regularly as were operations on less vital organs only a few years ago. Routinely, defective valves are replaced, abnormal openings in the walls of the chambers are mended, weakened ventricular walls are reconstructed, clogged coronary blood vessels are replaced so that the coronary blood supply is restored, blood vessels are patched, and hearts are transplanted. Totally artificial hearts also are being developed.

The heart-lung machine   Central to the new techniques in heart surgery is the heart-lung machine. This device allows blood to bypass the heart while surgeons work on it. The heart's pumping actions are stopped, and the heart is temporarily emptied of blood, as the machine oxygenates the blood, removes its wastes, and pumps it throughout the body.

Heart transplants   One of the most dramatic forms of surgery performed on individuals with very severely diseased or deformed hearts is the transplantation of the whole heart from a person who has just died (donor) to the critically ill heart patient (recipient). This new heart must be healthy and must come from a person who has very recently (only minutes before) died from causes unrelated to the heart.

There are requirements involved in the question of heart transplantation. The first is that the heart of the donor be removed only when physicians are certain that he is dead. Firm indicators must be used to confirm the legal death of the donor. In some countries a person is considered dead when he stops producing brain waves, as seen on an *electroencephalogram*. In other countries there are several requirements: brain waves are no longer being produced, breathing has stopped, and the heart is no longer pumping blood.

Once a person is pronounced dead, the heart must then be removed as quickly as possible; it cannot be allowed to degenerate. Irreparable cell damage to a heart begins within 30 minutes. This damage can be slowed by cooling the body artificially. If there is any delay, physicians may connect the donor heart to the heart-lung machine. In that case blood is circulated only through the heart.

Another requirement is similar *blood-tissue type* between the donor and recipient. Good type-matching greatly reduces the chances that the body of the recipient will reject the new tissue of the donor heart.

White blood cells in the body protect against foreign materials that may enter the body. Unfortunately, our *lymphocytes* (a kind of white blood cell) are unable to tell the difference between "wanted" and "unwanted" foreign materials—between a transplanted heart and a disease pathogen. To avoid the danger of losing a new heart, the recipient is given a drug, anti-lymphocyte globulin (ALG), to suppress the rejection actions of the lymphocytes. However, in taking this drug the recipient becomes more susceptible to any infection. Thus he must be kept in a sterile room. Enough ALG must be given to prevent rejection of the new heart, but not so much that his body loses *all* of its ability to protect him against infection.

The heart of the donor is detached by cutting off portions of the walls of both the right and left atria, and severing the pulmonary artery and aorta. It is then placed in the recipient's body, where similar cuts have been made, and is attached. The donor heart may then begin beating of its own accord, or it may require the stimulus of electric shock.

Heart transplantation is another surgical breakthrough that provides promise for the victims of coronary heart disease.

Drugs

Along with new surgical techniques has come the development of new drugs. As mentioned above, ALG is being used to suppress the rejection action against implanted hearts. Many drugs are available for reducing blood pressure. Anticoagulants prevent the formation of blood clots or reduce existing clots. Certain other drugs suppress abnormal heart rhythms that may follow a heart attack. In addition, there are drugs that dilate the arteries to reopen circulation. Further research and development continue.

SUMMARY

I. Circulatory system
   A. Circulatory system provides cells of the body with food and oxygen and eliminates wastes.

B. Heart
   1. Structure:
      a. four chambers—right and left atria; right and left ventricles.
      b. three-layered wall—endocardium, myocardium, and epicardium.
      c. four valves—tricuspid and mitral (atrioventricular valves), and pulmonary and aortic (semilunar valves).
   2. Physiology of the heart
      a. cardiac cycle—contraction phase (systolic phase), creating "lub-dub" heart sounds; relaxation phase (diastolic phase).
      b. action regulated by a nervelike conduction system in the heart—sinoatrial node (pacemaker), atrioventricular node, and bundle of His.
C. Blood vessels carry blood to all parts of the body.
   1. Arteries—carry blood, under great pressure, away from the ventricles.
   2. Capillaries—small, thin-walled tubes which lie between the arterioles (at the supply end) and the venules (at the delivery end).
   3. Veins—carry blood from all parts of the body into the venae cavae.
D. Lymphatics
   1. A system of tubules carrying lymph, made up of certain fluid portions of blood that bathe all cells of the body.
   2. Begin as blind ducts and converge into larger ducts which enter veins of the neck.
   3. Are lined with series of filters called lymph nodes.
E. Fetal circulation
   1. Fetal oxygen supply obtained from the mother's blood through the placenta.
   2. Fetal blood largely bypasses the lungs by means of the foramen ovale and ductus arteriosus (both of which normally close shortly after birth).
F. Blood
   1. Plasma.
   2. Red blood cells.
   3. White blood cells.
   4. Platelets.
G. Blood types and transfusions
   1. Based on various types of protein antigens in the blood:
      a. group A.
      b. group B.
      c. group AB.
      d. group O.
   2. Plasma may contain antibodies, which in some cases will agglutinate with a given type of antigen.
   3. Rh factor another significant blood protein.
H. Blood count—determines the ratio of white to red blood cells (normally about 1:700–800).
I. Blood disorders
   1. Anemias—reduction either in number of red blood cells or amount of hemoglobin in these cells.
   2. Leukocytosis—increase in the number of white blood cells. *Leukemia* is an extreme leukocytosis.

3. Leukopenias—reduction in white blood cells below the normal level.

4. Hemophilia—disruption of normal coagulation.

J. Pulse and blood pressure

1. Pulse is expansion and contraction of an artery wall due to the pressure of the blood following each heartbeat.

2. Blood pressure is the pressure of the blood in the arteries.

3. Factors influencing the pulse rate.

4. Factors influencing abnormal blood pressure.

K. Elimination of blood wastes

1. By means of the kidneys.

2. In relation to the role of exercise.

II. Cardiovascular diseases

A. Congenital heart diseases—those occurring before birth.

1. Kinds most commonly include:

a. septal defects.

b. patent ductus arteriosus.

c. stenosis.

d. tetralogy of Fallot.

2. Future for congenital deformities is medically to prevent them.

B. Degenerative diseases—those affecting a person some time after birth.

1. Rheumatic heart disease.

2. Coronary heart disease.

3. Heart block.

4. Atherosclerosis.

5. Hypertension.

6. Cerebrovascular accidents.

7. Vascular disorders—aneurysms, hemorrhage, shock, varicose veins, and phlebitis.

C. Incidence of cardiovascular diseases

1. They account for more than 50 percent of all deaths from all causes among all age groups in the United States.

2. Majority due to coronary heart disease, stroke, and hypertension.

3. Mortality incidence in the past several decades remains about the same for those between the ages of 25 and 65.

III. Environmental complications—considered the main causes of the major cardiovascular diseases, although no one factor can yet be considered the *most* important.

A. Serum-cholesterol levels.

B. Blood-pressure levels.

C. Smoking.

D. Obesity

E. Sugar intake.

F. Social factors.

G. Other factors: chronic diseases and combinations of the preceding factors.

IV. Symptoms and treatment of heart attacks

A. Symptoms—vary according to the nature of the illness; may be common to other conditions; should be called to immediate attention of physician.

1. Breathlessness.

2. Severe pain in the neck, shoulder, and arm areas, especially after exertion.

3. Edema—swelling due to abnormally large amounts of fluid in the body tissues.
4. Persistent fatigue.
5. Other symptoms may include cyanosis, loss of consciousness, palpitations, and recurrent bronchitis.
B. Treatment
1. Emergency care.
2. Long-term care.
V. Advances in heart research
A. Surgery—performed routinely today to replace defective valves, abnormal heart openings, clogged vessels; hearts are transplanted.
1. Heart-lung machine is central to new techniques in heart surgery; it allows blood to bypass heart while surgery is performed.
2. Heart transplants have been performed experimentally on some patients who would have died very shortly. Accurate blood-tissue cross-typing essential.
B. Drugs—development of new drugs essential to heart surgery by reducing blood pressure, preventing undue coagulation, suppressing abnormal heart rhythms, dilating blood vessels, and reducing tissue rejection.

Glossary

If you cannot find the word you wish in this glossary, check the index for text and glossary references.

abscess (ab′ses) (L. *ab-*, from; *cedere*, to go). Swollen, inflamed area of body tissues, in which pus gathers.

anemia (ə nē′mē ə) (G. *an-*, not; *haima*, blood). A condition in which there is a decrease in the number of red blood cells or in the amount of hemoglobin or in both.

aneurysm (an′yə rizm) (G. *aneurysma*, a widening). A saclike bulging of the wall of an artery or vein, resulting from weakening of the wall by disease or abnormal development.

angina pectoris (an jĭ′nə pek′tə ris) (G. *anchein*, to squeeze; L. *pectus*, breast). Pains in the chest, and often in the left arm and shoulder, arising from insufficient blood supply to the heart muscle.

antigen (an′ti jen) (G. *anti-*, against; *gennan*, to produce). A substance that induces the production of antibodies.

aorta (ā or′tə) (G. *aorte*, lift). The main artery of the body, carrying blood from the left ventricle of the heart to all parts of the body except the lungs.

aortic valve (ā or′tik). The valve at the junction of the aorta and the left lower chamber of the heart; formed by three cup-shaped membranes. Also called a *semilunar valve*.

apex (ā′peks) (L. *apex*, summit). The blunt rounded end of the heart, directed downward, forward, and to the left.

apoplexy (ap′ə plek sē) (G. *apo-*, down; *plessein*, to strike). Sudden paralysis with partial or total loss of consciousness and sensation, due to breaking or obstruction of a blood vessel in the brain. Also called a *stroke*.

arteriole (ahr tē′rē ōl) (L. *arteriola*, small artery). The smallest arterial vessels resulting from repeated branching of the arteries.

artery (ahr′tə rē). Any one of a system of tubes or vessels carrying blood from the heart to all parts of the body.

atherosclerosis (ath′ə rō sklə rō′sis) (G. *athere*, gruel; *skleros*, hard). A disease of the arteries in which the inner layer of the wall becomes thick and irregular by deposits of fat; these deposits decrease the inside diameter of the vessel.

atrioventricular block (ā′trē ō ven trik′yə lər) (L. *atrium*, hall; *venter*, belly). Interference with conduction of electrical impulses from upper to lower chambers of the heart and throughout the lower chambers. Also called *heart block*.

atrioventricular node. Small mass of special muscular fibers in septum between right atrium and ventricle which forms beginning of bundle of His; it receives electrical impulse from sinoatrial node. Abbreviated *AV node*.

atrium (ā′trē əm). One of the two upper chambers of the heart.

AV node. See *atrioventricular node*.

biscuspid valve (bī kus′ pid) (L. *bi-*, twice; *cuspis*, pointed end). A valve of two cusps located between the upper and lower chambers in the left side of the heart. Usually called *mitral valve*.

blood pressure. The pressure of the blood in the arteries.

bronchitis (brong kī′tis) (G. *bronchos*, windpipe; *-itis*, inflammation). Inflammation of the mucous lining of the bronchial tubes.

bundle of His (his) (Wilhelm His, Jr., German physician, 1863–1934). A bundle of specialized muscular fibers running from the atrioventricular node along the septum down to the lower heart chambers. It serves to conduct electrical impulses to the ventricles.

capillary (kap′i ler ē) (L. *capillus*, hair). One of the very small tubes or vessels forming a network between the arterioles and the venules; through its walls materials leave and enter the blood.

cardiovascular (kahr′dē ō vas′kyə lər) (G. *kardia*, heart; L. *vasculum*, a vessel). Pertaining to the heart and blood vessels.

cholesterol (kə les′tə rol) (G. *chole*, bile; *stereos*, solid). A fatlike substance found in animal tissue. An excess amount in the blood is often associated with high risk of coronary atherosclerosis.

chordae tendineae (kor′dē ten din′ē ē) (G. *chorde*, string; *tendene,* to stretch). Fibrous chords which serve to hold the valves between the upper and lower chambers of the heart secure when they are forced shut by pressure of blood in the lower chambers.

circulatory (sur′kyə lə tor ē) (L. *circulari*, to form a circle). Pertaining to the heart, blood vessels, and the circulation of the blood.

coagulation (kō ag yə lā′shən) (L. *co-*, together; *agere*, to move). Process of changing from a liquid to a thickened or solid state; the formation of a clot.

coarctation (kō ahrk tā′shən) (L. *co-*, together; *arctare*, to make tight). A pressing together or a narrowing of a blood vessel, usually the aorta.

collateral circulation (kə lat′ə rəl) (L. *co-*, together; *lateralis*, lateral, side). Circulation of the blood through nearby smaller vessels when a main vessel has been blocked.

congenital (kən jen′i tal) (L. *con*, together; *genere*, to beget). Pertaining to presence at birth, resulting from heredity or prenatal environment.

coronary artery (kor′ə ner ē) (G. *korone*, wreath). One of two arteries, arising from the aorta, arching over the top of the heart, and conducting blood to the heart muscle.

coronary disease. A destructive process involving the blood vessels conducting blood to the heart muscle.

coronary occlusion (ə kloo′zhən) (L. *ob-*, toward; *clausere*, to shut). An obstruction (generally a blood clot) in a branch of a coronary artery which hinders the flow of blood to some part of the heart muscle.

corpuscle (kor′pus əl) (L. *corpusculum*, little body). A blood cell.

cross-match. A determination of the compatibility of the blood of a donor with that of the recipient before transfusion, by placing red blood cells of donor in serum of recipient and red blood cells of recipient in serum of donor; absence of agglutination indicates that two blood specimens are compatible.

cyanosis (sī ə nō′sis) (G. *kyanos*, blue). Blueness of the skin caused by insufficient oxygen in the blood.

deoxygenated blood (dē ok′si jə nā ted). Blood that has lost or been deprived of oxygen.

diastole (dī as′tə lē) (G. *diastole*, dilation). In each heartbeat, the period of dilation of the heart.

ductus arteriosus (duk′təs ahr tē′rē ō sis) (L. *ducere*, to lead). A small duct in the heart of the fetus between the artery leaving the left side of the heart (aorta) and the artery leaving the right side of the heart (pulmonary artery); this duct normally closes soon after birth.

edema (i dē′mə) (G. *oidein*, to swell). Swelling due to abnormally large amounts of fluid in the tissues of the body.

electrocardiogram (i lek′trō kahr′dē ə gram) (G. *elektron*, amber; *kardia*, heart; *gramma*, mark). A graphic record of the electric currents produced by the heart. Abbreviated *ECG* or *EKG*.

embolus (em′bə ləs) (G. *embolos*, plug). A blood clot (or other substance such as air, fat, tumor) inside a blood vessel, which is carried in the bloodstream to a smaller vessel, where it becomes an obstruction to circulation.

endocarditis (en′dō kahr dī′tis) (G. *endon*, within; *kardia*, heart; *-itis*, inflammation). Inflammation of the inner layer of the heart (endocardium), usually associated with acute rheumatic fever or some infectious agent.

endocardium (en′dō kahr′dē əm). A thin, smooth membrane forming the inner surface of the heart.

epicardium (ep′i kahr′dē əm) (G. *epi*, upon; *kardia*, heart). The outer layer of the heart wall. Also called *visceral pericardium*.

erythrocyte (e rith′ro sīt) (G. *erythros*, red; *kytos*, cell). A red blood corpuscle.

fibrin (fī′brin) (L. *fibra*, fiber). An elastic protein which forms the essential portion of a blood clot.

fibrinogen (fībrin′o jən) (L. *fibra*, fiber; G. *gennan*, to produce). A soluble protein in the blood which, by the action of certain enzymes, is converted into the insoluble protein of a blood clot.

foramen ovale (fo rā′mən ō vā′lē) (L. *forare*, to bore; *ovum*, an egg). An oval hole between the left and right upper chambers of the heart of the fetus, which normally closes shortly after birth.

gamma globulin (gam′ə glob′yə lin) (G. *gamma*, greek letter g; L. *globulus*, globule). That portion of serum with which most of the immune antibodies are associated.

heart block. Interference with the conduction of the electrical impulses of the heart; blockage can be either partial or complete.

hemiplegia (hem′i plē′jē ə) (G. *hemi*, half; *plege*, a stroke). Paralysis of one half of the body caused by damage to the opposite side of the brain; it is sometimes caused by a blood clot or hemorrhage in a blood vessel in the brain.

hemocytometer (hē′mō sī tom′ə tər) (G. *haima*, blood; *kytos*, hollow vessel; *metron*, measure). An instrument used in counting the blood corpuscles.

hemoglobin (hē′mə glō′bin). The oxygen-carrying red pigment of the red blood corpuscles.

hemophilia (hē′mə fil′ē ə) (G. *philein,* to love). A hereditary condition in which the blood fails to clot quickly enough, causing prolonged, uncontrolled bleeding from even the smallest cut.

hypertension (hī′pər ten′shən) (G. *hyper,* over; L. *tendere,* to stretch). An unstable or persistent elevation of blood pressure above the normal range. Commonly called *high blood pressure.*

inferior vena cava (in fēr′ē ər vēnə kā′və) (L. *inferus,* low; *vena,* vein; *cava,* hollow). The venous trunk for the lower extremities, pelvis, and abdominal viscera which empties into the right atrium.

interatrial septum (in′tər ā′trē əl sep′təm) (L. *inter,* between; *atrium,* heart; *septum,* partition). The muscular wall dividing the left and right upper chambers, or atria, of the heart.

interventricular septum (in′tər ven trik′yə lər sep′təm). The muscular wall, thinner at the top, dividing the left and right lower chambers, or ventricles, of the heart.

lacteal (lak′tē əl) (L. *lacteus,* milky). Any one of the intestinal lymphatics that take up digested fats.

leukemia (loo kē′mē ə) (G. *leukos,* white; *haima,* blood). A fatal disease of the blood-forming organs, characterized by a marked increase in the number of leukocytes in the blood.

leukopenia (loo′kə pē′nē ə) (G. *leukos,* white; *penia,* poverty). Reduction in the number of leukocytes in the blood.

lipid (lip′id) (G. *lipos,* fat). Fat.

lymph (limf) (L. *lympha,* water). A tissue fluid confined to vessels and nodes of the lymphatic system.

lymphatic (lim fat′ik). Pertaining to or containing lymph.

lymph node (limf nōd) (L. *lympha,* water; *nodus,* knob). Small oval collection of lymphatic tissue interposed in the course of lymphatic vessels.

lymphocyte (lim′fə sīt) (G. *kytos,* hollow). A variety of small colorless corpuscles found in lymph.

lymphoid tissue (lim′foid) (L. *eidos,* form). Connective tissue infiltrated with lymphocytes.

mitral valve (mī′trəl) (G. *mitra,* headband). Sometimes called biscuspid valve. A valve of two cusps located between the upper and lower chambers in the left side of the heart.

murmur (L. *murmurare,* murmur). An abnormal heart sound, sounding like fluid passing an obstruction, heard between the normal "lub-dub" heart sounds.

myocardial infarction (mī ō kahr′dē əl in fahrk′shən) (G. *mys,* muscle; *kardial,* heart; L. *infarcire,* to stuff in). The damaging or death of an area of the heart muscle (myocardium) resulting from a reduction in the blood supply reaching that area.

myocardium (mī ō kahr′dē əm). The muscular wall of the heart; the heart muscle; the thickest of the three layers, lying between the endocardium (inner) and epicardium (outer).

occlusion (ə kloo′zhən) (L. *occlusus,* to shut). The closing or blocking of a passage, such as of a blood vessel.

palpitation (pal pi tā′shən) (L. *palpitare,* to feel). A fluttering of the heart of abnormal rate or rhythm, experienced by the person himself.

patent ductus arteriosus (pā′tənt duk′təs ahr tē′rē ō′sis) (L. *patens,* open). A congenital defect in which the ductus arteriosus fails to close. See *ductus arteriosus.*

patent foramen ovale (pā′tənt fo rā′mən ō vā′lē). A congenital defect in which the foramen ovale fails to close. See *foramen ovale.*

pathogen (path′ə jən) (G. *pathos*, disease; *gennan*, to produce). A microorganism or substance capable of producing a disease.

phlebitis (flə bī′tis) (G. *phlebos*, vein; *-itis*, inflammation). Inflammation of a vein, often in the leg; a blood clot may be formed in the inflamed vein.

plaque (plak) (Fr. *plak,* a disc). A flat or patchlike deposit of lipid (fat) in the inner walls (tunica media) of the arteries.

plasma (plaz′mə) (G. *plasma,* form). The cell-free fluid portion of uncoagulated blood. See *serum.*

platelet (plāt′lit). Roundish discs, smaller than red blood cells, found in the blood and associated with clotting.

pulmonary artery (pul′mə ner ē ahr′tə rē) (L. *pumo,* lung). The large artery which conveys unoxygenated (venous) blood from the lower right chamber of the heart to the lungs.

pulmonary circulation. The circulation of the blood through the lungs, flowing from the lower right chamber of the heart through the lungs, back to the left upper chamber of the heart.

pulmonary valve. The valve formed by three cup-shaped membranes at the junction of the pulmonary artery and the right lower chamber of the heart; also called a *semilunar valve.*

pulmonary vein. One of four veins (two from each lung) which conduct oxygenated blood from the lungs into the left upper chamber of the heart.

pulse (puls) (L. *pulsus,* stroke). The expansion and contraction of an artery which may be felt with the finger.

Purkinje fibers (pər kin′jē) (Johannes Purkinje, Bohemian physiologist, 1787–1869). Atypical muscle fibers lying beneath the endocardium of the heart which constitute the impulse-conducting system of the heart.

rheumatic fever (roo mat′ik) (G. *rheuma,* a flow). A disease, usually occurring in childhood, which may follow, a few weeks later, a streptococcal infection.

rheumatic heart disease. The damage done to the heart, particularly the heart valves, by one or more attacks of rheumatic fever.

SA node. See *sinoatrial node.*

sclerosis (skla rō′sis) (G. *skleros,* hard). A hardening of body tissues, usually as the result of an accumulation of fibrous tissue.

semilunar valves (sem ē loo′nər) (L. *semis,* half; *luna,* the moon). Cup-shaped valves; the aortic valve at the entrance to the aorta, and the pulmonary valve at the entrance to the pulmonary artery are semilunar valves; they consist of three cup-shaped flaps which prevent the backflow of blood.

septum (sep′təm) (L. *septum,* partition). A dividing wall; the atrial or interatrial septum is a muscular wall dividing the left and right upper chambers of the heart; the ventricular or interventricular septum is a muscular wall dividing the left and right lower chambers of the heart.

serum (sīr′əm) (L. *serum,* whey). The fluid portion of the blood which remains after the cellular elements have been removed by coagulation; it is different from plasma, which is the cell-free liquid portion of uncoagulated blood.

sinoatrial block (sī nō ā′trē əl). Also called a *heart block;* interference with conduction of electrical impulses throughout the upper chambers of the heart and to the atrioventricular node.

sinoatrial node. A small mass of specialized cells in the right upper chamber of the heart which give rise to the electrical impulses that initiate contractions of the heart. Also called the *SA node* or *pacemaker.*

sphygmomanometer (sfig′mō mə nom′ə tər) (G. *sphygmos,* pulse; *manos,* thin; *metron,* measure). An instrument for measuring blood pressure in the arteries.

stenosis (sti nō'sis) (G. *stenosis,* narrowing). A narrowing or stricture of an opening; mitral stenosis or aortic stenosis indicate narrowing of those valves.

stethoscope (steth'ə skōp) (G. *stethos,* chest; *skopein,* to examine). An instrument for listening to sounds within the body.

stroke (strōk). An impeded blood supply to some part of the brain caused by a clot, hemorrhage, embolus, or tumor. Also called apoplectic stroke, cerebrovascular accident, or cerebral vascular accident.

superior vena cava (sə pēr'ē ər vē'nə kā'və). The venous trunk for the upper extremities, thorax, head, and neck which empties into the right atrium.

systemic circulation (sis tem'ik) (G. *systema,* to set together). The circulation of the blood through all parts of the body except the lungs, the flow being from the left lower chamber of the heart, through the body, back to the right upper chamber of the heart.

systole (sis'tə lē) (G. *systole,* to draw together). In each heartbeat, the period of contraction of the heart; atrial systole is the period of contraction of the atria; ventricular systole is the period of contraction of the ventricles.

tetralogy of Fallot (te tral'ə jē uv fa lō') (G. *tetra-,* four; *logos,* word; E.-L. A. Fallot, French physician, 1850–1911). A congenital malformation of the heart involving four defects.

thoracic duct (tho ras'ik dukt) (G. *thorax,* chest; L. *ducere,* to lead). The largest lymphatic vessel of the body; originates in the abdomen, passes upward through the thorax, and empties into the left subclavian vein.

thrombocyte (throm'bə sīt) (G. *thrombos,* clot; *kytos,* a hollow). A blood platelet.

thrombus (throm'bəs) (G. *thrombos,* clot). A blood clot which forms inside a blood vessel or cavity of the heart. See *embolus.*

transfusion (tranz fyoo'zhən) (L. *trans,* across; *fundere,* to pour). The introduction of whole blood, plasma substitutes, or other solutions directly into the bloodstream.

tricuspid valve (trī kus'pid) (L. *tri-,* three; *cuspis,* a point). A valve consisting of three cusps located between the upper and lower chamber in the right side of the heart.

tunica externa (tyoo'ni kə ek'stər nə) (L. *tunica,* coating; *externus,* on the outside). The outer layer of wall of artery or vein.

tunica intima (tyoo'ni kə in'ti mə) (L. *intimus,* within). The inner layer of wall of artery or vein.

tunica media (tyoo'ni kə mē'dē ə) (L. *medius,* middle). The middle (intermediate) layer of wall of artery or vein.

valve (L. valva, leaf of a folding door). A structure in a canal or passage which prevents the backflow of the contents, such as the valves of the heart.

varicose veins (var'i kōs) (L. *varix,* enlarged vein). An abnormally or irregularly swollen vein.

vasoconstriction (vas'ō kən strik'shən) (L. *vas,* vessel; *con,* together; *stringere,* to draw). The narrowing of blood vessels, especially constriction of arterioles, leading to decreased blood flow; such narrowing may be caused by nervous or chemical stimulation.

vasodilation (vas'ō dī lā'shən) (L. *dilatare,* to bring apart). The enlarging of blood vessels, especially dilation of arterioles, leading to increased supply of blood to the part; such enlarging may be caused by nervous or chemical stimulation.

vein (vān) (L. *vena,* vein). Any of a series of vessels of the vascular system which carries blood from the various parts of the body to the heart.

vena cava (vē'nə kā'və). See *inferior* and *superior vena cava.*

ventricle (ven'tri kl) (L. *ventriculus*, little belly). One of the two lower chambers of the heart.

venule (ven'yool) (L. *venula*, vein). A very small vein.

vessel (ves'əl) (L. *vas*, a vessel). A tube circulating a body fluid, as a blood vessel or a lymph vessel.

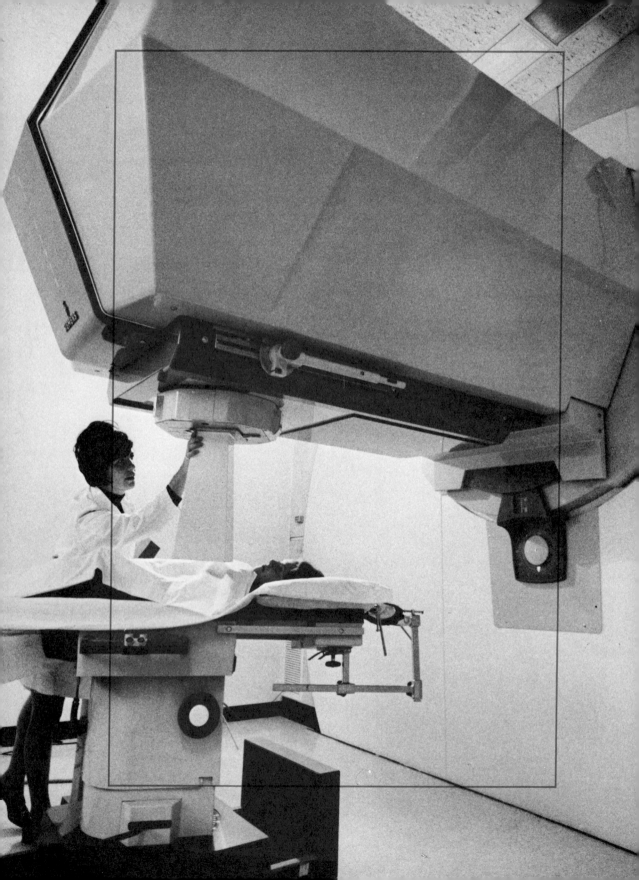

Cancer as a health problem

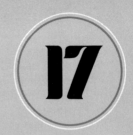

17

One of the great generalizations of science is the *cell theory*—that all living plants and animals consist of cells and cell products. This theory implies that the basic unit of living organisms is the cell. Cells, however, are not all alike. They vary in size, shape, and structure, according to the functions they perform. In spite of these differences new living cells can arise *only* when pre-existing cells reproduce them. Thus life is a continuous process.

WHAT IS CANCER?

The human begins life as a single cell, which is the product of fertilization between an ovum and a spermatozoon (see Chapter 11). This cell then grows by adding new cells through *mitosis*. This addition of cells is very rapid and random at first, and up to a point all the cells appear the same. Upon reaching this point the cells undergo the process of *differentiation*, wherein they begin to take on identity. Some become bone, others skin, and others nervous tissue; thus the complex structure of the human takes shape. After a time, limiting processes come into play, and growth begins to taper off slightly throughout infancy; it becomes more slow in childhood and finally stops in old age (except for the replacement of worn-out, injured, or shed shells).

From birth to death each living thing is constantly changing. It is growing, degenerating, being injured, repairing damage, reproducing, and adjusting. All of this activity normally involves the death and orderly replacement of millions of cells every day. If for any reason a disorderly replacement of these worn-out cells continues as an abnormal growth, the individual has cancer. Such uncontrolled, cancerous growth may appear in man or in any animal or plant.

Cancer, the *uncontrolled* growth of cells, does not heed the signals that govern normal cell and tissue behavior within the body. Normally, when a finger is cut, growth and cell division occur to a point and then stop as soon as healing is complete. But cancer cells grow abnormally and have a tendency to invade adjacent structures and spread to distant parts of the body. Such growth often leads to death.

Cancer cell structure

Cancer cells, like normal cells, consist of a nucleus, cytoplasm, and a cellular membrane which separates the cell from other cells and from its surroundings. (These subcellular structures, which also make up the normal cell, are discussed in Chapter 11.) Cancer cells are structurally similar to normal cells, but they show clear differences.

The nucleus in cancer cells, as in normal cells, is the site of the genetic material DNA, the center of cellular reproduction; it directs the cell's overall functions. Cancer cells are, however, distinguished from normal cells principally by the nucleus. Their nuclei are usually larger than those of comparable normal cells and may vary significantly in size and shape within a group of cancer cells. These large nuclei deviate from the normal in the number and appearance of chromosomes and also in the number of nucleoli present. Cell division is abnormal, resulting in the deviations in chromosomes.

The cytoplasm is similar in cancer and normal cells. No single cytoplasmic difference (structural or chemical) that would specifically characterize a cancer cell has been identified.

The normal cell membrane has the ability to allow the inward passage of nutrients and the outward passage of products of cell metabolism and secretion; the cancer cell membrane appears to differ from that of healthy cells in this ability. Cancer cell membranes adhere to each other less firmly than normal cells, and the cells tend to shed very readily.

In time the amount of cytoplasm increases, altering the size and shape of the cell; these changes may take months or even years. While the cancerous growth remains confined to the epithelium the cancer cells show fewer abnormalities than those in advanced tumors; see Fig. 17.1. At the cellular level the cancerous changes are slight. The earliest detectable sign of cancer is an increase in the number of chromosomes produced. Often *tetraploid cells*, those having twice the normal number of chromosomes, are found in cancerous organisms. Advanced invading cancers show odd and irregular numbers of chromosomes as well as abnormally shaped chromosomes.

Cancer cell processes and behavior

The processes of cell growth and behavior have been studied through tissue cultures. In such studies living cells are put into glass vessels containing sterile (germ-free) nutrient solutions. From time to time they are given new nutrients. Periodically the excess cells are removed and discarded. A tissue culture of cells from the embryonic heart of a chicken was started in 1912 under the direction of Alexis Carrel (early cellular physiologist at the Rockefeller Institute) and lived for twenty-seven years.

Cells of any kind grown in a tissue culture outside the body are described as being grown *in vitro* (within glass). Cells growing within the body are *in vivo* (within the living body).

The in vitro growth of cells is of great value to research. Cells grown in this manner may be observed growing and undergoing mitosis. The effects of substances added to the medium, which would normally kill or harm an individual, may also be observed. When cells growing in vitro touch each other, the normal active movement of the cell membrane is inhibited. There is at the same time a pronounced decrease in the synthesis of protein, RNA, and DNA within the cell, resulting in slower growth. Under certain conditions cell growth can be speeded up. For example, in skin the normal rate of cell division can be *increased* up to 90 times by removing successive layers of epidermal cells (with the aid of cellulose tape). But how does the cell "know" when new cells are needed, and how does it "know" when to stop growing?

In a normal human every cell is compressed against other cells, and each has a fluid medium that brings nutrients to the cell from the blood and carries away waste materials. This body fluid is also a chemical communication system. Special chemicals, when released into this fluid, may turn on or off specific chemical activities in the cells they enter. One group of chemicals, called *hormones,* has been found to control the whole body by such activity. But it is also believed that there exists a *general chemical feedback mechanism* among all cells, which may be used to control either a cell's own functions or the functions of other cells, or both. Although the mechanisms of feedback are not now readily understood, the outstanding feature of cancer cells appears to be their failure to obey signals of the normal cells in the body and their lack of such a feedback, self-controlling mechanism. They start to grow, produce large amounts of DNA, RNA, and protein, but their growth never stops.

Tumors

A growth which persists, grows, and serves no useful purpose is called a *tumor* or *neoplasm.* Tumors are divided into two classes: *benign tumors* and *malignant tumors,* or *cancers.*

Benign tumors Benign tumors are growths that may increase slowly in size, are usually surrounded by a fibrous membrane, and remain localized. Such a growth does not invade other tissues or produce secondary growths in other parts of the body. Benign tumors may, however, cause discomfort by pressure on adjacent structures.

Common benign tumors occur on the skin as *warts, wens,* and *birthmarks,* in the uterus as *fibroid tumors,* on the skeleton as growths of bone tissue, and in the breast or ovary as *cysts.* Some benign tumors, if subjected to certain harmful effects (explained later), may change into malignant tumors.

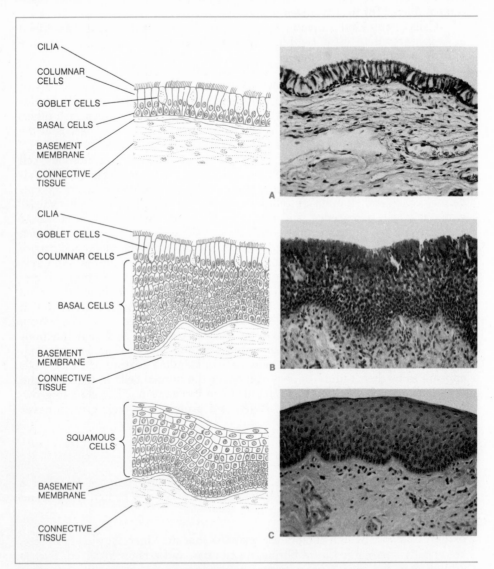

Figure 17.1 Progression of cancer through epithelium. Bronchial epithelium is the original site of almost all lung cancer, which often develops as shown in the photomicrographs. (A) normal bronchial epithelium. (B) one of the first effects of smoking becomes evident, an increase in the number of basal cells, termed *hyperplasia*. (C) The epithelium is lost, and the cells become *squamous*, or flattened, and show atypical (darkened) nuclei. (D) This stage

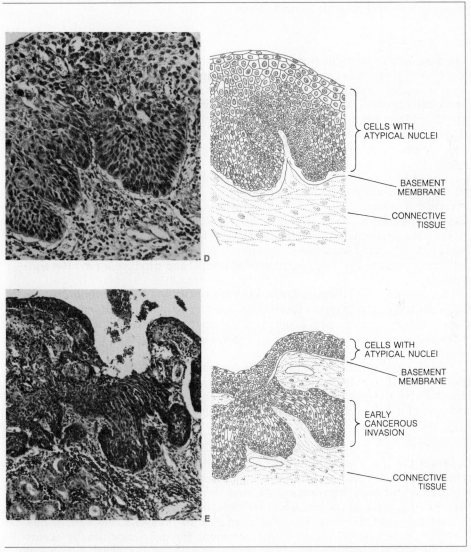

CELLS WITH
ATYPICAL NUCLEI

BASEMENT
MEMBRANE

CONNECTIVE
TISSUE

D

CELLS WITH
ATYPICAL NUCLEI

BASEMENT
MEMBRANE

EARLY
CANCEROUS
INVASION

CONNECTIVE
TISSUE

E

is termed *carcinoma in situ*, which refers to a preinvading cell. (E) A fully developed *cancer;* when these cells break through the basement membrane, the cancer may spread through the lungs and to the rest of the body. (From *The Effects of Smoking,* by Cuyler Hammond; copyright 1962 by Scientific American Inc.; all rights reserved. Photomicrographs by Dr. Oscar Auerbach of the Veterans Administration Hospital, East Orange, N.J.)

Malignant tumors (neoplasms) Cancer is the term commonly used to designate all malignant tumors, or neoplasms, regardless of their origin. Cancers are divided into two main classes: those arising from epithelial tissue are called *carcinomas,* and those arising from connective or supportive tissue are called *sarcomas.* Table 17.1 lists the more common cancers, their sites of origin, names, and possible complications.

How cancer spreads

The most serious complication in trying to cure cancer is the tendency of cancer cells to spread. This spreading may occur in one of three ways, as follows.

· INVASION   Malignant tumors, having no surrounding capsule or limiting membrane, possess an unlimited ability to enlarge, extend, and invade the spaces between the normal cells of the tissues in which they are located. Such growths (primary cancer growths) may remain unnoticed until, because of enlargement, they interfere with the functions of important structures and organs of the body.

· METASTASIS   Metastasis is the process of transferring disease from one organ or part of the body to another. This results in the formation of new (secondary) sites of disease. Rapidly growing and invading cancer cells shed very easily and may be filtered into the lymphatic system and thereby transported into the regional lymph nodes; see Fig. 17.2. Or they may actually invade an adjacent blood vessel, as shown in Fig. 17.3, be carried to remote parts or organs, lodge there, become established, and produce a new (secondary) site of cancer.

· IMPLANTATION   Because cancer cells are so easily shed, they may become dislodged easily and implant themselves in some adjacent organs, where they will continue to grow and produce their destructive effects. This type of spreading occurs quite frequently in cancers of the abdominal and thoracic cavities.

Malignant tumors, at the beginning, are always localized and often remain so for a time. Early diagnosis, while the growth is still localized, and complete removal offer the greatest chance of a cancer cure, but may be impossible after widespread metastasis or implantation has taken place.

How cancer kills

In cancer patients the inability or failure of cancer cells to obey the normal feedback of body signals results in a number of deficiencies that seriously interfere with bodily functioning. At least three deficiencies are important in the resulting death of an individual: *anemia, infection,* and *debility.*

Anemia and infection are closely related to bone-marrow deficiencies. Complete bone-marrow failure is not common; the deficiency usually occurs from the victim's inability to produce specific cells of the usual number or quality needed by the body. In anemia the primary effect of cancer is its causing either insufficient production of red blood cells or defective red cells that do not survive long in circulation. In chronic lymphocytic leukemia and Hodgkin's disease (Table 17.1) the red-cell life span is shortened by some factor which produces premature red-cell destruction.

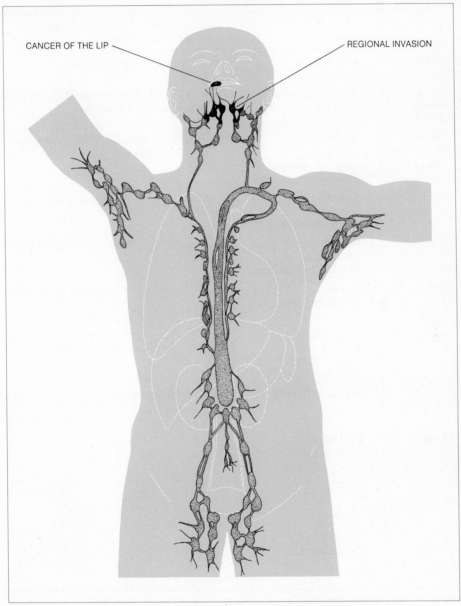

CANCER OF THE LIP

REGIONAL INVASION

Figure 17.2   Lymphatic system of the body showing cancerous regional invasion (metastasis) of the lip.

Table 17.1 *Common sites and types of cancer*

site	types of cancer	warning signal when lasting longer than two weeks—see your doctor
Breast	Carcinoma	Lump or thickening in the breast
Colon and rectum	Adenocarcinoma	Change in bowel habits; bleeding from the rectum; blood in the stools
Oral (including pharynx and larynx)	Squamous-cell carcinoma; adenocarcinoma; basal-cell carcinoma	Sore that does not heal; difficulty in swallowing; hoarseness
Lung	Squamous-cell carcinoma; adenocarcinoma	Persistent cough or lingering respiratory ailment
Skin	Squamous-cell carcinoma; basal-cell carcinoma	Sore that does not heal, or change in a wart or mole
Uterus	Adenocarcinoma; adenocanthoma	Unusual bleeding or discharge from vagina
Kidney and bladder	Squamous-cell carcinoma; Wilms' tumor; adenocarcinoma	Difficulty in urinating; bleeding or blood in urine, in which case consult your doctor at once
Prostate gland	Adenocarcinoma	Difficulty in urinating
Blood	Leukemia	
Lymph	Lymphomas	

SOURCE: *1973 Cancer Facts and Figures*, American Cancer Society, Inc., 1973.

Table 17.1 (*continued*)

safeguards	additional information
Annual checkup; monthly breast self-examination	Leading cause of cancer death of women
Annual checkup, including proctoscopy	Considered highly curable when annual physical checkups include proctoscopic examination
Annual checkup, including mirror laryngoscopy	Many more lives should be saved because the mouth is easily examined visually by physicians and dentists
Best safeguard is prevention by not smoking; annual physical checkup and chest x-ray	Leading cause of cancer death of males; largely preventable
Annual checkup, avoidance of over-exposure to the sun	Readily detected by observation and diagnosed by simple biopsy; few deaths result
Annual checkup including pelvic examination and Papanicolaou ("pap") smear	Mortality declined 50 percent during last 25 years with wider use of "pap" smear; many thousands more of lives can be saved
Annual checkup with urinalysis	Some linkage with cigarette smoking
Annual checkup including palpation of the prostate gland	Mainly in men over 60; can be detected by palpation and urinalysis at annual physical checkup
	Cancer of blood-forming tissues, characterized by abnormal production of immature white blood cells; *acute leukemia* mainly strikes children, is treated by drugs that have extended life and sometimes apparently cured; *chronic leukemia* strikes usually after age 25 and progresses less rapidly[a]
	Arise in lymph system; include *Hodgkin's disease* and *lymphosarcoma*; some can lead normal lives for many years[a]

[a] Cancer experts believe that if drugs or vaccines are found which can cure or prevent cancers they will be successful first for *leukemia* and *lymphomas*.

Intestinal bleeding, another cause of anemia, may result directly from a tumor or indirectly from cancers of the bone marrow, which may reduce the production of platelets. Platelets control clotting; when they are markedly reduced, as in the leukemias, hemorrhage results. Also, when growth of the cancer involves the blood supply of a specific tissue or organ, bleeding may result, as in lung cancer.

Any of these conditions may cause a depression of the host's defenses against infection; consequently, serious infections frequently occur in cancer patients. In patients with acute leukemia infection is the most common direct cause of death. Bacterial, fungal, and viral diseases are common in people who have had massive damage to their lymphocyte-producing tissues, as is caused by Hodgkin's disease and the leukemias.

The other example of physical damage is *debility*, the wasting away of the body. This is quite common in cancer patients. It may result from simple undernutrition, as might occur in a specific cancer that causes damage of the mouth or stomach and restricts what a person can eat, or it may result from treatment by drugs, surgery, or radiation. Loss of appetite because of continuous pain or emotional depression arising from neglect or loss of hope is common in cancer patients.

DIAGNOSIS IS NOT DEATH

Many cancers can be cured if they are diagnosed and treated in the early stages. One of the most serious deterrents to cancer control is that many patients do not seek medical advice during the time the disease can be cured.

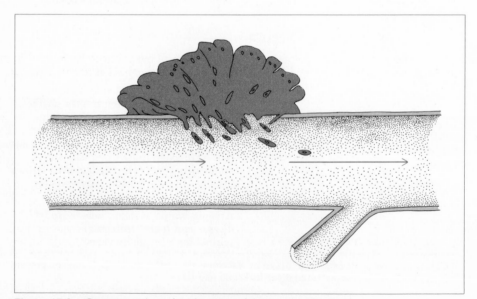

Figure 17.3   Cancerous invasion (metastasis) of a blood vessel.

The greatest need in the cancer program is to minimize the time between the appearance of early symptoms, their diagnosis, and the taking of corrective action. *The most important single weapon in detecting cancer before any symptoms appear is the painstaking periodic health examination of the presumably well individual.* Since no age group is totally without cancer, regular cancer examinations are essential for everyone.

Age is an important factor in the overall diagnosis of cancer. Studies have revealed that the death rate from cancer for females under 10 years of age is less than 10 per 100,000 population. At age 40 it is 100, and over 85 it is 1,000 per 100,000.[1] On this basis a lump in the breast of a girl under 10 is almost certainly *not* cancer, in a woman aged 40 there is a *chance* it may be cancer, and in a woman aged 85 it is very likely cancer. Further, different types of cancer appearing at selected body locations tend to have a maximal incidence within definite age groups. The most frequent sites of cancer according to the age of the individual affected are shown in Table 17.2. Everyone should keep these facts in mind and have regular—at least yearly—physical examinations that investigate the common sites of cancer for his age group.

Prevention of cancer

Many kinds of cancer may be prevented by avoiding or correcting long-continued irritations that may produce cancer. This prevention includes

Table 17.2 *Most frequent types of cancer by age groups*

age	most frequent types of cancer[a]
0 to 15	Cancer of bone, kidney, brain; leukemia; lymphosarcomas
15 to 34	
Male	Cancer of brain, genitals; leukemia; Hodgkin's disease, lymphosarcomas
Female	Cancer of uterus, breast, brain; leukemia; Hodgkin's disease
35 to 54	
Male	Cancer of lung, colon, rectum, brain, pancreas, stomach
Female	Cancer of breast, uterus, colon, rectum, ovary, lung
55 to 74	
Male	Cancer of lung, colon, rectum, stomach, prostate gland, pancreas
Female	Cancer of breast, colon, rectum, ovary, lung, uterus, pancreas
75 and older	
Male	Cancer of prostate gland, colon, rectum, lung, stomach
Female	Cancer of colon, rectum, breast, stomach, uterus, pancreas

SOURCE: Adapted from *1973 Cancer Facts and Figures*, American Cancer Society, Inc., 1973.
[a] Cancer of the skin is omitted from this table because there is seldom adequate reason for failure to diagnose it correctly and early.

[1] *A Cancer Source Book for Nurses*, New York, American Cancer Society, 1968, pp. 16–17.

avoiding both unnecessary exposure to x-ray radiation (as used in medicine) and excessive exposure to ultraviolet radiation (as found in strong sunlight). Using safeguards in occupations involving exposure to known cancer-producing chemicals and dusts, and avoiding exposure to tobacco—particularly cigarette smoke, which has been proven to play an important part in causing cancer of the lip, mouth, larynx, and lung—are important in preventing cancer.

Early symptoms

The identification of the earliest detectable signs of cancer is extremely important. A knowledge of the seven danger signals of cancer cannot be overemphasized. No one symptom or group of symptoms is invariably characteristic of the onset of cancer. But certain symptoms, which can be easily recognized, frequently tend to show themselves as the *first* expressions of the commonest forms of cancer. These "Seven Danger Signals of Cancer" include:

1. Any sore that does not heal, particularly those about the mouth, tongue, or lips.
2. A lump or thickening in the breast or elsewhere, such as on the lip or tongue.
3. Unusual bleeding or discharge from the nipple of the breast or irregular bleeding from any of the natural body openings.
4. Any change in a wart or mole, such as a progressive change in color or size.
5. Persistent indigestion or difficulty in swallowing, which may be followed by a sudden, unexplained loss of weight.
6. Persistent hoarseness or cough.
7. Any change in normal bowel habits.

Recognition of one or more of the seven signals may or may not indicate the beginning of cancer—but it is too dangerous to wait and find out. The person who shows any of these danger signals should consult a physician as soon as possible. Table 17.1 may give some insight into the formation, characteristics, and complications of the early symptoms of cancer.

The absence of pain in early cancer has been overemphasized. This is a generalization which is not always the case. A pain, or sensation of discomfort, which lasts more than a few weeks, always in the same place, and which can be localized with the tip of the finger, may be regarded with suspicion and calls for a medical examination.

Every woman should inspect her breasts monthly, immediately after the end of her menstrual period. Examination during the menstrual period is unsatisfactory because of the temporary changes and tenderness which normally may occur in the breasts at that time. Fig. 17.4 illustrates breast examination, which is performed in two stages. The *first stage* is performed while the woman is sitting before a mirror (A in the figure). With her arms at the sides and posture erect, she examines her breasts for symmetry in size and shape, noting any changes in *dimpling of the skin* or *depression of the nipple*. Then, with the arms overhead, she repeats this procedure. The *second stage* is performed while she is reclining on a bed. During this portion of the examination she places a flat pillow or folded towel under her shoulder on the same side as the breast to be examined. This prop raises the side of the body and distrib-

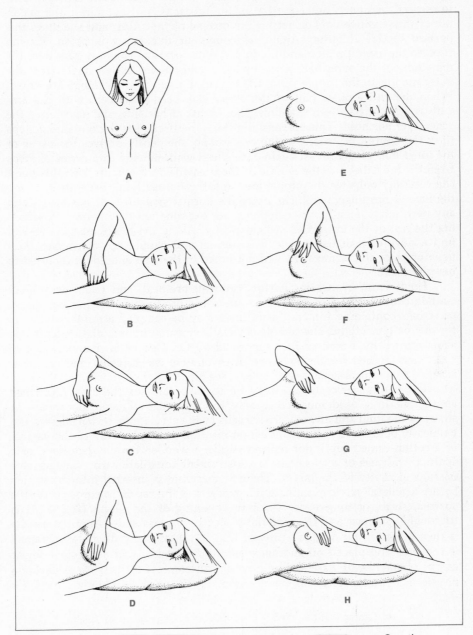

Figure 17.4 Steps for the systematic self-examination of the breast. See the text for description. (From National Cancer Institute.)

utes the weight evenly over her chest wall. Now, with one arm at her side, she systematically examines the flat, sensitive portions of the breast, extending her examination well into the armpit area (B in the figure). She now proceeds to inspect the upper, outer portion of the breast (C in the figure). She makes use of the sensitive flats of her fingers instead of their tips, and she gives this portion special attention. Again, any lump or thickening is noted. Having covered the armpit region and the upper, outer portion, she now goes over the remainder of the outer half of the breast, feeling in successive stages from the outer margin to the nipple (D in the figure). Lumps or thickenings are noted. When the entire outer half of the breast has been examined, with the arm with which she has been examining her breast at her side, she now raises the other over her head. This spreads and thins the tissue for the remaining steps (E in the figure). Beginning at the breastbone, she gently presses the tissue of the inner half of the breast against the chest wall, moving in a series of steps from the breastbone to the middle of the breast (F in the figure). At this point she carefully palpates the nipple area and the tissues lying beneath it. Using the flats of her fingers still, she notes the normal structures of her breast and any new lumps. Finally, she completes her examination of this breast by feeling the rest of the inner half systematically. Along the lower margin she will find a ridge of firm tissue, which is normal and should not alarm her. Any new lumps or thickenings she had not noted in the past should be reported to her physician.[2]

Fluids from bronchial, uterine, cervical, urethral, and rectal areas may contain cancer cells if these regions are either producing or being bathed by secretions containing tumors. Such fluids may be sampled a number of ways for microscopic study. The sample is usually smeared upon a glass microscope slide, stained by a method first suggested by Dr. George N. Papanicolaou in 1942, and studied for the presence of exfoliative cancer cells. Such a smear is called a Papanicolaou or "pap" smear; see Fig. 17.5.

The pap smear technique may be used for any of the areas described above, but it is used most commonly for diagnosis of cervical cancers. A smear of the fluid and any exfoliative cells of the cervix may be harmlessly and painlessly obtained by the introduction into the cervix, by way of the vagina, of a cotton-tipped applicator (cotton swab), a wooden tongue depressor, or a spatula, with use of a speculum (an instrument for dilation for viewing of a passage or cavity of the body). The dry speculum is inserted into the vagina before a general pelvic examination is made, and the cervix is exposed. With a spatula, swab, or tongue depressor the opening of the cervix (Fig. 17.5) is thoroughly scraped and the material placed on a glass slide. Another spatula is then placed in the vagina's interior (Fig. 17.5), and any discharge obtained is removed and placed on another glass slide.[3] Such a uterine-vaginal smear can be obtained with ease and without any discomfort to the patient during a physician's routine physical examination. If the smear is obtained carefully

---

[2] National Cancer Institute, Public Health Service, Department of Health, Education and Welfare.

[3] D. N. Holvey, Ed., *The Merck Manual*, 12th ed., Rahway, N.J., Merck & Co., 1972, p. 1826.

and the material adequately spread on the slides, sufficient diagnostic evidence usually is obtained for staining by the Papanicolaou method to produce either a negative or positive diagnosis of cervical cancer.

Sufficient evidence has accumulated at this time to indicate that *invasive epidermoid* or *squamous cervix cancer* (Fig. 17.1) develops from a diseased, cancerous surface epithelium known as *in situ carcinoma*. If all carcinomas of the cervix could be discovered and treated while still in this readily curable, in situ (preinvasion) stage, the possibility of eradicating cervical cancer as a cause of death would be very good indeed.

Unfortunately, in situ carcinoma may not produce alterations of the cervix visible to the naked eye, and their discovery cannot be left to a chance biopsy. The diagnosis of in situ carcinoma can be established only by a microscopic examination of tissues of cells derived from the cervix. A cytologic examination of Papanicolaou smears from the cervix is a reliable and accurate means of diagnosis of cancer of the cervix in its early stages.

It is generally assumed that the average age at the time of discovery of in situ carcinoma is from 5 to 10 years less than the average age of the time of discovery of the invasive carcinoma. This fact is of considerable importance, inasmuch as it indicates a very good chance of discovery of cancer of the

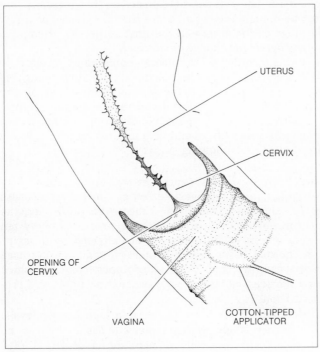

Figure 17.5   The cervix of the uterus. The "pap smear" is taken with a cotton-tipped stick.

cervix, in the in situ stage, if a systematic search for the disease is conducted along with annual physical examination from the teens on through middle age.

Cancer therapy

Many types of cancer can be successfully treated if detected early enough. When a physician speaks of "curing cancer," he means that the patient has not had a sign of the disease for five years after diagnosis and treatment. The three major types of cancer therapy are *surgery, radiation* and *chemotherapy.*

Surgery   Surgery in the treatment of cancer is an attempt to remove completely all the cancerous tissue in the involved organ. Because of the spreading nature of cancer large amounts of normal tissue are always removed along with the malignant growth. Surgery is used to remove certain endocrine glands (ovaries, pituitary or adrenal glands) in an effort to check the growth of cancer in organs which depend on the hormones produced by those glands for growth. It is also used to relieve pain in cases of incurable cancer by severing nerves serving the site of pain.

Numerous recent improvements in cancer surgery permit modern operations to be performed with far more safety than in the past. Even as early as 1953 the operative mortality rate had decreased considerably; today, the five-year-surgical-cure rate for some types of cancer has been greatly improved. However, it must be remembered at all times that the chance of a cure is still dependent on the stage of the disease at the time surgery is attempted. *The earlier the diagnosis the better the chance of survival.*

Surgery, radiation, and chemotherapy are being combined in an effort to find the most effective cancer cures possible. Chemicals are now being fed directly into the surgical wound to prevent the spread (metastasis) of any remaining cancer cells into the blood or lymph. Preoperative radiation to prevent implantation and growth of tumors in areas adjacent to the surgical area is being used. It is hoped that such preoperative radiation may materially reduce the degree of spread of cancer following surgery.

Radiation   Radiation has been used as a cancer treatment for about fifty years. Amounts of radiation that seem to have no effect on normal tissue cause a great deal of damage to cancerous tissue, sometimes even destroying the cancer completely. Radiation now is used to treat about six out of every ten cancer patients. Some types of cancer, however, are not affected by doses of radiation that are safe for normal tissue. Three sources of radiation are used in cancer therapy: high-voltage x-ray machines, radioisotopes (elements which release energy and nuclear particles as they change to other elements at a predictable rate), and laser radiation.

X-rays are controlled beams of electrons at variable high-energy levels. X-rays of extremely high energy levels readily penetrate tissue and can be used to arrest the growth or kill cancerous cells in deep internal organs. X-rays of relatively low energy are used for superficial cancers, such as skin growths.

Radioisotopes give energy in the form of alpha and beta particles and gamma rays. The advantage of such radioisotopes is that they are picked up by the body through the digestive system like other chemicals. A physician may select the radioactive isotope according to the area or organ he wishes to reach. Certain glands and organs tend to collect specific chemicals. Small, harmless doses of a radioisotope introduced into the body will then accumulate at such sites. The thyroid gland, for instance, tends to collect and accumulate iodine. Consequently, in treatment of cancer of the thyroid a radioisotope of iodine, I^{131}, is introduced into the body and is accumulated by the thyroid. Its destructive energy is thus in a strategic spot to attack the tumor with a controlled dose.

Radioactive cobalt also is used, the procedure being similar to that used in x-ray therapy. Cobalt therapy involves a carefully calculated placement of the patient in such a position that he or the cobalt can be rotated during exposure to the radiation beam so that the tumor is at the center of rotation in line with the radiation beam. This placement and rotation permits a maximal amount of radiation to be given to the tumor and a much smaller dosage to any one area of intervening tissue. An example of a cobalt machine is shown in Fig. 17.6.

Chemical compounds are now being used in conjunction with radiation. These drugs markedly increase the radiosensitivity of cancer cells. In some conditions the doses of radiation in combination with drugs are much smaller than those required when radiation is used alone.

Laser radiation is a relatively new type of light energy, which was first made available for biomedical research in the later 1950s and early 1960s. In cancer therapy the beams are focused on an accessible tumor or focused internally through special glass rods. This radiation has to some degree produced death in cancerous cells. The extent of such tumor control is dependent upon the amount of pigmentation of the tumor. The more highly pigmented the tumor, the greater the damage by lasers. Lesions that have been readily affected are basal-cell carcinoma, squamous-cell carcinoma, adenocarcinoma of the breast, and superficial and deep melanomas. Reduction of such tumors, followed by their surgical removal, has been successful. After laser radiation the cells have shown chromosomal changes, which emphasizes that cellular changes induced by lasers are more than just heat reactions.

Chemotherapy Although surgery and radiotherapy can often remove or arrest localized cancers, rarely can they cure cancers that have spread beyond their point of origin. These methods cannot be used to cure cancers of the blood or blood-forming tissues, such as leukemia, which are widespread throughout the body. For many years scientists believed that the only way to treat such cancers would be with drugs or chemicals that would destroy cancer cells and yet not harm normal cells. The treatment by the use of such drugs or chemicals is called *chemotherapy*.

The majority of cancers still are not curable by chemotherapy. Cancers such as those of the lung, colon-rectum, and breast—the three most common types of cancer in the United States—are not usually treated with drugs unless the conventional methods (surgery and radiotherapy) have failed or cannot be used at all. Often these diseases are treated with drugs to effect relief

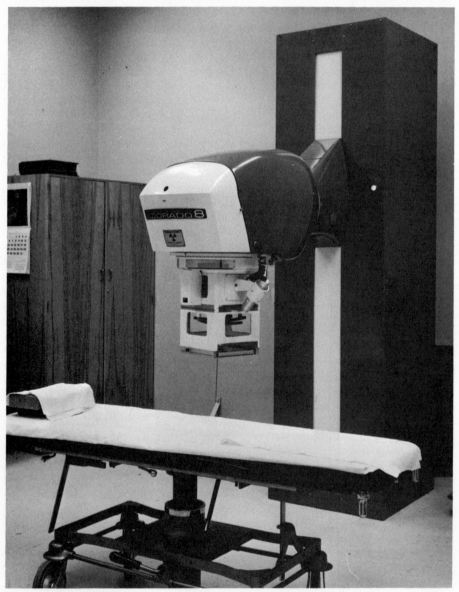

Figure 17.6   Cobalt machine for radiation therapy. (From UCLA Center for Health Sciences.)

from pain, produce a temporary lessening of the symptoms, or, in some instances, increase the individual's survival time.

The first success in chemotherapy came as a byproduct of wartime research during World War II. In the early 1940s accidental exposure of defense workers to nitrogen mustard gas was found to lead to a fall in the white-cell count in the blood. Since leukemia results in an overproduction of malignant white cells, nitrogen mustard gas was tested as a means of controlling this overproduction. The chemical proved more successful than anything previously tried.

Today some thirty drugs are being used in the treatment of cancer, and many more are being tested. None of these agents is a sure cure, but they all temporarily stop the growth of certain cancers, relieve pain, and allow the patient to live longer. Six or eight of these drugs have been found to be particularly promising in the treatment of leukemia, and several have been shown to be highly effective in producing complete remissions or cures in advanced Hodgkin's disease. These drugs were effective when used in combinations with one another and in conjunction with radiotherapy from x-ray machines. The results lead many to think that a combination of chemotherapy and radiotherapy may prove to be a greater benefit than either method of treatment alone.

The drugs currently being used in chemotherapy are of six main types: *alkylating agents, antimetabolites, hormones, plant alkaloids, antibiotics,* and *synthetic compounds.*

· ALKYLATING AGENTS   This is a large group of chemical compounds, which includes nitrogen mustard gas and urothane, that are in general cell poisons. They are called alkylating agents because they are capable of "alkylating"— that is, reacting and combining with a number of chemical groupings of which many are of vital importance in cell functions. Research in how these chemicals function within cells suggests that they act by cross-linking sections of DNA (see Chapter 11), inhibiting its replication, and thus stopping cell division. Consequently, these cell poisons interfere with the cell division of cancer cells and stop their growth. However, they also damage normal cells in the same manner and have had limited use until recently.

· ANTIMETABOLITES   Antimetabolites, or metabolic antagonists, are drugs very similar to the essential materials cancer cells need in synthesizing DNA. Flooding the cancer site with these drugs keeps the cells from building the chemicals needed to form DNA, thereby blocking cell division and slowing or stopping the growth of the cancer. Antimetabolites are effective in treating Hodgkin's disease and leukemia in children, often producing remissions that last several months.

· HORMONES   As explained earlier (Chapter 11), hormones are chemicals produced and secreted by the endocrine glands of the body. These chemicals influence or control many of the body's activities, such as growth and reproduction. Many cancers occur in hormone-controlled organs, such as the breasts, prostate gland, and uterus. Cancer tends to appear in these organs at a time in life when the body hormones are changing. These changes seem to produce an environment very suitable to cancerous growth. The importance in hormone chemotherapy lies in the fact that cancers arising from tissues modified by body hormones may retain some of the hormonal responsiveness they once had. Thus administration of hormones to re-alter the hormonal imbalance in the body of a cancer victim may cause regression of the cancer.

Male sex hormones (*androgens*) cause temporary regressions in about 20 percent of individuals with breast cancer, especially in premenopausal women. Female sex hormones, such as *estrogen*, are useful at times in reducing cancer of the prostate in males and metastatic breast cancer in postmenopausal women.

· PLANT ALKALOIDS   Plant alkaloids are a group of chemical compounds found in plants. The precise action of these drugs is not well understood, but they appear to act by inhibiting cell division. They do not appear to react with the DNA, but they actually block cell division and keep it from happening. Their effectiveness lies in the fact that many of these agents can easily enter specific cells without affecting others in the body. Some are able to produce a reduction in white-cell counts by stopping their production in the bone marrow. This is highly effective in the treatment of acute childhood leukemia.

· ANTIBIOTICS   Antibiotics have been used for years in the treatment of bacterial infections. In recent years they have been found to be effective in the treatment of certain types of cancer. This use is so new that extensive data on the duration of remissions produced are not yet available.

Certain antibiotics, such as *actinomycin D* and *Daunomycin*, seem to be effective in their control of cancer by being able to inhibit the enzyme needed for synthesis of RNA (transfer RNA) and thus block DNA synthesis.

· SYNTHETIC COMPOUNDS   Synthetic compounds are those produced in chemical laboratories. Some seem to act as general cell poisons, others, such as methyl GAG, interfere with protein metabolism; still others such as *o-p'*-DDD, a derivative of the insecticide DDT, are believed to be able to suppress hormone production and other body activities by inhibiting certain enzyme systems in the body.

CANCER INCIDENCE

It is not known how many people actually have cancer. Some cancers as, for example, skin cancer are observable shortly after the malignant growth begins, but many forms remain undetected until late in the course of the disease. In addition, some individuals fail to seek medical care even after the disease is noticeable. These conditions make the total number of persons who actually have cancer much larger than the number with diagnosed cancer. All published statistics are based on the number of persons who have been diagnosed as having cancer.

The magnitude of any disease problem is measured by (1) incidence, the number of new cases per year; (2) mortality, the number of deaths per year; and (3) prevalence, the number of cases under treatment or care at any one time during a given year. With information such as the incidence and mortality for all diseases it is possible to estimate what proportion of the population may be expected to develop cancer (or any other disease) during life or at any specified age. A projection of the increase in death from lung cancer is shown in Fig. 17.7.

Cancer is a disease that can affect people of any age. It occurs in children as well as in adults; however, it strikes and kills with increasing frequency with advancing age. And, as explained in Chapter 9 our older population is greatly increasing in size. More than 52 million Americans now living will eventually have cancer (or about one in every four). Two out of every three families in the United States will have someone who will contract cancer.

Cancer is a universal disease and respects no one. As early as 1968 the National Cancer Institute showed that the overall cancer incidence in the United States was increasing; see Fig. 17.8. According to this source, in 1930 less than 200 individuals per 100,000 population contracted cancer; by 1985, if current trends continue, almost 400 per 100,000 will contract cancer each year.

The one ray of hope in all of this is shown in Fig. 17.8. The incidence of cancer is indeed increasing, but the mortality rate both projected and present, remains almost stationary, making it clear that survival rates and cures of cancer are definitely improving. This is not true of all forms of cancer; the trend varies greatly with different types. As shown in Fig. 17.7, deaths from lung cancer are increasing at an alarming rate, while the mortality rate from

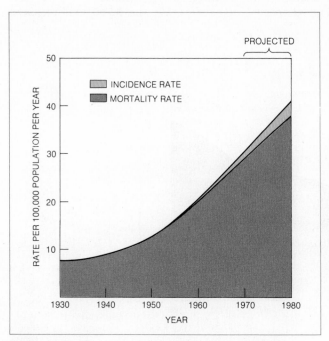

Figure 17.7   The upward trend of deaths from lung cancer is sharper than that from any other type of cancer. Although the cause is known, antismoking drives remain ineffective. Projection of the increase in lung cancer deaths through 1980 assumes that present trends will continue. (From National Cancer Institute.)

uterine cancers has fallen steadily for years and is expected to continue to fall; see Figs. 17.9 and 17.10. Except for deaths from cancer of the lung and the pancreas, and from leukemia, mortality rates in general are leveling out or, as discussed above, in some cases dropping off.

Of every six persons who contract cancer currently, two will be saved and four will die. The first two of the six will be saved by an early diagnosis and prompt treatment; the third will die but might have been saved had proper treatment been received in time; the last three will die of cancers that cannot yet be controlled and that only the results of further research could save. But *half* of the people who contract cancer can and should be saved—by known treatment—through *early diagnosis* and proper use of acceptable cancer therapy.

Cancer in children

Cancer as a cause of death in children in the United States has increased since 1930. At that time only 0.7 percent of all deaths under age 15 were attributed to cancer. In 1973, cancer accounted for 3,760 childhood deaths. More schoolchildren die of cancer each year than from any other disease.

Since 1955 cancer deaths in this country among children under 15 have been recorded according to specific body sites. Of the 3,760 children who

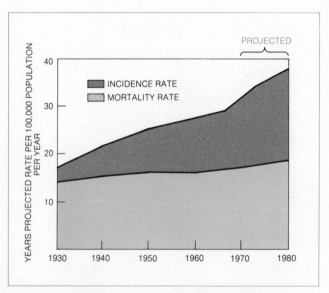

Figure 17.8 Incidence of cancer compared with increasing mortality from cancer: the general incidence is rising faster than the population, but the mortality rate has remained almost level. (From National Cancer Institute.)

died from cancer in 1973, for example, 1,387, or nearly half, died of leukemia. Other cancers that cause significant numbers of deaths in that age group are cancer of the brain, the lymphosarcomas, cancer of the bone, and cancers of the kidney, such as Wilms' tumor.

Cancer in males

The ten most common causes of death by cancer in males are shown in Table 17.3. Cancer of the lung is now the leading cause of cancer death in men, and it is increasing at an alarming rate (Fig. 17.7). Over the last fifty years cancer of the lung has shown a much greater rise in frequency than any other type of cancer; the rate today is more than fifteen times what it was only thirty-five years ago. This is within the lifetime of the average smoker today. In 1973 it was approximated that 150 deaths a day occurred because of lung cancer. As will be explained in Chapter 18, the single most important factor related to the control of lung cancer is cigarette smoking. To overcome lung cancer there must be a continuing intensification of the effort to educate Americans regarding the health hazards of cigarette smoking. Other effects of cigarette smoking and related diseases will be discussed in separate sections in this and other chapters.

The majority of lung carcinomas arise in the main bronchi or their immediate divisions, as shown in Fig. 17.11. Further extension of these cancers

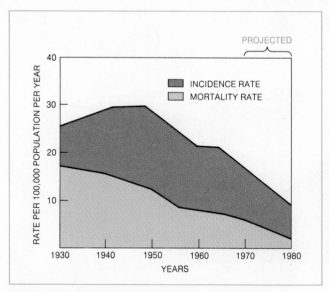

Figure 17.9 Incidence and mortality rates of cancer of the cervix: mortality is markedly lower, mainly because of "pap smear" examinations and prompt treatment. This trend is expected to continue. (From National Cancer Institute.)

gives rise to lymphatic metastases in their course by involving the regional lymph nodes very early. Cancer cells move upward to the nodes of the neck and downward to nodes around the abdominal aorta and on to the liver and adrenal glands. Metastasis by way of the bloodstream is frequent, so that brain cancer often is an outcome of lung cancer.

Carcinoma of the prostate accounts for 5 percent of the total cancer death rate and 9 percent of male deaths from cancer. It is the second commonest cancer in men, the first being cancer of the lung. Over 90 percent of cases of prostate cancer occur after the age of 60 (only one in five cases of enlarged prostate is malignant). The chief symptoms of the latter disease are the same as those for benign enlargements—frequency, urgency, and difficulty in urination. Later there is pain, especially during urination. The primary carcinoma is slow growing, but it gains early access to the surrounding venous and lymphatic channels, giving rise to metastases in the spine, pelvis, or regional lymph nodes.

Cancers of the oral cavity and pharynx are the tenth commonest types of cancer in men, yet they account for 3 percent of the male deaths from cancer (Table 17.3). *There is a strong link between these cancers and smoking.*

A few simple observations and safeguards practiced by all individuals could help in the prevention of mouth cancer. A heavy smoker in whose mouth white patches develop and persist should give up smoking. Any dental

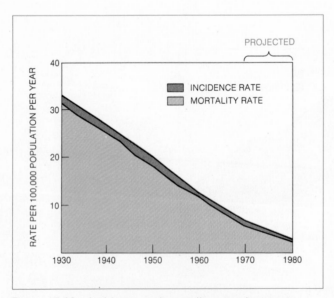

Figure 17.10   Incidence and mortality rates for cancer of the stomach: both have fallen steadily for years. What will happen in the future is not predictable. (From National Cancer Institute.)

Table 17.3 *Cancer deaths by sex and ten major sites, 1973*

site	no. of deaths	percentage of all cancer deaths
Male		
Lung	57,900	30
Prostate	17,800	9
Colon[a]	17,100	9
Pancreas	10,900	6
Stomach	8,700	5
Lymphomas[b]	11,100	6
Leukemia	8,600	5
Bladder and urethra	10,500	6
Rectum	5,800	3
Oral cavity	5,550	3
Total 10 major sites	153,900	82
Total of all sites	190,000	100
Female		
Breast	32,000	20
Colon[a]	19,900	12
Uterus[c]	11,800	8
Lung	14,100	8
Ovary[d]	10,500	7
Pancreas	8,300	5
Lymphomas[b]	9,200	6
Stomach	6,000	4
Leukemia	6,700	4
Liver and biliary passages	4,000	3
Total of 10 major sites	115,800	77
Total of all sites	160,000	100

SOURCE: Adapted from *1973 Cancer Facts and Figures*, American Cancer Society, Inc., 1973.
[a] Excluding rectum.
[b] Including lymphosarcoma, Hodgkin's disease, multiple myeloma.
[c] Corpus uteri and cervix.
[d] Including fallopian tube and broad ligament.

condition such as pyorrhea, gingivitis, decaying teeth, or ill-fitting dental prostheses should be corrected before they cause irritation, sores, or other damages to appear upon the gums, tongue, or lip. If, after removal of the cause, an irritated area should fail to heal promptly, the persistent sore may be an early cancer; thus medical advice should be sought. A crack in the skin of the lip which fails to heal or any growth or patches on the tongue or in the mouth which enlarge, thicken, or bleed should be regarded as danger signals, and medical advice should be sought immediately.

People with head and neck cancer are often undernourished by the time they seek treatment. They have neither taste nor desire for food, and for them eating may be difficult, uncomfortable, or even painful. This group of cancers produces constant discomfort from excessive salivation, sensations of obstruction, difficult swallowing, soreness, and pain.

Tumors of the bladder occur about twice as frequently in men as in women. Many of these growths seem to be benign when they first appear but have a pronounced tendency to become malignant and to recur. The natural course of bladder cancer is very prolonged, but treatment is quite successful. The average age of patients diagnosed as having bladder cancer is about 57 years, and it accounts for 3 percent of the total cancer death rate. Metastasis to the pelvic lymph nodes is not uncommon, but distant metastasis is rare. The symptoms and complications are listed in Table 17.1.

Cancer in females

As shown in Table 17.3, cancer of the breast accounts for almost one in every five female deaths from cancer. It is more common in women who have not

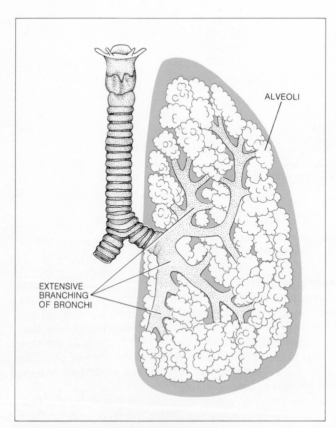

Figure 17.11   Respiratory system.

had children; the average age of patients is 51, which approximates the menopausal phase of life.

Most carcinomas of the breast arise in the small ducts leading from the glands. Skin nodules may occur at any time and usually develop over the breast in the untreated individual or around the scar in those operated upon. Cancer of both breasts is not uncommon, although it is difficult to say whether one is a metastasis from the other breast or a new primary growth. Some tumors metastasize so early and spread so widely that they often prove fatal within one year of onset.

The factors causing cancer of the breast seem to be as diverse as the various forms the disease may take. Endocrine factors often seem important, and occasionally inherited susceptibility appears significant. There is, however, no known way in which cancer of the breast can be prevented, making it very important that a tumor be detected at the earliest possible stage. Detection is accomplished by Breast Self-Examination (BSE), shown in Fig. 17.4 and explained elsewhere in this chapter, or by mammography or xerography; see Fig. 17.12.

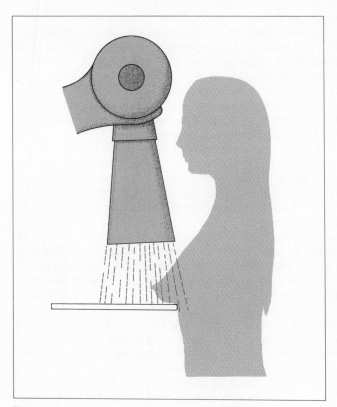

Figure 17.12　Mammography, or examination of the breast by x-ray.

Cancer of the uterus may be divided into cancer found in two areas, the cervix and the body of the uterus (*corpus uteri*). Cancer of the cervix is the second most common cancer in women; deaths are distributed by age in a manner similar to that for breast cancer. This cancer is more common in women who have borne children than in women who have not.

A possible association, proposed by some cancer researchers and disputed by others, is that between cervical cancer and a woman's sexual history. It has been reported that the incidence of cervical cancer is higher among women who begin sexual intercourse at younger ages and those with a history of many sexual partners. The incidence of uterine cancer is low among virgins, women with later onsets of sexual intercourse, and women with histories of one or few sexual partners.

Many factors associated with early intercourse or multiple sexual partners could account for such an association. Genetic mutation of the cervical cells is one possibility; the cause of such a mutation might be the repeated mechanical trauma during coitus or some carcinogenic chemical in semen, though the latter seems extremely unlikely. Another possible stimulus of cancer production is irritation of the cervical tissues by chronic infection with one or more of the many sexually transmitted organisms.

Herpes simplex, virus particles, are often found within cancerous cells of the uterus, but no cause-and-effect relationship has been established. Assuming that the statistical relationship between early coitus and uterine cancer is valid, the causive factor may be a sexually transmitted herpes simplex virus. Since the incidence of actual uterine cancer increases with age, and herpes simplex is noted for its ability to lie dormant (latent) for many years, it is possible that the cells of the younger woman are more susceptible to infection but that the dormant organism, unable to initiate cellular changes for many years, effects no actual cervical cancer until later in life.

The growth usually begins as a node near the opening of the uterus, an ulceration soon appearing. In the early stages of the disease the only outward symptom may be a slight watery discharge or an occasional spotting of blood between menstrual periods. Lengthening of menstrual periods may be an early symptom and, of course, any bleeding after the menopause is suspicious and demands immediate examination.

The degree of growth at the time of diagnosis and treatment is of great significance in the outcome of cancer of the cervix. The Cancer Committee of the League of Nations in 1929 initiated an international classification of carcinoma of the cervix, dividing the degree of involvement of the disease into four stages. The clarification of these stages is shown in Fig. 17.13 and is as follows.

In stage I, carcinoma of the cervix is established when a growth is found that is strictly confined to the cervix; only about 10 percent of the patients first seen are at this stage. In stage II the growth has spread into the upper part of the vagina or into the second layer of tissue of the cervix, but at no point has it reached the pelvic wall; about 30 percent of the patients are in this stage when treated. In stage III the growth has reached the pelvic wall at one point, so that no operation can remove such a growth; about 40 percent of the patients are in this stage when first seen. In stage IV the growth has invaded the bladder or rectovaginal area and may have filled the pelvis or given rise to distant metastases; about 20 percent of the patients are in this very advanced stage on their first examination.

When this criterion for the four stages of uterine cancer was established, it made no provisions for a flat, noninvading type of cancer cell that seemed to exist for years before spreading began. Since that time this noninvading cancer has been called *in situ epidermoid carcinoma* and is now designated

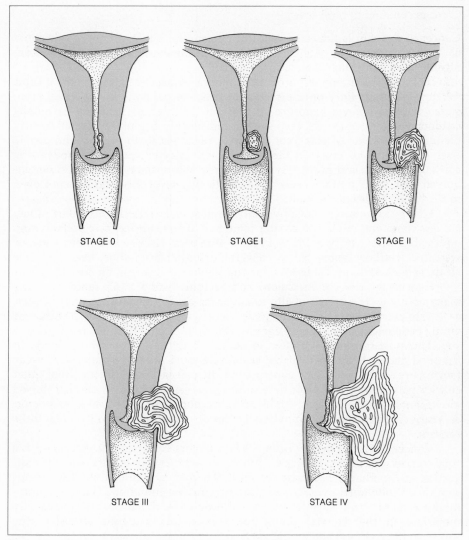

STAGE 0   STAGE I   STAGE II

STAGE III   STAGE IV

Figure 17.13   International classification of carcinoma of the cervix.

stage O in the international classification of carcinoma of the cervix. Such early cases of cancer are now discovered very frequently in women as a result of finding cast-off (exfoliate) cells in Papanicolaou smears. When found in this preinvasion stage (in situ carcinoma), the disease is always curable. For this reason *every* woman should be examined and have a "pap" smear once a year.

Cancer of the body of the uterus is uncommon and usually occurs in older age groups (early sixties). Such cancers arise from the endometrial lining, where frequently a preexisting growth has been present.

Cancers common to both sexes

Cancer of the skin is the commonest of all cancers, but its frequency does not show in mortality statistics because it seldom involves vital organs, is recognizable in an early stage, and is easily cured.

The most common type of skin cancer is basal-cell carcinoma (Table 17.1). It occurs mainly on the face and, in some patients, seems to be associated with prolonged exposure to the sun. Its highest incidence is among outdoor workers. It grows very slowly and usually begins as a small, pearly plaque in the skin. After a year or two it ulcerates in the center and covers over with a scab or crust. In the late stages it may extend to the underlying cartilage or bone and ultimately will destroy the nose, eye, or any other involved part. Unlike other cancers, it practically never metastasizes, not even to the lymph nodes in the immediate area.

Other skin cancers are physically similar to basal-cell carcinoma. They are less common but show a greater tendency to metastasize to regional lymph nodes after a year or two. Many of these skin cancers arise in a mole, wart, or wen that has been subjected to constant irritation by a shoe, belt, brassiere strap, and so on. (See Table 17.1 for suggestions in controlling such cancers.)

Cancers of the cecum, colon, and rectum (Table 17.1) taken together make up about 15 percent of the total cancer death rate. Although these diseases are seen mostly in older age groups, 4 percent of the cases occur in young people under 30 years of age.

The most common symptom of cancer in the large intestine is blood in the fecal material. The patient has usually ignored the early minor symptoms (such as repeated attacks of constipation, increased mucus in the stool, mild colicky pain before and after defecation, or a sensation of incomplete bowel movements), but he regards the bleeding as more serious and sees his doctor. A yearly proctoscopic examination is the best method of controlling these cancers.

Cancer of the stomach (Table 17.1) accounts for about 10 percent of the total cancer mortality. Its early symptoms are very indefinite—slight indigestion and, perhaps, a distaste for meat. The persistence of these two symptoms in an individual over 40 demands an x-ray examination. The later symptoms are mainly pain, anemia, and loss of weight. By this time there are usually metastases in the regional lymph nodes, soon followed by a spread of the cancer to the liver and abdominal walls.

The leukemias generally run a chronic course in adults, the average length of life from onset being from two to five years. In older men it may be five to ten years or longer. Some cases of lymphoid leukemia may have very long periods of remissions, when all symptoms may disappear. There is an acute form of leukemia which affects young children, especially those about 2 to 5 years old; it causes a rapid wasting away, and death may ensue in a few months.

Hodgkin's disease has several forms. The term is usually used to designate malignant growths of the lymph nodes and the spleen not affecting the bone marrow, liver, and other organs. Hodgkin's disease, along with some forms of leukemia, mainly affects young adults in the 20–30 age group. Since 1949 the International List of Diseases, Injuries, and Causes of Death has included the leukemias and Hodgkin's disease as forms of cancer,[4] leukemia has accounted for about 4 percent of the cancer mortality and Hodgkin's disease for 1 percent.

RESEARCH TRENDS

For many years researchers have probed the nature of cancer; now they share an attitude of optimism concerning the eventual understanding of these complex diseases.

Chemical carcinogens

Knowledge of the role of the chemical compounds in cancer comes primarily from clinical observation of the occurrence of certain types of cancer in men engaged in particular occupations. A limited number of human cancers are unquestionably caused by exposure to particular *chemical carcinogens*. Examples of such occupational carcinogens are (1) soot, tar and creosote, (2) petroleum-based oils, (3) aniline dyes, (4) metals and ores (notably chromates and nickel), and (5) asbestos.

Chemical studies have led to the identification of at least one powerful carcinogen in coal tar, 3:4-benzpyrene; the other carcinogenic compounds of coal tar have not yet been identified. Substances in the aniline dyes are among the best known of human carcinogens. The mining and processing of chromates is associated with a high incidence of carcinoma of the lung, and nickel refining is associated with carcinoma of the sinuses. Asbestos particles are proven to cause lung cancer.

In cancers related to occupational exposure the carcinogenic hazard is pinpointed by studies of the occurrence of specific tumors and then proved by studies of animals, in which similar types of cancer are induced by exposure to the suspected carcinogenic compounds whose carcinogenic activity is measurable only in laboratory animals. These compounds are being introduced into the environment in steadily increasing numbers as a result of industrialization, urbanization, and the other changes of modern living. This pollution of our environment has created an urgent need to identify, characterize, and

[4] World Health Organization, Geneva, Switzerland.

assess the ability of chemical agents to induce human cancer. In the meantime the agents that are proven to be carcinogenic should be regarded as hazardous. Such was the procedure in establishing the dangerous role of cigarette smoking in lung cancer (see Chapter 18).

Radiation

Cancer induced by exposure to radiation was first reported more than sixty years ago. Since then the ability of radiation to induce tumors in laboratory animals and human beings has been well documented. Studies of irradiated animals and men indicate that radiation of almost any part of the body increases the incidence of malignancy roughly in proportion to dosage. But it is impossible to say how much human cancer is induced by radiation, x-ray, or radionuclides lodged in the tissues.

Viruses

More than fifty years ago the relation of viruses to cancer in fowl was first demonstrated. Research since then has yielded numerous viruses that induce tumors in various animals, including mammals. Research into the development of leukemia in mice led to the discovery of a viral cause of that disease. Human leukemic tissues yield particles very similar to mouse leukemia viruses, and other particles from human leukemia and cervical cancer have the characteristics of herpes viruses (common herpes viruses cause diseases such as cold sores, shingles, and fever blisters) and are believed to be true viruses; they have been seen in other human cancers.

The task of solving the puzzle of tumor-producing viruses assumes a degree of urgency because of the role of these viruses in the leukemias of birds and rodents and in man. The infecting virus, upon entering the cell, takes over the cell's protein-synthesizing machinery. Then the cell synthesizes viral DNA and protein—instead of normal cell DNA and protein—just long enough to produce a crop of new complete viruses, after which the cell dies. These cell-destroying viruses are called *cytolytic* viruses. With viruses that do not destroy cells the cell does not turn off the synthetic processes; rather, it produces a slightly different DNA, which transforms the cell into a type that differs in some respects from the original infected cell. This infected cell is very probably malignant. The viruses that have been shown to perform this transformation are termed *oncogenic* (tumor-producing).

The precise role of the invading virus in the transformation of normal host cells into cancerous cells remains to be established, but the stage has now been set for such investigations. It is possible that all animals, including humans, are carriers of viruses with tumor-inducing potential. Research suggests that this potential requires activation by some other agent or agents, such as radiation, chemicals (carcinogens), another virus, hormonal imbalance, or an immunologic response. Many more of the intermediate steps between cell penetration by a virus and the actual cancer transformation must be clarified before science can move beyond the "suggestive" stage.

Endocrine factors

The suspicion that endocrine factors participate in cancer in man has long interested researchers. Observations have shown that hormones profoundly influence the rates of biochemical and physiological processes within the body. However, no evidence is available that cancer in man arises as a primary result of the production in the body of one or more hormones. Tumors, in both experimental animals and man, may regress to some degree after endocrinologic therapy.

Human malignancies such as cancer of the prostate, breast, and uterus and the lymphomas and leukemias can be inhibited by hormone changes. Although life has been prolonged, cures have never been obtained through the use of hormones.

Genetic factors

A few uncommon types of human cancer are considered to be hereditary. These include *xeroderma pigmentosium,* a recessive condition in which the skin is quite sensitive to sunlight, so that exposure may result in skin cancers. *Retinoblastoma,* a type of cancer of the eye, follows a dominant pattern of inheritance. Children with mongolism, a commonly inherited condition, have 20 times more leukemia than nonmongoloid children.

Information from studies of the more common types of cancer is difficult to analyze genetically because of the general makeup of the population. A family's tendency to cancer in a particular site is suggested when statistical studies show a frequency greater in one family than would be expected in the general population. Family tendencies have been reported for cancer of the breast, uterus, prostate, stomach, colon-rectum, and lung. However, these hereditary factors are not considered to be strong.

Immunity to cancer

Studies concerning the general immunities of the cancer patient are being made, as are intensive efforts to find specific antigens in human tumors. A patient does have some body defenses against his own cancer, but he also has certain immunity problems. Cancer patients are highly susceptible to infection. In the leukemias and similar diseases infection may be related to the advance of the disease, tumor invasion, and replacement of the tissues that produce white blood cells (which normally ingest foreign material).

Research in the future may attempt to stimulate body defenses by utilizing cancer vaccines made from a patient's own tumor or other patients' tumors.

SUMMARY

    I. What cancer is
       A. An uncontrolled, disorderly replacement of worn-out cells, which continues as an abnormal growth.

B. Cancer cells distinguished by the nuclei.
1. Usually larger than those of comparable normal cells.
2. Vary significantly in size and shape within a group of cancer cells.
3. Deviate in number and appearance of chromosomes.
C. Cellular processes and behavior
1. Cancer cells fail to obey feedback and self-controlling mechanisms.
2. They produce large amounts of DNA, RNA, and protein.
D. Tumors—growths which persist, grow, and serve no useful purpose
1. Benign tumors are growths that increase in size slowly, are surrounded by a fibrous membrane, and remain localized.
2. Malignant tumors are growths that increase in size rapidly, are not surrounded by a membrane or capsule, and tend to spread and invade other tissues:
   a. cancer—usually used to designate all malignant growths.
   b. carcinomas—malignant tumors arising from epithelial tissues.
   c. sarcomas—malignant tumors arising from connective tissues.
E. Spread of cancer
1. Invasion—extension into spaces between normal cells.
2. Metastasis—process of transferring cancer from an organ or part of the body to another, forming secondary cancer sites.
3. Implantation—dislodged or shed cancer cells that implant themselves in adjacent organs, grow, and produce their destructive effects.
F. How cancer kills
1. Anemia:
   a. insufficient production of red blood cells.
   b. production of defective cells that do not survive long in circulation.
   c. intestinal bleeding either directly from a tumor or indirectly (example: bone-marrow deficiencies).
2. Infection—frequently occurs because of the reduction of white blood cells, which causes a depression of the body's defenses against infection.
3. Debility (wasting away of the body) which might result from:
   a. damage to mouth or stomach.
   b. treatment by drugs, surgery, or radiation.
   c. loss of appetite from pain or emotional depression.
II. Diagnosis not death
A. Cancer can be cured if diagnosed and treated in early stages.
B. Prevention of cancer
1. Periodic health examination of the presumably well individual.
2. Avoidance of long-continued irritations or inflammations.
3. Knowledge of symptoms of the commonest forms of cancer, the Seven Danger Signals of Cancer.
C. Cancer therapy
1. Surgery—used to remove completely all of the cancerous tissue in an involved organ.
2. Radiation—used to damage or destroy cancerous tissues.
3. Chemotherapy—use of drugs or chemicals to destroy cancer cells without harming normal tissues.
III. Cancer incidence
A. Actual number of cases is not known; all statistics based on number of persons diagnosed as having cancer.

B. Cancer in children has increased since 1930.

C. In males the most common sites are lungs, prostate, colon, and pancreas.

D. In females most common sites are breast, colon, uterus, and lung.

IV. Research trends

A. Chemical carcinogens are chemical compounds unquestionably causing cancer.

B. Radiation has cancer-producing qualities.

C. Viruses can invade and transform normal cells into cancerous areas.

D. Genetic factors have produced only a few uncommon types of human cancers.

Glossary

If you cannot find the word you wish in this glossary, check the index for text and glossary references.

anemia (ə nē′mē ə) (G. *an*, negative; *haima*, blood). A condition in which the blood is deficient either in quantity or quality.

benign tumor (bi nīn) (L. *benignus*, well-born). An abnormal swelling or growth that is not malignant or cancerous.

birthmark (burth′mark). Some peculiar mark or blemish found on the body at birth and retained throughout life.

cancer (kan′sər) (L. *Cancri*, "crab"). A cellular tumor showing uncontrolled growth; the natural course is fatal and usually associated with formation of secondary growths.

carcinogenic (kahr si nō jen′ik). Causing or producing cancer.

carcinoma (kahr si nō′mə) (G. *karkinōma*, from *karkinos* crab, cancer). A new tumorous growth made up of epithelial cells invading the surrounding tissues and giving rise to secondary growths throughout the body.

cell poison (sel poi′zn) (L. *cella*, compartment; L. *potio*, to drink; G. *toxicum*, toxin). Any substance which by its chemical action may cause damage to the structure or function of the cell.

cervix (sur′viks) (L. *cervix*, neck). The lower and narrow end of the uterus.

chemotherapy (kem′ō ther′ə pē) (G. *chemeia*, chemistry; *therapeia*, treatment). The treatment of disease by administering of chemicals which affect the causative factor unfavorably but do not injure the patient.

chromosome (krō′mə sōm) (G. *chromo*, color; *soma*, body). A small dark-staining and more or less rod-shaped body which appears in the nucleus of a cell at the time of cell division; it contains the genes, or hereditary factors, and is constant in number in each species.

cobalt (kō′bawlt). A metal with atomic number 27; a radioactive isotope of the element cobalt is used in the treatment of cancer.

cyst (sist) (G. *kystis*, sac, bladder). Any vesicle or sac of membranous tissue.

debility (de bil′i tē) (L. *debilis*, weak). Lack or loss of strength.

endocrine glands (en′də krin) (G. *endo*, within; *krinein*, to separate; L. *glans*, acorn-like). Glands or organs whose function is to secrete into the blood or lymph a substance (hormone) that has a specific effect on another organ or part.

endocrinologic therapy (en′dō krin′ə loj′ik ther′ə pē). Treatment of disease by the administration of endocrine preparations (hormones).

endometrial lining (en′dō mē′trē əl) (G. *endo*, within; *metra*, womb.) The mucous membrane that lines the cavity of the uterus.

epithelium (ep i thē'lē əm) (G. *epi*, on, upon; *thele*, nipple). The covering of internal and external surfaces of the body, including the lining of vessels and other small cavities.

fibroid tumor (fī'broid), **fibroma** (fī brō'mə). A tumor composed mainly of fibrous or fully developed connective tissue.

hormone (hor'mōn) (G. *hormon*, excite). A chemical substance secreted into the body fluids by an *endocrine gland*, which has a specific effect on the activities of other organs.

incidence (in'si dəns) (L. *incidens*, falling upon). The range of occurrence of a disease.

infection (in fek'shən) (L. *infectio*, to dip in). Invasion of the body by pathogenic microorganisms and the reaction of the tissues to their presence and to the toxins generated by them.

in situ (in sī'too) (Latin term meaning "in the natural place"). In situ epidermoid carcinoma is a changing of the surface epithelium of the cervix which histologically resembles cancer but shows no evidence of invasion of the underlying fibromuscular stroma.

in vitro (in vē'trō) (L.). Within a glass; observable in a test tube.

in vivo (in vē'vō) (L.) Within the living body.

laser (lā'zər) (Light, Amplification, by Stimulated Emission of Radiation). An instrument for producing an enormously intense and sharply directed beam of light.

lymphoma (lim fō'mə) (L. *lympha*, water; G. *oma*, from *onkoma*, a swelling). Any tumor made up of lymphoid tissue.

lymphomatosis (lim'fō mə tō'sis). The development of multiple lymphomas in various parts of the body.

malignant (mə lig'nənt) (L. *malignans*, acting maliciously). Ability to invade the tissues of an individual; tending to go from bad to worse.

metabolic antagonist (met ə bol'ik an tag'ə nist) (G. *metabolos*, changeable; G. *antagonistes*, to struggle against). A substance which reverses or inhibits the physical or chemical processes by which living organisms produce and maintain life.

metastasis (mə tas'tə sis) (G. *meta*, after, beyond; *stasis*, stand). The transfer of disease from one organ or part to another not directly connected with it; it may be due either to the transfer of pathogenic organisms or to transfer of cells, as in malignant tumors.

mortality (mor tal'i tē) (L. *mortalis*, mortal, living). The death rate; the ratio of total number of deaths to the total population.

mucous membranes (myoo'kəs) (L. *mucosus*, slimy). The lining membranes of the body.

nucleus (nyoo'klē əs) (L. *nucleus*, a little nut). A spheroid body within a cell which controls the cell's activities.

platelet (plāt'lit) (G. *plate*, flat). Discs found in the blood of all mammals, which are concerned in coagulation of the blood and formation of clots.

prostate gland (pros'tāt) (G. *prostates*, one who stands before). A gland which in the male surrounds the neck of the bladder and the urethra.

radiation (rā dē ā'shən) (L. *radiatio*, to emit rays). The giving off of electromagnetic waves such as light, or particulate rays such as the alpha, beta, and gamma rays.

radioisotopes (rā'dē ō ī'sə tōp) (L. *radius*, ray; G. *isos*, equal; *topos*, place). An element, with radioactive properties, of chemical character identical with that of another element occupying the same place in the periodic table but differing from it in its atomic characteristics. Radioisotopes are used as tracers or indicators by being added to the stable compound under observation, so that the course of the compound in the body can be detected and followed by the radio-activity thus added to it. The stable element so treated is said to be "labeled" or "tagged."

radiosensitivity (rā′dē ō sen si tiv′i tē) (L. *radius*, ray; *-sensus*, to perceive). Being sensitive to, or destroyable by, radiant energy, as radium, x-ray, or electric radiations.

remission (ri mish′ən) (L. *remittere*, to send back). A decrease or abatement of the symptoms of a disease.

sarcoma (sahr kō′mə) (G. *sarkos*, flesh; *onkōma*, a swelling). A form of cancer arising from cells of nonepithelial tissue, such as connective tissue, lymphoid tissue, cartilage, bone.

tetraploid (tet′rə ploid) (G. *tetraple*, fourfold). Having four full sets of homologous chromosomes; they are found in cancerous organisms.

tumor (tyoo′mər) (L. from *tumere*, to swell). A mass of new tissue which persists and grows independently of its surrounding structures and which has no physiologic use (neoplasm).

ultraviolet (ul′trə vī′ə lit). Radiation beyond the violet end of the light spectrum; ultraviolet rays have powerful electrochemical properties.

wart (wort) (L. *verruca*, elevation). A small tumor on the skin.

wen (wen) (AS. wenn, *ultimate*). A lump on the body; a sebaceous cyst.

x-ray (*x*, unknown; L. *radius*, ray). Penetrating electromagnetic radiation discovered by German physicist Wilhelm Conrad Roentgen in 1895. Also called *roentgen ray*.

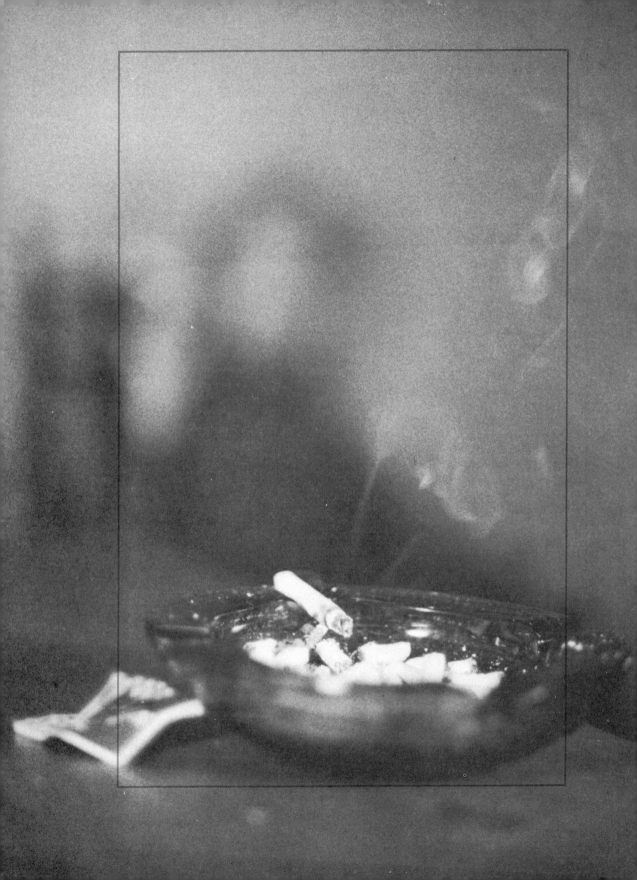

Smoking and the effects of tobacco

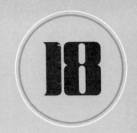

Cigarette smoking has become extremely common in our culture. To challenge an individual's smoking habit is to challenge a habit of nearly 70 million Americans. This has not always been the case. The cigarette consumption in the United States has increased tremendously since the turn of the century. In 1900 the per-person consumption rate for persons 18 years of age and over was less than 50 cigarettes per year. By 1967 this had reached the all-time high of 4,280 cigarettes consumed for every person over 18 years of age. In late 1967 and early 1968 a reduction in the per person consumption of cigarettes began; see Fig. 18.1. This trend continued through 1970, chiefly owing to the breaking of the habit by older individuals. Between 1968 and 1971 between 1.5 and 2 million Americans gave up smoking. By 1972 the trend had reversed and once again started upward, the per person consumption reaching 4,050 cigarettes a year. The increase reflects mainly a trend of the young people (between 17 and 24 years of age), who are starting to smoke for the first time.

Teenagers have never smoked to the extent that adults have. In 1953, 34 percent of the 17-year-old males and 25 percent of the 17-year-old females smoked. By 1968 this rate had dropped to 25 percent and 15 percent, respectively. Many of these individuals started smoking as early as 9 or 10 years of age. The majority of smokers, however, begin somewhere between 17 and 24 years of age, often during military service or as a result of the freedom and the pressures of the first years of college.

The sharpest increases in smoking have occurred during wars. A sharp rise began in 1914 during World War I. World War II produced another jump; the rise between 1942 and 1946 (the actual war years) was fantastic (Fig. 18.1). In the future we can expect to see some type of increase in cigarette smoking during any war or military conflict. The chief reason for this is that during such times as war an individual experiences increased tension. Knowledge that might ordinarily go unquestioned, moreover, such as the fact that smoking is harmful, no longer seems important when you are at war. Another reason for an increase during wartime is that young servicemen are introduced to smoking as a "tension reliever." Many of today's smokers were first introduced to cigarettes that were "donated" to them during wartime. Only in the late 1960s were free "gift" cigarettes removed from military hospitals. Tobacco companies also promote their brands to young adults by giving away millions of cigarettes on or near many of the college campuses.

COMPOSITION AND EFFECTS OF TOBACCO SMOKE

Tobacco contains more than a hundred known chemical compounds. Some of the substances found in tobacco remain in the ashes of a burned cigarette;

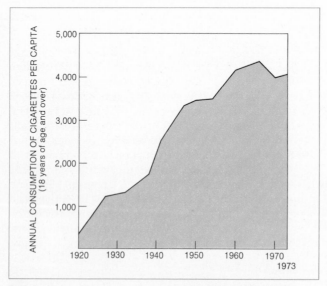

Figure 18.1   Trends in cigarette use. The consumption of cigarettes per person (including nonsmokers and smokers 18 years of age and over) from 1920 to 1973 (1972–1973 projected). (Adapted from reports from the Internal Revenue Bureau's *Statistics from Cigarette Sales* in 1972.)

others are greatly changed during the burning process. Additional compounds are produced during combustion. Primarily, scientists and physicians are concerned about the composition of the *cigarette smoke* that enters a smoker's body.

More than 270 chemical compounds have been identified in cigarette smoke. These include nicotine, tar, phenol, carbon monoxide, arsenic, and at least fifteen chemicals proven to be carcinogens (chemicals that have been proven to cause cancer, either in animal experiments or in observations of humans exposed to them). Table 18.1 lists these proven carcinogens in tobacco smoke.

Also present are *hydrocarbons*, which constitute many of the chemicals in general air pollution. Thus, tobacco smoking is an individual form of air pollution. Moreover, as explained in the "Solvents" section of Chapter 4, the long-term drug effects of hydrocarbon inhalation may also cause death.

When a person takes a puff of tobacco smoke, it first enters his mouth and throat. What happens next depends on whether he inhales the smoke or not. The more acrid, alkaline smoke of cigars and pipes is seldom inhaled deeply into the lungs. Cigarette smoke is deeply inhaled; consequently, the smoke passes down the trachea (windpipe) to the bronchial tubes and into the lungs.

Inspection of the lungs shows that each bronchial tube is wider at each fork. The air or smoke slows down as it enters this region of greater width and deposits chemicals that it contains. The exposure of the bronchial tubes to the substances, such as carcinogens, nicotine, and arsenic, contained in cigarette smoke is thus greatest at the points where the tube is widest. Autopsies of hundreds of human lungs have shown that it is precisely in these areas of maximal exposure that precancerous changes are most likely to take place—where lung cancers are most likely to appear (see Fig. 17.1 for an explanation of these changes).

As shown by Fig. 17.1, smoking also causes damage to the protective mechanisms in the lungs. The lining of the bronchial tubes is normally moist. It is covered with mucus that is produced by cells along the surface. These cells also contain small whiplike fringes called cilia (Fig. 17.1) which, with a back-and-forth waving motion, propel the mucus upward and outward to-

Table 18.1 *Carcinogenic chemicals extracted from cigarette smoke*[a]

Arsenious oxide	3:4-benzpyrene
1:2-benzanthracene	6:7-cyclopenteno—1:2 benzanthracene
3-4-benzfluoranthene	1:2–5:6 benzanthracene
10:11-benzfluoranthene	3:4–8:9 dibenzypyrene
11:12-benzfluoranthene	3:4–9:10 dibenzpyrene
1:12-benzprylene	3-methyl-pyrene
1:2-benzpyrene	2-naphthol
	Chrysene

[a] All these chemicals have been shown to cause cancer either in animal experiments or in observations of humans exposed to them.

ward the throat. Any irritating or poisonous particles, chemicals, or dust entering the bronchial tubes or lungs are trapped in the mucus and propelled by the
cilia out of the lungs and bronchial tubes into the throat. This protective
mechanism removes unwanted and irritating foreign materials from the easily
damaged lungs.

The alkaloid *nicotine* seems to be the compound that paralyzes the cilia,
causing the loss of ciliary action. This chemical and others cause changes to
occur in the lining of the tubes (Fig. 17.1) so that the cilia eventually disappear altogether. Then the carcinogen-saturated smoke, when inhaled, actually
reaches the cells that are the major sites of origin for the most prevalent types
of lung cancer.

Thus there are relationships between smoking, lung cancer, and many
other respiratory conditions due in part to the effects of smoke on the cilia
and the direct action of the carcinogens. Furthermore, cigarette smoke is itself
an irritant. Heavy smokers can feel this irritation in their throats and very
often develop "smoker's cough" after a few years of smoking.

Too few smokers realize the degree and extent of health damage associated with cigarette smoking. "Early morning hacking" and "smoker's coughs"
are so common that millions of Americans consider them "normal" rather
than signals that warn of damage to the body.

All of the effects of cigarette smoke on the tissues of the body are damaging. The actual role of cigarettes in the production of disease is felt to be of
great magnitude. There is a combination of harmful factors, any one of which
could be responsible for damage but together they are deadly.

SMOKING AND DISEASE

It is well established that cigarette smoking is injurious to health. Extensive
studies have shown that smokers of cigarettes have an increased risk of disability, illness, and death from a number of diseases or conditions. Fig. 18.2
shows some of the correlations of deaths from specific conditions for smokers
and nonsmokers. Elimination of cigarette smoking is, in fact, the single most
important health measure available today for the prevention of disease and
premature death in the United States.

The relationships between smoking and disease are being accumulated at
such a rapid pace that any summary can be only a temporary progress report.
The following are some of the major health hazards that have been linked
directly with smoking.

Cancer

The amounts of carcinogenic chemicals in tobacco are very small, in some
cases extremely small. But constant irritation over long periods of time allows
these carcinogens to change normal cells into cancerous cells.

The chances of cancer for nonsmokers and smokers, verified by scientific
investigations, are described and summarized in Table 18.2. This table also

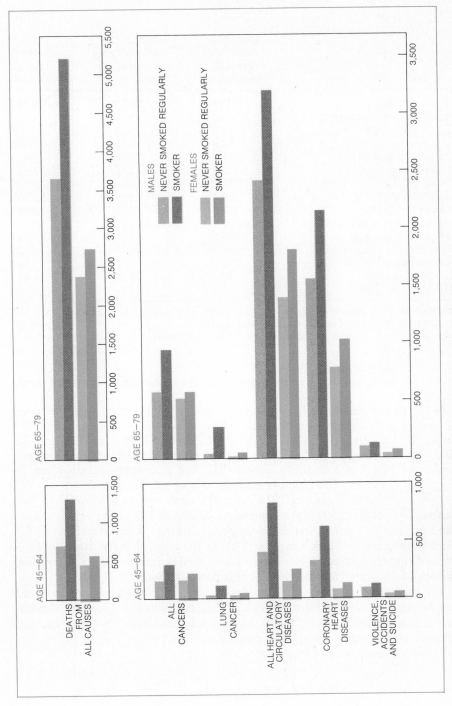

Figure 18.2 Death rates of smokers versus nonsmokers. (From U.S. Department of Health, Education and Welfare.)

Table 18.2 *Expected and actual deaths for smokers of cigarettes*

underlying cause of death	expected no. of deaths in general population	actual no. of smokers dying in general population	ratio of smoker deaths to expected deaths
Cancer of lung	170.3	1,833	10.8 to 1
Bronchitis and emphysema	89.5	546	6.1 to 1
Cancer of larynx	14.0	75	5.4 to 1
Oral cancer	37.0	152	4.1 to 1
Cancer of esophagus	33.7	113	3.4 to 1
Stomach and duodenal ulcers	105.1	294	2.8 to 1
Other circulatory diseases	254.0	649	2.6 to 1
Cirrhosis of liver	169.2	379	2.2 to 1
Cancer of bladder	111.6	216	1.9 to 1
Coronary artery disease	6,430.7	11,177	1.7 to 1
Other heart diseases	526.0	868	1.7 to 1
Hypertensive heart disease	409.2	631	1.5 to 1
General atheriosclerosis	210.7	310	1.5 to 1
Cancer of kidney	79.0	120	1.5 to 1
All causes of death[a]	15,653.9	23,223	1.7 to 1

SOURCE: Adapted from *The Health Consequences of Smoking*, Washington, D.C., U.S. Department of Health, Education, and Welfare, 1969.
[a] Includes all other causes of death besides those listed above.

shows the increased death rate from cancer expected of heavy smokers in any one year.

Dr. Oscar Auerbach has proven conclusively (Fig. 17.1) that carcinoma of the lung (epidermoid carcinoma) is caused by tobacco—largely by cigarette smoking. Dr. Alton Ochsner of the Ochsner Clinic, New Orleans, has said,[1] "After seeing more than 4,000 cases of cancer of the lung, I have become convinced that it is a hopeless disease. The five-year survival rate when the diagnosis of cancer of the lung is made is only about 8 percent."

In the United States in 1914 only 371 deaths were attributed to lung cancer. This number has since climbed to 72,000 in 1973. The rate is still on the rise, and if present trends continue, according to the American Public Health Association, "lung cancer will claim the lives of more than 1,000,000 present school children in this country before they have a chance of reaching the age of 70 years" (a projection of this trend is shown in Fig. 17.7).

Cancers of the tongue, lips, and larynx are also caused by tobacco, which can be cigar or pipe tobacco as well as cigarette tobacco. Cigarette smoking causes lung cancer, because the cigarette smoker inhales. The cigar and pipe smoker usually puffs rather than inhales—unless he has been a heavy cigarette smoker and switches to a pipe.

[1] *Diseases of the Chest*, Sept. 1968.

The incidences of cancer of the esophagus and urinary bladder are increasing, and usually patients with these conditions are smokers. The incidence of cancer of the bladder is definitely higher in people who use tobacco. When cancer is produced in animals by applying a carcinogen to the skin, not only will cancer develop at the site of application of the carcinogen, but it will develop in the bladder in a very high percentage of cases. The probable reason for this is that the carcinogen is absorbed into the bloodstream and is excreted in the urine, and the urinary bladder lining is particularly susceptible to cancerous changes.

Cardiovascular diseases

Cardiovascular disease is any condition that impairs the functioning of the circulatory system—the heart and blood vessels. The effects of smoking on the heart and blood vessels, both in man and in experimental animals, result from *nicotine* alone.

Recent studies of large groups of people have shown that cigarette smokers are more likely to die of certain cardiovascular disorders than are nonsmokers (Fig. 18.2). Diseases of the heart and blood vessels are the most common cause of death in our population. A definite cause-and-effect association has been established between cigarette smoking and the incidence of coronary attacks in humans (Table 18.2), especially in men between 35 and 55 years of age. The risk of death in male cigarette smokers in relation to nonsmokers is greater in middle age than in old age. Consequently, smokers are often struck down when they should be most active and enjoying life. Men who stop smoking have a lower death rate from coronary disease than those who continue to smoke.

Respiratory diseases

Smoking is being increasingly linked to the development and progression of respiratory (lung-connected) diseases such as *bronchitis* and *emphysema*. These two diseases severely disable large numbers of men of working age.

When healthy humans inhale cigarette smoke, pulmonary function is reduced. Airway resistance is increased and gas-transfer capacity is decreased. Smokers generally have a decreased ability to take in and utilize oxygen by the tissues of the body. This causes a lower fitness level in smokers, which reduces their ability to participate in active sports.

Air pollution and respiratory infections as well as smoking cause and aggravate chronic bronchitis and emphysema. Any pollutant, condition, or infection can cause permanent damage to the respiratory system and can be linked with these diseases. Smoking causes an increased irritation above and beyond the pollutants and irritants commonly encountered.

Chronic bronchitis   Bronchitis is an inflammation of the lining of the bronchial tubes. When the bronchi become inflamed, they are easily infected. Inflamed and infected bronchi impede air flow to and from the lungs, causing labored breathing and heavy mucus, or "phlegm," to be coughed up. A brief attack of acute bronchitis with fever, coughing, and spitting occurs in severe colds. *Chronic bronchitis* is the term applied to coughing and spitting that continues for months and returns periodically.

Cigarette smoking and air pollution are the most important causes of chronic bronchitis in the United States. Smoking also increases the chances of dying from chronic bronchitis. This disease seems, at first, just to hang on after a cold; the cough is usually dismissed as only "smoker's cough." But the colds become more frequent, the coughing and spitting last longer. After a while, without the individual's realizing it, the condition is lasting the year around. At this stage, without medical attention, the individual is open for a wide range of very serious respiratory diseases.

Pulmonary emphysema Pulmonary emphysema is a condition characterized by chronic shortness of breath and evidence of obstruction to the flow of air into and, particularly, out of the lung. Very advanced conditions show destruction of the alveoli.

The two chief complications are *ventilatory failure* and *congestive heart failure*. These constantly threaten an individual who has emphysema. Ventilatory failure occurs when the obstruction to breathing becomes so severe that air is not moved in and out of the lungs in amounts adequate to maintain a normal composition of gases (oxygen and carbon dioxide) in the arterial blood. Congestive heart failure is most commonly encountered in patients who have had ventilatory failure, which has made it impossible for the heart to maintain its increased activity.

The individual developing pulmonary emphysema is usually a male between 50 and 70 years of age who has smoked for years, has had colds accompanied by a heavy cough (sometimes amounting to chronic bronchitis), and begins to feel short of breath in the morning or evening. He may seek medical advice at this time, or he may wait until the coughing produces blood or until the obstruction and shortness of breath interfere with his normal daily activity. Unless the condition is promptly treated, the lungs may be permanently damaged, resulting in a day-in and day-out struggle to keep the lungs working. Every breath is labored and may be a major effort.

Doctors do not know how to prevent emphysema, but the best available advice is not to smoke and to clear up any infection of the respiratory system (mouth, nose, throat, sinuses, or lungs) as quickly as possible, because such infections set up a possible starting place for pulmonary emphysema.

Peptic ulcer

Studies indicate an association between cigarette smoking and peptic ulcer. Smoking's irritation of ulcers greatly interferes with the healing process.

Cirrhosis of the liver

The increased mortality of smokers from cirrhosis of the liver has been shown, but there is not sufficient evidence to support more than a suggestive association.

Maternal smoking, pregnancy, and infant birth weight

The expectant mother who smokes has more to worry about than the non-smoking woman. A British study of more than two thousand women showed that one in five spontaneous abortions would not have occurred had the mother not smoked regularly during her pregnancy. Smoking women also tend to have babies of lower birth weight. This may have further complications, because premature babies (children of low birth weight) are known to have a high incidence of neurological damage and a greater chance of dying during the first year of life.

There have been many studies showing the direct and indirect relationships between smoking and health. They are documented by scientists in countries throughout the world. Such reports as the "Smoking and Health" report of the Advisory Committee to the Surgeon General have made it quite clear that the habit of smoking is very injurious to health. But how does the general public feel about smoking? The sales of tobacco have diminished, but people are still dying at an increasing rate from lung cancer, emphysema, heart disease, and other diseases directly associated with smoking.

THE SMOKING HABIT

There is considerable evidence to support the conclusion that there are two distinguishable groups of smokers. In one group psychosocial factors appear to predominate; stopping smoking is relatively easy, and withdrawal symptoms are slight or absent. In the other group the dependence is harder to break, and withdrawal symptoms may be quite severe.

A person's first experiences with smoking tobacco are usually tied to psychological and social pressures. But if the use is continued, for some people it becomes habitual through the dependence-producing effect of nicotine on the body. These effects occur in a number of tissues and organs, including the central nervous system. The effect of nicotine on the smoker is that of a stimulant followed by depression. The "feelings" about smoking depend upon the person's real or imagined reaction to smoking. But whatever the particular reaction, nicotine-free tobacco or cigarettes made from other plant materials (such as lettuce) do not satisfy the smoker.

Within the two groups smoking produces widely differing responses in different individuals. Many describe the effects of smoking as stimulating; others say they obtain a soothing and tranquilizing effect. Smokers suggest that the soothing and calming effects are more important for the pipe and cigar smoker than for the cigarette smoker, who usually describes the effects of a cigarette as stimulating. Since most cigarette smokers inhale, the irritation to their bronchial tubes and lungs from inhaling cigarette smoke may have an important effect on their central nervous systems that helps to enhance the stimulant effects of the nicotine.

Smoking—a drug dependence

Throughout history plants containing chemicals that produce drug dependence have been abused habitually by large populations over long periods of time. Examples of these are *tobacco* (nicotine), *coffee, tea,* and *cocoa* (caffeine), *betel nut* (arecoline), *marijuana* and *hashish* (cannabinols), *khat* (pseudo-ephedrine), *opium* (narcotic alkaloids), *coca leaves* (cocaine) and, more recently, the many mood-modifying chemical compounds produced or ex-tracted in the chemical laboratory.

The drug dependence produced in some people by the use of tobacco should be defined as drug habituation rather than as drug addiction. Tobacco is not legally classified as a dangerous drug, because it does not cause the drastic mood modifications or behavior changes found among those who abuse the more potent drugs. But, although the immediate effects of tobacco are mild, the overall, long-range effects are very drastic. Because of continuing physical damage to the body and health of the individual, it is enough to justify classifying tobacco use as drug abuse.

Starting to smoke

As mentioned earlier, the years from the early teens to the early twenties are the years in which a majority of people begin to develop the habits and social patterns that will cause them to start to smoke or become smokers later in life.

Two factors help to explain why young people begin smoking: the desire to imitate and the wish for adult status. In many cases there is a relationship between smoking, a need for status among friends and peer groups, increased self-assurance, and a desire to feel or appear more mature. Psychiatrists see smoking as an accelerated striving for social status in the sense that the be-ginning smoker is often trying to show an adultlike need for personal and social standing.

As shown in Fig. 18.3, a strong relationship has been found to exist be-tween parents' and youngsters' smoking habits. It seems that parents' smok-ing influences the age at which their children take up smoking more than it influences whether the youngsters become smokers or nonsmokers. Conse-quently, many authorities believe that the most effective way to cut down smoking among young people is to decrease smoking among parents.

It should be noted here that many studies reveal that the health damage is greater among individuals who start cigarette smoking early in life than among those who start later. The ability of an individual to stop smoking when he desires to also is clearly related to how long he has been smoking and how dependent he is upon tobacco.

Personal and social aspects of smoking

There have been many scientific studies of the personal and social reasons for smoking. Some general conclusions can be used to explain the behavior of smokers. The following are some of the major personal and social characteris-tics that tend to be found among smokers as a group.

Social status   Evidence suggests that early smoking is linked with self-esteem and status-seeking in ambitious young people. The pattern or style of living an individual seeks within his family, town, and peer group seems to have a strong influence on his smoking behavior. A permissive cultural climate (one in which smoking is readily permitted) results in an increase of smoking among young people, especially those who tend to conform to the society's more liberal standards.

Personality and smoking   Although no "smoker personality" has been shown to exist, certain common personality traits among smokers have been reported. Smokers tend to be extroverted (outgoing) people who place, perhaps, too strong an emphasis on immediate pleasure. Because smokers often take a large part in various social activities, they are placed in situations that reinforce their smoking habits. They are also more open to suggestions from social influences and friends.

Generally, it seems that different personality types tend to establish specific smoking habits. The pipe and cigar smokers often look for sedation in smoking; the cigarette smoker more often wants stimulation. Consequently, very few cigarette smokers can change to pipes or cigars and be as satisfied as they were with cigarettes.

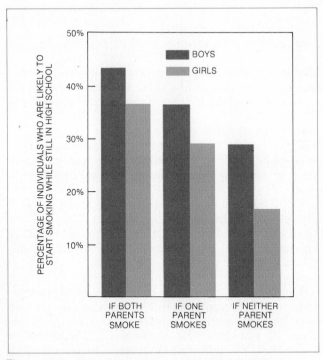

Figure 18.3   Parents and teenage smoking habits: a large majority of teenage smokers come from homes where one or both of the parents smoke.

Psychoanalytic theory of smoking Some psychoanalysts have set forth the theory that smoking, like thumb-sucking, is a return to an infantile (regressive) oral activity related to the infant's pleasure in sucking at his mother's breast. This theory claims that male thumb suckers are very likely to smoke, drink, or be overweight in later years. When these individuals stop smoking, they frequently show increased food consumption, weight gain, or dependence on chewing gum, to suppress this "oral need." However, other experts argue that this analysis is not in itself sufficient and that smoking patterns can be better explained by other psychological factors.

Smoking as a response to stress and tension Stress seems to be conducive to smoking, as it is to so many other habits. Tense or challenging situations contribute to the beginning of the smoking habit, its continuation, and to the number of cigarettes a person consumes. Increased stress among young people, together with social situations favorable to smoking, may set off first experiments with smoking. Later, tense or stressful situations (such as during war) tend to reinforce or strengthen the habit. By the time a smoker has developed a well-established dependence, he may respond to even the slightest tension by reaching for a cigarette.

Breaking the smoking habit

There is good evidence that the ability to stop smoking is related to the forces which led to the habit, the number of cigarettes smoked per day, and the duration of the smoking habit.

The ability of an individual to stop smoking has consistently been found to be highest among those who started late in life, those who have smoked for the least number of years, and those whose average cigarette consumption has been low.

The most frequent reasons for stopping smoking early, or not continuing to smoke after the first trials, are lack of enjoyment or actual dislike of smoking. These reasons are interesting, because they are not the reasons young people give for not taking up smoking: their reasons are connected with health, aesthetics, and morals.

Among adult smokers who quit the most frequent reason given is "various health reasons"; relatively few refer to specific diseases such as lung cancer, emphysema, or cardiovascular diseases. Other reasons for quitting include the expense of cigarettes, moral considerations, and "a test of willpower."

If you must smoke Anything a person does short of quitting smoking completely is merely a compromise. If a person is unable or unwilling to quit, he should at least try to reduce his consumption of cigarettes as a means of decreasing the harmful effects of smoking. The National Clearinghouse for Smoking and Health recommends the following five steps to reduce one's intake of cigarette smoke;[2] see also Table 18.3.

[2] *If You Must Smoke.* UPHS Publication No. 1786, U.S. Government Printing Office, Washington, D.C., 1968.

Table 18.3 *Tar and nicotine content of cigarettes. 134 brands are shown in increasing order of tar content.*

brand	type	tar (mg/cig.)	nicotine (mg/cig.)
Carlton 70's[a]	reg. size, filter	1	0.1
Carlton	king size, filter, menthol	3	0.3
Sano	reg. size, filter	3	0.2
Carlton	king size, filter	3	0.3
Marvels	reg. size, filter	3	0.2
Marvels	king size, filter, menthol	5	0.2
Marvels	king size, filter	5	0.3
King Sano	king size, filter	6	0.3
King Sano	king size, filter, menthol	7	0.3
Iceberg 10	king size, filter, menthol	9	0.6
Lucky Ten	king size, filter	9	0.7
Kent	reg. size, filter	9	0.6
Frappe	king size, filter, menthol	9	0.4
Life	100 mm, filter	10	0.6
Pall Mall Extra Mild	king size, filter (hard pack)	10	0.7
Benson & Hedges	reg. size, filter (hard wide pack)	10	0.7
Vantage	king size, filter	11	0.8
Vantage	king size, filter, menthol	11	1.0
Multifilter	king size, filter, menthol (plastic box)	11	0.9
Tempo	king size, filter	11	0.9
True	king size, filter	12	0.7
True	king size, filter, menthol	12	0.8
Marlboro Lights	king size, filter	14	1.1
Multifilter	king size, filter (plastic box)	14	1.1
Lyme	king size, filter, lime/menthol	14	1.0
Marlboro	king size, filter, menthol	15	1.0
Parliament	king size, filter (hard pack)	15	1.0
Alpine	king size, filter, menthol	15	1.0
Doral	king size, filter, menthol	15	1.1
Parliament	king size, filter	15	1.0
Doral	king size, filter	15	1.0
Silva Thins	100 mm, filter, menthol	15	1.1
Silva Thins	100 mm, filter	15	1.1
Belair	king size, filter, menthol	16	1.2
Parliament	king size, charcoal filter	16	1.1
DuMaurier	king size, filter (hard wide pack)	16	1.2
Parliament	king size, charcoal filter (hard pack)	16	1.1
Raleigh	king size, filter	16	1.2
Kent	king size, filter (hard pack)	16	1.0
Benson & Hedges	king size, filter (hard wide pack)	17	1.3
Kent	king size, filter	17	1.1
Viceroy	king size, filter	17	1.2
Kool	king size, filter, menthol	17	1.4
Virginia Slims	100 mm, filter	17	1.2
Lark	king size, filter	17	1.2

Table 18.3 (*continued*)

brand	type	tar (mg/cig.)	nicotine (mg/cig.)
L & M	king size, filter (hard pack)	17	1.2
Pall Mall	100 mm, filter, menthol	17	1.3
Virginia Slims	100 mm, filter, menthol	17	1.2
Eve	100 mm, filter	17	1.3
Eve	100 mm, filter, menthol	17	1.2
Kool	100 mm, filter, menthol	17	1.3
Viceroy	100 mm, filter	18	1.3
Belair	100 mm, filter, menthol	18	1.3
Marlboro	100 mm, filter	18	1.3
Adam (brown)	king size, filter	18	1.2
Raleigh	100 mm, filter	18	1.3
Lark	100 mm, filter	18	1.3
Marlboro	king size, filter (hard pack)	18	1.3
Marlboro	king size, filter	18	1.3
Kent	100 mm, filter, menthol	18	1.2
Chesterfield	king size, filter, menthol	18	1.2
Benson & Hedges 100's	100 mm, filter, menthol	18	1.3
Benson & Hedges 100's	100 mm, filter	18	1.3
Oasis	king size, filter, menthol	18	1.2
Chesterfield	king size, filter	18	1.3
Marlboro	100 mm, filter (hard pack)	18	1.4
Kent	king size, filter, menthol	19	1.2
Adam (white)	king size, filter	19	1.3
Parliament 100's	100 mm, filter	19	1.3
Montclair	king size, filter, menthol	19	1.4
Edgeworth Export	100 mm, filter	19	1.4
L & M	king size, filter	19	1.4
Tareyton	king size, filter	19	1.3
Edgeworth Export	king size, filter (hard pack)	19	1.3
Kent	100 mm, filter	19	1.3
Newport	king size, filter, menthol (hard pack)	19	1.2
L & M	100 mm, filter, menthol	19	1.3
St. Moritz	100 mm, filter, menthol	19	1.4
Sano	reg. size, nonfilter	19	0.6
Salem	king size, filter, menthol	19	1.3
Chesterfield	101 mm, filter	19	1.5
Galaxy	king size, filter	19	1.4
Peter Stuyvesant	100 mm, filter	19	1.5
L & M	100 mm, filter	19	1.5
Newport	king size, filter, menthol	19	1.3
Mermaid	100 mm, filter, menthol	19	1.4
Picayune	reg. size, nonfilter	19	1.5
Old Gold Filters	king size, filter	20	1.3
Winston	king size, filter (hard pack)	20	1.3
Pall Mall	100 mm, filter	20	1.4
Camel	king size, filter	20	1.3

Table 18.3 *(continued)*

brand	type	tar (mg/cig.)	nicotine (mg/cig.)
Newport[a]	king size, filter, menthol	20	1.4
Maverick	king size, filter	20	1.6
Pall Mall	king size, filter	20	1.3
Home Run	reg. size, nonfilter	20	1.5
Tareyton	100 mm, filter	20	1.4
St. Moritz	100 mm, filter	20	1.5
Winston	100 mm, filter	20	1.3
Winston	100 mm, filter, menthol	20	1.4
Peter Stuyvesant	king size, filter	20	1.5
Spring	100 mm, filter, menthol	20	1.2
Vogue (colors)	king size, filter (hard pack)	20	0.9
Winston	king size, filter	20	1.4
Newport[a]	king size, filter, menthol (hard pack)	20	1.5
Salem	100 mm, filter, menthol	21	1.5
Marvels	reg. size, nonfilter	21	0.8
Old Gold Straights	reg. size, nonfilter	21	1.2
Newport	100 mm, filter, menthol	21	1.4
Domino	king size, filter	22	1.3
Kool	reg. size, nonfilter	22	1.4
Lucky Filter	100 mm, filter	22	1.6
Philip Morris	reg. size, nonfilter	23	1.5
Old Gold Filters	100 mm, filter	23	1.5
Newport[a]	100 mm, filter, menthol	23	1.7
English Ovals	reg. size, nonfilter (hard wide pack)	23	1.8
Half & Half	king size, filter	24	1.7
Mapleton	king size, filter	24	1.3
Chesterfield	reg. size, nonfilter	25	1.5
Piedmont	reg. size, nonfilter	25	1.5
Camel	reg. size, nonfilter	25	1.6
Marvels	king size, nonfilter	25	1.0
Raleigh	king size, nonfilter	25	1.7
Old Gold Straights	king size, nonfilter	26	1.6
Domino	king size, nonfilter	27	1.5
Vogue (black)	king size, filter (hard pack)	29	1.2
Bull Durham	king size, filter	29	1.8
Lucky Strike	reg. size, nonfilter	29	1.6
Pall Mall	king size, nonfilter	29	1.8
Chesterfield	king size, nonfilter	29	1.8
Philip Morris Commander	king size, nonfilter	29	1.9
Herbert Tareyton	king size, nonfilter	29	1.8
English Ovals	king size, nonfilter (hard wide pack)	30	2.3
Fatima	king size, nonfilter	32	1.9
Players	reg. size, nonfilter (hard pack)	34	2.3

SOURCE: Federal Trade Commission, January 1973.

[a] Limited availability based on reduced sampling from Washington, D.C. only.

1. *Choose a cigarette with less tar and nicotine.* . . . Learn the tar and nicotine content of your cigarette. . . . See how your brand compares and find out how much you can reduce your tar and nicotine intake by switching to another brand, or to another version of the brand you are presently smoking. Will such a switch result in your smoking more? Probably not. Most smokers who make such a change either continue to smoke at their previous rate or even smoke less.

2. *Don't smoke your cigarette all the way down.* No matter which cigarette you smoke, the most tar and nicotine is found in the last few puffs. . . . So the sooner you put your cigarette out, the lower your dose will be of harmful ingredients. This same fact also points up the added risk of the new "longer" cigarettes. Their "extra puffs" are really "extra perils" for you.

3. *Take fewer draws on each cigarette.* . . . With practice, some people find they can substantially cut their actual smoking time without really missing it.

4. *Reduce your inhaling.* Easier said than done? Perhaps. But remember it is the smoke which *enters your lungs* that does most of the damage. . . . And it is this smoke that creates the cardiovascular changes which can bring on heart attacks.

5. *Smoke fewer cigarettes per day.* . . . Pick a time of day when you promise yourself not to smoke. It may be before breakfast. Or while driving to work. Or after a certain hour each evening. It's always easier to *postpone* a cigarette if you know you will be having one later. Maybe you're a pack-a-day smoker. Try buying your next pack an hour later each day. It may also help to carry your cigarettes in a different pocket. Or, at work, keep them in a drawer of your desk or in your locker—any place where you aren't able to reach for one automatically. The trick is to change the habit patterns you have established. Make a habit of asking yourself, "Do I really want *this* cigarette?" before you light up. You may be surprised at how many cigarettes you smoke you don't really want.

Cessation of smoking   Dr. Lawrence Stross of the Menninger Clinic in Kansas has said:

> In the face of the overwhelming medical evidence about the inevitable dangers and harmful effects of cigarettes, as a psychiatrist I would categorically say that anyone who continues smoking or begins smoking is acting in an irrational way and denying reality. I think cigarette smoking can properly be described as a kind of masochistic perversion in which people get pleasure out of hurting themselves and making themselves sick.[3]

Thus for a person to stop smoking he must first stop ignoring the health dangers of smoking and accept his smoking as a personal problem, which he must conquer. Then everything should be done to quit smoking, even if only for a limited time.

Stopping smoking has been done in a number of ways, but the most successful methods fall into the following categories: (1) individual medical care provided by physicians or psychologists, (2) self-help programs based on books, magazines, lectures, and pamphlets (such services are available from organizations such as the American Cancer Society, the Heart Association, and others), and (3) withdrawal clinics or a "smokers' clinic," often conducted by hospitals or medical or health organizations.

Withdrawal clinics, which are quite successful, are actually group-therapy

[3] *Diseases of the Chest*, Sept. 1968.

sessions in which physicians and health professionals conduct a series of sessions that explain the health hazards of smoking. They often have a psychologist who conducts part of the session to help reinforce the individual and suggest methods of stopping or reducing smoking. The participants are encouraged to explain how well they are doing and to make suggestions to other members of the group. Past participants also may conduct part of a session with small groups who identify with the problems this individual had when he stopped smoking.

Once the group has been established there are three goals to reach: (1) to assist the individual in building a strong motivation for stopping smoking, (2) constructively to confront the individual's attitudes toward smoking, especially those relating to events and feelings associated with the withdrawal experiences taking place within the group, and (3) to provide support and guidance during and immediately after the period of withdrawal.

The benefits for ex-smokers

Little is known of the relationships between not smoking and normal health. The main areas of study have, so far, been confined to the relationships between smoking and disease. These studies are just beginning to show which body changes, in response to cigarettes, are transitory and which are permanent.

On the basis of twelve years of experience in conducting smoking-withdrawal clinics Dr. Borje E. V. Elrup (Clinical Associate Professor of Medicine, Cornell Medical Center, New York) has been able to demonstrate the following anatomical and physiological changes in ex-smokers.

Digestive and eating patterns start to change even during withdrawal from cigarettes. Soon after a person stops smoking, intestinal motility decreases—often causing constipation for a short time. The absorption of food is greater, the appetite is better, and both the taste of food and the sense of smell are improved—all causing a weight gain.

Patterns of circulation also change. The ex-smoker is less tired. He often arises earlier in the morning and is more alert during the day. Skin circulation improves. The complexion of the face can be seen to change for the better, even during the process of stopping. Increased circulation helps to slow the pulse rate, reduce blood pressure, and increase heart efficiency—both at rest and after exercise.

Responses from the respiratory tract show a decrease in breathing rate (per minute) and an increase in maximal breathing capacity (per minute) and a better exchange of oxygen between the lungs and circulatory system. Respiratory conditions such as chronic bronchitis improve, and coughing disappears during withdrawal. Emphysema patients are able to breathe more easily, and many asthmatics improve substantially.

The age at which one stops smoking has a lot to do with the benefits. The younger a person when he stops, the greater the benefits. There have been studies showing increases in death rates for smokers as young as 11 years of age. An individual between 35 and 54 shows a marked decrease in the chances of dying from diseases associated with cigarettes if he stops smoking. However, a person between 55 and 74 shows only a slight decrease in his chances of dying from such diseases.

The longer since one has quit, the greater the benefit from nonsmoking. For the first year or so an individual may find that he is actually away from work or school more because of illness than he was while he was smoking. It takes time for the body to heal and adjust to a nonsmoking condition. In fact, the medical benefit from nonsmoking is relatively slight for the first five years (especially for those who have smoked 20 or more cigarettes a day). But studies of ex-smokers are showing significant changes in the patterns of disease. The cessation of smoking is firmly linked with decreased deaths—especially from coronary heart disease. The decrease in risk of dying from a heart attack is substantial even after just a year or two of not smoking. Moreover, the death rate after ten years of not smoking is equal to that of a person who has never smoked.

There is an impairment of breathing capacity as cigarette consumption increases over a length of time. Most smokers in the beginning are unaware of the injury to their lungs. This deterioration continues faster in heavy smokers than in lighter smokers, and before long wheezing and shortness of breath are common—until many individuals are unable to undertake any activity without unusual exertion. It is this inability to breathe properly which finally kills many smokers. If an individual does not stop smoking, this impairment of lung functioning ultimately becomes irreversible—the damage is permanent.

In conclusion, although quitting smoking is seldom easy, the effort required may be handsomely rewarded in added years of good health. If you smoke—quit now. If you don't smoke—don't start.

SUMMARY

I. Cigarette consumption trends in the United States
   A. Cigarette consumption increased steadily from 1900 until 1967.
   B. In late 1967 and early 1968 there began a reduction in the consumption of cigarettes; this trend reversed in 1972.
   C. Teenagers have never smoked to the extent that adults have.
II. Composition and effects of tobacco smoke
   A. More than 270 chemicals have been identified in cigarette smoke.
   B. Smoke causes damage to the cilia, which are part of the protective mechanisms of the lungs.
      1. Cilia remove unwanted and irritating foreign materials from the easily damaged lungs.
      2. Cigarette smoke paralyzes the action of the cilia in the bronchial tubes and may cause changes leading to the eventual disappearance of the cilia.
      3. The alkaloid *nicotine* seems to be the compound that paralyzes the cilia, causing their loss.
   C. Too few smokers realize the degree and extent of health damage associated with cigarette smoking.
   D. All the effects of cigarette smoke on the tissues of the body are damaging.

III. Smoking and disease
   A. It is well established that cigarette smoking is injurious to health.
   B. Elimination of cigarette smoking is the single most important health measure available today for the prevention of disease and premature death in the United States.
   C. The following are some of the major health hazards that have been linked directly with smoking.
      1. Cancer:
         a. the amounts of carcinogens in tobacco smoke are very small, but constant irritations over long periods of time allows these chemicals to change normal cells into cancerous cells.
         b. cancers of the tongue, lips, larynx, lungs, esophagus, and urinary bladder have been linked to tobacco smoking.
      2. Cardiovascular disease:
         a. a general term for any condition that impairs the functioning of the circulatory system.
         b. The effects of smoking on the heart and blood vessels result from nicotine.
         c. A definite cause-and-effect association has been established between cigarette smoking and the incidence of coronary attacks.
      3. Respiratory diseases—smoking is being increasingly linked to the development and progression of respiratory diseases such as *bronchitis* and *emphysema*.
      4. Peptic ulcer:
         a. there is a link between cigarette smoking and peptic ulcers.
         b. smoking's irritation of ulcers greatly interferes with the healing process.
      5. Cirrhosis of the liver—there is a suggestive association between cirrhosis of the liver and smoking.
      6. Maternal smoking, pregnancy, and infant birth weight:
         a. higher spontaneous-abortion rate with women who were heavy smokers during a pregnancy.
         b. smoking mothers tend to have babies of lower birth weight—children of lower birth weights (premature births) show a high incidence of neurological damage; these children have a greater chance of dying during the first year of life.
IV. The smoking habit
   A. Two basic groups of dependent smokers
      1. In one group psychosocial factors predominate:
         a. stopping smoking is relatively easy.
         b. withdrawal symptoms are slight or absent.
      2. The other group seems to be physically dependent on tobacco:
         a. the dependence is hard to break.
         b. withdrawal symptoms may be quite severe.
   B. *Nicotine* has effects that could produce the drug dependence associated with smoking that affects some people.
      1. First smoking experiences are usually tied to psychological and social pressures.
      2. Continued smoking is encouraged, continued, and made habitual by the drug-dependence effect of *nicotine*.
   C. Smoking—a drug dependence. The immediate effects of tobacco are mild, but the overall, long-range physical damage to health is enough to classify its use as drug abuse.

D. Starting to smoke
  1. Between the early teens and early twenties most people begin to develop habits and social patterns that will cause them to smoke.
  2. Two factors help to explain why young people begin smoking:
    a. the desire to imitate.
    b. the wish for adult status.
  3. A strong relationship exists between parents' and youngsters' smoking habits.
  4. The health damage is greater among individuals who start cigarette smoking early in life.
E. Major personal and social characteristics found among smokers
  1. Social status—early smoking is linked with self-esteem and status-seeking in ambitious young people
  2. Personality of smoker:
    a. tends to be extroverted.
    b. places too strong an emphasis on immediate pleasure.
    c. takes a large part in social activities and place themselves in situations that reinforce their smoking habits.
    d. is open to suggestions from social influences and friends.
    e. generally, different personality types tend to establish specific smoking habits.
  3. Psychoanalytic theory of smoking—links smoking, like thumb-sucking, to an infantile (regressive) oral activity related to the infant's pleasure in sucking at his mother's breast.
  4. Smoking as a response to stress and tension—stress and tension seem to be conducive to smoking, as they are to so many other habits.
F. Breaking the smoking habit
  1. The ability to stop smoking is related to:
    a. the forces which lead to the habit.
    b. the number of cigarettes smoked per day.
    c. the duration of the smoking habit.
  2. Among adults the most frequent reasons are:
    a. "various health reasons."
    b. the expense of cigarettes.
    c. moral considerations.
    d. "a test of willpower."
  3. If you must smoke—use the following five steps to reduce your intake of cigarette smoke:
    a. choose a cigarette with less tar and nicotine.
    b. don't smoke your cigarette all the way down.
    c. take fewer draws on each cigarette.
    d. reduce your inhaling.
    e. smoke fewer cigarettes per day.
  4. Cessation of smoking:
    a. stop ignoring the health dangers and accept smoking as personal problem.
    b. the most successful methods—individual care provided by physicians or psychologists; self-help programs based on books, magazines, lectures, and pamphlets; withdrawal clinics, or "smokers' clinics."

c. three goals to be reached—must build a strong motivation for stopping smoking; must confront his attitudes toward smoking; support and guidance during and immediately after the period of withdrawal from tobacco muse be provided.

d. The benefits for ex-smokers—changed digestive and eating patterns, leading to increased weight; changes in patterns of circulation; responses from the respiratory tract; decreased chances of dying from diseases associated with smoking.

Glossary

If you cannot find the word you wish in this glossary, check the index for text and glossary references.

arsenic (är'snik) (G. *arsen*, strong). A poisonous element; it is a brittle, lustrous, grayish solid with a garlicky odor.

bronchitis (bron ki'tis) (G. *bronchos*, windpipe). Inflammation of the bronchial tubes.

carbon monoxide (kär'bən mə näk' sīd) (L. *carbo*, coal). A colorless, poisonous gas, CO, formed by burning carbon with an insufficient supply of oxygen.

carcinogen (kär sin'ə jen) (G. *karkinos*, crab). Any cancer-producing substance.

carcinogenic (kär sin ə jen'ik). Causing or producing cancer.

cilia (sil'e ə). Very small, hairlike processes attached to a free surface of a cell.

cirrhosis (sə rō'sis) (G. *kirrhos*, orange yellow). A disease of the liver, marked by progressive destruction of the liver cells.

depression (di presh'ən) (L. *depressio*, *de*, down; *premere*, to press). A lowering or decrease of functional activity.

emphysema (em fə zē'mə) (G. *emphysema*, inflation). Presence of air in the tissues of the lungs as a result of distention and rupture of the pulmonary alveoli.

hydrocarbons (hī drə kär'bənz). An organic compound which contains hydrogen and carbon only.

nicotine (nik'ə tēn) (L. *nicotiana*, tobacco). A poisonous alkaloid; it is a colorless, oily fluid.

peptic ulcer (pep'tik ul'sər) (L. *ulcus*). An open sore in the esophagus, stomach, or duodenum, produced by a gradual disintegration of the lining membranes.

phenol (fē'nol). A colorless, crystalline compound; it is a powerful antiseptic and disinfectant and is extremely poisonous. Also called *carbolic acid*.

regressive (ri gres'iv) (L. *regressio*, a return). Going back or coming back; emotionally returning to a former state or age.

stimulant (stim'yə lant) (L. *stimulus*, to goad). Any agent temporarily increasing functional activity of the central nervous system.

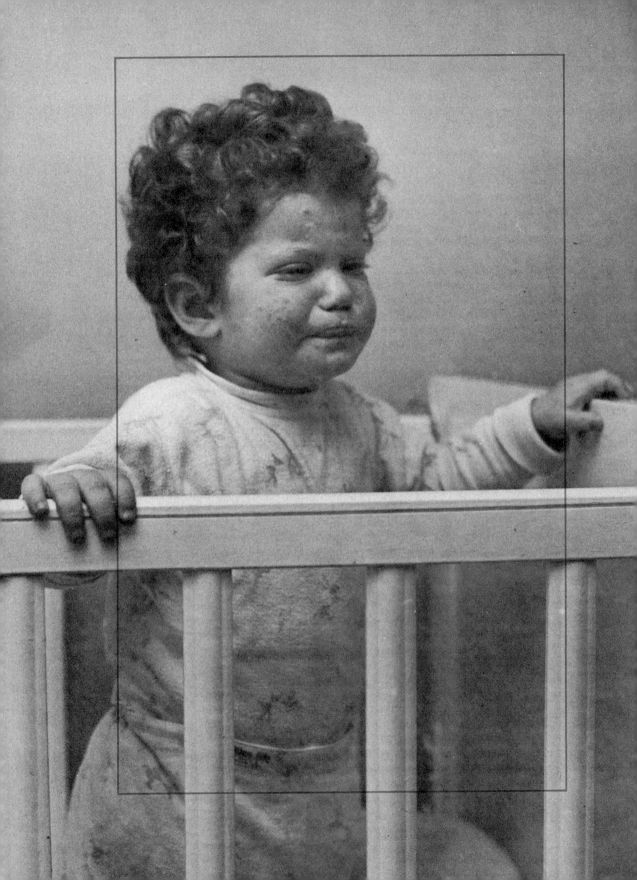

Infectious disease

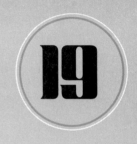

19

The term *infection* is applied to disease produced when the body is invaded by living organisms or parasites. Any disease that is *communicable*, or *contagious* (a disease that can be "caught"), is *infectious*. A disease is "caught" when a living parasite invades the human body.

PATHOGENS

Every communicable disease that causes illness in man is the result of the parasitism of man by some living organism. Disease-producing organisms are called *pathogens*, commonly "germs." Most, but not all, pathogens are microscopic in size and are therefore sometimes referred to as *microbes* or *microorganisms*. Only a small percentage of known microorganisms are human pathogens. Many others are highly beneficial to man, and still others produce diseases in plants and animals other than man.

A disease usually is due, not to the mere presence of the pathogen, but to some aspect of its life processes. A healthy man harbors many microorganisms; some are beneficial, such as the intestinal bacteria, which may produce vitamins; others are potential pathogens, capable of producing disease under the proper conditions; still others have been shown to be neither beneficial nor harmful. Since the organisms of the last category are able to derive their sustenance without producing any detectable harm to their host and therefore do nothing to lessen their own chances of survival, they may be said, biologically speaking, to be the most well adapted of parasitic microorganisms.

Organisms have been classified into several groups according to their basic characteristics. All known pathogens may be included in one of the following categories of living things (arranged in order from smallest to largest):

1. *Viruses:* subcellular, semiliving particles
2. *Bacteria:* single-celled, plantlike organisms
3. *Fungi:* unicellular and multicellular, plantlike organisms
4. *Protozoa:* single-celled animals
5. *Parasitic worms:* multicellular animals

Viruses

The viruses, although the smallest of all known pathogens, are responsible for much human misery; see Fig. 19.1. Viruses are the causative agents of such common diseases as colds and influenza and also of less common diseases such as poliomyelitis, rabies, and yellow fever. Viruses are not visible with even the most powerful light microscope, but they can be seen with electron microscopes. As many as a million virus particles could be placed within a bacterial cell.

Virus particles lack the more complex cellular structure that is characteristic of most plants and animals. A typical virus particle consists mainly of a central core of genetic material, either ribonucleic acid (RNA) or deoxyribonucleic acid (DNA), enclosed within a protein coating.

Viruses lie at the borderline between living and nonliving matter and lack some of the refinements of more typical living organisms. They are incapable of unassisted self-reproduction, growth, production of energy, and other vital processes of life. They must live and reproduce *within* the living cell of some host organism; thus they are all intracellular parasites. A host for a virus may be a plant, an animal, or even a bacterium. When a virus particle invades a suitable host cell, only the core of genetic material enters the cell; the protein shell of the virus remains outside. Once inside the host cell, the

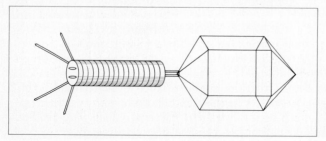

Figure 19.1   A typical virus, as enlarged with the electron microscope. Note the angular shape, characteristic of many viruses.

genetic material of the virus is believed to act as a "gene" which takes over the control of the cell and "tricks" the cell into manufacturing more virus material. The normal functioning of the cell is thereby disrupted, often with serious consequences. The cells may be only temporarily affected, producing such minor diseases as a common cold; or they may be permanently damaged, producing such serious diseases as polio and, possibly, cancer.

Bacteria

Bacteria are microscopic single-celled plants; see Fig. 19.2. Although much larger than viruses, they are still small enough for a million or more to be carried on the head of a pin. Unlike the viruses, however, most bacteria are neither parasitic nor pathogenic; in fact, many bacteria are quite beneficial to man. That most bacteria are not pathogenic is illustrated by the fact that in most states pasteurized milk may legally contain up to 113,550,000 bacteria per gallon. The water we drink and the air we breathe also contain numerous harmless bacteria.

Again unlike the viruses, most pathogenic bacteria rarely enter the indi-

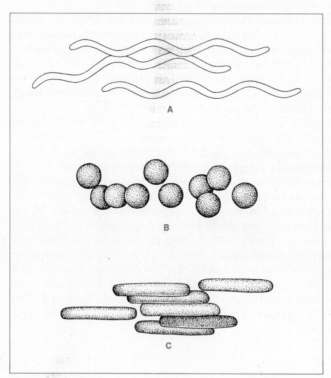

Figure 19.2 Bacteria in their three basic shapes: (A) spirilla, (B) cocci, and (C) bacilli.

vidual cells of man. Instead, they usually live on, around, and between the human cells. Of bacteria there are two families, the *Rickettsiaceae* and the *Chlamydiaceae*, that are in many respects between viruses and the larger bacteria. In appearance and structure these families resemble very small bacteria. However, like the viruses, they reproduce only within living host cells, which causes them to be called *obligate, intracellular parasites*. All rickettsiae are transmitted by insects and related animals (arthropods), such as fleas, lice, mites, and ticks. Some examples of rickettsial disease include typhus fever, Rocky Mountain spotted fever, and Q fever. Members of the Chlamydiaceae include the agents of lymphogranuloma venereum, a venereal disease (see Chapter 20) and trachoma, a severe infection of the eye often leading to blindness.

The harmful effect of pathogenic bacteria upon man is the result of their production of poisonous enzymes and *toxins*. Some of the bacterial toxins are among the most powerful poisons known to man—sometimes millions of times as toxic as cyanide. These toxins fall into two groups: the *exotoxins*, which diffuse out of the living bacterial cells into the surrounding human tissues, and the *endotoxins*, which are held within the bacterial cells and released only after the death of the cell. The significant difference between these two is in their abilities to cause production of *antibodies* in the host. The exotoxins of different pathogens stimulate the animal body to produce *specific* antibodies (discussed later in this chapter) that act upon the toxins to neutralize them; this action makes possible the production of immunizing substances against such exotoxin-caused diseases as tetanus and diphtheria. The endotoxins do not stimulate the production of specific antibodies by man or other animals, so it has not yet been possible to produce highly effective immunizing substances against them. Unfortunately, there are more endotoxin-producing bacteria than exotoxin-producing ones.

The enzymes and toxins of some bacteria have a localized effect, killing and dissolving the human cells near the site of infection. The contents of the damaged cells are then available as food for the bacteria. As further cells are killed, the infection spreads deeper into the surrounding tissue. Such is the condition in the development of an abscessed tooth, where bone and supportive tissues, at the apical end of the tooth, are lost as the abscess increases in size. Other toxins are produced at one point in the body, are carried by the blood, and act upon the body at some other point. Often some specific system is then affected as, for example, the nervous system in a tetanus infection.

There are three basic bacterial shapes (Fig. 19.2), and bacteria are often named for them: coccus, bacillus, and spirillum. The *cocci* are the spherical bacteria; they may occur singly, in pairs (*diplococcus*), in chains (*streptococcus*), or in irregular clusters like bunches of grapes (*staphylococcus*). The *bacilli* are rod-shaped bacteria. The *spirilla* are the spiral, or corkscrew-shaped, bacteria.

Fungi

The fungi are primitive plants; see Fig. 19.3. Some of the more common fungi are mushrooms, toadstools, and bread and cheese molds. Only a few fungi cause human diseases. The diseases range from bothersome skin infections, such as *ringworm* and *athlete's foot*, to the sometimes fatal *histoplasmosis*, a lung infection. Fungus infections of man are most commonly associated with the skin and lungs; they are frequently very difficult to treat or cure. Treatment forces adverse conditions upon the fungi; in response they form "spores," a dormant stage which is extremely resistant to heat (will survive boiling water for several hours as well as *dry* heat of 212° F.), drying, disinfectants, and powders or salves commonly used in treatment.

Protozoa

Protozoa are primitive single-celled animals. Although much larger than bacteria, most protozoa are still microscopic; see Fig. 19.4. Most protozoan diseases are associated with tropical areas, some examples being malaria, African sleeping sickness and amebic dysentery. Many protozoan diseases tend to be recurrent; that is, the patient suffers periodic relapses, and between attacks the pathogen remains inactive in the body.

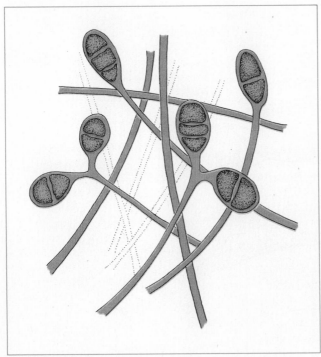

Figure 19.3   A typical fungus. This fungus is the cause of athlete's foot and similar skin infections. Note the spores, by which fungi reproduce.

Parasitic worms

The parasitic worms are multicellular animals ranging in size from about the size of the head of a pin (such as the worm causing trichinosis) up to many feet long (the tapeworms); see Fig. 19.5. Many parasitic worms include other animals as well as man in their life cycles. Such worms can be acquired by man through contact with these animals or through eating incompletely cooked meat; typical animal hosts are pigs, cows, fish, and snails.

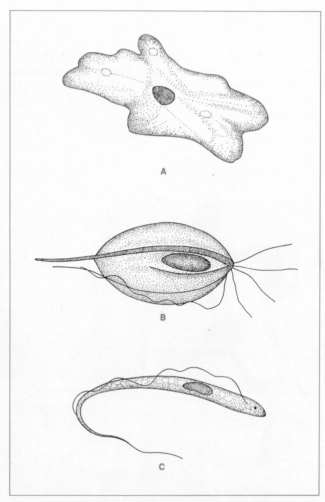

Figure 19.4   Protozoa, single-celled animals: (A) an amoeba, (B) a trichomonad, and (C) a trypanosome.

COURSE OF A COMMUNICABLE DISEASE

Communicable disease in general follows a characteristic pattern of development. The course is shown in Fig. 19.6 and explained in the following sections.

Transmission and infection

For a person to become infected—that is, to "catch" a communicable disease—the pathogen must be carried in some manner from the source or reservoir of the disease in sufficient number to overcome body resistance and successfully invade the body through one of its portals of entry. This movement of disease agents from the reservoir to the victim is called *transmission*. There are various methods of transmission of communicable diseases.

Person to person   An infection may be caused by transmission from one person to another. This may be by *direct contact*, the actual touching of an infected person through kissing, sexual intercourse, or other close personal contact, or by *indirect contact*, the touching of objects contaminated by an infected person, such as toys, drinking glasses, handkerchiefs, and soiled clothing or bedding. Indirect transmission may also be made by airborne droplets through the coughing, sneezing, talking, or singing of an infected person.

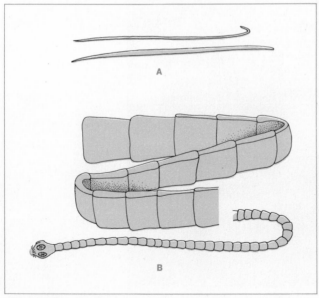

Figure 19.5   Parasitic worms: (A) roundworm and (B) tapeworm.

Contaminated water Diseases of the digestive tract are often acquired from contaminated water when sewage accidentally contaminates drinking water.

Contaminated food or milk Contaminated food or milk might result from infection in the animal food source (such as in meat or milk) or from the subsequent handling of food by an infected person.

Animal to person Although most diseases that affect animals do not affect humans, there are many diseases of animals to which humans are susceptible. Transmission from animals to humans can be described as either direct or indirect. *Direct transmission* can result from the handling or the bite of an infected animal. *Indirect transmission* can result from contact with fecal material or other residue from an infected animal.

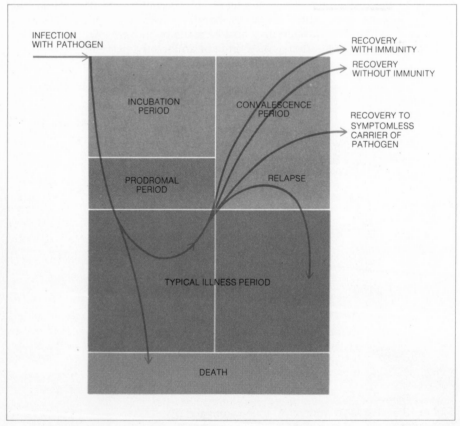

Figure 19.6   The course of a communicable disease, from infection to recovery or death.

Vectors   Some diseases are transmitted exclusively through the bites of arthropods or by contact with their feces. Insects and related animals that are capable of transmitting a disease are called *arthropod vectors*. The pathogens they carry usually cannot be transmitted directly from one person to another, except perhaps through blood transfusion, since the pathogen often completes part of its life cycle within the vector.

Portals of exit and entry   A pathogen generally leaves the patient by the same route (portal) as that by which it entered. The common portals of entry and exit include the *body orifices* (mouth, nose, eyes, anus, and urogenital canals) and the *skin* and *mucous membranes*. A few pathogens may pass through the unbroken skin or mucous membrane, but most require a cut or wound for passage.

Incubation period

After an infectious organism has entered the body, there is a period of time during which the pathogen is reproducing within the body, but no symptoms appear. This time of reproduction is called the *incubation period*.

Most diseases are not communicable during the incubation period, although some, such as measles and chickenpox, are contagious during the latter parts of their incubation periods.

Each disease has its characteristic incubation period, which depends upon the rate of reproduction of that particular pathogen and the area of the body in which the pathogen multiplies. Incubation near the surface of the body, as in gonorrhea and diphtheria, is usually rapid; incubation at remote sites, as in typhus fever and infectious hepatitis, requires a longer period of time.

During the incubation period a person's body may build up a defense against the invading pathogens. The speed with which such defenses are mobilized plays a role not only in the incubation period but also in the severity of the disease. The person who has previously come into contact with an organism will react faster and may be able to overcome the organism before it can become established. This fast reaction is indicative of *immunity* (discussed later in this chapter).

Communicable period

The time during which an infectious pathogen may be transmitted from an infected person to another person or from an infected animal to a person is called its *communicable period*. In diseases such as tuberculosis, syphilis, and gonorrhea, the communicable state may extend over a long period of time, intermittently recurring when unhealed *lesions* of the disease permit the discharge of infectious pathogens from the surface of the skin or through any body openings. Other diseases, such as measles and chickenpox, are communicable for only a short time during the late incubation period and early stages of the diseases. In diseases transmitted by arthropod vectors communicability lasts as long as the pathogen is in the blood of the infected person.

Prodromal period

The onset of nonspecific symptoms occurs during the *prodromal period*. During this time the patient may suffer from such discomforts as headache, watery eyes, nasal discharge, mild fever, irritability, and general aches. Often an individual suffering in the prodromal period of a serious disease believes that he has only a common cold. He may stay out in public and unknowingly expose a considerable number of people to the specific disease he has contracted. *During the prodromal period the individual is highly contagious.*

Typical illness stage

A short time after the prodromal period the first set of symptoms of a specific disease appears. Then we have the typical illness: measles, whooping cough, chickenpox, and so on. The diagnosis of the specific infectious disease is made principally by the physician's recognition of characteristic symptoms or groups of symptoms. A group of symptoms is termed a *syndrome*. Among the factors that help the physician make a diagnosis are the following:

Manner of onset—whether abrupt or gradual. When did the first symptoms appear?

Type of fever—whether continuous, remittent, or intermittent. How and when did the fever terminate?

Course of the disease—its duration, the presence of symptoms on certain days.

Incubation period—the time between exposure to the disease and the first appearance of symptoms.

Leukocyte count—the number and kinds of white blood cells that are present in the body.

Agglutination reaction—whether the patient's blood causes the organisms of the suspected disease to clump together.

Isolation of the organism—whether the organism suspected of causing the disease can be found in the blood, urine, feces, spinal fluid, pleural fluid, and so on.

The disease has now been recognized, and treatment can begin. The illness, now at its height, is still communicable, but since the patient is ill enough to be in bed, the danger of his spreading the disease at this stage is reduced. During this time the body's defenses begin either to defeat the invading pathogens or to succumb to them.

Convalescence

At termination of the typical illness the patient either has succumbed or is passing into the next period, the *convalescence*, or *recovery state*. During this time the patient begins to regain his health. However, if he overexerts himself at this time, he may weaken the body's defenses and give the invading organisms a fresh start, producing a rapid return of the symptoms. The body still contains large numbers of virulent organisms which, if multiplication recurs, soon reach symptomatic proportions. Such a return of disease is called a *relapse*. During recovery a period of recuperation is needed for the patient to regain normal strength and vitality.

Termination

The convalescent period is followed by one of three possible terminal states: *resusceptibility,* the *carrier state,* or *immunity.*

In one of these terminal states the person is *resusceptible:* he may immediately become infected again if he comes into contact with the pathogen. This is the case in diseases such as gonorrhea.

A person or animal who harbors a disease but does not show the clinical symptoms of the disease and is able to pass such a disease on to another person is called a *carrier.* Several different types of carrier exist. A person who transmits a disease during the communicable period of the disease is termed an *incubatory carrier.* A person who is able to pass a disease on while he is overcoming the disease (convalescence stage) or after all symptoms have disappeared and he is considered completely normal (postconvalescence period), is a *convalescent carrier.* A person whose carrier state occurs with an infection that has not been evident (a subclinical condition) is said to be a *healthy carrier.* Carrier states are common after the occurrence of typhoid fever, diphtheria, cholera, influenza, and cerebrospinal meningitis. The carrier is probably the main reservoir of infections.

The ability of a body to resist disease is called *immunity.* The persistence of immunity following infection varies within wide limits. After a number of the viral infections, such as measles and yellow fever, it is lifelong and does not depend on reinfection in order to be maintained. After staphylococcal infection, gonorrhea, or treated syphilis, any immunity that may develop is very short-lived. When many different organisms can produce a clinically recognized disease, such as pneumonia, it is difficult to determine the duration of immunity. Immunity conferred by influenza appears to persist less than a year.

The immunity that a vaccine gives against diseases such as smallpox is known to weaken with the passage of years; but if the disease is acquired even several years after vaccination, it is generally mild. This weakening of immunity is the general reason for "booster" doses.

Subclinical illness

The term *gradient of infection* refers to the variety of responses to an infection. At one extreme is the infection that produces a fatal illness, in the middle lie the illnesses, severe or mild, from which the person may recover, and at the other extreme is the unapparent infection, an infection so mild that it does not produce a "typical illness." The term *subclinical illness* has essentially the same meaning as *unapparent infection.* Such an illness is detectable only by laboratory means, such as the discovery of the organism in the person's body, the demonstration of antibodies in the person's bloodstream, or hypersensitivity to tests of the skin. This type of infection will still run the typical course of a communicable disease (Fig. 19.6), but nearly all of its periods are unrecognizable.

Types of disease outbreaks

When a communicable disease occurs in a single individual or in scattered cases throughout an area, it is termed a *sporadic outbreak*. On the other hand, when a disease is present more or less continuously in an area, it is said to be *endemic* to that specific area. An outbreak of a disease which is clearly in excess of the normal incidence for that size of a community, population, or area is an *epidemic*. Such an outbreak is frequently propagated from a single common source. A disease that sweeps over a large region (an entire country or continent) is termed *pandemic*. Influenza has been pandemic at times in the United States and throughout the world.

THE BODY'S DEFENSES AGAINST DISEASE

Skin and mucous membranes

Commonly referred to as the "first line of defense" are the *skin* and *mucous membranes*. Although the unbroken skin and membranes form an effective barrier against most pathogens, some organisms have the ability to penetrate the unbroken skin or membranes of the body.

The trachea and bronchioles are lined with countless microscopic hairlike projections, *cilia*, which clear bacteria from the lungs. These cilia, which constantly wave rhythmically, carry dust and bacteria (on a layer of mucus) from the lungs to the throat, where it is swallowed without conscious effort. These cilia are lost by the heavy smoker, who depends on his "smoker's cough" to rid his lungs of mucus and foreign matter.

The gastric juice of the stomach is highly acid. This acidity kills some, but not all, bacteria.

The eyes obtain some measure of protection against infection from the constant flow of tears, which washes away many bacteria and contains an enzyme (lysozyme) which kills bacteria.

Inflammation

When infection does become established, the body still has several means of defense. The second line of defense is *inflammation*, a local dilation of the capillaries in response to the infection. The area surrounding the infection becomes hot, red, and swollen as a result of increased blood supply. The increased blood supply brings an abundance of white blood cells, which engulf and destroy the bacteria.

Immunity

The third and most important body defense against disease is *immunity*, of which there are many types.

Natural immunity Natural immunity (also called "resistance") is merely an inherited lack of susceptibility. This immunity may be characteristic of the entire human species, of certain races of man, or of certain individuals, depending upon the disease in question.

Acquired immunity   Acquired immunity is always the result of *antibodies*. Antibodies are protective chemical substances produced by the body in response to the presence of an *antigen* in the body. The function of the antibody is to destroy or inactivate the antigen. (You will recall that an antigen is a foreign substance, usually a protein, which has been introduced into the body.) Antibodies are *specific*—that is, they will inactivate only the same type of antigen that caused the production of the antibody. Acquired immunity may be one of two types: active or passive.

1. *Active immunity* results when a person produces his own antibodies in response to the presence of an antigen. The antigen usually is a microorganism or its toxic product. Natural active immunity is obtained while the person is recovering from an actual case of the infectious disease. This type of immunity is often of very long duration. Artificial active immunity is the result of *vaccines* containing antigens which, when introduced into the body, cause the production of immunizing antibodies. Fortunately, for many diseases there are today vaccines and toxoids. A vaccine or toxoid consists of an antigen which has in some way been attenuated (weakened) so that it no longer causes disease but still stimulates the production of antibodies. A *vaccine* consists of a killed or weakened pathogen; a *toxoid* consists of a modified toxin.

2. *Passive immunity* results when antibodies are introduced into the body from some outside source. But since no antigen is introduced, there is no stimulus for the production of any new antibodies. As a result, passive immunity is of short duration, lasting only as long as the introduced antibodies remain active in the body. Like active immunity, passive immunity may be either natural or artificial.

Natural passive immunity is the *congenital* immunity conferred by the mother upon her unborn child. Antibodies are small enough to allow their diffusion across the membranes of the placenta from the mother's blood to that of the fetus. The newborn infant is thereby immune to most diseases to which the mother is immune. Since congenital immunity is passive, it lasts only as long as the original antibodies remain active, usually several months.

Sometimes a person is exposed to a communicable disease for which no vaccine or toxoid is available, or perhaps he has neglected to take advantage of an existing vaccine. In these cases it may be possible to confer upon that person artificial passive immunity through an injection of antibodies. The antibodies are usually concentrated from the blood of an animal that has been injected with the proper antigen. It must be emphasized that this type of immunity is temporary and results in no long-lasting protection. Passive immunity (of about two weeks' duration) for several virus diseases may be obtained through the injection of *gamma globulin*. Gamma globulin is a derivative of human blood in which a high concentration of antibodies exists. Some of these are specific antibodies, for specific diseases; others are more generalized and serve to protect the body from several diseases.

Interferon

Interferon is believed to be one of the body's principle defenses against viral diseases. It is a chemical substance (a protein) released from cells that have been infected with a virus or treated with one of several known interferon-inducing chemicals. The effect of interferon is to protect other cells from viral infection. Interferon is not specific against the same virus that induced its production; it protects against other viruses as well. Every species of animal apparently produces a slightly different form of interferon. When interferon is extracted from other animals and injected into humans it does not prevent viral infection. Research is currently underway in an effort to find methods of inducing interferon production in the human body by means of harmless viruses or chemicals. Interferon induction may someday be used to prevent a variety of viral diseases.

ALLERGY

Although *allergy*, also called *hypersensitivity*, is not an infectious disease, it seems appropriate to discuss it at this point, since an allergy is the result of an antigen-antibody reaction. When a person has an allergy, he has developed antibodies against some normal component of the diet or environment. Allergies are commonly developed against such varied substances as pollens, feathers, furs, dusts, cosmetics, and foods of all types. In fact, it is difficult to mention a substance to which no person would be allergic. An accurate description of an allergy might be "a reaction to a substance that may be harmless to other people."

The discomfort felt during allergic reactions is the result of a substance called *histamine*, which is released from the tissues in response to antigen-antibody reactions. Some of the effects of histamine include dilation of the small blood vessels (inflammation), sneezing, running nose, constriction of the bronchioles (*asthma*), and local swelling.

A severe allergic reaction, releasing much histamine, can lead to an often fatal condition called *anaphylaxis*, or *anaphylactic shock*, in which the blood pressure drops dangerously, owing to the dilated blood vessels. Nausea and convulsions often accompany this shock. It is through this mechanism that bee stings or penicillin reactions kill many people each year.

The cause of an allergy often can be determined through a series of skin-patch tests, in which small amounts of various antigens, such as foods and pollens, are scratched into the skin on the back. In these tests allergic reactions are indicated by local inflammation. Then the patient often can be desensitized by a series of injections of minute amounts of the offending antigen.

TREATMENT OF DISEASE

The treatment, or *therapy*, for a disease may be defined as any effort to cure the disease, arrest its course, lessen its severity, or alleviate the pain and inconvenience the disease causes. There are five types of therapy.

Dietary therapy is the treatment of disease by regulation of the food the patient eats. In the treatment of all diseases it is important that a patient have proper food and a proper amount of fluid.

Operative therapy is the surgical treatment, in which disease is removed with the scalpel and other instruments of the surgeon. It is a mechanical treatment of disease. The diseased organ or area is removed, repaired, opened, drained, or manipulated.

Physical therapy is the use of physical agents in the treatment of disease—heat, cold, light, other rays (x-rays, infrared and ultraviolet rays, and radiation), electricity, exercise, and body manipulation.

Psychotherapy is the treatment of emotional disorders. Its purpose is to remove or reduce the emotional factors in disease—to dispel the worries, doubts, and fears that are so often the cause of illness and that nearly always affect organic diseases (see Chapter 2).

Chemotherapy is the introduction, into the body, of drugs that are designed to cure a disease, affect its course, lessen its severity, or alleviate its pain and inconvenience. The majority of drugs exert actions that enable them to be divided into two major groups: those which work on the human body itself and those which exert their action against the pathogenic invaders of the body. Our concern in the following paragraphs is some of the latter group of drugs, the antimicrobial drugs.

The antimicrobial drugs, which act against the infectious invaders of the body, either are highly selective (working against only a single organism or group of organisms) or act against many types of pathogen. The two most widely used groups of antimicrobial drugs are the *antibiotics* and the *sulfa drugs*.

Antibiotics are produced during the normal growth of many types of soil-inhabiting microorganisms. They inhibit the growth of bacteria that compete with the soil microorganisms for the available food. They were first recognized by Sir Alexander Fleming, a Scottish bacteriologist, in 1929. Since that time several hundred antibiotics have been isolated and purified for use in controlling disease-producing bacteria.

The exact effect of antibiotics on bacteria is still not in every case known, but evidence indicates that the antibiotics interfere with various steps in cellular metabolism vital to bacterial growth. The antibacterial activity of antibiotics is highest during the period of greatest bacterial multiplication. Thus there is a good reason for early diagnosis of a disease and immediate treatment. When antibiotics are present in adequate concentrations, they kill bacteria; lower concentrations may only inhibit the growing organisms. Old cultures of bacteria beyond the stage of rapid growth show less response to antibiotics than do new cultures.

The administration of antibiotics is ordinarily by intramuscular or, occasionally, intravenous injection. Most antibiotics are readily absorbed after injection into the tissues. The simple antibiotics are prepared so as to be absorbed at different speeds for maximal blood concentration. Penicillin is absorbed within 30 minutes; other antibiotics, such as streptomycin and the tetracyclines, are absorbed in about 60 minutes. Preparations of some slowly absorbed antibiotics are available, so that the period of effective treatment following injection can be prolonged; that is, one dose of penicillin compound can be absorbed continuously for three days, whereas another is absorbed for nearly three weeks in smaller daily amounts.

When given orally, penicillin must be protected against the destructive secretions of the stomach. It is usually prescribed for use before meals, when there are less secretions in the stomach. However, even when it is protected, five times the intramuscular dose of penicillin must be administered orally to the patient for equivalent blood levels. Erythromycin, which may be substituted for penicillin, need not be given in such large doses, because it is absorbed adequately after oral administration. Tetracycline antibiotics and others are absorbed very readily from the digestive tract, but only about 10 percent of an oral dose of streptomycin is absorbed into the bloodstream, the rest of the dose remaining in the digestive tract, where it inhibits many kinds of bacteria and may upset the digestive processes and cause slight discomfort to the patient.

Most antibiotics can be distributed readily through the body, but not into the central nervous system in concentrations adequate for treatment of either sytemic or local infections there. Although they diffuse into the central nervous system with difficulty, very high concentrations of antibiotics in the bloodstream will promote diffusion even into the nervous tissues.

Antibiotics must be used cautiously, or their value will be lost. On the other hand, no patient should be deprived of the benefit of antibiotic therapy solely because of fear of inducing resistance in the disease germ.

The sulfonamides (sulfa drugs) were discovered in 1935. They have been very important in controlling bacterial diseases in man. Despite the subsequent introduction of the more effective and less toxic antibiotics, the sulfonamides continue to be widely used in the treatment of certain diseases.

The sulfonamides are produced by chemical synthesis; they are manufactured in tablets, which are administered orally. Since they have limited solubility in water and in the fluids of the body, there is sometimes difficulty in eliminating the drugs in the urine.

The sulfonamides inhibit bacterial multiplication during the growth phase. A bacterial cell has a complicated enzyme system for the satisfying of its nutritional requirements. This enzymatic activity involves a series of chemical reactions requiring vitaminlike compounds for its completion. The sulfonamide drugs interfere with the function of the enzymes, and this reduced function of the enzymes in turn damages the cell, resulting in its inability to produce energy and grow. If there is enough sulfa compound in the vicinity of a growing bacterial cell, this cell will incorporate this material in place of the vitaminlike material needed for normal growth. Consequently, the sulfonamides may be likened to "antivitamins" in their mode of action in controlling bacteria.

Because of the need for flooding a diseased area with sulfa, these drugs must be administered at regular intervals throughout a twenty-four-hour period for general effectiveness. The goal in sulfonamide therapy is to maintain an antibacterial concentration of sulfonamide continuously in all tissues of the body where the disease germs might multiply.

Anyone taking sulfa drugs should be certain to drink plenty of water, because water is the vehicle through which the kidney excretes these drugs from the body. If there is too little fluid intake, the drug may precipitate as crystals in the kidney, causing kidney damage.

Neither the antibiotics nor the sulfa drugs are effective against viral infections. These drugs are of no value against common colds, influenza, measles, mumps, and similar virus diseases—although they may effectively treat the secondary bacterial infections that may follow virus diseases. The drug *amatadine* has been successful in treating influenza viruses (such as the A2 virus of Hong Kong flu), returning the infected individuals to normal living within a day. Amatadine also has been shown able to prevent influenza when administered before an individual is exposed to the disease.

SUMMARY

I. Pathogens—disease-producing organisms
  A. Viruses—subcellular, semiliving particles.
  B. Bacteria—single-celled, plantlike organisms.
    1. Harmful effect is the result of their production of poisonous substances:
      a. exotoxins—substances which diffuse out of living bacterial cells into the surrounding tissues.
      b. endotoxins—substances released only after the death of the bacteria.
    2. Types of bacterial shape:
      a. cocci—spherical.
      b. bacilli—rod-shaped.
      c. spirilla—spiral or corkscrew-shaped.
  C. Fungi—primitive multicellular and unicellular plants.
  D. Protozoa—primitive single-celled animals.
  E. Parasitic worms—multicellular animals; the better known examples are roundworms, flukes, and tapeworms.
II. Course of a communicable disease
  A. Transmission and infection—the passing (transmission) of pathogenic organisms from one source or reservoir into the body of a victim (infection).
    1. Methods of transmission:
      a. person to person—which may be by direct or indirect contact.
      b. contaminated water—when sewage has accidentally been mixed with drinking water.
      c. contaminated food or milk—infection in the animal source or handling by infected individuals.
      d. animal to person—direct transmission through handling or the bite of an infected animal; indirect transmission through contact with fecal material or other residue from an infected animal.
      e. vectors—transmission exclusively through bites or fecal material of arthropods.
    2. Portals of exit and entry—pathogens usually leave and enter by the same route.
  B. Incubation period—after infection and before the appearance of symptoms, when the pathogen is reproducing within the individual.

C. Communicable period—when an infectious pathogen may be transmitted.
D. Prodromal period—period of nonspecific symptoms.
E. Typical illness stage—appearance and period of signs and symptoms.
F. Convalescence or recovery stage—when patient begins to regain his health.
G. Termination of a disease—three possible terminal stages after convalescence.
   1. Resusceptibility—person is resusceptible immediately after termination of the disease if he comes into contact with the pathogen.
   2. Carrier state—harboring a disease and having the ability to transmit it to another person without showing the clinical symptoms.
   3. Immunity—ability of the body to resist disease.
H. Subclinical illness—an infection so mild that it does not produce a "typical illness stage."
I. Types of disease outbreaks—terms used in reference to the number of cases of a particular disease in an area.
   1. Sporadic outbreak—a single or scattered occurrence of a communicable disease.
   2. Endemic—more or less continuous presence of a disease.
   3. Epidemic—outbreaks clearly in excess of the normal.
   4. Pandemic—the sweeping of a disease over large regions.
III. The body's defenses against disease
A. Skin and mucous membranes—the first line of defense; the unbroken skin and mucous membranes form an effective barrier against most pathogens.
B. Inflammation—the second line of defense; a local dilation of the capillaries in response to an infection.
C. Immunity—the third line of defense.
   1. Natural immunity (resistance)—inherited lack of susceptibility.
   2. Acquired immunity—the result of antibodies, produced in response to an antigen:
      a. active immunity results when a person produces his own antibodies in response to the presence in his body of an antigen—natural active immunity is obtained while a person is recovering from an actual case of an infectious disease; artificial active immunity results from the use of vaccines or toxoids.
      b. passive immunity results when antibodies are introduced into the body from an outside source—natural passive immunity (congenital immunity) is conferred by the mother upon her unborn child through the diffusion of antibodies across the placental membranes into the bloodstream of the fetus; artificial passive immunity results from the use of serums.
D. Interferon
   1. Produced by virus-infected body cells.
   2. Protects other cells from viral infection.
   3. Protects against many viruses (not specific).
   4. Interferon from other animals does not work in humans.
   5. May someday be important in disease prevention.
IV. Allergy—an antigen-antibody reaction which takes place within an individual who is hypersensitive to some normal component of the diet or environment.

V. Treatment of disease
  A. Kinds of therapy
    1. Dietary therapy—regulation of the food the patient eats.
    2. Operative therapy—surgical treatment, removal of diseased tissue or organ by the surgeon.
    3. Physical therapy—use of physical agents.
    4. Psychotherapy—treatment of emotional disorders by meaningful discussion between patient and therapist.
    5. Chemotherapy—introduction into the body of substances designed to:
      a. cure a disease.
      b. affect its course.
      c. lessen its severity.
      d. alleviate its pain or inconvenience.
  B. Antimicrobial drugs—act against pathogens.
    1. Antibiotics:
      a. produced by living microorganisms.
      b. interfere with cellular metabolism of bacteria.
    2. Sulfa drugs:
      a. produced by chemical synthesis.
      b. inhibit multiplication of bacteria.
      c. person taking sulfa drugs should drink plenty of water to prevent kidney damage.
    3. Neither antibiotics nor sulfa drugs are effective against viruses.
    4. Drug *amatadine* is effective in treating some viral diseases.

Glossary

If you cannot find the word you wish in this glossary, check the index for text and glossary references.

allergen (al′ər jen) (G. *allos,* other; *gennan,* to produce). A substance capable of producing an allergy.

allergy (al′ər jē) (G. *allos,* other; *ergon,* work). A hypersensitive reaction to a particular substance.

anaphylaxis (an ə fə lak′sis) (G. *ana,* up; *phylaxis,* protection). An exaggerated reaction to a foreign substance; an antigen-antibody reaction.

antibiotic (an′ti bī ot′ik) (G. *anti,* against; *bios,* life). A chemical produced by microorganisms which has the ability to inhibit the growth of bacteria or other microorganisms.

antibody (an′ti bod′ē). Chemical agents formed by the body to help destroy antigens.

antigen (an′ti jen). A foreign substance, usually a protein, which stimulates the production of antibodies.

attenuation (ə ten′yoo ā′shən) (L. *ad,* to; *tenuis,* thin). The act of weakening, such as the weakening of a pathogen or toxin.

bacillus (bə sil′əs) (L. *bacillus,* rod). A rod-shaped bacterium.

bacteria (bak tēr′ē ə) (G. *bakterion,* little rod). Microscopic, single-celled, plantlike organisms.

carrier (kar′ē ər). An individual who harbors disease organisms in his body without suffering from the disease.

chemotherapy (kem'ō ther'ə pē) (G. *chemeia,* chemical; *therapeia,* treatment). The treatment of disease with chemicals or drugs.

coccus (kok'əs) (G. *kokkos,* berry). A spherical bacterium.

communicable (kə myoo'ni kə bl). Capable of being transmitted from one person to another.

contagious (kən tā'jəs). Capable of being transmitted directly from one person to another.

disease (di zēz'). Any abnormality of the body; its parts, or its functions.

endemic (en dem'ik) (G. *endemos,* dwelling in a place). Present in an area at a low level at all times.

endotoxin (en dō tok'sin) (G. *endon,* within; *toxikon,* poison). A bacterial toxin released only after the death of the cell.

epidemic (ep i dem'ik) (G. *epidemios,* prevalent). A disease attacking many people at the same time.

exotoxin (ek'sō tok'sin) (G. *exo,* outside; *toxikon,* poison). A bacterial toxin released while the cell is still alive.

fungus (fung'gəs) (L. *fungus,* mushroom). A filamentous plant which lacks chlorophyll.

histamine (his'tə mēn). A chemical occurring in all tissues which, upon release, causes dilation of the capillaries and has other effects.

hypersensitivity (hī'pər sen si tiv'i tē). An allergy or abnormal sensitivity to a stimulus of any kind.

immunity (i myoo'ni tē) (L. *immunitas,* exemption). The power which an individual may acquire to resist an infection to which most members of the species are susceptible.

incubation (ing kyoo bā'shən) (L. *incubare,* to lie on). The interval between exposure to a disease and the appearance of the first symptom.

infection (in fek'shən) (L. *inficere,* to taint). Invasion of the body by pathogens.

infectious (in fek'shəs). Capable of being communicated by infection; capable of being transmitted.

inflammation (in flə mā'shən) (L. *inflammare,* to set on fire). A tissue reaction to injury.

interferon (in ter fēr'on). A protein produced by cells in response to a virus infection.

lesion (lē'zhən) (L. *laesio,* to hurt). An injury, wound, or infected area.

pandemic (pan dem'ik) (G. *pan,* all; *demos,* people). A widespread epidemic disease.

parasite (par'ə sīt) (G. *para,* alongside; *sitos,* food). A plant or animal that lives on or in another (host) organism at the expense of the host.

pathogen (path'ə jən) (G. *pathos,* disease; *gennan,* producing). A disease-producing organism or substance.

prodromal (prō drō'məl) (G. *prodromos,* forerunning). Indicating the approach of a disease.

protozoa (prō tə zō'ə) (G. *protos,* first; *zoon,* animal). Single-celled animals.

relapse (ri laps') (L. *relapsus,* slipping back). The return of a disease after the beginning of convalescence.

reservoir (rez'ər vwahr) (L. *reservare,* to keep back). A stockpile or pool; a reservoir of infection may be a symptomless carrier.

rickettsiae (ri ket'sē ə) (Howard T. Ricketts, American pathologist, 1871–1910). Microscopic bacterialike organisms transmitted by arthropods.

spirillum (spī ril'əm) (L. *spirillum,* coil). A corkscrew- or spiral-shaped bacterium.

sporadic (spo rad'ik) (G. *sporadikos,* scattered). Occurring only occasionally.

syndrome (sin'drōm) (G. *syndrome,* concurrence). A group of symptoms.

therapy (ther′ə pē) (G. *therapeia*, treatment). The treatment of disease.

toxin (tok′sin). A poison.

toxoid (tok′soid) (G. *toxikon*, poison, *eidos*, form). An attenuated (weakened) toxin which has lost its toxic properties while retaining its ability to cause production of antitoxins; used in immunization.

transmission (tranz mish′ən) (L. *trans*, through; *missio*, sending). Transfer of anything, as of a disease.

trauma (traw′mə, trou′mə) (G. *trauma*, wound). An injury or wound.

vaccine (vak sēn′) (L. *vaccinus*, of cows). A preparation of killed or attenuated microorganisms for use in immunization.

vector (vek′tər) (L. *vehere*, to carry). An animal, usually an arthropod, which transmits pathogens from one host to another.

virus (vī′rəs) (L. *virus*, poison). A minute infectious particle consisting of a core of DNA or RNA contained within a protein coat; all viruses are intracellular parasites.

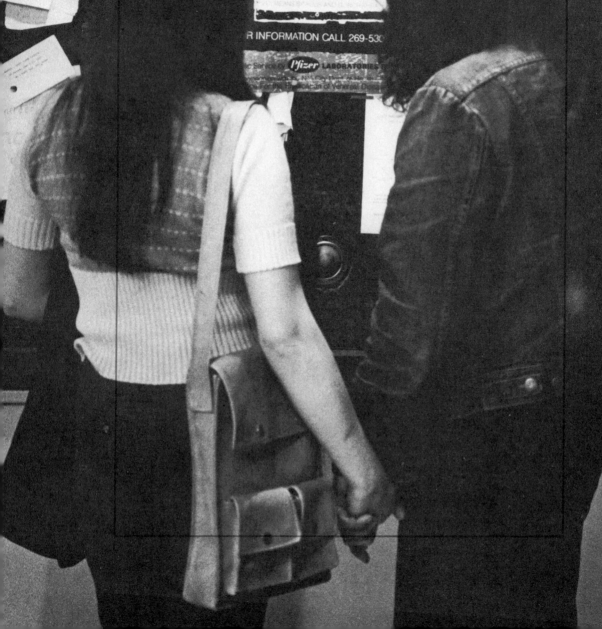

Venereal disease

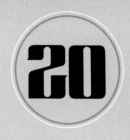

A number of types of organism infect both the male and female reproductive tracts. The organisms are transmitted during sexual contact between two people, contact that may be heterosexual or homosexual. Five of the diseases produced, if untreated, may lead to complications that are crippling or fatal; they are known as the venereal diseases. The word *venereal* refers to Venus, the Roman goddess of love.

The five venereal diseases recognized in the United States are syphilis, gonorrhea, chancroid, granuloma inguinale, and lymphogranuloma venereum. Although each disease varies as to the organism causing it and its particular symptoms, all have one thing in common: they are spread chiefly by sexual or other close physical contact.

Modern sanitation practices in the United States, along with modern medicine, have reduced the incidence of chancroid, granuloma inguinale, and lymphogranuloma venereum. Today these three are found mainly in large cities, and the total number of cases reported are far fewer than those of either syphilis or gonorrhea. Yet every effort should be made to detect these infections as long as they exist. It is, moreover, important to distinguish between these disorders and syphilis or gonorrhea for purposes of diagnosis and treatment. An individual may have more than one venereal disease at one time, and reinfection may occur at any time.

Syphilis and gonorrhea are the more significant because of their wide distribution. Syphilis is especially important because of its chronic nature and the

585

serious lesions, disabilities, and deaths that result from it. A review of reports on the trend of venereal diseases around the world indicates that both syphilis and gonorrhea are on the rise.

All venereal diseases are infectious communicable diseases (Chapter 19). The organisms that induce the diseases are very well known, and diagnosis, treatment, and cure are equally well known. The only common factor in venereal diseases is the manner in which they are contracted: mainly by sexual intercourse. If eradication of these diseases is ever to be accomplished, there must be a proper enlightenment among people about discriminate sexual relations. The diseases must be regarded in the same light as any other communicable disease, without undue reference to any moral implication. Shame or guilt must not discourage victims from seeking treatment, as it often has in the past.

INCIDENCE

Of the five venereal diseases gonorrhea is by far the most common. In fact, in the United States, *gonorrhea is the leading reported communicable disease* of the more than forty diseases which must, by law, be reported to health authorities. The incidence of gonorrhea has risen sharply in recent years. Currently over 600,000 cases are being reported each year. But the total number of cases of gonorrhea is actually much greater, since many cases are treated by private physicians without being reported, and many additional cases, particularly among females, never receive treatment. The actual incidence of gonorrhea is estimated at over 2 million cases per year. For syphilis it is estimated that there are more than a million people in the country with untreated syphilis, and more than 85,000 new cases are being added each year. Because so many cases are not treated, there exists in the United States a large reservoir of people who need treatment, probably about 1,200,000.

What would happen if more than a million people in the United States contracted smallpox? The answer is obvious: there would be mass panic. Yet syphilis can cause more permanent organic damage to the individual who survives the disease than smallpox can. Of untreated syphilitics 1 in 200 will become blind, 1 in 48 will develop *paresis* (paralysis caused by brain-tissue degeneration), 1 in 25 will become crippled to some extent, and 1 in 13 will develop syphilitic heart damage. Each year 1 in 400 (3,000 per year) will die of syphilis.[1]

As previously mentioned, the incidence of chancroid, granuloma inguinale, and lymphogranuloma venereum is low. In recent years their combined incidence has been only about 2,100 cases for the entire United States.

Who gets VD? Anyone, from the most respected professional to the laborer. It crosses all lines of race, creed, and color. Most of the infections occur in persons aged 15 to 24. According to Dr. Walter Smartt, past chief of Los Angeles County Venereal Disease Control Division of the Public Health

[1] P. E. Sartwell, *Preventive Medicine and Public Health*, 9th ed., New York, Appleton-Century-Crofts, 1965, pp. 274–278.

Department, the probability that a person will acquire VD by the time he is 25 is about 50 percent.

The victims are about equally divided between males and females. Most patients seeking treatment are male, because men show the symptoms that cause them to seek treatment. For every two women being treated for gonorrhea there are seven men being treated for it. The difference is more than made up by the large numbers of undiagnosed females whose disease does not produce apparent symptoms (asymptomatic). Tests for gonorrhea conducted on females coming to both private and public health clinics for birth-control information show that about one in ten girls between the ages of 15 and 25 has gonorrhea and does not know it.

Homosexuals are more likely to acquire a venereal disease than is any other identifiable group. It has been estimated that up to 50 percent of new cases of syphilis occur among male homosexuals.

Why have syphilis and gonorrhea emerged as the leading communicable diseases in young people? The following are a few of the major conditions which help to spread venereal diseases.

1. Millions of young people between the ages of 15 and 24 know little or nothing about these diseases; others are saturated with misinformation passed on from one person to another.

2. Parents and society may overemphasize the moral and social implications of venereal disease to such an extent that young adults will neither present themselves for treatment nor voluntarily submit to public-health interviews, which are the only means of eventually eradicating venereal disease.

3. To avoid embarrassment, many individuals seek treatment through "quacks" or self-medication.

4. The curative powers of the antibiotics and sulfa drugs have been so far overrated that widespread apathy among young people, physicians, and society in general has resulted. Consequently the reporting of cases and the resulting contact studies are not nearly as routine as they should be. Apathy and ignorance on the part of physicians lead to misdiagnosis, inadequate follow-up studies of treated patients, and a weak response to public-health pleas for reporting of venereal-disease patients to be screened for investigation and interviewing. With the advent of penicillin and its ease of administration and low cost much venereal-disease treatment is being given in the private physician's office.

5. Uninformed homosexuals may not realize that venereal infection can be transmitted by or contracted through homosexual or close physical contacts.

6. Greater sexual freedom among young people has contributed to the spread of venereal disease.

7. The increased use of alcohol and other drugs also has contributed to the increase of venereal disease among young people.

8. The use of oral contraceptive pills has reduced the use of the condom ("rubber"), which is a help in reducing the transmission of disease when it is used correctly. For a condom to be effective against the transmission of gonorrhea an individual must use it throughout all sexual contact, not just prior to orgasm, make sure it is intact and not damaged prior to its use, keep it intact

during use and check to see that it hasn't broken during use, and put it on fully and remove it carefully.

A condom does not cover the base of the penis, the pelvic area just above the base of the penis, or the thighs. These are the areas often bathed with a woman's vaginal secretions during the sex act, helping syphilis to become established.

9. The use of contraceptive pills increases the alkalinity and moisture of the female genital tract. The wearing of tight-fitting pants, panty hose, and "jeans" further increases the heat and moisture in the genital area. The conditions of alkalinity, increased moisture, and heat turn the genital tract into a virtual *culture medium*, causing all diseases of the female genital tract to increase (Candida, Trichomonas, herpes virus, and gonococcus). Some public-health officials feel that the risk of contracting gonorrhea for a woman engaging in a single act of unprotected intercourse with an infected male is about 40 percent; for one taking the pill the risk is nearly 100 percent.

10. The increased acceptance of genitooral play and genitorectal sex has caused a greater risk of infection and the spread of infections to new areas.

PREVENTION AND CONTROL

The successful control of any communicable disease depends upon the recognition and elimination of sources of infection, a process which is especially necessary in the control of venereal disease. Officers for the control of venereal disease agree that, to reduce the incidence, a much higher percentage of infected persons must be interviewed, so that *all* contacts may be found, examined, and treated if infected. If cases are not reported, it is not possible for health departments to provide trained interviewers to obtain the names of all the infected individual's close contacts. And, also, if cases are not reported, infected individuals will continue to spread the disease.

One infected individual, untreated, may infect two, three, or more people who, if not found and treated will in turn infect others. Every diseased patient interviewed should reveal at least one other case of infectious syphilis: the one who infected him.

Society's methods of controlling venereal disease

Interviewing procedure   The interviewing procedure will vary from area to area, but the following is the usual process.

As patients are diagnosed, they are interviewed and asked to name those people to whom they have been exposed sexually (from the beginning of the incubation period to the time that treatment renders them noninfectious) and also the names and addresses, if possible, of anyone made a sexual partner during the six months before the symptoms began. All these *contacts* are then located, examined and, if necessary, treated.

The interviewer makes these contacts by telephone or by visiting the individuals. He explains to them that they have been "exposed to a dangerous communicable disease" and asks that they please see either their own physician or the local public health clinic as soon as possible. This contacting is done without mentioning the reporting patient's name or identifying him in any manner. If the individual elects to see his own physician, the doctor's name is asked for, and the physician is informed of the suspected venereal disease and asked to conduct the tests and inform the public-health interviewer of the outcome. If the contact does not report to the public health clinic or to his physician within a reasonable period of time, the local police are asked to "pick up" the individual and bring him to the clinic for an examination. Under no condition is the reporting patient's name ever disclosed to anyone, including the police, the private physician, or the suspected contact.

Reporting by private physicians Unless more private physicians are brought into the control effort, venereal disease will remain a serious hazard to the health of the public. Private physicians hold the key to the eradication of venereal disease, but they must give more support to locating and examining all known contacts as well as to posttreatment followup examinations.

Cluster testing In addition to increasing the interviewing of contacts another method has been introduced for the control of venereal disease. Patients with infectious venereal disease are, as usual, interviewed for sexual contacts but are also asked to name other persons, of either sex, who move in the same sociosexual environment and who the patient thinks might benefit by an examination for syphilis, gonorrhea, or other venereal diseases. These other people include friends, acquaintances, neighbors, fellow employees, or anyone with sexual behavior approximating that of the patient. This type of interviewing is called *cluster testing*.

Personal responsibility in controlling venereal disease

The contracting of venereal disease depends wholly upon how an individual conducts his life. If one is never exposed to a disease, he will not contract it. The best preventive measure against venereal disease is *abstinence from casual sexual contact*. Such sexual contact may be either heterosexual (individuals of the opposite sex) or homosexual (individuals of the same sex); both contacts can transmit venereal disease to an equal degree. Married individuals having extramarital sexual relationships run the risk of exposing not only themselves but also their spouses to venereal disease.

If a person does place himself in a situation in which there is a possibility of contracting venereal disease, he can reduce his chances of infection by using a few precautions, during and immediately after exposure. None of these methods is 100 percent effective.

It used to be the male's responsibility to prevent both pregnancy and venereal disease by use of the condom. The emphasis in contraception has now shifted to the female through the use of pills, intrauterine devices, and foams —none of which prevents venereal disease. The male no longer favors nor understands the need of the condom, even when contraception is not the goal. The properly used condom should prevent almost all transmission of gonorrhea (male to female or female to male), though it will not protect completely against syphilis because it does not cover all of the skin of both sex partners.

Soap and water have disinfectant properties against the frail organisms of syphilis and gonorrhea. Both males and females can reduce the infective ability of the organisms by liberal use of soap and water to cleanse the genitalia and surrounding areas immediately after intercourse. The female can reduce her chance of infection by douching with an antiseptic douching solution. Males should urinate as soon as possible after intercourse, reducing the chance of infection from gonorrhea (though not from syphilis).

The ideal preventive product for venereal diseases would, of course, be a vaccine (no communicable disease has ever been truly "controlled" until a vaccine was developed). A vaccine for syphilis is now under development, although its perfection seems to be several years in the future. There currently seems to be little chance of an effective vaccine against gonorrhea.

The next best measure for the prevention of venereal disease is for all individuals to be aware of the problem and the necessity of prompt and proper medical treatment when signs or symptoms of infection appear.

Individuals also must recognize and dispel misconceptions concerning venereal disease. Mistakenly, some people believe that a genital sore that heals requires no further medical care, that venereal disease cannot be spread by homosexual contact, that venereal disease cannot be cured, or that some people are naturally immune. Many people mistakenly believe that a prophylactic device will absolutely prevent venereal disease or that both pregnancy and venereal disease can be prevented by douching with water or other liquids, such as a carbonated drink, after intercourse. Then there are those with no opinions—and, often, no knowledge whatsoever. Mistaken ideas transmitted in the home, the school, the church, and between individuals must be replaced with up-to-date information.

SYPHILIS

Syphilis is a body-wide disease produced by infection with the spirochete *Treponema pallidum*; see Fig. 20.1. There are two distinct forms of syphilis, venereal and nonvenereal.

Nonvenereal syphilis

Nonvenereal syphilis is referred to as *endemic syphilis* or *bejel*. It is spread by means other than sexual contact and is confined to parts of the world where economic, social, and climatic conditions favor its development; it is not found in the United States. Bejel is found mostly in Syria and surrounding countries. It is characterized by lesions of the skin and mucous membranes, usually without an initial primary lesion; these lesions may be indistinguishable from secondary lesions of venereal syphilis.

Venereal syphilis

Throughout this discussion the word *syphilis* will mean *venereal syphilis*.

Venereal syphilis is of worldwide occurrence. The spirochete that causes syphilis (*Treponema pallidum*) is a corkscrew-shaped organism (Fig. 20.1). This organism is extremely fragile and unable to resist drying. It is destroyed by many common antiseptics and can survive only *momentarily* on exposure to air. Its normal and preferred habitat is deep in the body tissues, but when it is deposited from an open lesion onto moist, warm skin, it can survive long enough to burrow through the surface, establish a colony, and eventually spread throughout the body. Because of these required conditions of intimate contact it is easy to recognize why syphilis is spread almost exclusively by sexual contact, either heterosexual or homosexual, during intercourse, through a lip wound or the oral cavity when kissing, or by close bodily contact with a secondary syphilitic rash. In few other circumstances is there the necessary combination of body surfaces and intimate contact necessary to transfer *Treponema pallidum* alive from one person to another.

Because of the great variety of potential signs and symptoms that occur in all stages of syphilis it has been called "the great imitator." There are at least 40 skin diseases that secondary syphilis may resemble, 23 that the mouth lesions may resemble, and at least 16 that resemble primary genital lesions.[2]

The course of the disease is divided into four distinct stages, each with its own signs and symptoms. This course is outlined in Figs. 20.2 and 20.3 and explained in more detail in the following sections.

Primary syphilis During sexual contact *Treponema pallidum* gains entry by burrowing into the body of the partner. After entry it reproduces at the site of entrance and within a few hours produces millions of spirochetes, which begin to spread by way of the blood and lymph throughout the body. This stage is the incubation period (Fig. 20.2), which ranges from ten to ninety days (the average is three weeks).

The first indication or symptom of the disease is the *primary lesion,* called a *chancre,* which appears at the site of entry of the spirochete within three to four weeks after exposure. This highly infectious lesion may be a typical

[2] Sartwell, *op. cit.,* p. 277.

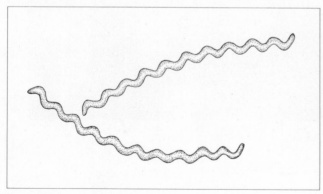

Figure 20.1 *Treponema pallidum,* the organism that causes syphilis.

chancre (a painless lesion, the size of a dime, pink, raised, ulcerated, and firm, with enlarged neighboring lymph nodes), or it may be so slight as to go unnoticed. Since primary syphilis may resemble many diseases, any lesion of the genital area of a male or female who has had prior sexual contact should be regarded as possible primary syphilis until it is proven, by medical consultation, to be something else. Any lesion anywhere on the body—particularly on the lips, tongue, tonsils, or fingers—which fails to heal in a reasonable length of time may be a primary syphilis lesion.

The primary lesion will disappear spontaneously without treatment before the appearance of the secondary stage. It usually leaves no scar, but the disease agents are still present in the body. Blood tests of victims are negative when the primary lesion appears but become positive one or two weeks after the chancre is first noted (Fig. 20.3).

Secondary syphilis   The spread of *Treponema pallidum* throughout the body before the primary lesion appears produces secondary syphilis symptoms in the skin, mucous membranes, eyes, and nervous system. The organism multiplies in these areas of the body, and in about four weeks to six months after the appearance of the primary chancre, the secondary signs and symptoms may appear; see Table 20.1. These include a rash, which does not itch, which may be all over the body or just on the palms of the hands or the soles of the feet, and which often is difficult to see. The victim may also have a sore throat, mild fever, or headache. Other more or less common symptoms

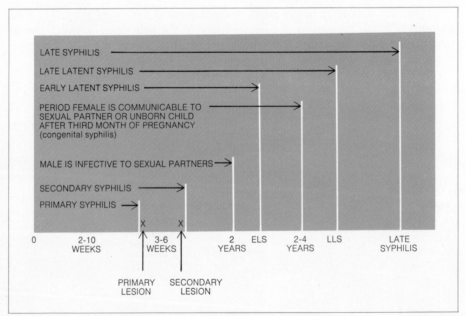

Figure 20.2   Stages of syphilis, including infectious periods.

are falling patches of hair, external or internal inflammation of the eyes, pain in the joints from bone involvement, and jaundice from liver involvement. (In very severe conditions, syphilitic meningitis with severe headache, convulsions, deafness, partial paralysis, and sometimes coma may occur.)

It is important for a person who is seeking medical examination for the symptoms described here to divulge whether he has been exposed or thinks he may have been exposed to syphilis in the past six months. The symptoms of secondary syphilis persist for a variable period of time, ranging from a few days to several months, and then disappear spontaneously. Secondary syphilis, which lasts three to six months, can always be diagnosed by blood tests (Fig. 20.3).

Latent syphilis Latency begins with the healing of untreated secondary lesions; it may extend from a few months to a lifetime. If we consider the first two years of an untreated infection the overall period of potential infectiousness, latency may be divided into two stages: the potentially infectious stage, or *early latent syphilis*, and a noninfectious later stage, or *late latent*

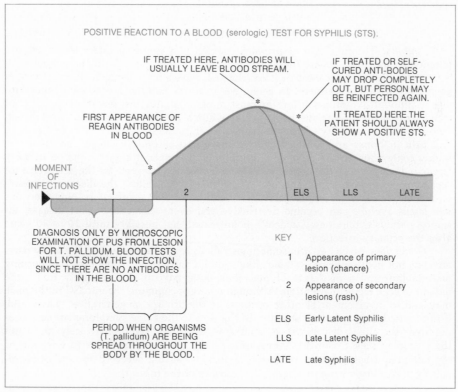

Figure 20.3   Course of syphilis, with effectiveness of blood serological tests.

Table 20.1 *Natural history of acquired syphilis and gonorrhea*

	syphilis	gonorrhea
Causative agent	*Treponema pallidum* (spirochete)	*Neisseria gonorrheae* (coccus)
Incubation period	10–90 days, usually 21 days after exposure	In 5 days for 85% of males after exposure; 2–8 days for females
Mode of transmission	Direct physical contact, usually during sexual relations	Sexual contact, usually sexual intercourse
Immunity	No immunizing agent (vaccine). Acquired immunity eventually may develop in absence of treatment. Though early treatment halts immunological process and readily permits reinfection, it also protects body against systemic advance of disease process.	No immunizing agent (vaccine). An attack of the disease does not afford protection against reinfection.

Syphilis: The first sign of *primary syphilis* is a single, painless lesion or sore (chancre), most often where the germs entered the body, usually in the genital area. Sometimes it does not appear or is overlooked, especially in women; if it appears, it goes away without treatment. In a few weeks to six months *secondary syphilis* appears; although symptoms differ, the most common are lesions, few or many, large or small, appearing on various body areas: whitish patches in the mouth or throat, "moth eaten" or "patchy" falling hair, low fever, painless swelling of lymph glands, and pain in bones and joints. In the *primary* and *secondary* stages the disease is highly contagious. When secondary symptoms disappear it enters a period of *early latency,* during which the degree of infectiousness is governed by the recurrence of secondary lesions. In any event, because of such a possibility, the disease is considered communicable for approximately 4 years after initial infection. Noninfectious *late latent syphilis* can become destructive and eventually cause heart disease, insanity, paralysis, blindness, or death, if untreated, but possibly until 10 to 30 years after the primary infection.

Gonorrhea, or GC as it is sometimes called, is a local disease of the body parts affected, not body-wide or systemic, like syphilis. In the *male* it manifests as burning on urination and a discharge of pus. It is quite painful and generally forces the patient to seek medical attention. Although not very common, chronic GC in the male may lead to involvement of other portions of the urinary or generative system and, if not treated early, produce sterility. In the *female* the early symptoms are less pronounced; the slight discomfort associated with urinary symptoms rarely motivates the person to seek treatment. Progression of the disease often leads to infection of the fallopian tubes, ovaries, and lower abdomen, causing severe pain, and often resulting in sterility, owing to scarring and closure of the tubes.

SOURCE: Adapted from Los Angeles County Health Department outline.

syphilis. These phases, commonly called "hidden syphilis," are not recognizable by visible signs or symptoms. They are uncovered only by blood tests (Fig. 20.1). Latent syphilis is usually discovered during routine blood examinations.

· EARLY LATENT SYPHILIS   If the disease goes untreated during the secondary eruptions, there may be a series of recurring infectious lesions of the skin or mucous membranes of the mouth for the first two to four years; this is the period of early latent syphilis. Because of these possible early lesions the disease is considered communicable throughout its early latency. During this long latent period the disease loses some of its infectiousness, and after the first two years a person can rarely transmit syphilis through sexual intercourse, although a syphilitic pregnant woman can still transmit it to her unborn child (*congenital syphilis*) for about two more years. A prenatally infected child is presumptive proof of the mother's latent infection.

· LATE LATENT SYPHILIS   After an individual has lost all capacity for infecting, the disease has entered the period of late latent syphilis. This period may last a few months or a lifetime. During this time there are no discernible signs of illness. If routinely examined, the individual will show a positive blood-test result but will have no further signs. In this latent stage progressive degeneration of the brain, spinal cord, hearing, sight, or bones may be going on unnoticed. If the symptoms of this degeneration appear, the individual then slips into the last stage, late syphilis.

Late syphilis   Of all persons acquiring syphilis many may be expected to develop, if untreated, a late manifestation that will incapacitate or kill them. Although almost any part of the body may be affected, only the most common manifestations are discussed below.

· CARDIOVASCULAR SYPHILIS   The lesions in most cases of cardiovascular syphilis are located in the thoracic aorta (Fig. 16.1). The elastic tissue is destroyed, and the aorta dilates, producing an aneurysm, or the infection may involve the aortic valve, causing an insufficient flow of blood. The symptoms of cardiovascular syphilis differ in no unique way from other heart and vascular disorders (Chapter 16).

· NEUROSYPHILIS   The process of neurosyphilis (syphilis affecting nervous tissue) may be detected by routine spinal-fluid examination years before the appearance of obvious changes in the behavior of the individual. *Paresis* (partial paralysis), a common late manifestation of syphilis, will be the eventual fate awaiting this victim.

The symptoms of neurosyphilis arise from a widespread destruction of the brain tissue by large numbers of *Treponema pallidum*. The mental changes vary, the most common being gradual changes in personality, decreased ability to work, and impairment of concentration and judgment. These changes produce abnormal behavior, including delusions, loss of memory, lack of insight, apathy or violent rages, convulsions, and disorientation. Neurosyphilis is responsible for many deaths besides much of the invalidism seen in mental institutions.

· TABES DORSALIS   Tabes dorsalis is a failure of muscular coordination within the body; it is the common outcome of the destruction of the spinal cord by large numbers of spirochetes. Similar degeneration of the optic and other cranial nerves is common. The usual diagnostic sign is a weakening or loss of ankle and knee reflexes. Occasionally all reflexes may be lost, including the ability to change pupil size, sense of position, or any irregularity of muscular coordination.

In treated cases life can be prolonged, but permanent care may be necessary because of the extreme degeneration that may have taken place prior to treatment.

· PRIMARY OPTIC ATROPHY   A degeneration of the optic nerve is usually first noticed as a loss of peripheral vision. Central vision may be lost in advanced cases, leaving the individual completely blind. Primary optic atrophy also results from glaucoma (Chapter 3) and other conditions affecting the eyes.

Syphilis in pregnancy

If a woman is infected with syphilis at the time of conception or shortly thereafter, the primary chancre appearing on her may be very mild or completely suppressed. Secondary symptoms in her skin are likely to be absent, and if she has not had blood tests during her pregnancy, she may have no indication that she has syphilis before the birth of her child. Infection of a fetus is caused by spirochetes of syphilis crossing the placental membranes. The infection of the fetus apparently does not occur before the fifth month of fetal life. Consequently, adequate treatment of a previously syphilitic pregnant woman before the fifth fetal month will ensure the child's safety. Treatment given a mother after the fifth month will also reach and cure the syphilitic fetus. Because of the aforementioned conditions and because syphilis can also be acquired during pregnancy, blood tests during the first half of pregnancy and during the seventh month are considered to be adequate for detecting this disease.

In a majority of instances the infection of the fetus takes place quite late in the pregnancy, and the more recent the mother's syphilitic infection, the greater the chance that the child will be born with syphilis. A severe infection is very likely to lead to the death of the fetus before birth. Thus syphilis is a rather common cause of stillbirths. Of the infants born alive to untreated syphilitic mothers approximately half will have syphilis at birth. Syphilis obtained in this manner is termed *congenital syphilis*.

Congenital syphilis

An infant born with syphilis may show secondary lesions at birth, may appear normal at birth and develop lesions within a few months, or may remain without symptoms until adolescence, when the symptoms of late syphilis may appear. As a rule, the earlier the symptoms appear, the more severe is the infection. Syphilis is capable of producing many different types of lesion, but never do all of them occur in one infant.

Of the various secondary lesions appearing at birth, *rhinitis* (inflammation of the nose) with a discharge of *Treponema pallidum* spirochetes is the most frequent. The discharge may interfere with breathing, is extremely infectious, and accounts for many infections of individuals who handle such children. If it is severe and continues over a long period, the growth of the nasal bones is disturbed, resulting in the deformity known as "saddle nose"; see Fig. 20.4. Skin lesions at birth are frequent and are often similar to the rash seen in secondary stages of venereal syphilis. In a high proportion of children the palms and soles or the skin about the mouth is reddened, inflamed, and thickened at birth or shortly after birth. When this occurs around the mouth, fissures may radiate in all directions. After the healing the lesions and radiating scars about the mouth are known as _rhagades_ and are considered signs of congenital syphilis; see Fig. 20.5.

After the secondary lesions, the course of untreated congenital syphilis is similar to that of venereal syphilis. The late symptoms may appear in a few months, at six or seven years, or late in the teens. Some of the more common are _keratitis_, a condition of the eyes that is uncommon in young children but very common in older children and may cause permanent blindness (neurosyphilis), bone and joint involvement, a lung condition that usually leads to death during the first few days or weeks of life, and Hutchinson's teeth, which are "notched" or screwdriverlike permanent central incisors; see Fig. 20.6.

Diagnosis and therapy

Early diagnosis followed by prompt and adequate treatment will completely cure syphilis.

Microscopic examination The lesions of early syphilis that may begin to appear at the points of physical contact within three to five weeks from contact are rich in _Treponema pallidum_, which provides the best means for the

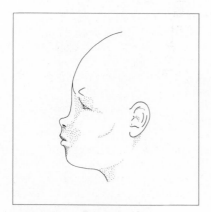

Figure 20.4   Saddle nose: destruction of the septum in congenital syphilis.

conclusive diagnosis of this disease. *Treponema pallidum* taken from such a chancre of primary syphilis or from skin lesions of secondary syphilis can readily be seen under a microscope by what is termed darkfield illumination. The more recent the lesion is, the more readily can the organism be discovered and the disease cured.

Blood (serologic) tests for syphilis (STS)   The blood tests show positive only after a general invasion of the body by the spirochetes. The underlying principle of a blood test is the appearance in the blood, after syphilis infection (and occasionally after some other conditions), of an *antibodylike* substance called *reagin*. All the blood tests for syphilis, based on reagin in the blood, are modifications of the original Wassermann test (a test for determining reagin in the blood, which was much less sensitive than the currently used tests).

Besides the reagin tests there are other blood tests for syphilis. These are for *Treponema pallidum* spirochetes and specific antibodies produced by the body in response to the syphilis infection. They are positive for syphilis only, are quite expensive, and involve complicated procedures that could not be used as easily as the reagin tests for screening numbers of individuals.

Therapy   The purposes of treatment are to destroy all spirochetes, to initiate the healing of existing lesions, and to prevent further damage to the body. Treatment of syphilis also serves to prevent the spread of the disease to others. The earlier this treatment is started, the more effective it is in accomplishing these purposes.

In the 1940s penicillin began to replace the long, expensive, and difficult treatment of syphilis with arsenical products and bismuth preparations. Since that time the use of penicillin alone in the treatment of syphilis has been standard all over the world.

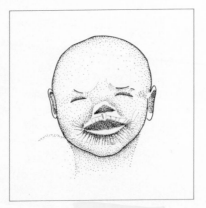

Figure 20.5   Rhagades (scars around mouth), due to congenital syphilis.

The primary consideration in treatment is the maintenance of a high penicillin level in the blood and tissues for a sufficient period of time to destroy all of the organisms in the body. Consequently, the treatment varies with the stage of the disease. Unfortunately, the widespread use of penicillin for the treatment of a variety of other disorders has frequently added some difficulties to the diagnosis of syphilis. Syphilitic infection may be masked completely or its course altered by smaller doses of penicillin than are necessary to treat syphilis adequately. When a patient's sensitivity to penicillin restricts the use of this preferable drug, the tetracyclines are good alternatives. No matter what drug is used, inadequate therapy may lead to a relapse.

GONORRHEA

Gonorrhea is an acute venereal disease that frequently progresses into a chronic state. It is initiated by a microorganism that prefers to live in the mucous membranes lining the genitourinary tract, the rectum, the mouth, and the eye. This organism is the gonococcus *Neisseria gonorrheae*; see Fig. 20.7.

All gonococcal infections, except the eye infections of newborn infants and occasional accidental eye infections of adults, are the result of direct physical contact. Although the gonococcus is rarely spread by circulation of the blood, it can cause serious infection of the heart or joints (arthritis) when it does enter the blood.

The gonococcus is quite sensitive to conditions outside the human body. Infection requires the direct depositing of *Neisseria gonorrheae* near the susceptible tissues. Occasionally the organism is accidentally deposited from the hand to an eye or into the eyes of a newborn as a result of its passage through an infected birth canal (*ophthalmia neonatorum*).

The incubation period of gonorrhea is usually three to five days, but

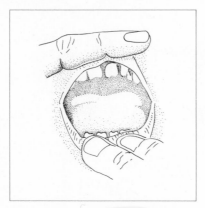

Figure 20.6 Hutchinson's teeth, due to congenital syphilis.

occasionally it varies from two to ten days. The signs, symptoms, and outcome differ between males and females. The course of the disease is explained in Table 20.1, and the significant factors are explained in the following discussion.

Male gonorrhea

In nine out of ten men a symptom of gonorrhea will appear in *two days to a week* after exposure. The tenth man will still have the disease but remain symptomless. The first symptoms of gonorrhea are a sensation of burning during urination and a discharge ("drip") of pus from the penis, which may be severe or so mild as to go unnoticed. Without treatment the organisms gradually work their way along the urethra and vas deferens into the internal organs of the male reproductive tract. Damage to the testes and the vas deferens can cause permanent sterility. Infections of the mouth are as common as infections of the urethra among those who perform orogenital acts (such infections are common in homosexuals).

Female gonorrhea

Most women are unaware they are infected with gonorrhea until their male partners tell them. The initial symptom of gonorrhea in the female, a slight vaginal discharge of pus, in most instances is so mild as to go unnoticed. Only when the infection has progressed into the fallopian tubes, generally months after infection, is a woman likely to be aware of gonorrhea. Then pain may occur in the lower abdomen and often is mistaken for appendicitis.

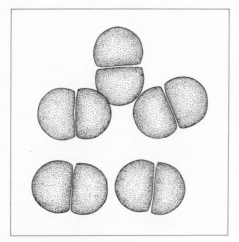

Figure 20.7   *Neisseria gonorrheae*, the organism that causes gonorrhea.

The "pill," while protecting a woman against pregnancy, actually helps her become infected with gonorrhea. The pill causes an increase in the moisture content of the vagina and changes the moisture from an acid to an alkaline environment, which is ideally suited for the growth of the gonococcus organism. By contrast, other contraceptive aids for women, such as the vaginal jelly and foam, are acidic and provide an environment antagonistic to the growth of the organism. A female on the pill who has intercourse with an infected male has no chance of escaping infection and will also suffer complications from the gonorrhea infection much sooner than if she were not on the pill.

When exposure to gonorrhea is suspected or when there is a vaginal discharge that may be caused by gonorrhea, the physician usually takes samples of secretions from the woman's uterus, cervix, and vagina for both smears and cultures. Many different organisms can cause vaginal discharge, and the job of establishing which are involved may take much time and effort. Prolonged exposure to infections may cause sterility from strictures that form within the fallopian tubes. Since different drugs are effective against different organisms, a correct diagnosis obviously is important.

Carriers

The problem of asymptomatic carriers (individuals who have disease without any visible symptoms) is an important part of the story of the gonorrhea epidemic. Carriers can pass on the disease without the knowledge of anyone, not even of themselves. Public Health Service studies show that between 1 and 8 percent of *all* women in the United States may be asymptomatic carriers of gonorrhea. Asymptomatic carrier males are also being recognized. Public Health investigators are reporting the recovery of gonococci from the urethra of males showing no symptoms of gonorrhea.

Diagnosis and therapy

In both men and women gonorrhea remains infectious until cured. Since in women the early symptoms are mild and commonly ignored, a woman may be infected for months or years. Gonorrhea in a woman is often not suspected until complications occur or until a sexual partner is infected and identifies her to the public health department as a sexual contact. The tracing of sex contacts is just as important for gonorrhea as it is for syphilis.

There is no blood test available for detecting gonorrhea, though current research shows some promise of the development of such a test. Diagnosis is currently a hit-or-miss procedure, based upon microscopic detection of the pathogen.

Gonorrhea is generally treated with antibiotics, of which penicillin was the drug of choice for many years, but recently *Neisseria gonorrheae* has become increasingly resistant to penicillin. In 1965, 2.4 units of penicillin provided a complete cure in almost every case. Today it may take as much as 6 million units. Especially resistant strains are found on the West Coast and in Asia. The importation of resistant Asian strains of gonorrhea by United

States troops returning from duty has become a major problem. Penicillin doses have now reached the maximum that can be given. Fortunately, other antibiotics and sulfa drugs are generally effective when penicillin fails or when the patient has a sensitivity (allergy) to penicillin.

Ophthalmia neonatorum

A condition causing blindness in the newborn children of mothers who are infected with gonorrhea at the time of birth is ophthalmia neonatorum. The source of infection is the mother's birth canal, which is infected with *Neisseria gonorrheae*. The organisms rub off onto the child while it is being born, incubate in 36 to 48 hours, and start destroying the tissue of the eyes.

The condition can be prevented by the use of preparations for the protection of the eyes of babies at birth. An established effective treatment is drops of silver nitrate solution put into the eyes of children shortly after birth. Such treatment has been a law in all states for many years. Many antibiotic solutions are as effective as silver nitrate and are now being used in some areas.

CHANCROID

Chancroid, also known as *soft chancre,* is an acute, localized, infectious communicable disease acquired through sexual contact; see Table 20.2. It is induced by an organism known as the Ducrey bacillus (*Hemophilus ducreyi*). Soft chancre was distinguished from the primary lesion of syphilis in 1850 and later named *chancroid*. In 1889 Augusto Ducrey, an Italian dermatologist, identified the microorganism that caused the disease. The genital ulcerations produced by the disease are variable in appearance and even yet are occasionally confused with the chancre of syphilis.

Usually the disease is self-limiting, but when a lesion is in an area that is hard to keep clean or is hidden, or where it cannot be properly exposed and treated, prolonged infection will cause severe tissue destruction. Spreading of the organisms to adjacent areas of the body may cause reinfection and multiple lesions.

Chancroid occurs throughout the world and is especially common in tropical and subtropical countries. In many countries it is not a reportable disease, and exact data as to its occurrence, distribution, and trends are not available.

About three to five days after exposure to *Hemophilus ducreyi* a small, red area appears at the site of infection; this enlarges into a pimplelike growth, which soon breaks down, forming an ulcer with ragged edges and oozing pus. The ulcers are very painful and bleed easily. In about half the cases a swelling develops in the local lymph glands within two weeks. It becomes inflamed, accumulates large amounts of pus, and may rupture spontaneously.

The key to prevention of chancroid is cleanliness. The use of soap and water immediately after exposure is a preventive measure. But better education, better living standards, and improved personal hygiene will eliminate the infection.

Table 20.2 *Natural history of chancroid, lymphogranuloma venereum, and granuloma inguinale (the "minor" venereal diseases)*

	chancroid[a]	granuloma inguinale[a]	lymphogranuloma venereum[a]
Causative agent	Hemophilus ducreyi (bacillus)	Donovania granulomatis (bacillus)	Miyagawanella lymphogranulomatosis (extremely small bacterium)
Incubation period	An average of 3 to 5 days	1 to 12 weeks	5 to 21 days
Mode of transmission	Sexual contact, usually sexual intercourse	Considered to be sexual contact, never completely proven	Sexual contact, usually sexual intercourse
Immunity	None	Acquired immunity depends on duration of untreated infection	Acquired immunity depends on duration of untreated infection

Chancroid: An acute, localized genitoinfectious disease characterized by a single, but sometimes multiple, ulcerative lesion. The ulceration is usually accompanied by painful swelling of lymph nodes in the groin. The disease is usually self-limited but may persist for a long time.

Granuloma inguinale: A chronic progressive disease, which begins as a small papule, vesicle, or nodule, ulcerates and gradually spreads to form a smooth, velvety surface. The lesion may occur in any genital area and quite often involves the lymph nodes in the groin. Extragenital lesions occur in 6 percent of all reported untreated cases.

Lymphogranuloma venereum: The first sign is usually a small, transient lesion followed by regional swelling of lymph nodes. Constitutional symptoms are often present, including chills, headache, fever and generalized aches. The disease may disappear spontaneously or progress to more consequences. Malignancy may occur in long-standing lesions.

SOURCE: Adapted from Los Angeles County Health Department outline.
[a] National and local morbidity rates not significant.

GRANULOMA INGUINALE

Granuloma inguinale is a chronic venereal disease that usually affects the genital and inguinal regions of the body (Table 20.2). It is initiated by a microorganism known as the Donovan body (*Donovania granulomatis*), a bacterium. Among the other names given this disease are ulcerating granuloma, granuloma pudendi tropicum, granuloma contagiosa, chronic venereal sore, and granuloma venereum.

The first report of a case was in India in 1882. The first case reported in the United States was in 1913. Exact data on its incidence and prevalence are not available, but it seems to be the least common of the venereal diseases. It is most frequent in the tropics but has been reported in all countries of the world. In the United States it is found quite often in the South, particularly among the lower socioeconomic groups, and is more frequent among males than females.

The incubation period has been stated to be from eight to twelve weeks, but it has run more than a hundred days. The initial lesions are on the genital organs and slowly spread to the inguinal regions. The lesion takes the form of a deep, red ulceration, which rarely heals and continues to enlarge. If secondary infections occur, pain and fever may appear. Ultimately, in most untreated cases, severe debility develops, ending in death.

LYMPHOGRANULOMA VENEREUM

Lymphogranuloma venereum (Table 20.2) is a sexually acquired infection of the lymph channels and lymph glands near the genital organs. It is known also as lymphogranuloma inguinale, climatic bubo, proadenitis, lymphopathia venereum, and Nicolas-Favre disease. It is relatively common, occurring throughout the world, especially in the tropical and subtropical areas. It is found in the southern part of the United States, especially among the lower socioeconomic groups.

The cause of lymphogranuloma venereum is an extremely small bacterium called *Miyagawanella lymphogranulomatosis*. The organism is so small that it was for many years grouped with the viruses. The primary lesion, an open ulceration, appears on the genital organs from 5 to 21 days after infection has taken place. The lesion is often of such short duration that it escapes notice; thus the first symptoms of the disease may be swollen, hot, tender groups of lymph glands in the inguinal region, appearing from 10 to 30 days after exposure. Fever, chills, headache, and joint pains may also be present. The inflamed lymph nodes frequently fill with pus and drain continuously. In females the initial lesion often is internal or absent, and the first symptoms are enlarged lymph glands that appear near the rectum.

OTHER INFECTIONS OF THE REPRODUCTIVE ORGANS

The reproductive organs are susceptible to several kinds of infection besides the true venereal diseases. The infections are not usually classified as venereal diseases because they are very commonly transmitted through nonsexual means, though each of the infections may also be transmitted through sexual contact.

Candida ("yeast")

One of the most troublesome infections of the sexual organs, and especially of the vagina, is caused by a yeastlike organism called *Candida albicans*; see Fig. 20.8. This organism is a normal inhabitant of the mouth, digestive tract, and vagina of many women, but it is usually held in check by the other organisms present and the body's natural defenses.

Various factors may allow candidiasis, as the infection is called, to erupt into a serious vaginal infection. Among these are antibiotic therapy, which kills the organisms that usually hold *Candida* in check, poor nutrition, and diabetes, which impairs the body's defenses against the infection. Frequently birth-control pills, other hormone therapy, and pregnancy cause severe infections. The changes in hormonal concentrations alter the vaginal environment, favoring the growth of *Candida*. A moist environment favors its growth; spending many hours in a wet swimsuit or in clothing that does not "breathe" freely sometimes leads to severe infections.

In treating vaginal candidiasis (the medical name for *Candida* infection), it is important to take prescribed medications, keep the vaginal area dry, and correct any contributing conditions such as poor nutrition. It is also important that male sex partners use condoms (rubbers) during the periods of infection to avoid "ping-pong" infections (in which the male is infected and later reinfects the female). Males should also be treated at the same time as their female partners.

Trichomonas

Another common vaginitis (inflammation of the vagina) is an infection caused by the protozoan *Trichomonas vaginalis;* see Fig. 20.9. *Trichomonas* lives in the vagina of many women without producing noticeable symptoms. Symptomless infections of the male prostate gland, urethra, and seminal vesicles also are common. Under certain conditions, however, *Trichomonas* can multiply enormously in either the male or female reproductive organs, causing serious infection.

The infection, called trichomoniasis, is common and is transmitted from person to person by contact with vaginal and urethral discharges of infected persons during sexual contact, during the birth process, and possibly by con-

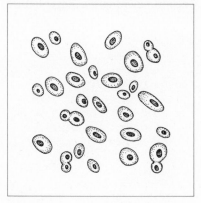

Figure 20.8 *Candida albicans*, a yeastlike organism that causes troublesome vaginal infections. Actual size is microscopic.

tact with infected articles. As with *Candida*, symptomless vaginal infections are often converted to troublesome vaginitis through the modification in the vaginal environment produced by the hormonal changes from birth control pills or pregnancy.

Trichomoniasis can be successfully treated by medically prescribed oral or vaginal medications. The simultaneous treatment of sexual partners is important.

Nonspecific urethritis

Usually nonspecific urethritis in the male is characterized by a milky, cloudy, or watery discharge from the penis. A male often mistakes this discharge for a symptom of gonorrhea. In fact, gonorrhea is another form of urethritis, gonococcal urethritis, and "nonspecific urethritis" means any urethral discharge in males that does not contain gonococci. A urethral discharge may result from an inflammation of the urethra (urethritis), of the prostate gland (prostatitis), or of the seminal vesicles (seminal vesiculitis).

The inflammation may be due to one or more of many conditions, and often the exact cause is never found. Urethritis is related to sexual activity in many ways. *Trichomonas vaginalis* and *Candida albicans*, passed to males from infected females during intercourse, are common causes. Some physicians think that nonspecific urethritis can be an allergic reaction of the male urethra to something normally present in their female sexual partner; this may be so when a female sexual partner has no genital or urinary disease. Urethritis also occurs after overactive or vigorous intercourse.

Genital herpes virus infections

Some of the most troublesome and persistent genital infections are caused by viruses from the *herpes simplex* group. Herpes simplex viruses are apparently carried by most people at all times, though usually in a state of latency (dormancy). They are associated, not only with genital sores, but also with cold sores, fever blisters, eczema, corneal infection, meningitis, encephalitis and possibly, uterine cancer, and other cancers.

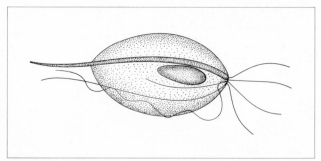

Figure 20.9 *Trichomonas vaginalis*, a microscopic, one-celled animal common in the vagina of women throughout the world.

Most people receive their initial infection with herpes virus during fetal development, across the placental membrane from the mother. Since the antibodies carried by most adults also are transferred across the placenta to the fetus, most infants are protected from infection during the first few months after their birth.

The genital sores in adults may result either from the reactivation of latent herpes infections or from newly acquired viruses transmitted through genital or orogenital sexual contact. The sores may appear on the labia or within the vagina of females or on the penis or within the urethra of males.

A possible, though still unproven, association is that between a herpes simplex virus and cancer of the uterine cervix. A herpes virus is often found within the cancerous cells, but no cause-and-effect relationship has been established. Further discussion of this will be found in Chapter 17.

Pubic lice (crabs)

Pubic lice, commonly called "crab lice" or "crabs," do not cause a venereal disease in the usual sense of the term. They are small insects (1/16 inch) that live as parasites on the body; see Fig. 20.10. They commonly infest pubic hair and the hair under the arms or in eyebrows or beards, but never scalp hair. These lice feed on human blood, causing an intense itching and discoloration of the skin. They often remain attached for days, with their mouth parts

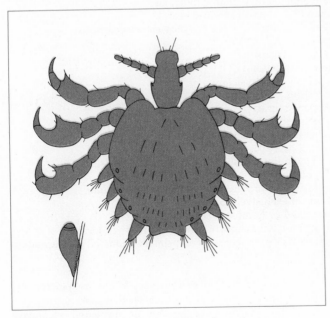

Figure 20.10   Pubic louse (crab louse), and an egg attached to human hair, lower left. Actual size of louse is 1/16 inch.

inserted in the host's skin. Female lice attach eggs—which hatch in 6 to 8 days—to the body hair.

Crab lice are transmitted mainly through sexual intercourse but, unlike the true venereal diseases, they can also be spread through other physical contact with infested persons or infested toilet seats, clothing, blankets, and so forth.

The crabs usually can be killed by washing the affected body parts with a special shampoo, such as Kwell; several applications are required. Infested hair need not be shaved. Exposed clothing need not be thrown away or given special laundering, although it should not be worn for at least two days.

SUMMARY

    I. Five venereal diseases—spread by sexual or close physical contact
       A. Syphilis
       B. Gonorrhea
       C. Chancroid
       D. Granuloma inguinale
       E. Lymphogranuloma venereum
    II. Incidence
       A. Gonorrhea
          1. Most common venereal disease.
          2. Estimated at more than 2,000,000 cases per year.
       B. Syphilis
          1. Physically more serious than gonorrhea.
          2. More than 85,000 new cases per year.
       C. Other venereal diseases—about 2,100 cases per year total.
    III. Prevention and control
       A. Public (social) methods
          1. Interviewing of patients.
          2. Case reporting by physicians.
          3. Cluster testing.
       B. Personal responsibilities
          1. Avoid casual sexual contacts.
          2. Use available prophylactic methods.
    IV. Syphilis
       A. Nonvenereal syphilis: called *endemic syphilis* or *bejel*.
       B. Venereal syphilis
          1. Body-wide disease produced by *Treponema pallidum*.
          2. Spread almost exclusively by:
             a. heterosexual or homosexual contact.
             b. a lip or oral-cavity chancre contracted through kissing.
             c. any close bodily contact with a "primary chancre" or "secondary rash."
          3. Four stages:
             a. primary syphilis—appearance of primary lesion or chancre.
             b. secondary syphilis—appearance of a rash that does not itch.
             c. latent syphilis—begins with healing of untreated secondary lesions; divided into two stages, early latent syphilis (ELS), the infectious stage, which may last for the first two to four years,

and late latent syphilis (LLS), the period after all powers of infection have been lost.

    d. Late syphilis—appearance of manifestations that incapacitate or kill.

C. Syphilis in pregnancy
1. Primary chancre may be mild or absent.
2. Secondary symptoms (rash) usually absent.
3. Spirochetes of syphilis cross the placental membranes into the blood of the child and produce congenital syphilis.

D. Diagnosis of syphilis
1. Microscopic examination of spirochetes from primary chancre or secondary lesions.
2. Blood (serologic) tests—positive results only after a general invasion of the body.

E. Syphilis therapy should:
1. destroy all spirochetes.
2. initiate healing of lesions.
3. prevent further damage to body.
4. prevent spread of disease to others.

V. Gonorrhea
A. Acute venereal disease initiated by *Neisseria gonorrheae.*
B. Male gonorrhea—sensation of burning during urination and a discharge of pus from the penis.
C. Female gonorrhea
1. Initial symptom—a slight vaginal discharge of pus, which may go unnoticed or be mistaken as part of the daily discharge.
2. Women likely to become aware of disease only after months of infection.
D. Carriers—asymptomatic female and male carriers transmit the disease without anyone's realizing it.
E. Diagnosis
1. In male by a microscopic study of discharge of pus from penis.
2. In women usually after complications or because an infected male sexual partner was interviewed by the public health department.
F. Ophthalmia neonatorum—condition causing blindness in newborns.

VI. Chancroid (soft chancre)
A. Localized, raised ulcer with ragged edges and oozing pus.
B. Self-limiting venereal disease induced by the Ducrey bacillus (*Hemophilus ducreyi*).

VII. Granuloma inguinale
A. Chronic venereal disease usually affecting the genital and inguinal lymph nodes of the body.
B. Initiated by a microorganism known as the Donovan body (*Donovania granulomatis*).

VIII. Lymphogranuloma venereum
A. Infection of the lymph glands and channels near the genital organs.
B. A disease caused by an extremely small bacterium named *Miyagawanella lymphogranulomatosis.*

IX. Other infections of the reproductive organs
A. Candidiasis—an infection of the sexual organs of males and females caused by the yeastlike organism *Candida albicans.*
B. Trichomoniasis (trichomonal vaginitis)—caused by the protozoan *Trichomonas vaginalis.*

    C. Nonspecific urethritis—characterized in the male by a milky, cloudy, or watery discharge from the penis that does not contain gonococci.
    D. Genital herpes virus infections
       1. Initial infection occurs during fetal development, across placental membrane.
       2. Genital herpes simplex sores in adults may result from reactivation of latent herpes infections or newly acquired viruses transmitted from person to person.
       3. Uterine cancer as a venereal disease—a possible association between a herpes simplex virus and cancer of the uterine cervix.
    E. Pubic lice (crabs)
       1. Infest the pubic hair and other body hair.
       2. Suck blood, causing intense itching.
       3. Transmitted mainly through sexual intercourse but also through infested toilet seats, etc.

Glossary

If you cannot find the word you wish in this glossary, check the index for text and glossary references.

arsenical (ahr sen′i kəl) (G. *arsen*, strong). A drug containing arsenic.

bismuth (biz′məth) (L. *bismuthum*). A silver-white metal, atomic number 83; its salts have been used for inflammatory diseases of the stomach and intestine and in the treatment of syphilis.

chancre (shang′kər) (L. *cancer*, crablike). The primary lesion of syphilis developing at the site of entrance of the syphilitic organism.

chancroid (shang′kroid). A nonsyphilitic venereal ulcer; also called *soft chancre.*

coma (kō′mə) (G. *koma*, a deep sleep). An abnormal, stuporlike sleep occurring in illness.

congenital (kən jen′i təl) (L. *congenitus*, born together). Existing at, and usually before, birth.

contact (kon′takt) (L. *contactus*, a touching together). In the control of venereal diseases, an individual who is known to have been sufficiently near an infected individual to have been exposed to a disease.

erythromycin (e rith′rō mī′sin) (G. *erythros*, red; *mykes*, fungus). An antibacterial substance produced by *Streptomyces erythreus.*

genital (jen′i təl) (L. *genitalis*, genital). Pertaining to the organs of reproduction.

gonorrhea (gon ə rē′ə) (G. *gone*, seed; *rhein*, to flow). A contagious inflammatory disease of the genitourinary tract, affecting either sex.

granuloma inguinale (gran yə lō′mə ing gwi nal′ē) (L. *granulum*, a little grain; *inguinalis*, in the groin). A venereal disease characterized by deep pus-containing ulcerations of the skin of the genital organs and groin areas.

heterosexual (het′ər ō sek′shoo əl) (G. *hetero*, other; L. *sexus*, sex). One having normal attraction for the opposite sex.

homosexual (hō′mō sek′shoo əl) (G. *homo*, like, same; L. *sexus*, sex). One sexually attracted to another of the same sex.

infectious (in fek′shəs) (L. *inficere*, to stain). Capable of being spread. Infectious disease—any disease caused by the entrance, growth, and multiplication of a disease-causing organism.

jaundice (jawn′dis) (G. *ikteros,* yellow). Condition characterized by yellowness of skin due to deposition of bile pigments.

lesion (lē′zhən) (L. *laedere,* to hurt). Any diseased condition of tissue.

lymphogranuloma venereum (lim′fō gran′yə lō′mə ve nĕr′ē əm) (L. *lympha,* water; *granulum,* a little grain; G. *oma,* a tumor; L. *venereus,* from Venus, the goddess of love). Specific venereal disease affecting chiefly the lymphatic tissues of the iliac and inguinal regions of the body.

paresis (pə rē′sis) (G. *paresis,* weakening). Partial or incomplete paralysis which can result from syphilis.

promiscuous (prə mis′kyoo əs) (L. *pro,* before; *miscere,* to mix). Engaging in indiscriminate, deviant or casual sexual intercourse.

reagin (rē ā′jin) (L. *re,* back, again; *agere,* to act). An antibody associated with many diseases such as syphilis, hay fever, and asthma.

reservoir (rez′ər vwahr) (L. *reservare,* to keep). The nonclinical source of an infection.

self-limiting. A disease that runs a definite limited course.

syphilis (sif′i lis) (from an eighteenth century poem about a shepherd boy named *Syphilis*). An infectious, chronic, venereal disease characterized by lesions which may involve any organ or tissue of the body.

syphilitic meningitis (sif i lit′ik men in jī′tis). Inflammation of the meninges due to a syphilitic infection.

tetracycline (tet′rə sī′klēn) (G. *tetra-,* four; *kyklos,* a circle). A yellow, odorless, crystalline powder, with antibiotic activity against a wide range of organisms.

venereal (və nĕr′ē əl) (L. *Venus,* the goddess of love). Due to or propagated by sexual intercourse.

Wassermann test (Wahs′ər mən) (after A. von Wassermann, 1866–1925, German bacteriologist). A test based on the *reagin* antibody in the serum of syphilitic patients. Used as a test for syphilis.

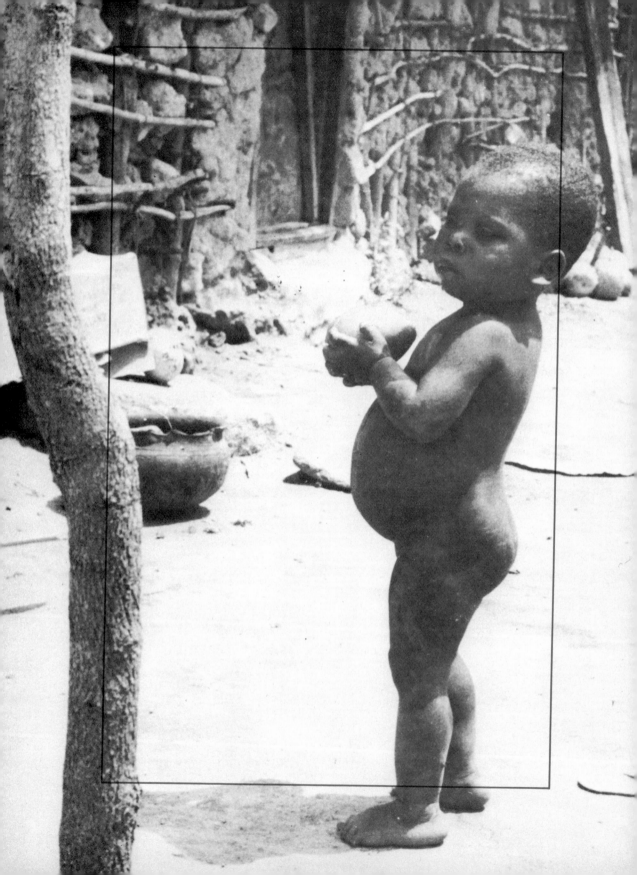

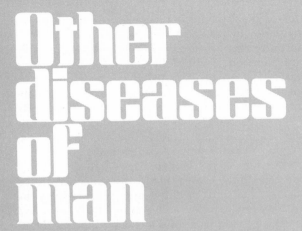

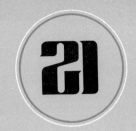

Other diseases of man

This chapter is concerned with some of the multitude of other diseases that afflict mankind, in addition to those previously discussed—emotional ills, heart diseases, cancers, and venereal diseases. Most of the diseases in this chapter are caused by living infectious agents, although some of the occupational diseases are the result of nonliving chemical and physical agents. The diseases have been chosen on the basis of either a high incidence or a great severity. Also discussed briefly is the World Health Organization, which has played an important role in reducing the incidence of many of the diseases discussed.

CHILDHOOD DISEASES

Infant mortality

Many authorities consider the infant mortality, or death, rate to be the best single index of the general health conditions of a given population. Infant deaths are defined as deaths occurring during the first year of life. Not many years ago infant mortality rates of 250 to 300 of every 1,000 babies born were fairly common. Infant mortality is the first vital rate to decline as health conditions in a region improve. Most of the world's countries have been able to reduce their infant death rates to considerably below the earlier figures.

(Unfortunately, the birth rates of many countries have not declined, which has resulted in tremendous population increases and famine.)

Since 1945 the infant mortality rate has declined rapidly throughout the world, owing largely to the introduction of antibiotic and sulfa drugs in the control of communicable diseases. The use of DDT to control malaria-bearing mosquitoes, and the World Health Organization's campaign to control small-pox also have been important factors in reducing infant mortality rates. By 1970 Northern Europe had dipped below 20 deaths per 1,000 births, while many developing nations, such as the United Arabic Republic, Costa Rica, and Mauritius, were still struggling to pull below 83 deaths per 1,000 births.[1]

By 1971 the infant mortality rate in the United States had dropped to 19.2 deaths per 1,000 births. In the United States the deaths are concentrated among the very youngest infants. One third of the deaths occur during the first day of life, another third between one day and one month of age, and the remaining third among those surviving from one to twelve months. Non-white infants die at the rate of 30.2, almost double that of white infants, 16.8.[2]

Because of the nature of their causes, the deaths of neonates (newborns, through the first month) have been more difficult to reduce than those of older infants and children. Of neonate deaths 70 percent are caused by pre-maturity, birth injury, congenital deformities, and lack of oxygen. That the infant death rate *can* be reduced even further is shown by the fact that fifteen other countries currently have a lower rate than the United States does. The steps necessary to reduce the infant death rate include improved prenatal care, especially for low-income mothers, and improved facilities and practices for the care of newborn infants.

Disease conditions

After the first year of life the child faces a completely new set of hazards from his expanding environment. His increased range of locomotion within and outside the home and his natural tendency to climb and investigate sets the stage for accidents. As he progresses, his expansion out of the home and into the neighborhood and school increases his exposure to communicable diseases. This section will deal with the common childhood diseases that predominantly affect the age group 1 through 15.

Appendix A also includes the more common childhood diseases. The appendix explains these diseases, their symptoms, when they may be passed on, the chances of recurrence, available immunizations, and other specific information valuable to a parent. Since this checklist is a very valuable aid to a family, it should be retained as a ready reference.[3]

[1] *The World Population Dilemma*, Population Reference Bureau, Washington, D.C., 1972.

[2] Monthly Vital Statistics, Annual Summary for the United States, U.S. Dept. of Health, Education and Welfare, Washington, D.C., 1971.

[3] Further information about any specific disease can be found in reference books such as *Control of Communicable Diseases in Man* (paperback), published by the American Public Health Association, 1790 Broadway, New York, N.Y., *The Merck Manual*, published by Merck and Company, Rahway, N.J., *Physicians' Desk Reference*, published by the Medical Economics Corporates, Oradell, N.J., and *Diseases of Children* (also in paperback), published by Davis Publications, Inc., 44 Portland St., Worcester, Mass.

Poliomyelitis

Poliomyelitis is a communicable disease caused by one of three types of polio-myelitis viruses. The polio viruses, if they gain entrance into the central nervous system, cause malfunction or death of nerve cells. Commonly, however, they do not enter the central nervous system but cause an infection centering around the digestive tract, where they produce no recognizable signs of destruction. Only in about 1 out of 100 infections do the viruses progress into the central nervous system. Polio infections may occur in several degrees. For convenience of study these are usually grouped into (1) the carrier state, wherein the individual excretes the viruses in his feces and urine with no evidence of a disease, (2) abortive infection, with symptoms of initial polio-myelitis (brief fever, headache, sore throat, mild diarrhea, abdominal pain, nausea, and vomiting) but with no involvement of the nervous system, (3) nonparalytic, similar to the foregoing, except that symptoms may be prolonged over several days, and there is evidence of some nervous-system involvement but no paralysis, and (4) paralytic poliomyelitis, the most severe outcome of the disease, which produces some degree of permanent crippling or involvement of the respiratory mechanisms, which leads to respiratory failure, the usual cause of death in this disease.

The intensive administration of polio vaccines has effected a marked reduction in the incidence of polio in the United States. However, the immunization of every child remains extremely important, because the viruses are still present in this country. Two vaccines are available: one is an *inactivated poliovirus vaccine* (IPV) developed by Jonas Salk, and the other, an *attenuated live oral poliovirus vaccine* (OPV) developed by Albert Sabin.

Inactivated polio vaccine is made from live types I, II, and III poliomyelitis viruses that have been killed and placed in a single vaccine, which is then injected into the individual to be immunized. This was the first immunizer successfully developed.

After much debate the Sabin idea of using unkilled poliomyelitis viruses for purposes of immunization was accepted. Since this was an oral dose, taken with a cube of sugar, it had great appeal to the public. Both IPV and OPV are effective and acceptable, but the oral, live, attenuated poliovirus vaccine has certain advantages such as ease of administration and longer-lasting immunity.

Diphtheria

Diphtheria is induced by the growth of the bacillus *Corynebacterium diphtheriae* on skin or mucous-membrane surfaces. The growth produces a drainage of pus cells and fibrin (an insoluble protein formed in a clotting process). The fibrin coagulates into a pseudomembrane, which seems to grow across the infected body surface. This membrane is at first grayish-white but later becomes a dirty gray, and forcible removal of it results in its spreading in all directions. The most frequent locations of the infection and the membrane are in the throat (particularly on the tonsils), nose, larynx, and trachea, sometimes on the skin.

Diphtheria produces a toxin that has severe destructive effects locally and systemically. The toxin causes degeneration and death of tissue; degeneration of the heart muscle (myocarditis) is one of the most serious effects. Diphtheria toxin also causes degeneration of nerves, producing paralysis, malfunctions of organs, and respiratory involvement, which may result in death.

Transfer from an infected to a noninfected individual may occur by many means, since the organism survives for hours and even days outside the body. The diphtheria bacillus will grow in milk very well without appreciably changing its flavor or appearance. Unpasteurized milk has been the occasional source of diphtheria outbreaks.

The toxoid that prevents diphtheria has been available since 1935, yet diphtheria is still found in all large communities because of the apathy of parents about having their children immunized. Although it occurs to some degree in all seasons, it increases in winter, sometimes to the extent of an epidemic, and declines in late spring. Diphtheria occurs at all ages but has the greatest frequency in children between 1 and 14 years of age. All children should be protected prior to their first birthday.

Although a single injection of toxoid may give satisfactory immunity, three or four smaller injections a month apart each give more reliable protection and fewer unpleasant reactions. The time required to produce immunity varies from two weeks to six months; most children are immune within two months. Even among those vaccinated it is desirable to verify the presence of immunity by means of a Schick test, which consists of injecting into the skin a small amount of toxin. A *positive*, or *nonimmune*, reaction consists of redness, swelling, and tenderness around the area of the injection, the reaction reaching its maximum usually within a few days after the injection. If there is no reaction, the individual has obtained immunity from diphtheria. Booster injections of toxoid are usually necessary to maintain immunity into adulthood.

Diphtheria toxoid is sometimes efficiently used in combination with other disease antigens. Commonly today the combination of diphtheria toxoid, tetanus toxoid, and whooping cough (pertussis) vaccine, called DPT, is used for young children.

Whooping cough (pertussis)

Whooping cough is caused by the bacillus *Bordetella pertussis*. It commonly occurs in children under 6 years of age and rarely in those over 10. Very young infants are susceptible, for immunity is not transmitted across the placenta. One attack may be expected to confer lifelong immunity, although it does not do so in all instances, second attacks of the disease occasionally occurring.

The typical stage of severe cough, called a *paroxysm*, consists of a series of explosive coughs rapidly repeated on a single expiration with no time for a breath between them. When the breath is expired to such an extent that no more coughing is possible, there is a rapid intake of air, and the coughing continues. Each inspiration during the paroxysm is accompanied by a peculiar crowing sound or "whoop." The course of the disease is from six weeks to several months.

There is no natural immunity to whooping cough, and 70 percent of the deaths from this disease occur before the age of 1 year. Consequently, the infant is desperately in need of vaccine protection as soon as possible. In unprotected children whooping cough can have serious consequences: coughing can rupture lungs, permanently enlarge the bronchial tube, or even burst small blood vessels in the brain.

Immunization of infants against whooping cough is usually given in combination with diphtheria and tetanus toxoids (DPT). Three injections are given at intervals of four to eight weeks starting at 3 or 4 months of age. Single reinforcing injections should be given one year later and again before the child enters school.

Measles (rubeola)

Measles is a highly communicable disease induced by the rubeola virus. The disease is manifested by symptoms of a cold, bronchitis, fever, and *Koplik's spots*—bluish-white, pinpointed, surrounded by a red, circular area on the mucous membranes of the mouth—which are important in the early diagnosis of measles before the rash appears on the skin. Following the spots, a rash consisting of small dark-red papules, which increase in size and grow together, produces the appearance characteristic of measles.

During the active stage of the disease the measles virus is present in the nose, the mouth, the throat, and the eyes. It is spread through contamination of the discharges of these areas from an infected person. It is communicable from the beginning of the respiratory symptoms, before the appearance of the rash, and slowly diminishes in communicability as the respiratory symptoms disappear.

Measles occurs chiefly in the late winter and the early spring. Infants under 6 months of age usually do not become infected with measles because of acquired congenital immunity from the mother. After about 6 months the child's susceptibility at any age is very great, but the disease is most often contracted between 2 and 8 years of age. One attack usually protects permanently against a second attack.

Until 1963 there was no way to avoid measles. Indeed, it was considered by most to be one of the hazards of growing up. Overlooked was the fact that measles may have many side effects. Before the introduction of the measles vaccines, which have proven to be some of the most effective vaccines ever developed, an average of 4 million children per year suffered from measles. Of infected children, 1 in every 15 will suffer serious side effects from middle-ear infections, which may cause lifelong deafness, pneumonia, and encephalitis, which is a brain inflammation that will send many children to mental institutions for the rest of their lives. One in each 1,000 infected children, according to the American Medical Association, dies of complications from this "hazard of growing up."

Measles vaccine should be given to infants at or soon after 12 months of age. Congenital immunity will protect them for a few months after birth; in fact, early injections of vaccine may be inactivated by congenital immunity.

Two types of measles vaccine have been developed—live, attenuated virus vaccine and inactivated virus vaccine. The live, attenuated measles vaccine is recommended by the majority of physicians. With this vaccine a single dose induces active immunity by producing a mild measles infection.

German measles (rubella)

German measles, or "three-day measles" is a contagious virus disease characterized chiefly by a skin eruption and mild associated symptoms. The disease itself is relatively unimportant because of the slight incapacity produced. It does not commonly occur in the first 6 months but usually is found in the age group 2 to 15. The immunity produced by the disease is permanent; recurrences are rare.

The only complications of importance are congenital malformations of a fetus when the mother develops German measles. If a pregnant woman develops German measles during the first six months of pregnancy, the fetus may develop congenital cataracts, deafness, or malformities of the heart, spinal cord, or extremities. It was previously believed that this damage was limited to the first three months of pregnancy, but studies of infants born after the 1965 German-measles epidemic showed that many infants had been deformed as a result of German measles having been contracted by the mother during the second three months of her pregnancy.

In 1969 a highly effective vaccine against German measles was released for public immunization. In the United States this vaccine is recommended principally for the immunization of children, since its safety for use during pregnancy has not been established. It is believed that through immunizing the majority of school-age children the chances that a child will bring the German measles virus home to his pregnant mother can be minimized.

As explained in Chapter 11, many physicians believe that a mother's having German measles in the first months of pregnancy is reasonable grounds for a therapeutic abortion. This is now legal, although it was not during the 1965 epidemic.

Roseola (baby measles)

Roseola is a communicable disease of infancy and early childhood. The causative agent has not been identified, but it probably is a virus. Roseola is also known as *roseola infantum* and *exanthema subitum*.

The disease occurs predominantly in infants, nearly always in those under 3 years of age; a few cases in older children have been reported. The onset is abrupt, with a fever which rises to between 102 and 105° F in a few hours and continues for approximately four days, with some morning remissions. When the fever ends, the characteristic eruption appears; then the child seems to be as well as ever. No isolation is required, because the communicability of the disease seems to disappear by the time the rash appears and the diagnosis is made. There are no known complications, but the disease is often confused with measles or scarlet fever.

Chickenpox

Chickenpox is a highly communicable disease produced by the varicella virus. The chief feature is a generalized breaking-out of a characteristic mature lesion, which is a small blister filled with clear fluid and surrounded by a red area. This vesicle dries gradually, becoming depressed at the center; later a flat crust forms. The crust falls off in one to three weeks. The period of communicability is from about one day prior to the breaking-out to when the vesicles dry up. Since infectivity precedes the onset of symptoms, little is gained by the isolation of patients, but they should be kept out of school for about one week after the appearance of the rash.

The disease is usually induced at the first exposure after 6 months of age. It is most frequent between 2 and 8 years of age. The principal serious complications, which are rare, are encephalitis and pneumonia.

The chief public-health importance of chickenpox lies in its possible confusion with smallpox. The virus also seems identical with the virus that causes *herpes zoster*, also known as *shingles*, an inflammation of certain nerve ganglia, which produces small vesicles on the skin in the areas supplied by the infected nerves. The differences in response to the same virus seem to depend in some way upon localization of the virus and its persistence in the tissues.

Mumps

Mumps is an acute virus disease that chiefly affects the salivary glands, especially the parotid salivary glands. The swelling of these glands appears abruptly and slowly subsides over one or two weeks. The disease produces moderate symptoms of fever, headache, and vomiting, which precede the swelling by one or two days. The swelling causes pain in the back and the neck when the victim opens his mouth.

The infectious process of mumps may affect not only the salivary glands but also the pancreas, testes, and ovaries, as well as the central nervous system and other organs. Symptoms of extension to other glands and structures usually develop from four to seven days after the onset of the swelling of the salivary glands, when this swelling is beginning to subside. Such extensions most often occur in males 15 to 25 years old. An affected testis may shrink to some extent and lose its ability to produce sperm, but complete sterility seldom is produced, since both testes are rarely involved. The analogous infection of the ovaries in mature females is much less frequent, but it does occur.

The largest number of children are attacked by mumps in the early school years, owing to their greater opportunity for exposure at this time. The age distribution of mumps is somewhat older than that for the other childhood diseases, and it is not unusual for individuals to escape infection until young adult life. Contracting of mumps in adult life is dangerous because of the greater risk of infectious extension at this time. Immunity is generally lifelong, but a second attack is reported frequently.

The early forms of mumps vaccine were not generally recommended, because their protection was of limited duration and could have merely delayed mumps infection until the adult years. But the currently available mumps vaccine is believed to offer lifetime immunity and is now highly recommended for the routine immunization of all children and any young adults who have not yet had mumps.

Hemolytic streptococci

The streptococci are a large group of bacteria which have in common the properties of roundness and the ability to form chains during the process of reproduction; see Fig. 21.1. These organisms are of great importance in human disease, particularly in childhood diseases.

The streptococci that are of major importance in disease produce *hemolysis*, the separation of hemoglobin from red blood cells, with the destruction of the red cell. The hemolytic streptococci have been subdivided into about a dozen groups (Groups A, B, C, etc.). Only the ones in Group A are important in human disease.

There are approximately forty-six types of Group A hemolytic streptococcal bacterium; they cause a wide variety of diseases, which are usually differentiated according to (1) portal of entry, (2) the tissue in which the infectious agent is localized, and (3) the presence of a scarlatinal rash. The more

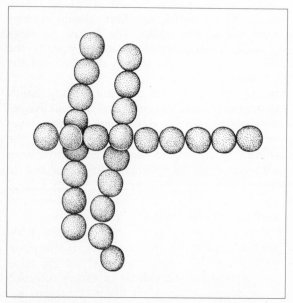

Figure 21.1   Streptococci. Members of this group of bacteria are responsible for scarlet fever, rheumatic fever, strep throats, and other infections.

important conditions are *scarlet fever* and *streptococcal sore throat* (streptococcal tonsillitis, streptococcal pharyngitis). Rheumatic fever also is caused by this group of bacteria.

Scarlet fever (scarlatina) and streptococcal sore throat   Scarlet fever is a streptococcal sore throat in which the infectious organism is capable of producing a toxin which in turn produces the characteristic scarlet-fever rash. If the patient is immune to the toxin, there will be no rash or scarlet fever, but a streptococcal sore throat will result.

Scarlet fever rarely occurs in the first year of a child's life. Most commonly it occurs between 5 and 8 years of age, after which it decreases in incidence. It occurs chiefly in the fall and winter months, rarely in summer.

The onset of scarlet fever is sudden, with sore throat, vomiting, and fever. The child's temperature remains elevated continuously for several days and then gradually declines, reaching normal in from 10 to 14 days after the onset. Great variations in the severity of scarlet fever have been observed. In one instance the disease may be so mild that it is difficult to recognize it; in another, so severe that the child dies in a few days, sometimes before a rash appears. There are also many complications from the high fever, the toxins, and the streptococcal bacteria. In general, scarlet fever is less severe today than it was in former years; few deaths now result directly from its effects.

The isolation period should be based on the persistence of streptococci in the throat. In uncomplicated cases transmission is possible mainly during the incubation and fever stage of the disease, which is approximately ten days; adequate treatment with penicillin will eliminate, within 24 hours, the ability to transmit the disease, although the streptococci may still be present much longer. With the occurrence of complications the child remains a source of infection for months or even years.

The toxin which produces the rash in scarlet fever is *erythrogenic* (rash-producing); it is sometimes called Dick toxin. Consequently, a small amount of it may be injected under the skin and, if a small local rash occurs, the result is positive, and the person is susceptible to scarlet fever. This test gives information only on the susceptibility to the rash and associated scarlet fever; it does not indicate the person's susceptibility to streptococcal infections in general.

Rheumatic fever   Rheumatic fever is a systemic disease that causes characteristic involvement of many organs and tissues. The most important effects of rheumatic fever are on the heart (see Chapter 16). Other common characteristics are joint pains, various skin eruptions, and chorea (St. Vitus' dance), a convulsive nervous condition.

The primary underlying factor in rheumatic fever is infection in the throat with a Group A hemolytic streptococcus. Continued infection or repeated reinfection by these organisms causes the body to become sensitized. After sensitization repeated infection leads to allergic response, the response varying in nature and degree according to the degree of sensitization. Before sensitization the throat infection has no systemic effects. All or any one of these streptococcal infections may be inevident or unrecognized before the onset of rheumatic fever.

Because of the process needed to produce this disease it is rare in the first years of life—not because infections are uncommon, but because the development of the allergy requires time. The incidence increases from about 5 years of age to between 7 and 10 and then declines. The disease is most prevalent in the temperate zones of the world and in those seasons of the year during which respiratory infections are most frequent. Rheumatic fever has a high family incidence, occurs more frequently in lower socioeconomic groups, and is affected by environment, living conditions, and nutrition.

Unlike many other communicable diseases, rheumatic fever carries with it the threat of future additional heart damage or other complications. Consequently, an individual who has it must maintain a high degree of vigilance for the greater part of his life. Prophylactic doses of antibiotics should be taken before any type of medical or dental work is performed upon him; otherwise he may become contaminated with streptococcal organisms. Colds, influenza, and sore throats are also constant threats of reinfection.

Immunizations

Disease prevention through immunization may be achieved in two ways. *Active immunity* is produced through the injection of weakened or killed antigens, which stimulate the body to produce antibodies against a specific disease (see Chapter 19). This method is used before a person is exposed to the disease in question, in order to impart long-lasting protection against that disease. *Passive immunity* is achieved through the injection of antibodies that have already been produced by some other animal or person. This is strictly an emergency procedure useful when a person has already been exposed to a disease. The immunity thus obtained is of relatively short duration, since no natural production of antibodies occurs, but it is very useful in certain situations.

Schedules of immunizations

Immunization should be started at the proper age. Since some infants will have limited immunity response, the recommended booster doses are intended to ensure or maintain immunity. The current practice is to begin active immunization during the second month of life with a triple vaccine (DPT injection) and a concurrent oral polio vaccine (OPV, or Sabin vaccine). These four immunizations should be given in a series, and a routine for recall, or booster, injections throughout life is recommended also; see Appendix C.

Unfortunately, deaths from whooping cough still occur among infants from birth up to 2 months of age, which is about the earliest date DPT injections can be safely started. Consequently, the best protection for the very young infant is to be sure all older children are properly immunized.

Recall, or booster injections

Recall, or booster, injections give very rapid reincreases in antibody level, in contrast with the slow increases during and after the initial series. The first recall injection after the initial series is of such great importance that it may be considered part of the basic immunizations.

When children up to 6 years of age who have received DPT as infants are exposed to whooping cough, booster injections of whooping cough vaccine should be given. Administration of booster doses of diphtheria toxoid, poliomyelitis, or smallpox vaccine is to be given according to the standard schedule at any age.

Immunization history   Because of the constant movement of families, each family should take it upon itself to originate and maintain an immunization record for each child. This will serve as a reference in an emergency situation and also as a means of keeping all immunizations up to date. Physicians' records of individual immunizations may not always be forwarded when a family changes doctors or moves to another locality. Consequently, the establishment of a personal health record, such as that in Appendix C, will prove to be a valuable tool.

Precautions in immunizations   Under some conditions immunizations should be delayed. Injections should be postponed when a person has an acute respiratory infection. Children with eczema or other acute dermatitis ordinarily should not be vaccinated against smallpox because of the risk of generalized vaccinia (cowpox infection).

The initial vaccination against smallpox and poliomyelitis preferably should be done in cool weather, during the latter half of the year. An interval of a month or more is desirable between doses of live virus antigens such as smallpox, measles, and poliomyelitis.

Isolation and quarantine

A child who is suspected of having a contagious disease should be separated from others until a diagnosis can be made. One who has the disease should be isolated until the danger of transmitting it to others no longer exists.

There is a distinction between isolation and quarantine. Quarantine consists of compulsory stoppage of travel or movement from, or into, the place of confinement. A ship coming into port is held in quarantine until the port health officer is satisfied, through inspection, that communicable disease is not present; passengers and crew are confined to the ship, and no visitors are permitted. Such a strict quarantine is employed in homes for very few diseases. Home quarantine is of less value than port quarantine, since it is seldom strictly enforced. In the case of diphtheria, the members of the household commonly are quarantined until they are shown not to be carriers. For certain other diseases, such as whooping cough, measles, chickenpox, mumps, and scarlet fever, exposed children are merely excluded from school.

Isolation is the separation from contact with others of patients having a contagious disease. An appropriate period of isolation depends on the duration of communicability of the disease (Appendix A). For some diseases, this period is determined by the presence or absence of the causative agents. Statistical studies have shown that after a certain time has elapsed, a child no longer transmits a disease to susceptible persons. By means of such observations suitable isolation periods have been established for each disease.

DISEASES OF ANY AGE GROUP

The common cold

The common cold stands today as the most common infectious disease in the United States and probably in the entire world. No other infectious disease causes as much absenteeism from work and school, personal inconvenience, and discomfort. Yet the cold remains the least preventable and treatable of infectious diseases.

It is believed that fifty or so different viruses can cause the symptoms known as "the common cold"—sore throat, stuffy and runny nose, sneezing, coughing, and watery eyes. The first symptoms usually include a scratchy feeling in the throat, a chilly feeling at a normally comfortable temperature, and a fatigued feeling. A high fever is *not* a normal symptom of a cold; when it accompanies cold symptoms, a physician should be consulted, as it may indicate a dangerous secondary infection.

Colds are "caught" by transfer of the virus from the nose and mouth discharges of an infected person. This transfer may be through direct contact, through droplets released in sneezing, coughing, or talking, or indirectly through contact with eating utensils or other articles contaminated by an infected person. Colds often seem to arise quickly after chilling or rapid cooling off after overheating. Such environmental factors may act by causing changes in the mucous membranes, which allow invasion by viruses already present. Colds are most contagious during their early stages, especially the first day. No transmission occurs beyond five days after the onset of symptoms. In fact, any cold symptoms remaining after five days are usually not the result of the original cold virus but of secondary bacterial infection of the virus-damaged mucous membranes.

Prevention   Unfortunately, no suggestions can be given that will guarantee the prevention of the common cold. Even if all reasonable precautions were taken, the average person could expect at least one cold a year and possibly two or three. It is only common sense, however, to take certain precautions such as avoiding unnecessary contact with people having colds, maintaining general good health through adequate rest and nutrition, and dressing for the weather—neither too much clothing nor too little. No effective immunization against colds has been developed so far, probably because of the number of viruses that can cause colds, the high incidence of mutations among these viruses, and the slight degree of active immunity, if any, which results from actually having a cold.

Treatment   Despite the introduction each year of "miraculous" nonprescription cold remedies, there is still no specific cure for the common cold. The apparent effectiveness of the cold remedies stems from their psychological effect and from the fact that many colds terminate spontaneously while still in the early stages. Most of the folk remedies (they are too numerous to list) prove worthless upon scientific investigation.

Although we commonly speak of "fighting a cold," the best advice to the person with an early cold is "don't fight it." The best treatment for a cold is still to stay in bed during the early stages. Aspirin often helps relieve some of the discomfort at this time. The result of "fighting" a cold is often severe secondary bacterial infection, especially of the ear or sinuses. The symptoms of these secondary infections may linger for weeks. Though antibiotics are useless against the virus stage of a cold, they may be necessary to clear up the secondary bacterial infections.

Influenza

The word *influenza*, "flu," is commonly applied to many conditions as well as to the actual disease. Virus infections of many types and even bacterial intestinal infections are sometimes incorrectly called "flu." The true influenza is a virus infection of the respiratory tract characterized by very rapid onset of fever, chills, headache, muscular aches, and severe coughing; see Fig. 21.2. Marked prostration is typical, and after several days the symptoms may resemble those of a cold. Recovery usually occurs in two to seven days. Influenza often occurs in massive epidemics, sometimes sweeping over the entire world. The importance of influenza lies in the great numbers of people disabled at the same time—so many that the functioning of the community is disrupted. Uncomplicated influenza rarely leads to the death of an otherwise healthy person, but the death rate always rises during epidemics. A recent epidemic in the

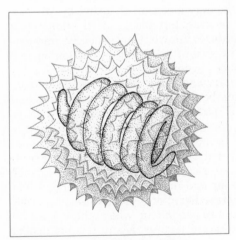

Figure 21.2 Influenza virus. Many strains of viruses produce influenza-type diseases.

United States resulted in 57,000 deaths in excess of the normal death rate, mostly of elderly persons or those already suffering from some chronic disease. In such persons influenza often leads to bacterial pneumonia, which is the actual cause of death.

Many types and strains of viruses have been associated with influenza. The types are called A, B, and C. Types A and B are the most common; several strains of each type have been isolated. The Asian influenza virus is one of the type A viruses. Influenza is transmitted through virus contained in the discharges from the nose and mouth of infected persons.

The best prevention of influenza is vaccination, followed by annual booster vaccinations. Vaccination is especially important for older persons, pregnant women, persons with chronic diseases, persons who have much public contact, and persons engaged in essential community services.

Tetanus (lockjaw)

Tetanus (lockjaw) is a disease resulting from an exotoxin produced by the bacterium *Clostridium tetani*. This bacillus is commonly found in the soil and fecal discharges of man and animals.

The organism is harmless when growing in the digestive tract but, when introduced into the body by way of a wound, it is able to grow and induce the disease tetanus. Its growth in a wound produces no local tissue damage and no characteristic lesion, but it does produce the exotoxin. This exotoxin has a special affinity for nervous tissue, finds its way into the central nervous system, and induces the characteristic signs and symptoms of tetanus. The effects of the toxin are shown by an early difficulty in opening the mouth (lockjaw), convulsions, spasms in the back muscles, and later a rigid neck. One half to two thirds of the victims die.

Tetanus is not contagious nor transmissible directly from one person to another. Contamination of a wound is the only means of inducing the disease. There is no natural immunity against tetanus, but the artificial immunizing process is one of the most effective procedures known. Consequently, immunization of all children and adults, with the goal of providing protection against tetanus for the entire population, should be encouraged.

The duration of immunity is temporary and varies from person to person. However, it is recommended that routine booster injections of tetanus toxoid be administered with diphtheria (adult TD) booster every ten years.

The spores of the tetanus bacillus are highly resistant; they may survive in nature for years. Tetanus bacilli are found in the intestinal tract of many animals, even occasionally in man, and that accounts for their abundance in the soil, especially if it has been manured. Because of their great abundance and small size, spores are blown in the air and may settle in household dust or street grime or on a sharp object, a refuse heap, or a great variety of other objects. Burns, compound fractures, or *any wound* in which there may be soil or dust contamination is likely to produce tetanus. Many tetanus deaths occur among auto accident victims who are not immunized. Cases of tetanus in women are on an increase because of the greater activity of women in outdoor sports.

Nonimmunized individuals may be prevented from developing tetanus by an injection of an antitoxin as soon as possible after an injury. A decision about which wounds require antitoxin is sometimes difficult to make; in case of doubt the antitoxin should always be given. The antitoxin is prepared in horses; the fluid portion is the serum of the blood of the horse. Unfortunately, horse serum often causes violent and, at times, deadly allergic reactions. Consequently, an individual should always be tested for his sensitivity to horse serum before the antitoxin is given. A *human donor blood* antitoxin is now available that reduces the effect of reactions; unfortunately, this human serum is more expensive. In the long run an initial series of tetanus injections and *routine boosters* provide the easiest and cheapest means of tetanus protection.

Infectious hepatitis

Infectious hepatitis is a virus infection of the liver, which leads to symptoms that include fever, loss of appetite, nausea, and general ill feeling; it may be followed later by jaundice (yellowing of the skin). Infectious hepatitis is more severe in adults than in children but is rarely fatal. Many cases in children are probably not diagnosed, owing to the mildness of the symptoms. Severe cases in adults are often followed by a long convalescent period. This disease is of worldwide occurrence.

The sources of infection are the feces, urine, blood and, probably, the nose and throat discharges of infected persons. Transmission is through close personal contact, blood transfusions, or contaminated needles used for injections. Epidemics have been traced to sewage contamination of water, milk, or food, especially raw oysters and clams.

A similar disease, serum hepatitis, is characterized by the same symptoms but is transmissible only through blood or blood products (including contaminated injection needles). The incubation perod of serum hepatitis is usually 80 to 100 days, that of infectious hepatitis is about 25 days. Apparently two different viruses are involved.

The preventive measures for infectious hepatitis will also provide protection against serum hepatitis. Good personal hygiene and sanitary sewage disposal are important in the prevention of infectious hepatitis. Careful selection of blood donors and thorough sterilization of syringes, needles, and finger-puncture stylets is important in the prevention of either type. Skin-tattooing instruments are often responsible for hepatitis transmission, as are the injection needles and instruments of drug abusers. Exposed persons can be temporarily protected from infection through the use of gamma globulin.

Infectious mononucleosis

Infectious mononucleosis is a viral infection centering in the lymph glands and characterized by sore throat, fever, and swelling of the lymph glands. The white blood cell count rises markedly, especially the count of the large monocytes. The disease is rarely fatal, but it often results in a general weakness lasting from a few weeks to several months. In children the disease is generally mild and difficult to recognize. The most severe cases usually occur in young adults. Infectious mononucleosis is worldwide in distribution, occurring most commonly in college students and military personnel.

Infectious mononucleosis is believed to be transmitted through contact with the respiratory discharges of infected persons. Infected people may continue to shed the virus, transmitting the disease for up to 16 months after their symptoms disappear. Since kissing is one good method of transmission, and since the disease is rather common on college campuses, it is sometimes called the "kissing disease." No preventive methods are known.

Bacterial meningitis

Bacterial meningitis is an infection of the meninges (membranes covering the brain and spinal cord) by the meningococcus *Neisseria meningitidis*. The symptoms include a sudden onset of fever, intense headache, nausea, and often a rash. Delirium and coma often follow. The previous fatality rate of 40 to 50 percent has been reduced to about 5 percent through antibiotic therapy.

Meningitis is of worldwide occurrence. Sporadic cases are reported throughout the year, epidemic waves starting every seven to eleven years and lasting two to three years. Meningitis reaches its highest incidence among military personnel and other persons living under crowded conditions, such as in barracks and institutions.

A high degree of natural resistance exists among the general population, such that many exposed persons become *symptomless carriers*. During nonepidemic periods it is estimated that from 10 to 25 percent of the population are healthy carriers; during epidemics more than half of the members of a military command may become carriers. Symptomless carriers are important as sources of infection, since their nose and throat discharges carry the bacteria. Transmission of the disease requires direct or fairly close contact, since the meningococcus (like the closely related gonococcus) is rapidly killed through chilling or drying.

Preventive measures include avoiding direct contact and droplet infection and prevention of overcrowding in living quarters, working places, and public transportation. During epidemics mass treatment with protective drugs is sometimes used to reduce the incidence, but drug-resistant strains of meningococcus are reducing the effectiveness of such treatment.

Staphylococcal infections

The many strains of *Staphylococcus aureus* are among the most widespread and common bacteria infecting man; see Fig. 21.3. The staphylococci produce a great variety of infections ranging from tiny skin pustules to massive blood-borne infections of the entire body, leading to death. Staphylococcal ("staph") infections are usually characterized by the formation of pus and abscesses (pus-filled cavities). The infective ability of each strain of staph depends upon the type and quantity of enzymes and toxins it produces. The known strains range from the nonpathogenic to the highly virulent.

Some commonly occurring staphylococcal infections of the skin are *boils, abscesses, carbuncles, impetigo,* and *infected cuts and abrasions.* In more severe cases the bacteria may infect the lungs or be carried by the blood to infect the bones, joints, inner lining of the heart, or even the brain.

Staphylococcal infections are a major problem in hospitals, especially in nurseries and surgical sections. If a pathogenic strain is introduced into the hospital nursery, it may spread rapidly through the highly susceptible population. Most infants suffer only skin infections, but more serious infections sometimes occur. Staphylococcal infection following operations has increased in importance as surgical procedures have become more complex and the patients more elderly. The patient who has a chronic illness is often highly susceptible to staph infection.

Hospital-acquired staph infections are often introduced into the home, where infections may alternate between members of the family for many months. Newborn infants are more likely to bring home such infections than are adults. A major obstacle in treating hospital-acquired staph infections is their high degree of resistance to drugs. More than 90 percent of such infections involve strains of bacteria that are resistant to penicillin or other commonly used antibiotics.

The most important source of infectious staphylococci is the pus and other discharges from staph infections. Transmission may be direct or through contact with contaminated articles. Potentially dangerous staph organisms can be found almost everywhere, since 30 to 40 percent of all healthy persons carry pathogenic staphylococci in their nasal cavities. Such persons may infect themselves or others.

Preventive measures applicable in the home include strict personal cleanliness (soap and water), avoidance of shared use of towels or other toilet articles, prompt treatment of any infections that appear, and careful disposal of dressings or other objects contaminated with discharges from infections.

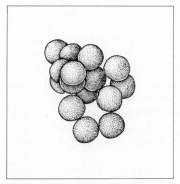

Figure 21.3   Staphylococci. Strains of staph cause many common infections such as boils, abscesses, impetigo, and wound infections.

Hospitals should strictly enforce rules (too numerous to elaborate here) designed to reduce the danger of infection, and patients and visitors should respect and follow these rules. Certain highly potent antibiotics should be reserved for use only for resistant staphylococcal infections, as their widespread use would hasten the development of staph strains resistant even to these drugs.

DISEASES OF WORLDWIDE IMPORTANCE

Trachoma

Trachoma is a chronic infection of the eyes, which, because of its serious threat to vision, is the world's most important eye infection; see Fig. 21.4. Trachoma is worldwide in occurrence. High prevalence is usually associated with poverty, poor sanitation, and crowded living conditions, especially in dry, dusty areas. In the United States today the disease remains a problem only among North American Indians and Mexican immigrants in the Southwest.

Trachoma is caused by unusually small, intracellular bacteria called *Chlamydia trachomatis*, which are spread through the eye discharges of infected persons. The disease produces extreme inflammation of the eye, with deformity of the eyelids and damage to the cornea, leading to visual disability and blindness. In some parts of the world 5 percent of the population are blind or near-blind as the result of trachoma.

The prevention of blindness includes the finding and prompt treatment of all infected persons; see Fig. 21.5. In addition, improved basic sanitation is required, including the use of soap, water, and clean personal towels and other toilet articles. Children should be taught always to wash their hands before touching their faces.

Malaria

Although great strides have been made in the control of malaria in many countries, including the United States, it is still a major problem in many tropical and subtropical areas, such as parts of Africa, Asia, Central and South America, and the Southwest Pacific. Malaria is the result of infection by protozoa (several species of *Plasmodium*), which are transmitted from man to man only by certain species of *Anopheles* mosquitoes; see Fig. 21.6. The mosquitoes are common almost everywhere in the world. No direct man-to-man transmission is possible, except through blood transfusions or contaminated hypodermic needles.

An untreated case of malaria may last for years and is characterized by repeated cyclic attacks. Each attack is usually accompanied by weakness, chills, fever, headache, nausea, and profuse sweating. Long-term results include anemia and general weakness, with as much as a 10 percent fatality rate. However, fatalities are rare in treated cases. Many effective drugs are available for treatment, but the development, by some strains of *Plasmodium*,

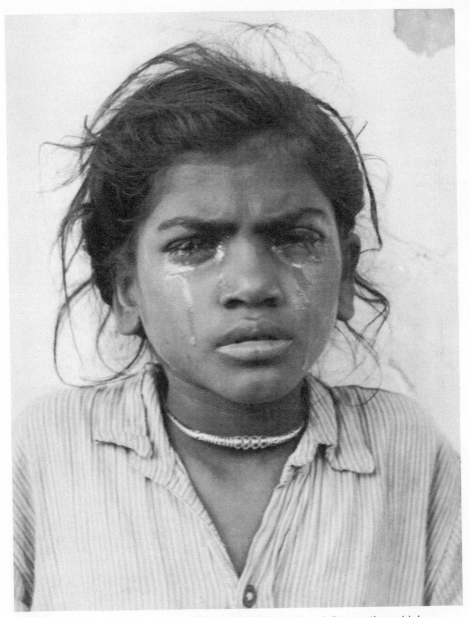

Figure 21.4   Untreated trachoma. The eyes show serious inflammation which, if untreated, may lead to permanent blindness. (From *World Health, the Magazine of the World Health Organization*.)

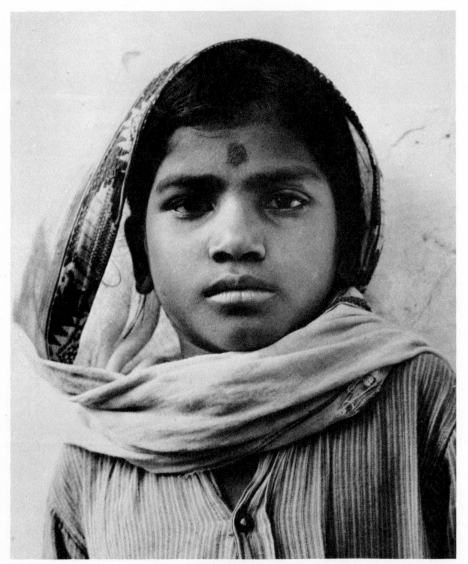

Figure 21.5   Treated trachoma. The eyesight of this child has been saved by prompt treatment with antibiotics. (From *World Health, the Magazine of the World Health Organization.*)

of resistance to the newer antimalarial drugs has forced a return to the older drug, quinine, in treating some cases of malaria.

The prevention of malaria is primarily through mosquito suppression, including elimination of breeding places, chemical control of larvae and adult mosquitoes, screening of houses, and use of repellents; see Fig. 21.7. In certain situations antimalarial drugs are used as a preventive measure.

Yaws

Yaws, also known as *frambesia,* is a tropical disease, particularly common in equatorial Africa, the Philippines, Southeast Asa, Indonesia, and throughout the South Pacific islands. Yaws is usually contracted during childhood; an untreated case lasts for many years. The infective agent of yaws is a spirochete very similar to that of syphilis. Although a nonvenereal disease, yaws is in some ways similar to syphilis. Infection occurs through direct contact with the skin of an infected person. About a month after contact a lump called a "mother yaw" appears at the point of infection. Within a few weeks or months mild, generalized lesions develop over the skin and bones. Successive crops of such lesions occur for several months or years. After five or ten years the late stage occurs, with permanently destructive lesions of the skin and bones, resulting in crippling and disfiguration. Unlike

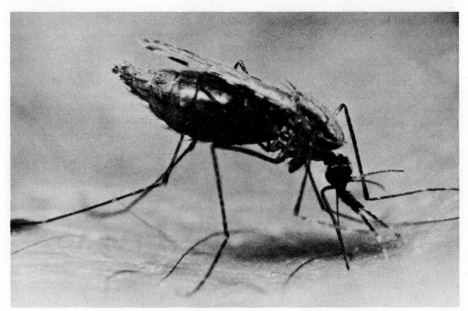

Figure 21.6 *Anopheles* mosquito. This mosquito, shown puncturing the skin of a person, is of a malaria-transmitting species. (From *World Health, the Magazine of the World Health Organization.*)

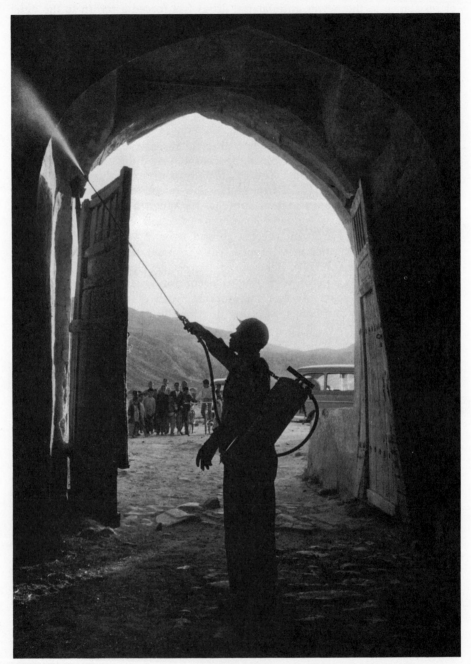

Figure 21.7 Malaria control. A mosquito-spraying operation in Persia for the control of malaria-transmitting mosquitoes. (From *World Health, the Magazine of the World Health Organization.*)

syphilis, the central nervous system and other vital organs are not involved, and there is no congenital transmission. Yaws is not usually fatal.

The most successful approach to the control of yaws has been through mass treatment of all persons in heavily infected communities and selective treatment of infected persons and their contacts in less heavily infected localities. A single injection of long-acting penicillin can cure yaws. Also important in prevention of yaws are improved sanitation and social and economic conditions.

Tuberculosis

Historically tuberculosis has been a major cause of death in most of the countries of the world. For many years tuberculosis (then called *consumption*) was the number one cause of death in the United States. Today the death rate from tuberculosis has been reduced to a low level in the United States and in many other economically fortunate countries because of improvements in housing, nutrition, working conditions, and the general standard of living of most people. But tuberculosis remains a major cause of death in countries and regions with a low standard of living and among the underprivileged classes of many other countries.

Tuberculosis is a chronic infection by a rod-shaped bacterium, *Mycobacterium tuberculosis*. The usual site of infection is in the lungs, but *any* part of the body may be infected. The principal source of infection is bacteria carried by the respiratory discharges (through coughing, sneezing, or talking) of infected persons. These bacteria are more resistant to drying and chemical agents than are most pathogens, but they can be destroyed by exposure to direct sunlight, high temperature (not lukewarm dishwater), and certain disinfectants. They can remain alive for long periods of time in dried sputum in a dark place. Dried respiratory droplets containing the bacteria may be suspended in the air as dust. Infection most commonly occurs when the bacteria are inhaled into the lungs. Drinking unpasteurized milk from tuberculous cows may cause infection of the digestive system.

Following lung infection, the disease may take one of several courses. Rarely does the infection spread rapidly through the lungs, leading to the swift death of the person; more commonly it spreads slowly through the lungs and, if left untreated, leads to death after a period of years. Many people have the ability to confine a tuberculosis infection to a small area of the lung, where the bacteria may remain alive but inactive for several years. Such resistive ability is thought to depend upon many factors, including nutritional state, general health, and race. Inactive cases sometimes become active at a later time, when the physical condition of the infected person is weakened.

Despite the reduced incidence of tuberculosis in the United States, it remains an important personal responsibility to prevent or detect tuberculosis infection. Personal prevention today consists mainly of avoiding contact with known or suspected active cases and avoiding places frequented by such individuals. Skid-row alcoholics have a very high incidence of tuberculosis; any place frequented by these derelicts is likely to be contaminated with tuberculosis bacteria. Maintenance of a high level of general health and nutrition is important for resisting infection when exposure does occur.

Several tuberculosis vaccines have been produced and have had widespread use in several countries, but they have never been extensively used in the United States, owing to their limited effectiveness, possible hazards, and interference with skin tests for tuberculosis (see below). The use of BCG (bacille Calmette-Guerin) vaccine is, however, recommended for high-risk individuals, such as nurses and children in contact with active tuberculosis cases.

Diagnosis   There are two methods of tuberculosis screening in common use today, each having its advantages and limitations. These are chest x-rays and skin tests. Chest x-rays are important in detecting tuberculosis and other lung disorders, although they may not reliably distinguish tuberculosis from other disorders nor the active from the inactive tuberculosis. Nor will chest x-rays detect tuberculosis in other areas of the body.

In tuberculin testing a purified extract of killed tuberculosis bacteria, called *tuberculin,* is injected into the skin. If the person has, *or has ever had,* tuberculosis, a local inflammation will occur at the point of the injection. The tuberculin reaction becomes positive about four to six weeks after the first tuberculosis infection and remains positive; thus tuberculin testing cannot distinguish between active and inactive cases. The tuberculin test described above is the Mantoux test, the most widely used of the tuberculin tests. In other variations of tuberculin testing the material is scratched or punched into the skin. When both the x-ray and tuberculin tests indicate possible tuberculosis, the confirming test for active tuberculosis is the bacteriologic examination of the sputum or other secretions for the presence of tuberculosis bacteria.

Treatment   Despite the vast improvement that has been made in the treatment of tuberculosis, its complete cure remains a very slow process. Active cases should be isolated and preferably hospitalized, to prevent infection of family and other contacts. The sputum usually becomes free of bacteria within six months after treatment begins; the person is then no longer infective. A complete cure takes much longer, however.

Yellow fever

Yellow fever is an often fatal virus disease transmitted only by certain mosquitoes. Fortunately, yellow fever has been entirely eliminated from many countries where it was once common or epidemic. Many years have passed since the last epidemic occurred in the United States. Yellow fever occurs today primarily as sporadic cases in the jungle areas of Mexico, Central and South America, and Africa, with occasional outbreaks in cities bordering upon jungles.

Yellow fever is an acute disease, lasting just a few days but having a 5 to 40 percent fatality rate. The higher death rate is characteristic of persons born in areas where yellow fever does not occur and who travel into a yellow-fever area. Apparently over the years a selection for yellow fever tolerance has taken place among native populations of disease areas.

The yellow-fever virus attacks the liver, causing severe jaundice; there is bleeding from many areas of the body, possibly through a destruction of the platelets necessary for the clotting of blood. There is typically bleeding from the nose and mouth and vomiting of blood. Those persons surviving yellow fever are left with a lifelong immunity to the disease.

The reduction in the incidence of yellow fever has been partly the result of intensive control measures directed against its mosquito vectors, especially *Aedes aegypti;* see Fig. 21.8. This mosquito, which breeds primarily in con-

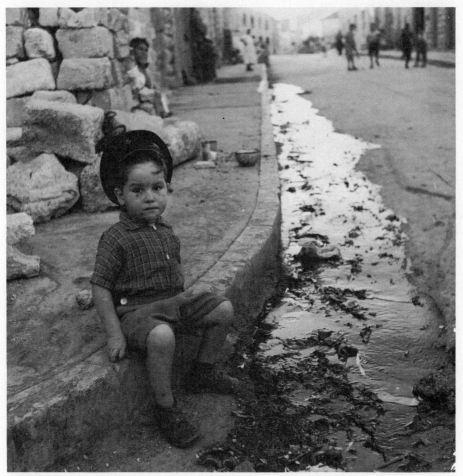

Figure 21.8   *Aedes* breeding situation. *Aedes aegypti* is the most domesticated of all mosquitoes. This mosquito multiplies abundantly in small quantities of water resulting from human activities. Notice the bites on this small body. (From *World Health, the Magazine of the World Health Organization.*)

tainers of water around human dwellings, has been completely eliminated from some areas. Also of prime importance in the reduction of yellow fever has been the widespread use of effective vaccines, which provide an immunity lasting at least seventeen years. Vaccination is important for all persons living in or traveling through yellow-fever areas and is required by law by many countries for travelers coming from or through yellow-fever zones.

Dengue (dengue fever)

Dengue is a virus disease transmitted by mosquitoes of the genus *Aedes*. Explosive epidemics of this disease occur in the Pacific islands, Southeast Asia, Indonesia, India, and northern Australia. The last outbreak in the United States was in the Rio Grande Valley of Texas in 1942.

The fatality rate of dengue is very low, but the disease is quite disabling, the suffering intense, and the recuperation period long. Symptoms of dengue include fever, rash, and pain in the muscles and joints.

Dengue is currently best prevented by control of *Aedes* mosquitoes. Research is being done on vaccines, but none is yet commercially available.

Smallpox

It is hard to visualize the terror in which people must have lived when smallpox raged unchecked. Smallpox was once as common throughout the world as chickenpox is today, but with a death rate of 30 to 40 percent of all cases. After its introduction into the Western Hemisphere by the Spaniards it wiped out 50 percent of all American Indians. Periodic epidemics throughout the world killed millions (an estimated 60 million Europeans died of smallpox during the seventeenth century).

In 1972 the World Health Organization embarked on the final phase of a global campaign to eradicate smallpox. Because of the success of this program public health services in the United States and the United Kingdom decided to discontinue recommending routine smallpox vaccination in their countries. This has caused some concern among physicians, but in recent years in the United States there have been between six and ten deaths a year from the smallpox vaccination whereas there hasn't been a case of smallpox for more than ten years. At the same time the countries of Europe and North America agreed that the international certificates of vaccination (see Appendix B) would no longer be routinely required to travel between and within these areas.

Smallpox is still a major threat in parts of Asia and Africa. There are nearly 200,000 cases a year in those areas, leading to more than 50,000 deaths. The problem lies in the need of revaccination every three to five years for maximal protection. One out of every three who contract smallpox die, and the other two are left either badly disfigured or blind; see Figs. 21.9 and 21.10. There is no specific cure for the disease.

Smallpox is a highly communicable disease caused by the variola virus, which is present, during the course of the disease, in lesions of the skin and mucous membranes of the nose and throat and in the digestive tract, the blood, the feces, and the urine.

This disease is contagious from the beginning of the earliest symptoms until all the lesions have healed. It is transmitted by direct contact with the skin lesions, by droplets from the nose and throat lesions that are projected from the respiratory tract of an infected individual in breathing, coughing, or spitting, and also by dried infectious material from healing lesions that is suspended in airborne dust particles. Indirect transmission takes place through contamination of bed clothes, drinking glasses, eating utensils, or other personal articles.

Smallpox may be contracted by any exposed person, regardless of age,

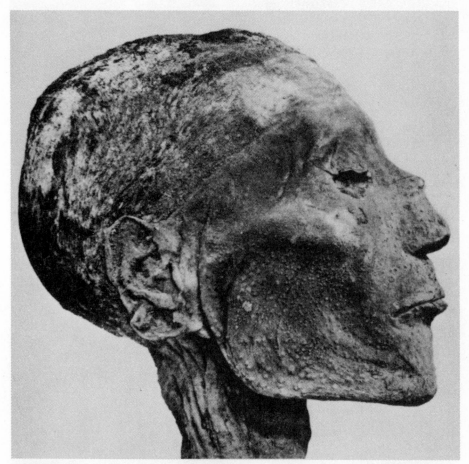

Figure 21.9   Smallpox. Smallpox struck not only the common people but also the great. The mummified face of the Egyptian Pharaoh Ramses V shows clear traces of smallpox. (From *World Health, the Magazine of the World Health Organization*.)

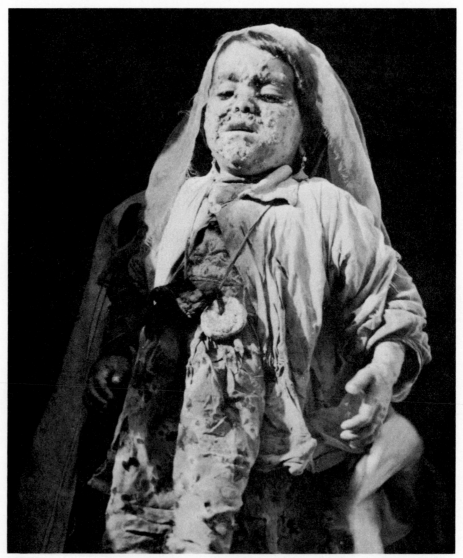

Figure 21.10   Smallpox. A young girl struck by smallpox in Afghanistan. Her parents have dressed her in her finest clothes as if to protect her from evil. (From *World Health, the Magazine of the World Health Organization.*)

who is not immune because of a previous attack or by vaccination. If it were not for vaccination, smallpox would be chiefly a disease of childhood.

Three major types of the variola-vaccinia virus group have been recognized: variola major, or smallpox, variola minor, or alastrim, and vaccinia, or cowpox. The viruses are closely related, evincing essentially the same physical characteristics and properties; they may be distinguished by the reactions they produce in man and experimental animals. Exposure to any one of the three produces immunity for the complete group. Consequently, the vaccination for smallpox consists of introducing vaccinia virus into the skin for the purpose of inducing cowpox in order to prevent smallpox. Cowpox, a disease normally affecting cattle but communicable to man, is less virulent and less serious for both cattle and man than is smallpox for man.

Cholera

Cholera is a very serious, acute disease resulting from the infection of the digestive tract by a bacterium, *Vibrio cholerae*, also called *Vibrio comma*. In past centuries cholera has swept over most of the world. Today it is still a great scourge in parts of India, Iraq, and southern China, and in recent years epidemics have occurred in parts of Egypt, Thailand, Indonesia, the Philippines, Hong Kong, Macao, Korea, Taiwan, and Malaysia. No cases have been reported in the United States for many years.

The incubation period for cholera is only a few hours or days. The disease is marked by a very profuse diarrhea, persistent vomiting, cramps, and profound sweating. The stools consist of little more than water with flakes of mucus and occasionally streaks of blood. In many outbreaks most of the patients die, although proper care reduces the fatality rate. Death is the result of dehydration.

The source of infection of cholera is the feces and vomitus of infected persons, transmitted through contaminated water, contaminated food, flies, and direct contact.

Prevention of cholera involves sanitary sewage disposal, protection and purification of water supplies, pasteurization of milk, sanitary preparation of foods, and fly control. Cholera vaccine is available for use in epidemics, for persons traveling into cholera areas, and for those subject to unusual risk. The immunity produced, however, is of short duration—not more than six months.

Typhoid fever

Typhoid fever has a worldwide distribution and is a major public health problem in many countries. In the United States its incidence has dropped considerably, to about 300 or 400 cases a year. Typhoid fever is caused by the bacterium *Salmonella typhosa*. This bacterium invades the entire body, producing fever, general ill feeling, loss of appetite, and headache. The pulse is slow, and rose-colored spots appear on the body. A fatality rate of about 10 percent can be reduced to 2 or 3 percent with antibiotic therapy.

The source of infection is the feces and urine of infected persons. Symptomless carriers are a problem with this disease. The bacteria may live in the gallbladder for many years, being passed with the feces. Transmission of the bacteria is through direct or indirect contact with patients or carriers, contaminated food or water, and flies.

Prevention of typhoid fever involves sanitary sewage disposal, safe water supplies, fly control, and vaccination.

Leprosy (Hansen's disease)

The fear of leprosy is almost without parallel, owing to the body mutilations produced by the advanced disease, exaggeration of its infectiousness, and ignorance of the benefits of modern treatment. Leprosy is a chronic, moderately communicable, bacterial infection of the skin, with infiltration of nerves, muscles, and bones; see Fig. 21.11. Atrophy and deformity of the extremities occurs in advanced cases; see Fig. 21.12. The progress of the disease is very slow, and death seldom results from it.

The number of cases of leprosy (also called Hansen's disease) is estimated at 5 to 12 million. Most of these cases occur in the tropics and subtropics, especially in Africa and Asia. A small number of cases occur in the United States, primarily in Hawaii and southeastern Texas.

The infectious agent of leprosy is the bacterium *Mycobacterium leprae*, related to the one which produces tuberculosis. Leprosy is transmitted through contact with the bacteria-laden discharges from the lesions of infected persons. Among persons living in the same household with a leprosy victim, about 30 percent of the males and 15 percent of the females will contract the disease. Leprosy is unique in its long incubation period—usually three to five years or longer.

In controlling leprosy the old policy of isolating infected persons in hospitals or colonies is being replaced with outpatient treatment. Drugs are available which render a person noninfective in a short period of time and which over a longer period often lead to a complete cure; see Fig. 21.13. The compulsory segregation of infected persons formerly acted as an obstacle to leprosy control, since leprosy was often concealed to avoid forced separation of the sufferer from home and friends.

PARASITIC WORMS

The majority of all persons living on earth today are infected by one or more types of parasitic worms. Such parasites are partially responsible for the slow rate of development of many of the nations of the world. Parasitic worms seldom cause the total disability or sudden death of a person but, instead, sap him of the strength necessary for progress—individual or national. The infected person needs all his available strength just for the day-to-day processes of living. His life span is decreased considerably, as is his ability to enjoy life while it lasts.

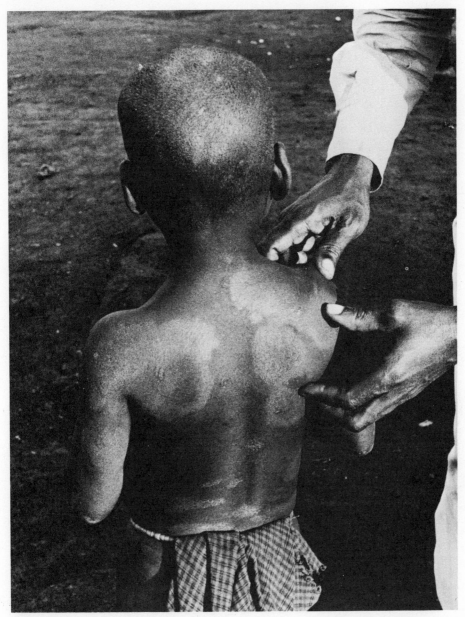

Figure 21.11   Early leprosy. Like many other diseases, leprosy is more easily cured if detected in its early stages. (From *World Health, the Magazine of the World Health Organization.*)

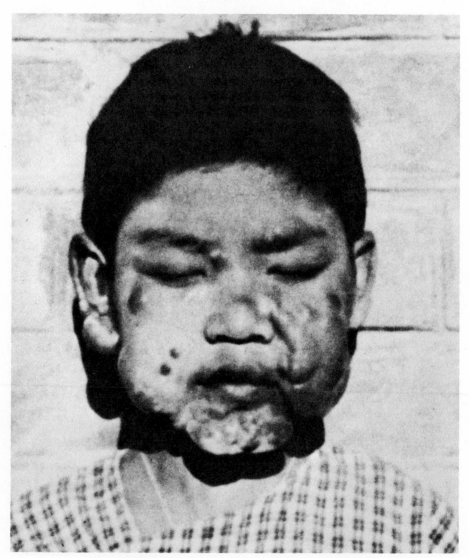

Figure 21.12   Advanced leprosy. This 8-year-old in Burma has an advanced, seemingly hopeless case of leprosy. (From *World Health, the Magazine of the World Health Organization*.)

Fortunately, most of the parasitic worms we shall discuss are now relatively scarce, localized, or totally absent in the United States. But with international travel so commonplace and rapid there is always the possibility that some kinds of parasitic worm will turn up in any town in the United States. The factors that help to minimize the worm problem in the United States include a temperate climate (many worms are favored by tropical climates), good nutrition (important in resisting worm infection), education (knowing what is dangerous and why), sanitary water supplies, sewage, and garbage disposal, decent housing, wearing of shoes, and elimination of insect vectors or carriers of the worms. If parasitic worms are to be reduced in importance in other countries, these are the problems which must be solved. People will have to change their eating and living habits. Practices such as eating raw fish and meat or using the same river for bathing, ex-

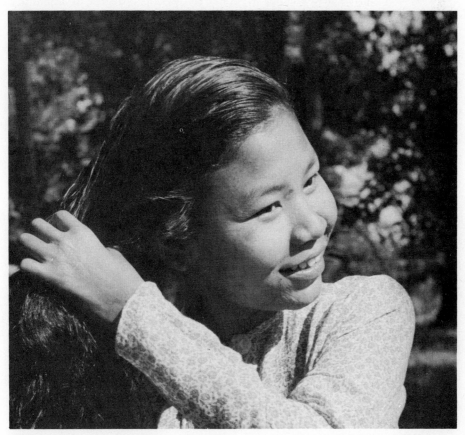

Figure 21.13   Treated leprosy. This is the same girl seen in Figure 21.12, now 13 years old and entirely free of symptoms after several years of drug treatment. (From *World Health, the Magazine of the World Health Organization.*)

creting, and drinking will have to be stopped. Certain religious practices and beliefs may have to be revised.

A few of the parasitic worms of great world importance will be discussed below. These discussions are arranged by the method of transmission to man—from person to person, from insect vectors, and from animals to man.

Worms transmitted from person to person

Hookworms   Hookworms are small roundworms, less than a half-inch long and quite slender, which attach themselves by oral hooks into the inner lining of the small intestine. There they remain for five or ten years, constantly sucking blood and laying eggs. The effect on man of hookworm infection is chronic anemia and weakness. These symptoms are usually serious only when the infected person is poorly nourished. A good diet not only prevents anemia from developing but also enables a person to develop a degree of immunity that results in resistance to infection and loss of worms already harbored.

The eggs of hookworms pass from the intestine with the feces, hatch in the ground, and develop into an infective larval (immature) form. The larvae wait in the soil or vegetation until a barefooted person comes by. The larvae burrow through the skin of the foot into a blood or lymph vessel. They are carried by the blood to the right side of the heart, then into the capillaries of the lungs, where they burrow out into the air sacs. The larvae are then carried by the cilia of the bronchial tubes or coughed up into the throat, where they are swallowed. When they reach the intestine, they attach themselves, develop into adults, and the cycle repeats itself.

The prevention of hookworm infection thus involves three phases: good diet, sanitary disposal of feces, and wearing of shoes. Hookworms remain a problem today only in the economically depressed areas of the southeastern United States, where diet is apt to be poor, sewage disposal inadequate, and shoes worn only occasionally.

Ascariasis   Ascariasis is the infection of man by large worms of the genus *Ascaris*. This roundworm often exceeds a foot in length; see Fig. 21.14. About two thirds of the world's population is infected by ascaris worms, probably the most widespread worm infection. The adult ascaris normally lives in the small intestine, where it feeds on partly digested foods and probably sucks some blood. The infected person suffers from loss of appetite and weight; when the worms are abundant (thousands have been removed from a single person), the intestine may be completely blocked, leading to death if the worms are not surgically removed. Toxic products of the worms cause such conditions as nervousness, swelling, convulsions, delirium, and coma. Other complications occur when the worms "wander" into ducts and cavities. They often invade the bile and pancreatic ducts and may travel to the gallbladder or liver.

Ascaris worms lay tremendous numbers of eggs (two hundred thousand per female per day), which pass from the intestine with the feces. In moist soil the eggs remain alive for up to six years. Infection of man usually occurs when the eggs are swallowed with raw vegetables or from contaminated hands. The eggs hatch in the small intestine, but the larvae take a little tour of the body before settling down. They burrow into the blood vessels of the small intestine, are carried with the blood to the liver, the heart, and the lungs, burrow out into the air sacs, travel up to the throat, and are swallowed—a route similar to that of hookworms. When the small intestine is reached the second time, the worms mature into adults, living for nine months to a year.

Like hookworm infection, ascariasis is most common in moist tropical countries. In the United States the disease is most prevalent in the South. The prevention depends upon the use of sanitary toilet facilities and the training of children to wash hands after defecation and before eating and not to eat food dropped on the floor. Washing of raw vegetables is of some importance. Similar worms infect many dogs and almost all pigs, but their infection of man is believed to be uncommon.

Pinworms   Pinworms, or seatworms, are the most common parasitic worms infecting children in the United States. The Caucasian race is the most susceptible to pinworm infection. Few members of this race manage to get through life without being at some time infected with pinworms. Pinworms are very slender, white roundworms an eighth to a half of an inch in length;

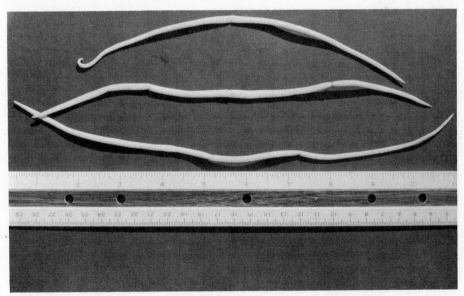

Figure 21.14 *Ascaris* worms. Reaching 1 foot or more in length, these worms infect more than two thirds of the world's population.

see Fig. 21.15. The worms live in the large intestine and rectum. Mature females emerge from the anus at night, lay eggs around the anus, and retreat back into the rectum, although some worms remain on the skin around the anus.

Pinworm infections are acquired through ingestion of the eggs. An infected child usually scatters the eggs throughout his environment. His hands, clothing, and bed linen are all likely to be contaminated. Carpets, draperies, and furniture are also frequently contaminated. The microscopic eggs are even airborne as dust particles. The air in classrooms containing infected children has been found to carry *hundreds* of pinworm eggs. It is not unusual for an entire family or class to become infected.

The results of a pinworm infection are usually more irritating than serious. The migration of the worms in the anal region causes intense itching, leading to loss of sleep, restlessness, nervousness, and even hysteria. In girls the worms may cause vaginal inflammation. Contrary to popular belief, pinworms are not a common cause of appendicitis.

Suspected cases of pinworms are sometimes diagnosed by pressing

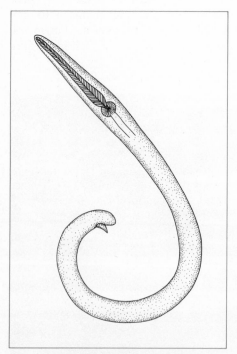

Figure 21.15   Pinworm. Very common in children in the United States, these small worms range from ⅛ to ½ inch in length.

Scotch tape around the anal region early in the morning. If worms are present, the physician can detect the eggs stuck to the tape and will prescribe an effective treatment. All members of the family should be tested.

Pinworm prevention must include use of sanitary toilet facilities and teaching children to wash hands after defecation and always before eating. Children should be discouraged from nail biting or otherwise putting fingers in the mouth or nose. When there is a known infection in a family, all clothing and bed sheets should be laundered daily in *hot* water (washing with warm water can spread the infection). Floors should receive frequent washing or vacuuming. Some authorities feel, however, that extreme efforts to eliminate pinworms completely may lead to a "pinworm neurosis" that is worse than a mild pinworm infection.

Worms transmitted by insect vectors

Filariasis   Filariasis leads to the condition that most people call *elephantiasis;* see Fig. 21.16. This disease is common in many tropical countries but is not present in the United States. Filariasis is caused by microscopic, hairlike roundworms called filaria, which are transmitted from man to man only by mosquitoes of several species. These minute worms live in the lymph ducts and lymph glands of man, causing an allergic reaction that produces chills, fever, aches, and pains. In old infections the flow of lymph through the lymph ducts is blocked, causing fluid to build up in the tissues. The result is elephantiasis—a tremendous and grotesque swelling of the arms, legs, breasts, and particularly the scrotum. If left untreated for several years, this swelling becomes permanent.

Filaria worms cannot complete their life cycles without mosquitoes. The female worms give birth to living young, which are carried in the bloodstream of the infected person, but these young worms cannot mature into adults without being taken up by a mosquito. Thus, to become heavily infected a person must be bitten by many infected mosquitoes. Since filariasis is transmitted only by mosquitoes, its control is through elimination of mosquitoes and their breeding places, control of adult mosquitoes, screening of houses, and use of insect repellents. Prompt treatment of infected persons also helps to break the chain of infection.

Worms transmitted from animals to man

Tapeworms   Few human parasites are the subject of as much folklore and misinformation as the tapeworms. Tapeworms (Fig. 19.5) are almost paper-thin flatworms, each of which possesses a head bearing hooks and suckers plus a long chain of segments. Some species attain a length of over thirty feet. The adult forms of most species of tapeworm infecting man live in the small intestine, causing digestive disturbances, loss of weight, insomnia, nervousness, and abdominal pain. Each of the several species of tapeworm that commonly infect man will be discussed individually below.

· PORK TAPEWORM   The pork tapeworm (*Taenia solium*) infects man in any part of the world where pork is eaten without being cooked thoroughly. The adult pork tapeworm lives in the small intestine of man. The larval (immature) worms form cysts (knotlike structures) in the flesh of pigs. The cysts are oval, whitish bodies from a quarter to a half of an inch long. When such cysts are eaten by man in poorly cooked pork, the larva attaches itself to the wall of the small intestine and in two or three months grows into a

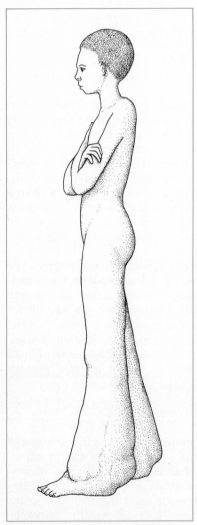

Figure 21.16   Elephantiasis. This disease is caused by microscopic filaria worms, which block the lymph ducts.

mature tapeworm. A man infected with a pork tapeworm passes several hundred mature segments per month with the feces, each segment containing thousands of eggs. If the eggs are consumed by a pig, then the cycle is completed, and the flesh of that pig will become infected with cysts. The pork tapeworm is particularly dangerous because, if the eggs are consumed by man, as on contaminated vegetables, cysts are formed in the muscles, brain, eye, heart, or other vital organs of man. This condition commonly occurs in Mexico and other countries where sanitation is poor. In heavy infections the fatality rate is high. Thorough cooking of all pork will prevent infection in man.

· BEEF TAPEWORM The beef tapeworm (*Taenia saginata*) has a life cycle similar to the pork tapeworm's, except that cattle rather than pigs serve as the larval host, and only the adult worms, not the larvae, will infect man. The distribution of this tapeworm is worldwide. Thorough cooking will kill the larvae in beef, as will thorough salt curing.

· DWARF TAPEWORM The dwarf tapeworm (*Hymenolepis nana*) is the smallest adult tapeworm found in man, seldom exceeding four inches in length, but is the most common tapeworm infecting man. Its distribution is worldwide. This worm differs from almost all other tapeworms in its ability to complete its entire life cycle in the same host. In addition to man, rats and mice are commonly infected. Most human infections are believed to result from contamination of food with rat, mouse, or human feces. The worm eggs consumed with these feces will hatch in the small intestine, pass through several larval stages, and mature into adults. The eggs of this worm sometimes hatch while still in the intestine of an infected man, and this may result in massive secondary infection. The dwarf tapeworm does form minute cysts in fleas or grain beetles which have eaten worm eggs from rat or mouse feces. Consumption of these insects by man in contaminated food can lead to an intestinal infection of adult worms. Prevention of infection by the dwarf tapeworm is mainly through control of rats and mice, especially where their feces might contaminate food.

· DOG TAPEWORM The dog tapeworm (*Dipylidium caninum*) is an extremely common parasite of dogs and cats all over the world. Its cysts are formed in fleas and mature into adults when the fleas are eaten by a dog or cat. Most human infections are in children who have accidentally eaten fleas while playing with a dog or cat. Children are sometimes infected by having their faces licked by a dog just after the dog has nipped a flea. Therefore, it is important that pets be kept free of fleas.

· FISH TAPEWORM The largest tapeworm infecting man is the fish tapeworm (*Diphyllobothrium*) which often exceeds thirty feet in length. The number of worms infecting a single person may be more than a hundred. The infection is acquired by eating raw or poorly cooked fish infected with the larvae of this worm. Infected fish are found primarily in the cold, fresh waters of the northern hemisphere, including the Great Lakes region of the United States. In some parts of Alaska nearly 100 percent of the population is infected. Fortunately, the symptoms of infection are usually mild or absent, although some persons develop severe anemia or toxic symptoms. The fish species commonly infected include pike, salmon, trout, perch, pickerel, turbot, and eel. The life cycle of the fish tapeworm is complex. The adult worm lives in the small intestine of man or other fish-eating mammals. Eggs passed with the feces hatch in fresh water, releasing a larva that must be swallowed by a small crustacean to continue its development. The crustacean must in turn be eaten by a fish, in the flesh of which the worm larva forms a cyst. If the fish is eaten by a man or other mammal, the cycle is complete. The obvious prevention of a fish tapeworm infection is to cook all fish before eating it. As an alternative, freezing of fish for several days at 0° F will kill the encysted larvae. Inspection of fish for cysts is impractical.

Trichinosis Trichinosis is the invasion of human flesh by the larvae of a parasitic roundworm, *Trichinella spiralis*. Man is infected by eating the poorly cooked flesh of animals containing the encysted larvae of the worm. The usual source of infection is pork, although bear or any meat-eating mammal may carry these larvae. After a man or any flesh-eating mammal has eaten diseased flesh, the larvae are freed from their cysts by the digestive juices, pass into the small intestine, become sexually mature, and give birth to living larvae, which penetrate the walls of the intestine. The larvae are then carried by the blood to all parts of the body. Almost every organ and tissue is invaded, but further development of the larvae takes place only in the muscles, where cysts are produced, which completes the cycle.

The severity of the symptoms of trichinosis in man depends upon how many larvae are consumed. The disease may be mild or fatal. The first symptoms occur as early as 24 hours after ingestion of infected meat; they include nausea, diarrhea, and abdominal pain, resulting from the intestinal activity of the worms. Beginning about seven to nine days later and continuing for several weeks, the larvae penetrate the muscles and other organs. It is during this period that the serious or fatal symptoms may appear. These symptoms commonly include fever, weakness, muscle soreness and pain, swelling of eyelids, chills, sweating, and difficulty in breathing. When death results, it is usually the result of invasion of the heart muscle. Muscular pains and weakness may continue for several months.

Trichinosis is worldwide in occurrence and is particularly common in the United States. Many Americans are infected at some time during their lives. The most effective and cheapest preventive measure is the thorough cooking of all pork or pork products. Butchers should carefully clean pork from meat grinders before grinding beef. Uncooked garbage fed to pigs may be infected by infected pork scraps contained in the garbage; most states outlaw this practice, but enforcement on small farms is virtually impossible. Meat inspection for trichinosis is impractical, costly, and not reliable. Freezing of pork at very low temperature effectively kills the larvae, but home freezers cannot be depended upon to reach these temperatures (20 days at 5° F, 10 days at −10° F, or 6 days at −20° F).

Schistosomiasis About 150 million persons are currently infected with schistosomes, or *blood flukes*. These are small, slender flatworms, a quarter or half an inch long; see Fig. 21.17. Blood flukes are common in Africa, South America, and the Orient but do not occur in North America. There are several species of blood flukes, each of which tends to live in specific veins, usually those leading from the large intestine, rectum, and bladder. The symptoms of infection depend upon the veins infected and may be slight or severe. Among the more typical symptoms are fever and dysentery.

The life cycle of each species of schistosome requires a snail for its completion; see Fig. 21.18. The worm eggs leave the body of an infected person with the urine or feces. The egg hatches in water, and the larva must then burrow into a suitable species of fresh-water snail. After several weeks the larva begins to produce thousands of larvae of another form (*cercariae*), which leave the snail and swim freely through the water. A man entering the water will be infected by the cercariae, which penetrate directly through the skin. The larvae enter the bloodstream, grow to maturity in the blood vessels of the liver, then migrate as adults into the abdominal veins. Through destruction of tissues the eggs escape into the urinary bladder or large intestine, to leave the body with the urine or feces. Infection of man is also possible through drinking of water containing the cercariae.

Preventive measures include sanitary disposal of feces and urine, drain-

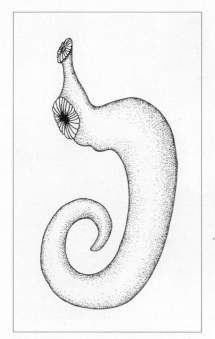

Figure 21.17 Blood flukes (schistosomes). Actual size ¼ to ½ inch long.

age of swamps, chemical control of snails, pure water for drinking and bathing, protective clothing for persons who must enter contaminated water, and education for persons living in areas of contaminated water.

Liver flukes   A serious health problem in many areas of the Far East, especially Japan, Korea, and China, is *clonorchiasis*, Oriental liver-fluke disease. Liver flukes are slender, oval flatworms half or one inch long that live in the bile ducts of the liver. In light infections the symptoms may be mild or absent. Severe infections may cause digestive disturbances or liver damage but seldom lead to death. Infection sometimes lasts twenty years or more. Man is infected with liver flukes through eating incompletely cooked fish (fresh, dried, salted, or pickled). The life cycle, like that of blood flukes, involves snails; see Fig. 21.19. Worm eggs laid in the bile ducts leave the body of man with the feces. The eggs hatch after being eaten by fresh-water snails, which are in turn eaten by fish. The worm larvae form cysts in the flesh of the fish, and man is infected by the infected fish. The best preventive measure, obviously, is to cook thoroughly all fresh-water fish before eating them.

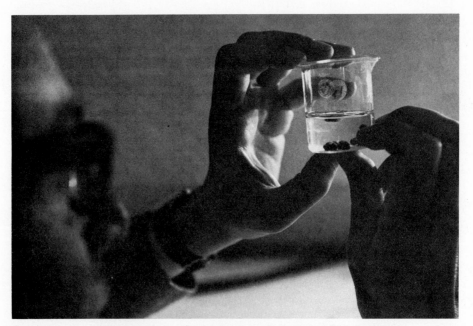

Figure 21.18   Schistosomiasis. A scientist examines one of the species of water snails serving as hosts for the larvae of blood flukes. New irrigation projects in some parts of the world are increasing the problem of schistosomiasis. (From *World Health, the Magazine of the World Health Organization*.)

OCCUPATIONAL DISEASES

The past

Occupational diseases are diseases that arise as a result of occupational exposure to some harmful element. In the strictest sense this term applies only to those diseases which are specific to a given occupation and are not found among the general public. In a broader sense, many diseases which do occur in the general population may be considered occupational diseases if their incidence is greatly increased within a given occupation.

In years past it was accepted that many occupations had particular hazards, and persons working within those occupations accepted the probability that eventually they would suffer from that occupational disease. Naturally, they did not like the idea—but such hazards were considered to be an unavoidable aspect of the struggle to make a living. Miners, for example, accepted lung diseases as an inevitable part of their way of life. Corporations, large and small, either showed no concern for the health of their employees or lacked the technical ability to overcome occupational hazards.

The present

The incidence of occupational diseases has dropped considerably during the past forty to fifty years. This fortunate decrease may be attributed to several important developments. First, technical advances have been made that have either eliminated certain hazardous occupations completely or have increased the safety of the employee. Second, industrial safety laws have been passed to force the improvement of working conditions, and labor unions have often been successful in correcting occupational hazards for their members. Perhaps the most important development has been the realization by most corporation administrators that the health of their employees has a great influence upon the corporation's profit. An experienced, vigorous employee is worth much more to an employer than the same man weakened by an occupational disease or than his inexperienced replacement, if he becomes completely disabled.

Despite the improvements that have been made, many occupational-disease hazards remain in the United States today. They may be classified in the following manner.

Chemical hazards Many occupational diseases result from exposure to chemical substances, such as solvents, dusts, and gases. Almost every occupation involves some exposure to potentially dangerous chemicals. Even the office secretary is exposed to such solvents as type cleaners and duplicating fluids. The main portals of entry into the body for occupational chemicals are the lungs, for the dusts, gases, and vapors, and the skin, for many of the solvents. Although the employer is responsible for providing ventilation and other basic protections against chemicals, it is the duty of the employee to *learn* and *follow* the safety precautions for every chemical with which he has

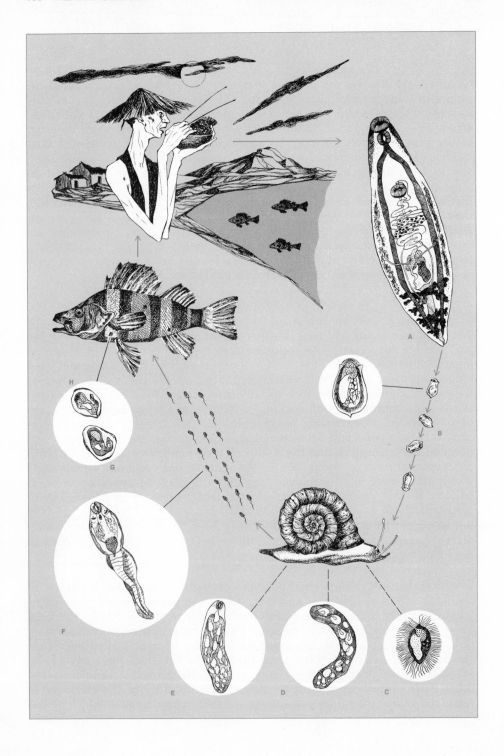

contact. Absence of poisoning symptoms is not proof of adequate protection, since many chemicals will cause *permanent damage to vital organs* long before any noticeable symptoms of poisoning develop.

Physical hazards Certain occupational diseases result from physical factors of the environment, such as temperature, noise, and radiation. The effects of temperature extremes depend upon how high or low the temperature is, the humidity, the length of exposure, and the degree of exertion. Exposure to extreme noise, such as that which occurs in factories of many types, may cause a temporary hearing impairment, recovery from which may take days or months or may result in permanent hearing loss, which reaches a maximum after five to ten years of exposure. The degree of hearing loss depends upon the pitch (frequency) of the sound and its intensity (measured in decibels). Damage begins to occur at 90 to 120 decibels, depending upon the pitch. Some typical noise intensities are listed in Table 10.4.

Among those types of radiation from which protection must be provided for the employee are gamma ray, x-ray, ultraviolet ray, intense visible light, infrared ray, laser, microwave, and the atomic or particulate radiations. As the industrial use of many of these forms of radiation has become widespread, it has become important for the individual employee to learn and observe carefully all safety precautions relating to their use. Some of the harmful effects of overexposure to the forms of radiation are the following:

Gamma rays, x-rays, atomic particles. All have same effect; all are ionizing radiations causing permanent damage or death of cells. Chromosome damage leads to abnormal division. Effects of repeated small doses are cumulative. Mutations and cancer are produced. Any tissue of the body may be damaged. Large doses are always fatal.

Ultraviolet rays. Little penetrating ability. Affects only skin and eyes. Burns skin, produces tanning, thickens skin. Causes skin cancer. Inflammation of conjunctiva of eye. Clouding and ulcers of the cornea (usually temporary).

Clouding of lens (cataract) not proven.

Intense visible light. Inflammation of conjunctiva and cornea. Temporary or permanent loss of vision through damage to retina.

Infrared rays. Burning of skin. Temporary or permanent damage to retina of eye. Possible cataracts of lens of eye.

Laser beams. Skin burns. Heat injury to any part of eye, especially the retina.

Microwaves (radar and others). Main effect is the production of heat in tissue where absorbed. Cataracts produced.

Figure 21.19   Life cycle of the liver fluke: (A) the adult fluke lays eggs in the human liver, and these eggs pass through the bile duct to the intestine and thence to the outside; (B) when the eggs are eaten by a certain species of water snail, they hatch and go through stages (C to E) in the snail's body; (F) the tadpole-like cercariae leave the snail and form cysts (G) and (H) in the muscles of the fish. These cysts infect human beings who eat the infected fish. (From W. G. Whaley et al., *Principles of Biology*, New York, Harper & Row, 1964, p. 583.)

The precautionary measures that apply to these types of radiation are too numerous and specific for discussion at this point. Any person working with or near any radiation should *learn and observe* the precautions applying to that type of radiation.

Mechanical factors Among the mechanical factors that may lead to occupational disease are exposure to high or low atmospheric pressure, physical strain, and unusual movements. In exposure to high or low pressures the considerations must include, not only the effect of the unusual pressure, but also the effect of a sudden *change* in pressure. The effect of a sudden decrease in pressure may be the development of nitrogen bubbles in the blood, causing severe pains (called "the bends") and leading to possible rapid death or permanent physical damage. The nitrogen cannot be held in solution at the lower pressure, so the bubbles appear just as bubbles appear in a bottle of soda after it is opened.

Certain vibrating tools such as drills, grinders, riveters, and sanders may cause spasms of the blood vessels or inflammation of the joints. The most damaging vibrations are those of 2,000 to 3,000 cycles per minute. Improper lifting and carrying of loads is the most common cause of back trouble. The back should never be bent when lifting but should be held straight while the knees are bent. Other problems can result from prolonged work in one position, especially prolonged standing or bending.

Infectious agents Some jobs, especially in agriculture, expose a person to infectious disease agents. Several diseases can be contracted from animals or animal products. Certain lung-invading fungi are commonly contracted by agricultural or construction workers through airborne spores of the fungi. Most of these infectious diseases are discussed at other points in this book.

Psychological factors Often underrated as occupational diseases are the psychological factors inherent in certain types of employment. Few generalizations can be made here, because a job might be ideally suited to the psychological makeup of one person yet be totally unacceptable to another. The person who is very shy or withdrawn might suffer greatly from a job requiring a great deal of public contact or persuasion. Conversely, a very outgoing person would suffer from a job involving constant isolation. Fortunately, there are both types of person and both types of work, but it is important that they be suitably matched. Much of the illness for which people miss days of work is believed to be the psychosomatic result of jobs that are either consciously or subconsciously disliked: as an escape mechanism the person develops a physical illness, which rescues him from his misery for a few days. Industrial accidents are another common result of psychological problems: the accident-prone person may subconsciously want to be hurt. Many large corporations now hire psychologists or psychiatrists to deal with the emotional problems of their employees.

The future

New technical advances will bring solutions for many of the occupational hazards of today but will, at the same time, produce new hazards. Increased use of various types of radiation and of new and more exotic chemicals will require the observance of safety precautions more rigid than those in the past. More than ever before the hazards will be obscure or invisible to many employees, who will blindly have to follow regulations that often will seem needless to them. Precautions will require an almost military discipline.

WORLD HEALTH ORGANIZATION (WHO)

The World Health Organization, an agency of the United Nations, was organized in 1946 and formally established in 1948, in recognition of the fact that diseases do not respect national boundaries. With today's large numbers of international travelers and the speed of such travel, a disease outbreak may jump from continent to continent in a few hours' time. In addition to fighting infectious diseases, the World Health Organization seeks the improvement of the general level of health of the world's population. Since the infectious diseases have been reduced in importance, the WHO, to achieve its goal, has put greater emphasis upon the problems of modern life, particularly heart disease, cancer, mental illness, drug abuse, suicide, venereal diseases, accidents, and the problems of the developing nations.

The constitution of the World Health Organization states its purpose as follows:

1. To assist governments upon request in strengthening health services.
2. To promote improved standards of teaching and training in the health professions.
3. To provide information, counsel, and assistance in the field of health.
4. To promote improvement in nutrition, housing, sanitation, working conditions, and other aspects of environmental hygiene.
5. To promote among scientific and professional groups cooperation related to health.
6. To promote maternal and child health and welfare.
7. To promote activities in the field of mental health, especially those affecting the harmony of human relations.
8. To promote and conduct research in the field of health.
9. To study social techniques affecting public health.

As world health problems have changed through the years, the World Health Organization has correspondingly shifted the emphasis of its programs and has played an important role in improving the health of the world's population.

SUMMARY

    I. Childhood diseases
      A. Infant mortality (death during first year of life)

1. United States is sixteenth among nations, with a rate of 19.2 per thousand births.
2. One third of infant deaths occur during the first day of life, another third during remainder of first month.
3. Rate for nonwhite infants is twice that for white infants.
B. Disease conditions
C. Poliomyelitis
1. Caused by one of three types of virus.
2. Preventable through immunization.
D. Diphtheria
1. Caused by the bacillus *Corynebacterium diphtheriae.*
2. Prevention is by immunization with DPT vaccine.
E. Whooping cough (pertussis)
1. Caused by the bacillus *Hemophilus pertussis.*
2. Prevention through DPT vaccine.
F. Measles (rubeola)
1. Caused by the rubeola virus.
2. Protection by immunization.
G. German measles (rubella)
1. Caused by the rubella virus.
2. Preventable through immunization.
3. May cause congenital malformations if contracted by a woman in the first six months of pregnancy.
H. Roseola (baby measles)—probably caused by a virus.
I. Chickenpox
1. Caused by the varicella virus.
2. Same virus is the cause of shingles.
J. Mumps
1. Causative agent is a virus.
2. Vaccines are now effective.
K. Hemolytic streptococci
1. Streptococci bacteria that destroy red blood cells are *hemolytic.*
2. Important results of these bacteria include:
a. scarlet fever.
b. "strep" throat.
c. rheumatic fever.
L. Immunizations
1. Active immunity—produced through the injection of antigens that stimulate the body to produce its own antibodies.
2. Passive immunity—achieved through the injection of antibodies produced by some other animal or person.
3. Schedules of immunizations:
a. should be started at the proper age.
b. recall or booster injections should be given according to the schedule in Appendix C.
c. every family should maintain an immunization record for each member of the family (a form for this purpose is provided in Appendix C).
II. Diseases of any age group
A. Common cold—remains as the most common and least preventable communicable disease.
B. Influenza—a virus infection of the respiratory tract characterized by fever, chill, headache, muscular aches, and coughing.

    C. Tetanus (lockjaw)
       1. Result of an exotoxin produced by the bacterium *Clostridium tetani*.
       2. Immunization with tetanus toxoid provides highly effective protection.
       3. Booster injections at ten-year intervals are necessary to maintain immunity.
       4. Nonimmunized individuals may be given temporary protection after an injury with injection of tetanus antitoxin.
    D. Infectious hepatitis—virus infection of the liver.
    E. Infectious mononucleosis—virus infection of the lymph glands, showing a marked rise in white blood cell count.
    F. Bacterial meningitis—infection of the meninges by the meningococcus *Neisseria meningitidis*.
    G. Staphylococcal infections
       1. Boils.
       2. Abscesses.
       3. Carbuncles.
       4. Impetigo.
       5. Infected cuts and wounds.
III. Diseases of worldwide importance
    A. Trachoma—chronic bacterial infection of the eye.
    B. Malaria
       1. Result of infection by protozoa of the genus *Plasmodium*.
       2. Transmitted only by mosquitoes of the genus *Anopheles*.
    C. Yaws—a nonvenereal tropical disease caused by a spirochete similar to that of syphilis.
    D. Tuberculosis
       1. Caused by the bacillus *Mycobacterium tuberculosis*.
       2. Remains a major cause of death in countries and regions with low standard of living.
    E. Yellow fever—an often-fatal virus disease transmitted only by the mosquito *Aedes aegypti*.
    F. Dengue
       1. A virus disease.
       2. Transmitted by *Aedes* mosquitoes.
       3. Epidemics are explosive, but fatality is low.
    G. Smallpox
       1. Caused by the variola virus.
       2. Effective vaccine has been available since about 1800.
       3. Revaccination is necessary every ten years.
    H. Cholera—results from the infection of the digestive tract by the bacterium *Vibrio cholerae* (*Vibrio comma*).
    I. Typhoid fever
       1. Cause is the bacterium *Salmonella typhosa*.
       2. Symptomless carriers are a problem with this disease.
    J. Leprosy (Hansen's disease)—results from an infection by a bacterium related to the tuberculosis organism.
IV. Parasitic worms
    A. Worms transmitted from person to person
       1. Hookworms—roundworms living in the small intestine.
       2. Ascariasis—infestation of the intestine of man by the ascaris worm.

3. Pinworms:
   a. commonly infect children in the United States.
   b. live in the large intestine and deposit eggs at the anus.

B. Parasitic worms transmitted by insect vectors—filariasis (elephantiasis)
   1. Microscopic roundworms transmitted by mosquitoes.
   2. Worms live in the lymph ducts, causing grotesque swelling of the arms, legs, breasts, and scrotum.

C. Parasitic worms transmitted from animals to man
   1. Tapeworms:
      a. pork tapeworm—man infected by eating larval cysts in poorly cooked pork.
      b. beef tapeworm—man infected by eating larval cysts in poorly cooked beef.
      c. dwarf tapeworm—infection of man usually through food contaminated with rat, mouse, or human feces.
      d. dog tapeworm—most human infections are in children who have accidentally eaten fleas from a dog or cat.
      e. fish tapeworm—infection of man is through eating poorly cooked fish containing the larvae of this worm.
   2. Trichinosis
      a. invasion of human flesh by the roundworm *Trichinella spiralis*.
      b. man infected by eating animal flesh containing the encysted larvae of the worm.
   3. Schistosomiasis (blood flukes)—man infected when he enters infected water, drinks such water, or eats contaminated water plants.
   4. Liver flukes—man infected through eating incompletely cooked fish.

V. Occupational diseases—diseases which arise as a result of occupational exposure to some harmful element.
  A. Occupational diseases once accepted as an unavoidable aspect of the struggle to make a living.
  B. Despite improvements that have been made, occupational-disease hazards remain in the United States today.
  C. New technical advances will bring solutions for many of the occupational hazards of today but will also produce new hazards.

VI. World Health Organization (WHO)
  A. An agency of the United Nations, organized in 1946 and formally established in 1948.
  B. Goal is improvement of the general level of health of the world's population.

Glossary

If you cannot find the word you wish in this glossary, check the index for text and glossary references.

abscess (ab′ses) (L. *ab*, away; *cedere*, to go). A localized collection of pus in a cavity formed by the disintegration of tissues.

Aedes (ā ē′dēz) (G. *aedes*, unpleasant). A genus of mosquitoes that includes many important vectors of yellow fever, dengue, and encephalitis.

Anopheles (ə nof′ə lēz) (G. *anopheles,* hurtful). A genus of mosquitoes that includes many vectors of malaria.

anoxia (an ok′sē a) (G. *a-,* absence; oxygen). Absence or lack of oxygen.

Ascaris (as′kə ris) (L. *ascaris*). A genus of roundworms living as intestinal parasites in man and other animals.

booster dose. An injection of vaccine or toxoid administered at some time after primary immunization in order to maintain immunity.

Bordetella (bor də tel′ə) (Jules Jean Bordet, Belgian bacteriologist, 1870–1961). A genus of bacteria to which belongs the organism causing whooping cough.

carrier (kar′ē ər). An individual who harbors somewhere in his body the pathogens of a specific disease without suffering symptoms of that disease.

cercaria (sər kair′ē ə) (Pl. *cercariae*) (G. *kerkos,* tail). The final free-swimming larval stage of certain parasitic flukes.

cholera (kol′ə rə) (G. *chole,* bile). A serious condition marked by severe diarrhea and vomiting.

clonorchiasis (klō nor kī′ə sis) (G. *klon,* branch; *orchis,* testis). The state of being infected with liver flukes of the genus *Clonorchis.*

Clostridium (klo strid′ē əm) (G. *kloster,* spindle). A genus of rod-shaped, spore-forming, generally anaerobic bacteria that includes species responsible for tetanus, botulism, and other diseases.

Corynebacterium (kor′ə nē bak tēr′ē əm) (G. *koryne,* club; *bakterion,* little rod). A genus of bacteria that includes the organism producing diphtheria.

cyst (sist) (G. *kystis,* sac). A sac.

Diphyllobothrium (dī fil ō both′rē əm) (G. *di,* two; *phyllon,* leaf; *bothrion,* pit). A genus of tapeworms that includes the fish tapeworm.

Dipylidium (dī′pi lid′ē əm) (G. *dipylos,* having two entrances). A genus of tapeworms that includes the common dog tapeworm.

eczema (ek′zə mə) (G. *ekzein,* to boil out). A skin-inflammation disease, characterized by lesions with watery discharge and the development of scales and crusts.

elephantiasis (el ə fən tī′ə sis) ("elephant disease"). A common name given to the enlarging of body parts resulting from filariasis of the lymphatic ducts.

encephalitis (en sef′ə lī′tis) (G. *enkephalos,* brain; *-itis,* inflammation). Inflammation of the brain.

erythrogenic (e rith′rō jen′ik) (G. *eryehros,* red; *gennan,* to produce). (1) Producing erythrocytes. (2) Producing a rash.

exanthema (ek san thē′mə) (G. *exanthema*). Any disease characterized by eruption or breaking out of the skin.

filariasis (fil ə rī′ə sis) (L. *filum,* thread). A diseased state due to the presence of filaria (thread-like parasitic roundworms) in the body.

hemolysis (hē mol′i sis) (G. *haima,* blood; *lysis,* dissolution). The separation of the hemoglobin from red blood cells.

hepatitis (hep ə tī′tis) (G. *hepar,* liver; *itis,* inflammation). Inflammation of the liver.

herpes (hur′pēz) (G. *herpes*). An inflammatory skin disease characterized by the formation of clusters of small vesicles.

Hymenolepis (hī mə nol′ə pis) (G. *hymen,* membrane; *lepis,* rind). A genus of tapeworms to which belongs the dwarf tapeworm.

jaundice (jawn′dis) (Fr. *jaune,* yellow). Deposit of bile pigment in the skin with resulting yellow appearance of the patient.

Koplik's spots (Kop′liks) (Henry Koplik, pediatrician, 1858–1927). Small, irregular, bright red spots on the tongue and mouth lining, each with a minute bluish-white speck in the center, indicative of early measles.

larva (lahr′və) (L. *larva*, early stage). An immature stage in the life history of an animal in which it is unlike the parent.

Mantoux test (man too′) (Charles Mantoux, French physician, 1877–1947). The injection of tuberculin into the skin as a diagnostic procedure for tuberculosis.

meninges (mə nin′jēz) (G. *meninx*, membrane). The three membranes that cover the brain and spinal cord.

meningitis (me nin jī′tis) (G. *meninx*, membrane; *itis*, inflammation). Inflammation of the meninges.

Mycobacterium (mī′kō bak tēr′ē əm) (G. *myces*, fungus; *bakterion*, little rod). A genus of rod-shaped bacteria, to which belong the organisms causing tuberculosis and leprosy.

papule (pap′yool) (L. *papula*). A small, solid elevation of the skin.

paroxysm (par′ək sizm) (G. *paroxysmos*, attack). A sudden attack or recurrence of symptoms.

Plasmodium (plaz mō′dē əm) (G. *plasma*, anything formed; *eidos*, form). A genus of protozoa, parasitic in red blood cells; the malaria parasites.

pneumonia (nyoo mō′nē ə) (G. *pneumon*, lung; *-ia*, pertaining to). Inflammation of the lungs.

pseudomembrane (soo′dō mem′brān) (G. *pseudes*, false). A false membrane.

quarantine (kwor′ən tēn) (It. *quarantina*, 40 days). To detain or isolate in order to prevent transmission of a disease.

roseola (rō zē ō′lə) (L.) In its general sense, any rose-colored rash; specifically, roseola infantum (baby measles).

rubella (roo bel′ə) (L. *ruber*, red). German measles.

rubeola (roo bē ō′lə) (L. *ruber*, red). Measles.

Schistosoma (shis′tə sō′mə) (G. *schistos*, split; *soma*, body). The blood flukes—formerly called *bilharzia*.

schistosomiasis (shis′tə sō mī′ə sis) (G. *schistos*, split; *soma*, body). The state of being infected with flukes of the genus *Schistosoma*—formerly called *bilharziasis*.

Taenia (tē′ nē ə) (L. *taenia*, tape). A genus of common tapeworms to which belong the pork and beef tapeworms.

tetanus (tet′ə nəs) (G. *tetanos*, stretched). (1) Continuous steady contraction of a muscle; (2) an acute infectious disease caused by the toxin of *Clostridium tetani*, resulting in spasms of various body muscles.

toxin (tok′sin) (G. *toxikon*, poison). A poison.

toxoid (tok′soid). A weakened bacterial toxin which has lost its toxic properties while retaining its ability to cause production of antitoxins; used in immunization.

trachoma (trə kō′mə) (G. *trachoma*, roughness). A disease of the conjunctiva and cornea of the eye, leading to visual disability and blindness.

Trichinella (trik i nel′ə) (G. *trichinos*, of hair). A genus of parasitic roundworms to which belongs the worm causing trichinosis.

trichinosis (trik i nō′sis). A disease condition due to the infection of the body by *Trichinella spiralis* worms.

tuberculin (tyoo bur′kyə lin) (L. *tuberculun*, a small nodule). A liquid extracted from the tuberculosis bacillus for use in tuberculosis skin testing.

vaccine (vak sēn′) (L. *vaccinus*, of cows). A preparation of killed or attenuated microorganisms for use in immunization.

vaccinia (vak sin′ē ə). A virus disease (cowpox) of cattle communicated to man in order to confer immunity against smallpox.

variola (və rī̄ə lə) (L.) Smallpox.

Vibrio (vib'rē ō) (L. *vibrare,* to shake). A genus of short, curved, rod-shaped bacteria, species of which cause cholera and similar diseases.

yaws (yawz). Infection of man by *Treponema pertenue,* resulting in destructive lesions of the skin and bones.

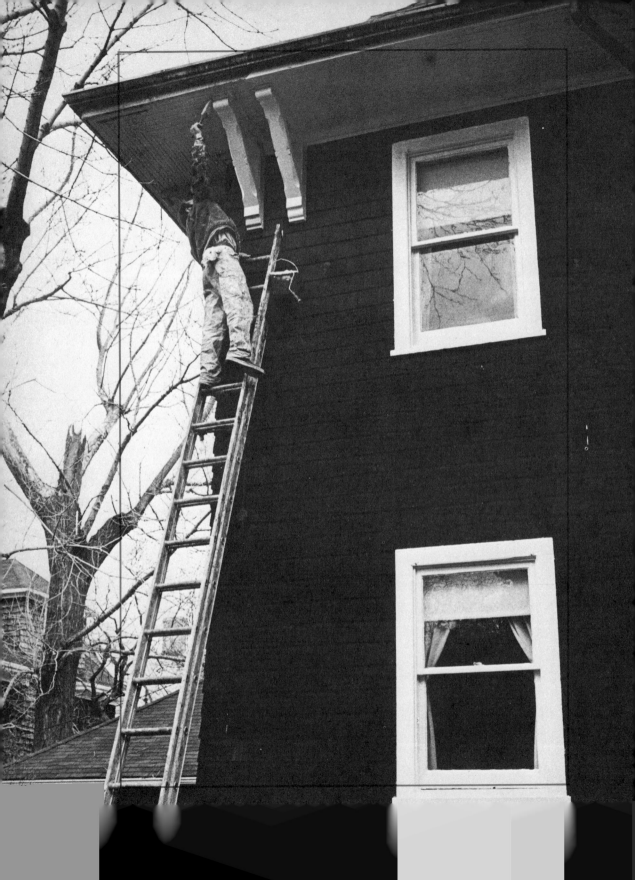

Accident prevention

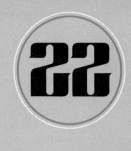

22

Accidents stand among the greatest public health problems in the United States today. They are important not only as causes of death but also as agents of temporary and permanent disability. The total cost of accidents, in terms of dollars and human suffering, is tremendous. Yet the vast majority of accidents could be entirely avoided if the level of safety-consciousness of the nation could be increased. Even now, an individual can materially reduce his own chances of being involved in an accident by being able to recognize potentially dangerous situations and by maintaining attitudes of concern toward accident prevention.

THE ACCIDENT PROBLEM

The scope of the accident problem can be measured in many ways, such as numbers of deaths, persons disabled for life, time lost from work, and dollar loss to the individual or to society. By any scale of measurement the accident problem in the United States is tremendous.

Accidental deaths

Accidents stand today as the third leading cause of death in the United States, following circulatory disorders and cancer. Accidents are currently killing about 115,000 persons per year in the United States alone. Not only is the number of persons killed in accidents great, but the average age of these persons is also much younger than that of people who die of heart disease or cancer. Thus each accidental death represents a greater loss in terms of years of remaining life expectancy.

Motor-vehicle accidents head the list of causes of accidental death, followed by falls, fires, and drownings. The numbers of deaths per year from these and other leading accidental causes are compared in Table 22.1.

Accidental injuries

Every year about 51 million people in the United States are injured seriously enough to require medical attention. This represents 1 in every 4 persons. About half of these injuries are serious enough to require restriction of activities and more than 11 million accident victims must spend some time confined to bed each year—2 million require hospitalization. Over 400,000 persons are left with permanent physical impairments annually. While there is no way to measure the pain and inconvenience suffered by these accident victims, it is obvious that few persons escape being seriously injured at some time during their lives and that the total human suffering is immense. The types of accident causing these injuries are summarized in Table 22.2.

Table 22.1 *Number of accidental deaths per year in the United States, by cause*

cause	approximate number of deaths per year
Motor-vehicle accidents	54,700
Falls	17,900
Drowning	7,300
Fires and burns	6,700
Suffocation on food or other solid objects	3,500
Poisoning by solids and liquids	3,500
Firearms (accidental)	2,400
Poisoning by gases and vapors	1,600
Boats	1,600
Aircraft	1,500
Blow from falling object	1,400
Mechanical suffocation	1,200
Electrocution	1,000
Railway	800

SOURCE: *Accident Facts,* 1972 ed., National Safety Council, 425 N. Michigan Ave., Chicago Ill., 60611. Revised annually, sold for $2.65 per copy.

Table 22.2 *Number of injuries requiring medical attention per year in the United States, by cause*

type of accident	bed cases	total cases
Home	3,955,000	19,748,000
Work	1,879,000	8,426,000
Motor vehicle	1,284,000	3,551,000
Other[a]	4,720,000	18,710,000
Total	12,014,000	51,229,000

SOURCE: *Accident Facts*, 1972 ed., National Safety Council.
[a] Includes recreational accidents, transportation other than motor vehicles, accidents in public buildings, etc.

Dollar cost of accidents

The total dollar cost of accidents in the United States during a recent year was estimated to be at least $29,500,000,000 (29.5 billion). This staggering cost is borne not only by those directly involved in accidents but also by practically everyone else—through increased insurance premiums, taxes, and higher prices of items purchased. The factors contributing to this financial loss are summarized in Table 22.3.

FACTORS IN ACCIDENT DEVELOPMENT

Accident research has revealed that certain general factors are common to all types of accident. At the root of almost every accident lies one or more of these generalized causes.

Table 22.3 *Estimated costs of accidents in the United States in 1971*

item	cost
Wage losses due to temporary or permanent inability to work	$ 7,800,000,000
Medical and hospital bills	3,100,000,000
Insurance administrative costs	7,300,000,000
Property damage in motor-vehicle accidents	5,000,000,000
Property destroyed by fire	2,200,000,000
Other costs of work accidents	4,100,000,000
Total	$29,500,000,000

SOURCE: *Accident Facts*, 1972 ed., National Safety Council.

The accident-prone person

Certain individuals have long been observed to have "more than their share" of accidents. While the laws of probability alone would account for some of these unfortunate persons, many such individuals can today be identified as being *accident-prone*. Psychiatrists and psychologists have been able to identify certain personality traits with accident-proneness. For example, many authorities believe that the accident-prone person often subconsciously desires to have accidents. There are several possible motivations behind this desire:

1. There may be subconscious guilt for which the accidents serve as "punishment," thereby relieving the guilt feelings.
2. Accidents may provide a means of escape from anxieties or unwanted responsibilities.
3. Accidents may provide desired attention or sympathy.

When accident-proneness is motivated by one of the above or similar factors, it is easy for a pattern of repeated accidents to develop as a form of life-adjustment. Such a pattern of accidents can best be broken by psychotherapy.

The personality traits common, though not universal, among accident-prone persons include resentment of authority, extreme pleasure-seeking, difficulty in interpersonal relationships, impulsive acts, and avoidance of responsibility.

It is well established that an individual's safety record can be improved with psychotherapy or reeducation toward accident prevention. Many corporations conduct effective safety-education programs and employ psychologists to counsel personnel with poor safety records.

Temporary emotional states

Many accidents are the result of temporary emotional upsets or anxieties, which lead to carelessness or aggressiveness or divert the attention from hazards. For example, the man who has just finished a heated argument with his wife or boss before driving his car stands a greatly increased risk of accident. His mind may be on the argument rather than his driving, or he may attempt to reassert his masculinity through aggressive or competitive driving. Similarly, industrial accidents are often associated with temporary emotional stresses.

Physical factors

Human physical factors play a role in many accidents. Many studies, for example, have clearly related the risk of highway and occupational accidents with fatigue. The risk of highway accidents rises sharply in relation to the number of hours of consecutive driving. Federal and state laws wisely limit the number of hours a commercial truck or bus driver can work each day, generally allowing a maximum of 12 hours for trucks and 10 hours for passenger vehicles. Further, it is important to take a "break" from driving about every two hours to maintain mental alertness. Periodic "breaks" are also essential in the prevention of occupational accidents.

Illness is another physical factor in accidents. Persons working or driving during periods of illness have an increased accident rate. The accident rate of children, too, increases when their mother is ill or pregnant; this increase has been related to lack of supervision and, in some cases, to the use of accidents by children as attention-getting devices, especially when the mother is pregnant.

Physical defects are often implicated in accidents, particularly among the elderly. Rather common defects leading to accidents include poor vision or hearing and temporary loss of equilibrium (dizziness). Less commonly involved are heart attacks and epileptic-type seizures.

Physical factors of prime importance are drug and alcohol influence (see Chapters 4, 5, and 6). The hazards in drug abuse are well known. Less widely appreciated are the hazards that may lie in the legitimate use of prescribed medications and nonprescription drug preparations. Many such drugs produce drowsiness, dizziness, and other conditions that may interfere with driving and other hazardous operations. Label warnings on medications must not be ignored. Few people realize that they can be arrested and prosecuted for driving under the influence of legitimately prescribed drugs.

Taking stimulant drugs in order to stay awake for night driving is particularly dangerous. Among the many hazards presented are hallucinations and other disturbances in perception that may develop after many hours without sleep, the chance of suddenly falling asleep, and all of the hazards inherent in self-medication.

Equipment factors

Sometimes accidents result directly from equipment failures (which can often, in turn, be traced back to human failures). Accidents may result from poorly designed equipment with built-in hazards. Or equipment that was originally safe may be allowed to deteriorate into a hazardous condition because of poor maintenance. Another human failure is the improper application of equipment, such as overloading beyond design capacity or the use of inappropriate equipment for a given job. Many industrial accidents result when inexperienced personnel are inadequately instructed in the use of equipment.

Environmental factors

Weather conditions are common contributors to many types of accident. Rain, snow, fog, and ice are particularly hazardous conditions. In addition to the natural environmental factors of weather are such man-made conditions as poorly lighted work areas and accumulations of carbon monoxide and other toxic gases.

ACCIDENT PREVENTION

Safe attitudes

The most basic step toward the prevention of all types of accident is the development of an attitude which is generally called "safety-consciousness." Safety-consciousness includes being watchfully *alert* for potential hazards plus being *concerned* for the safety of yourself and others. The incidence of almost every type of accident could be markedly reduced by raising the public's level of safety-consciousness.

Motor-vehicle accidents

Motor-vehicle accidents are of great concern because they currently kill more Americans than does any other class of accidents. It seems likely that this will remain the case for some years to come. Efforts at reducing the motor-vehicle accident rate must be directed toward vehicle factors, driver factors, highway factors, and legal factors.

Vehicle factors   The vehicle factors in accident prevention include both design and maintenance. The automotive industry has, unfortunately, stressed speed and styling in the design of its products, the safety considerations often receiving a low priority. Many safety features have been incorporated into automobiles only when required by law. So far most of the government regulations have related to protection of the occupants in case of accident— through safety belts and harnesses, padded dashboards, telescoping steering columns, and plastic control knobs. Cars are still being marketed which provide very poor visibility to the sides and rear, have inadequate brakes, handle poorly in emergencies, and have many other accident-causing design deficiencies.

Equally essential to accident prevention is proper maintenance. Even the safest new car can develop serious hazards in a short time without adequate maintenance. For continued safety the engine must be kept tuned for adequate acceleration and to avoid stalling. The transmission, universal joints, and other members of the drive train must be in good condition. Steering gear, wheel alignment, and wheel balance are important. Shock absorbers must be replaced periodically, as worn shocks can lead to loss of control of the car. Good tires are essential (industry sources indicate that 90 percent of tire failures occur in the last 10 percent of tread wear). The exhaust system must be free of leaks; even small amounts of carbon monoxide may result in drowsiness. Brakes must be in top condition. Glass must be clean and free of damage. All lights must be operating and headlights properly aimed. It is important that the driver frequently inspect his car for such deficiencies as burned-out lights and worn or underinflated tires. Mechanical features such as brakes and shock absorbers should be periodically inspected by properly trained mechanics.

Driver factors   Essentially the same human factors are involved in auto accidents as in other types of accident. Included are psychological factors such as a concern for the safety of oneself and others, freedom from aggressive and competitive driving tendencies, and freedom from emotional disturbances.

Physical factors, previously discussed, include freedom from fatigue or illness, adequate hearing and vision, and not using alcohol and any prescribed or nonprescribed drugs or medication that might influence driving ability.

Highway factors   A third step toward increased auto safety is the improvement of roads and highways. Studies have clearly indicated that accident rates can be reduced by half or more through road improvements. But even some of the newest highways have design deficiencies that lead to unnecessary loss of life. For example, entry and exit ramps may be poorly marked or poorly lighted, concrete pillars and abutments may be inadequately guarded with railings and other protective devices, and signs and light standards may be of such rigid construction as to inflict fatal injuries when struck. Inadequate or poorly located signs—such as those indicating exits—create confusion, hesitation, and sudden lane changes by drivers, leading to accidents. Traffic lanes are still often marked only with painted lines which are not visible when it rains, while raised reflective indicators have been available for several years. The list of highway defects is long indeed.

Highway maintenance is also deficient in many areas, leading to dangerous road surface conditions, illegible or missing signs, intersections obscured by weeds, and many similar defects.

Legal factors   Rigid traffic laws, strictly enforced, *can* help reduce the auto accident rate. This was clearly shown in England when an intensive campaign against drunken driving led to a sharp decrease in the accident rate. Similar decreases in accidents are often observed in the United States when particular highways or areas are strictly patrolled. But intensive law enforcement costs money, and few taxpayers seem anxious to support enforcement efforts that might lead to their getting ticketed. Too many drivers still think of patrolmen as "the enemy" rather than as important factors in reducing the accident rate.

One problem in traffic-law enforcement is the variation in laws from state to state, which leads to confusion for the interstate driver and to resentment against lawmen. Citizens can help achieve uniformity in traffic laws by letting their state and federal representatives know of their support for this movement.

Another problem in many areas is that speed limits and other traffic regulations are inadequately posted, again leading to accidents, confusion, and resentment.

Driver-licensing regulations in some states are so lax that unqualified drivers can obtain a driver's license that is good not only in the state issued but also anywhere in the United States. Further some states allow a driver to retain his license despite a record of repeated traffic violations and accidents.

Home accidents

The greatest number of injury-producing accidents occur in the home. In a typical home dozens of accident hazards can be readily identified.

Falls   The greatest number of these injuries and deaths occur in falls. Especially likely to fall are the very young and the elderly. Small children commonly fall from high places where they have climbed, while elderly persons more commonly trip and fall as a result of poor vision, dizziness, and reduced muscle coordination.

The risk of falls in a home can be materially reduced by the elimination of such hazards as clutter on floors, small rugs which can slip or trip a person and faulty steps and stairs; see Fig. 22.1. Safe ladders should be available for reaching high places, rather than climbing on chairs and similar makeshifts. Proper lighting of halls, stairways, and doorways, as well as the use of only approved nonslip waxes on floors are important.

Elderly people are especially likely to fall while they are away from the familiar surroundings of their own homes. It is therefore important when

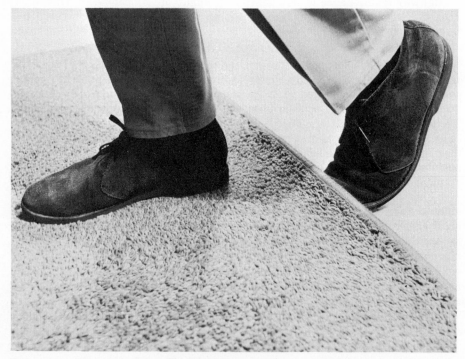

Figure 22.1   Small rugs can cause serious falls by tripping or slipping; they are especially dangerous for elderly people.

entertaining elderly guests to inspect the home for hazards and to assist them with steps, doorways, and similiar potential hazards.

Fires   Fires are the number two cause of home deaths and injuries. The greatest single cause of home fires is careless smoking, with thousands of fires starting every year in beds and upholstered furniture. Other major causes of home fires include the use of gasoline or other flammable solvents for cleaning parts and clothing; overheated cooking oils; defective furnaces; children playing with matches; and overloaded electrical wiring; see Fig. 22.2.

The wiring in many older houses is inadequate for modern electrical appliances. When the rewiring of such houses is not feasible, utmost care must be taken by residents to avoid overloading electrical circuits. Overloaded wires can heat to the point that nearby dry and dusty wood bursts into flame.

Other steps toward reducing the chance of fire include annual service and inspection of furnaces and other heating equipment and the elimination of fire hazards such as piles of paper and other trash.

Despite all efforts at fire prevention, fire may still break out. Almost every fire starts as a small fire which a prepared resident can often extinguish before extensive damage occurs. Every home should be equipped with a good fire extinguisher of adequate size and approved type and properly maintained.

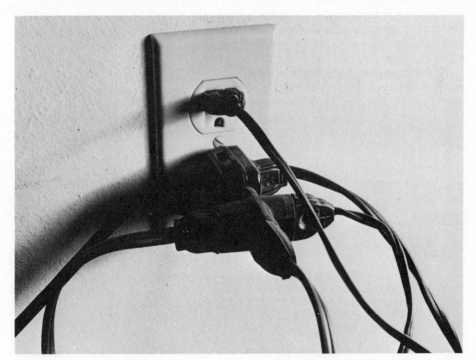

Figure 22.2   Overloaded wiring can become hot enough to cause nearby wood to burst into flames.

Family members should know for which type of fires the extinguisher is approved and understand its operation. Of course, the resident must not become so engrossed in fighting the fire that he neglects to call the fire department.

Family members should also be instructed and drilled in emergency procedures to be followed in case of fire—such as calling the fire department and various alternate routes for evacuating burning rooms.

Poisonings Poisonings rank high among types of home accident; about three-fourths of all poisonings occur in the home. Children are especially likely to ingest poison as a result of their great curiosity and the tendency to put things into their mouths. Parents must be constantly alert to the importance of keeping all medicines, cleaning products, and other hazardous materials out of the reach of children. Many products, such as cleaning solutions, are not toxic enough to require labeling as poisons, but they are toxic enough to cause serious illness or even death to a child who ingests large quantities. Parents must never underestimate the ability of their small children to climb and reach high cupboards; see Fig. 22.3. The best location for toxic materials is in a *locked* cabinet.

Even adults can be poisoned when empty food or beverage containers are reused to contain toxic materials. It is quite common for an unsuspecting child or adult to consume a poison that has been placed in a food container.

Entire families can be killed by carbon monoxide fumes from improperly installed or maintained gas appliances. Since carbon monoxide is colorless and odorless, the first sign of its presence may be the drowsiness of a family member.

Many persons have taken accidental overdoses of sleeping pills or other medications kept near their beds—where they could be reached while they were drowsy. Dangerous medications should never be kept near the bed.

The life of a poison victim often depends upon the emergency procedures followed in the first few minutes after ingestion of the poison. Proper procedures include the following:

1. *Most poisons.* If victim is conscious, give large quantities of water or milk, then induce vomiting by gagging (insert a finger into the throat). Give more fluid and repeat vomiting. CALL PHYSICIAN IMMEDIATELY.

2. *Acids.* DO NOT INDUCE VOMITING. Give baking soda in water or milk to neutralize in stomach. CALL PHYSICIAN IMMEDIATELY.

3. *Alkalies (lye, drain cleaners, etc).* DO NOT INDUCE VOMITING. Give vinegar or lemon juice in water to neutralize in stomach. CALL PHYSICIAN IMMEDIATELY.

4. *Strychnine.* Do not induce vomiting if there are any signs that the poison has entered the system. If poison has been ingested within the past few minutes, give fluid and induce vomiting. CALL PHYSICIAN IMMEDIATELY.

5. *Gasoline, kerosine, and other petroleum distillates.* DO NOT INDUCE VOMITING. CALL PHYSICIAN IMMEDIATELY.

In any case of poisoning, as soon as the first-aid procedures have been followed, if a physician is not readily available the victim should be taken to the nearest hospital that has emergency facilities. A sample of the poison

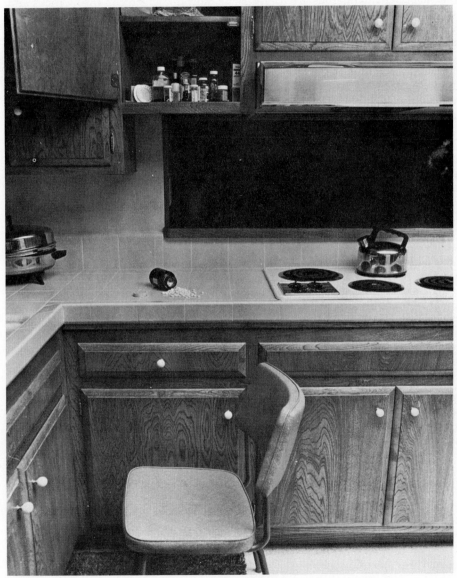

Figure 22.3   Medicines should be stored in locked cabinets. Parents often underestimate the ability of children to climb and reach high places.

should be taken to the physician along with the patient so that the substance can be definitely identified and proper antidotes administered.

Other home hazards   Although every home presents some of its own unique hazards, some common hazards are the following:

1. *Power mowers.* Any power lawn mower demands extreme care in its use. Especially dangerous are rotary blade mowers, which can throw rocks and other objects at great force. Nonoperating persons should remain at a safe distance while these mowers are in operation. Goggles should be worn with such garden tools as power edgers.

2. *Power tools and appliances.* Many power tools and appliances present the dual hazards of electrical shock and physical injury. All such devices must be either grounded with a three-wire cord plugged into a grounded receptacle or built with the newer "double insulation" techniques. Operating instructions should be read and followed carefully. Goggles should be worn while one is operating grinders and similar devices.

3. *Hot liquids.* Every year thousands of children are killed or permanently scarred by hot liquids. Many such accidents could be prevented by simply turning the handles of cooking pots toward the rear of the stove, out of the reach of small children; see Fig. 22.4.

4. *Glass doors.* Both children and adults are commonly injured by walking into closed glass doors. Glass doors should be of safety glass and well marked with decals or other devices to minimize the chance of this type of accident.

5. *Swimming pools.* The home swimming pool should be enclosed with a six-foot fence fitted with self-closing, self-locking gates. Children should be allowed to use the pool only under adult supervision. Many pool accidents involve small children who wander alone into untended pools. Safety pool covers can prevent this kind of accident. Roughhousing in or around pools should be strictly forbidden.

Recreational accidents

The number of such accidents has risen as more people have had the time and money necessary to engage in hazardous forms of recreation. Recreational accidents are particularly common among youths and young adults and among novices in any particular sport.

A great many sports involve water. Thus it is important that every child be given swimming lessons at an early age. Persons operating boats must learn and obey the rules of safe boating.

Many sporting accidents involve persons who are attempting an activity in which they have had inadequate training. Skiing, in particular, is often attempted by untrained novices with disastrous results.

The proper protective gear should always be used for each particular sport. This would include a flotation belt or jacket for water skiing, properly adjusted safety bindings for snow skis, and similar devices.

Occupational accidents

In the United States every year more than 14,000 persons are killed in occupational accidents and almost 2 million receive disabling injuries. The degree of hazard varies tremendously from industry to industry, and no job is absolutely free of hazard. Mining, construction, and agriculture, in that order, are the three most hazardous industries, while trade, manufacturing, and service jobs present far less hazard.

The death rate from occupational accidents has been considerably reduced since 1935; in that year the death rate was about 40 per 100,000 workers, in recent years this rate has dropped below 20. Intensified efforts could produce even a further drop in this rate.

An important step is the recognition by management of the high cost of accidents. Realizing the profitability of accident prevention, many corporations have achieved outstanding safety records. One chemical plant in Tennessee actually recorded over 45.8 million continuous man-hours without a single disabling injury. Such a record is achieved through intensive efforts in safety education and supervision.

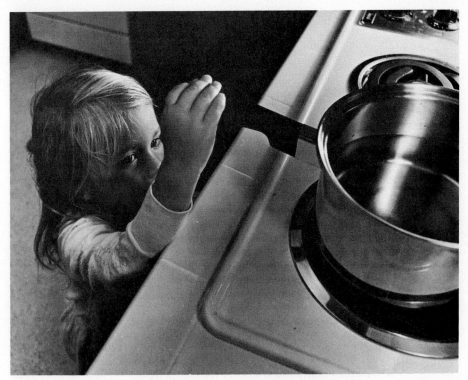

Figure 22.4   The handles of pots and pans should be turned to the rear of the stove to prevent children from pulling hot liquids onto themselves.

One requirement is the safety engineering of plant premises and equipment. Not only can obvious hazards be eliminated, but equipment can often be designed to "forgive" serious employee errors. In cases in which management does not voluntarily take safety precautions (generally in marginally profitable industries or corporations), rigid industrial safety laws can be enacted and enforced to assure employee safety. In cases in which hazards cannot be eliminated, they should be clearly marked or posted with proper precautions.

New employees should be thoroughly trained and made aware of any hazards to which they will be exposed. All employees should receive a periodic review of safety regulations in order to refresh their memory and maintain their safety-consciousness.

Supervisory personnel should be constantly alert to accident-producing factors in their subordinates—such as fatigue, illness, drunkenness, or drug influence.

SUMMARY

I. The accident problem
   A. Third leading cause of death in the United States; about 115,000 deaths per year.
   B. Fifty-one million persons injured each year (1 in 4).
   C. Dollar cost estimated at 29.5 billion.
II. Factors in accident development
   A. The accident-prone person
      1. Certain individuals have "more than their share" of accidents.
      2. Many psychiatrists believe that the accident-prone person subconsciously desires to have accidents:
         a. there may be subconscious guilt for which the accidents serve as "punishment."
         b. accidents may provide a means of escape from anxieties or responsibilities.
         c. accidents may provide desired attention or sympathy.
         d. repeated accidents may become a form of life-adjustment.
      3. Certain personality traits are common (but not universal) among accident-prone persons:
         a. resentment toward authority.
         b. pleasure seeking.
         c. poor interpersonal relationships.
         d. impulsive behavior.
         e. avoidance of responsibility.
   B. Temporary emotional states—many accidents are the result of temporary emotional upsets or anxieties which lead to carelessness or divert the attention from hazards.
   C. Physical factors
      1. Fatigue—studies have clearly related increased highway and occupational accidents with fatigue.
      2. Illness:
         a. persons working or driving during periods of illness have an increased accident rate.

      b. the accident rate of children increases when their mother is ill or pregnant (possible factors include lack of supervision and attention).

    3. Physical defects:

      a. poor vision or hearing.

      b. temporary loss of equilibrium (dizziness).

      c. sudden heart attacks.

      d. uncontrolled epilepsy.

    4. Alcohol and other drugs:

      a. alcohol—see Chapter 5.

      b. drug abuse—see Chapter 4.

      c. prescribed medication—many prescription (and nonprescription) drugs cause drowsiness, dizziness, and other conditions that may interfere with driving and other operations. Label warnings should not be ignored.

  D. Equipment factors

    1. Poor design—built-in hazards.

    2. Poor maintenance, allowing hazards to develop.

    3. Improper application of equipment—overloaded or inappropriate equipment.

    4. Worn-out equipment.

    5. Lack of instruction or training in use of equipment.

  E. Environmental factors

    1. Weather conditions—rain, snow, fog, ice.

    2. Poor lighting.

    3. Carbon monoxide and other toxic gases.

III. Accident prevention

  A. Safe attitudes

    1. Alertness to potential hazards.

    2. Concern for safety of self and others.

  B. Motor-vehicle accidents

    1. Vehicle factors:

      a. design

        (1) adequate visibility

        (2) adequate brakes

        (3) emergency handling characteristics

        (4) protection of passengers in collisions

      b. maintenance

        (1) engine and drive train

        (2) steering gear and wheel alignment

        (3) shock absorbers

        (4) tires

        (5) exhaust system

        (6) brakes

        (7) glass

        (8) lights

    2. Driver factors:

      a. psychological factors

        (1) concern for safety of self and others

        (2) freedom from emotional disturbances

      b. Physical factors

        (1) freedom from fatigue

        (2) adequate vision and hearing

(3) freedom from alcohol, drugs, or illnesses that might affect driving

3. Highway factors:
   a. safety engineering.
   b. proper maintenance.
4. Legal factors:
   a. need for uniformity of traffic laws.
   b. adequate posting of laws.
   c. strict enforcement.
   d. rigid driver-licensing regulations.

C. Home accidents
   1. Falls:
      a. supervision of young and elderly.
      b. elimination of environmental hazards such as clutter on floors, throw rugs, and faulty steps and stairs.
      c. safe ladders for reaching high places.
      d. proper lighting.
      e. nonslip waxes on floors.
   2. Fires:
      a. care when smoking.
      b. extreme care with flammable liquids such as gasoline and solvents.
      c. never overload electrical wiring.
      d. approved-type fire extinguisher in kitchen for grease and other cooking fires.
      e. annual service and inspection of heating equipment.
      f. elimination of hazards such as piles of paper and other trash.
      g. instruction of family members in emergency procedures such as calling fire department and evacuation of building.
   3. Poisoning:
      a. all medicines, cleaning products, and other hazardous materials out of reach of children (children have great climbing ability).
      b. no nonfood materials in food or beverage containers.
      c. proper handling of foods to avoid food poisoning.
      d. gas appliances of approved type, properly installed, and routinely inspected.
      e. no medications such as sleeping pills near bed where drowsy person could take accidental overdose.
      f. emergency procedure to follow in poisonings—*most poisons,* induce vomiting after giving large volume of water or milk and repeat; *acids,* do not induce vomiting, give baking soda in water or milk to neutralize; *alkalies,* do not induce vomiting, give vinegar or lemon juice in water to neutralize; *strychnine,* do not induce vomiting if any signs that poison has entered system; *gasoline, kerosine, etc.,* do not induce vomiting; *in any case, get immediate medical aid.*
   4. Other home hazards include:
      a. power mowers.
      b. power tools and appliances.
      c. hot liquids.
      d. glass doors.
      e. swimming pools.

D. Recreational accidents are reducible.
1. Swimming lessons for children.
2. Adequate instruction before skiing or engaging in any such sport.
3. Proper protective gear for particular sport.
E. Occupational accidents are reducible.
1. Safety engineering of premises and equipment.
2. Management recognition of the cost of accidents.
3. Enforcement of industrial safety laws.
4. Thorough training of new employees.
5. Periodic review of safety regulations for old employees.
6. Existing safety hazards clearly marked or posted.
7. Special attention to the physical factors such as fatigue, use of alcohol or drugs, and illness.

Diseases in brief

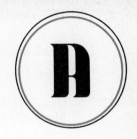

This appendix provides condensed information on many infectious diseases for quick reference or review. For more complete information refer to Chapters 19, 20, and 21 of this text.

Chancroid

Caused by:	*Hemophilus ducreyi*, a bacillus.
Usual age infected:	15 to 30.
Mode of transmission:	Predominantly through sexual intercourse.
Incubation period:	Usually 3 to 5 days.
Early signs:	An open, red sore, oozing pus, painful, on or near the genitalia; swelling of local lymph glands.
Length of disease:	Usually self-limiting within 1 month; may be chronic.
Contagious period:	Until healed.
Permanent aftereffects:	None.
Immunity:	None.
Prevention:	Chancroid can be definitely prevented by the proper use of soap and water immediately after exposure.

Chickenpox

Caused by:	Varicella virus. Same virus causes herpes zoster (shingles) in adults.
Usual age infected:	2 to 8 years.
Mode of transmission:	Direct or indirect contact with discharges from skin lesions or nose or throat of infected person, or airborne.
Incubation period:	10 to 21 days, usually 14 to 16.
Early signs:	Slight fever, skin eruption.
Length of disease:	9 to 14 days.
Contagious period:	From 1 day before eruption until 6 days afterward.
Permanent aftereffects:	Very rare—death due to encephalitis or pneumonia.
Immunity:	One attack confers long immunity.
Prevention:	None.

Common cold

Caused by:	Over 50 types of virus.
Usual age infected:	Any.
Mode of transmission:	Direct or indirect contact with nose or throat discharges of infected persons.
Incubation period:	12 to 72 hours, usually 24 hours.
Early signs:	Sore throat, running nose, chilliness, aches.
Length of disease:	3 to 5 days.
Contagious period:	From 24 hours before onset until 3 to 5 days after.
Permanent aftereffects:	None.
Immunity:	Little or none.
Prevention:	Avoid infected persons.

Diphtheria

Caused by:	*Corynebacterium diphtheriae*, the diphtheria bacillus.
Usual age infected:	Under 15 years.
Mode of transmission:	Contact with nose or throat discharges of a patient or carrier.
Incubation period:	1 to 6 days.
Early signs:	Sore throat, mild fever, running nose.
Length of disease:	Highly variable—possibly several weeks.
Contagious period:	Variable—usually from 3 days before until 10 days after onset of symptoms.
Permanent aftereffects:	5 to 10 percent of cases fatal; toxin may permanently damage heart or nervous system.
Immunity:	Congenital immunity lasts for several months; the actual disease sometimes confers lasting immunity.

Diphtheria (continued)

Prevention:	Immunization with DPT shots according to the schedule in Appendix C.

German measles (rubella)

Caused by:	Rubella virus.
Usual age infected:	2 to 15 years.
Mode of transmission:	Direct or indirect contact with nose or throat discharges of infected person, or airborne.
Incubation period:	10 to 28 days, usually 14 to 21.
Early signs:	Slight fever, swelling of lymph glands, rash.
Contagious period:	From one week before until end of rash.
Length of disease:	1 to 4 days.
Permanent aftereffects:	Rare, except for damage to fetus in early pregnancy.
Immunity:	One attack usually confers permanent immunity.
Prevention:	Immunization with German-measles vaccine.

Gonorrhea

Caused by:	*Neisseria gonorrheae*, a gonococcus.
Usual age infected:	15 to 30 years.
Mode of transmission:	Sexual intercourse; infection of eyes of newborn during childbirth.
Incubation period:	3 to 5 days, sometimes 9 days or longer.
Early signs:	Male—discharge of pus from urethra, burning urination. Female—slight discharge from vagina, slight burning in urination.
Length of disease:	Indefinite—until properly treated.
Contagious period:	Indefinite—as long as discharges persist.
Permanent aftereffects:	Sterility in male or female; occasional damage to joints or heart lining.
Immunity:	None.
Prevention:	Avoidance of casual sexual contacts, case-finding programs, antibacterial drops in eyes of newborn infants; personal prophylaxis before, during, and after exposure is of some value.

Granuloma inguinale

Caused by:	*Donovania granulomatis*, a bacillus.
Usual age infected:	20 to 40 years.
Mode of transmission:	Sexual intercourse.
Incubation period:	From 8 to 100 days.
Early signs:	Deep, red, open sores, starting on the genitalia and spreading to surrounding areas.
Length of disease:	Indefinite—until treated.
Contagious period:	As long as skin lesions persist.

Granuloma inguinale (continued)

Permanent aftereffects:	The untreated disease may lead to destruction of the genital organs; on rare occasions the disease may become generalized and lead to death.
Immunity:	None.
Prevention:	Avoidance of casual sexual contacts, personal cleanliness, case-finding programs.

Infectious hepatitis

Caused by:	A virus.
Usual age infected:	Any.
Mode of transmission:	Fecal contamination, contact with patient, contaminated food or water.
Incubation period:	2 to 7 weeks, commonly 3 to 4 weeks.
Early signs:	Fever, mild headache, chilliness, fatigue, jaundice.
Length of disease:	Variable—often 2 to 4 weeks.
Contagious period:	Unknown—believed to be from 1 week before onset until 1 week after.
Permanent aftereffects:	Rarely, death or permanent liver damage.
Immunity:	Second attacks are rare.
Prevention:	Good sanitation and sewage disposal, sterile injection syringes and needles, gamma globulin after exposure to disease.

Infectious mononucleosis

Caused by:	A virus.
Usual age infected:	2 to 20 years.
Mode of transmission:	Unknown—believed to be direct contact with nose or throat discharges of infected person.
Incubation period:	2 to 6 weeks.
Early signs:	Fever, sore throat, fatigue, enlarged lymph nodes.
Length of disease:	Variable—1 week to several months.
Contagious period:	Probably from several days before symptoms until end of sore throat.
Permanent aftereffects:	None.
Immunity:	Infection with or without symptoms is believed to confer lasting immunity.
Prevention:	None.

Influenza

Caused by:	Several types of influenza virus; new strains frequently develop.
Usual age infected:	Any.
Mode of transmission:	Direct or indirect contact with nose or throat discharges of infected persons, possibly airborne.
Incubation period:	1 to 3 days.

Influenza (continued)

Early signs:	Sudden fever, chills, headache, muscular pain, marked prostration, dry cough.
Length of disease:	3 to 10 days.
Contagious period:	1 day before onset until 4 days after.
Permanent aftereffects:	Rare, but predisposes elderly or weakened persons to pneumonia; the general death rate rises during epidemics.
Immunity:	Infection produces immunity, of unknown duration, to the infecting virus but not necessarily to other influenza viruses.
Prevention:	Annual immunization with vaccine based upon prevailing strains of viruses.

Lymphogranuloma venereum

Caused by:	*Miyagawanella lymphogranulomatosis,* a bacterium.
Usual age infected:	15 to 30.
Mode of transmission:	Primarily through sexual intercourse, also indirectly through contaminated articles and clothing.
Incubation period:	Usually 7 to 12 days, may be several months.
Early signs:	Small lesion on genitalia, swelling of lymph nodes and genitalia.
Length of disease:	Indefinite.
Contagious period:	Variable—from weeks to years.
Permanent aftereffects:	Rarely fatal, but may cause great disability.
Immunity:	Recovered persons may be immune.
Prevention:	Avoidance of casual sexual contacts, cleanliness.

Measles

Caused by:	Rubeola virus.
Usual age infected:	2 to 8 years.
Mode of transmission:	Direct or indirect contact with nose or throat discharge of infected person; also airborne.
Incubation period:	7 to 14 days, usually 10 to 12.
Early signs:	Gradually increasing fever, cold symptoms, severe cough, conjunctivitis, running nose; rash appears on third or fourth day.
Length of disease:	6 to 12 days.
Contagious period:	From 4 days before until 5 days after rash appears.
Permanent aftereffects:	Occasional death and brain damage due to encephalitis.
Immunity:	Congenital immunity lasts a few months; the disease usually confers permanent immunity.
Prevention:	Immunization with live measles vaccine.

Meningitis (bacterial)

Caused by: Neisseria meningitidis, a meningococcus, several types.

Usual age infected: Any.

Mode of transmission: Direct contact with patient or carrier; indirect contact not important.

Incubation period: 2 to 10 days, commonly 3 to 4.

Early signs: Fever, headache, nausea, irritability, delirium, coma.

Length of disease: Usually 1 to 3 weeks.

Contagious period: Until 24 hours after treatment with proper drug.

Permanent aftereffects: Fatality rate about 5 percent with proper treatment, 40 to 50 percent without treatment; brain damage is frequent.

Immunity: Over half of the population exhibits natural immunity, becoming healthy carriers upon exposure; degree and duration of immunity after attack unknown.

Prevention: Personal hygiene, prevention of overcrowding, mass treatment in epidemics.

Mumps

Caused by: Mumps virus.

Usual age infected: 2 to 14 years.

Mode of transmission: Direct or indirect contact with nose or throat discharges of infected person.

Incubation period: 12 to 28 days, usually 16 to 20.

Early signs: Fever; swelling and tenderness of salivary glands.

Length of disease: 4 to 10 days.

Contagious period: 7 days before swelling until end of swelling.

Permanent aftereffects: Very rarely, brain damage; atrophy of one testis (rarely both) in about 25 percent of males over age 15; ovarian infection in females much less frequent.

Immunity: The disease usually confers lifelong immunity.

Prevention: Immunization with live mumps-virus vaccine.

Poliomyelitis (Polio)

Caused by: Three types of polio virus.

Usual age infected: Any, but most common among children.

Mode of transmission: Direct contact or close association with infected persons, indirectly through fecal contamination or nose or throat discharges of infected person.

Incubation period: 3 to 28 days, usually 7 to 12.

Early signs: Fever, headache, sore throat, nausea, muscle pain, and weakness.

Poliomyelitis (Polio) (continued)

Length of disease:	Highly variable—up to several months.
Contagious period:	Maximum period from 1 week before to 3 months after onset of symptoms; usually from 3 days before to 10 days after onset.
Permanent aftereffects:	2 to 10 percent fatality rate in paralytic cases; paralysis may be permanent.
Immunity:	Most cases are nonparalytic and result in immunity to the specific type of virus responsible, but not to the other two types.
Prevention:	Oral polio vaccine administered according to the schedule in Appendix C.

Rabies

Caused by:	Rabies virus.
Usual age infected:	Any.
Mode of transmission:	Bite or scratch of infected animal (all mammals are susceptible); airborne spread from bats to man in bat caves has been reported.
Incubation period:	Usually 4 to 6 weeks, may be shorter or longer.
Early signs:	Headache, anxiety, fever, muscular pain.
Length of disease:	About 1 week.
Contagious period:	Not contagious from man to man, except possibly through saliva.
Permanent aftereffects:	Almost always fatal.
Immunity:	No natural immunity; few survivors.
Prevention:	1. Vaccination of bitten person for 14 to 21 consecutive days, beginning soon after bite; passive immunization with serum is often also used.
	2. Vaccination of all dogs.
	3. Avoidance of contact with infected bats or other mammals.

Scarlet fever

Caused by:	Over 40 types of group A hemolytic streptococcal bacteria.
Usual age infected:	1 to 9 years.
Mode of transmission:	Direct or indirect contact with patient or carrier.
Incubation period:	1 to 5 days.
Early signs:	Fever, sore throat, nausea, rash.
Length of disease:	4 to 10 days.
Contagious period:	Highly variable—from 1 week to several months.
Permanent aftereffects:	Kidney disease or rheumatic heart disease.
Immunity:	Second attacks of scarlet fever are rare, but repeated attacks of streptococcal infection are common.

Scarlet fever (continued)

Prevention: Prompt treatment of streptococcal infections; pasteurization of milk, strict sanitary precautions in doctors' offices and hospitals.

Smallpox

Caused by: Smallpox or variola virus.

Usual age infected: Any.

Mode of transmission: Direct or indirect contact with throat or skin discharges of infected person; airborne transmission over short distances.

Incubation period: 7 to 16 days.

Early signs: High fever, headache, prostration, skin eruption.

Length of disease: 1 to 7 weeks.

Contagious period: From 4 to 5 days before rash until rash disappears.

Permanent aftereffects: From 1 to 40 percent of cases die; blindness, brain damage, scars.

Immunity: Second attacks are rare.

Prevention: Vaccination according to the schedule in Appendix C; see also Appendix B.

Syphilis

Caused by: *Treponema pallidum,* a spirochete.

Usual age infected: 15 to 30 years.

Mode of transmission: Sexual intercourse, other close direct contact; congenital transmission across placenta.

Incubation period: 10 days to 10 weeks, usually about 3 weeks.

Early signs: The chancre.

Length of disease: Usually persists until proper treatment.

Contagious period: During primary and secondary stages (see Chapter 20).

Permanent aftereffects: Death; damage to brain, heart, other vital organs.

Immunity: Develops only after long-term infection.

Prevention: Avoidance of casual sexual contacts, premarital and prenatal blood testing, intensive case-finding programs; personal prophylaxis before, during, and after exposure.

Tetanus

Caused by: *Clostridium tetani,* the tetanus bacillus.

Usual age infected: Any.

Mode of transmission: Tetanus spores infect the body through a wound.

Incubation period: Commonly 4 days to 3 weeks.

Tetanus (continued)

Early signs:	Painful contractions of muscles.
Length of disease:	Variable—several weeks.
Contagious period:	Not contagious directly from man to man.
Permanent aftereffects:	Fatality rate averages about 35 percent; usually no permanent damage in patients who recover.
Immunity:	Second attacks are known to occur.
Prevention:	Immunization according to the schedule in Appendix C.

Tuberculosis

Caused by:	*Mycobacterium tuberculosis,* the tubercle bacillus.
Usual age infected:	Any.
Mode of transmission:	Contact with patients, airborne, indirect contact through contaminated articles, unpasteurized milk.
Incubation period:	4 to 6 weeks.
Early signs:	None.
Length of disease:	Indefinite.
Contagious period:	As long as disease is active.
Permanent aftereffects:	Death; destruction of lungs, bones, kidneys, skin.
Immunity:	Immunity conferred by healed infection is very limited.
Prevention:	Avoidance of crowding, proper nutrition, intensive case-finding programs, testing of cattle, pasteurization of milk, BCG vaccine for high-risk individuals.

Whooping cough (pertussis)

Caused by:	*Bordetella (Hemophilus) pertussis,* the pertussis bacillus.
Usual age infected:	Birth to 10 years.
Mode of transmission:	Direct or indirect contact with nose or throat discharges of an infected person.
Incubation period:	5 to 16 days, usually 7 to 10 days.
Early signs:	Gradually increasing dry cough, especially at night.
Length of disease:	2 to 10 weeks, usually 4 to 6 weeks.
Contagious period:	Variable—usually first two weeks.
Permanent aftereffects:	In infants, death or brain damage.
Immunity:	No congenital immunity; second attacks of the disease occasionally occur.
Prevention:	Immunizaton with DPT shots according to the schedule in Appendix C.

Tips for international travelers

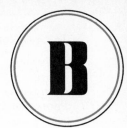

INTERNATIONAL CERTIFICATE OF VACCINATION

When you are planning to travel outside the United States there are certain laws pertaining to health that you should be aware of. You must obtain the *International Certificate of Vaccination* (a small, yellow booklet). You must have this certificate validated by the local public health department before you leave the United States. It is important, because it records special health information such as all inoculations, blood type, allergies, and prescriptions for glasses.

Americans do not have to show this yellow vaccination certificate when returning from a trip outside the United States, unless they have stopped, even briefly ("touched down," by air), or resided or traveled in a country where *smallpox* has been reported within the preceding 14 days or *yellow fever* within the preceding 6 days. But the *International Certificate of Vaccination* is required for entry into most countries of the world.

The following sections list recommendations for immunization. A *medical kit* is described at the end of this appendix.

Smallpox

A smallpox vaccination is no longer needed to reenter the United States, but you should check to see whether it is needed for other countries on your itinerary. Many countries still require it for entry. A smallpox vaccination is considered to be good for 3 years. See under "Yellow Fever" below for more recommendations concerning smallpox.

Yellow fever

Yellow fever is still present in all of Africa below the Sahara, in Central and South America from southern Mexico to midway of South America, and in the Caribbean. United States travelers who have come from or passed through an area considered to harbor yellow fever are required to present a valid certificate of vaccination against yellow fever upon reentering the United States. Yellow-fever vaccine is administered only at official yellow-fever vaccination centers; be sure to have your International Certificate stamped when receiving the vaccination. Some governments will not accept the certificate as valid until 10 or 12 days after you have been vaccinated. A yellow-fever vaccination is good for 10 years. If you are pregnant or allergic to eggs, or if you plan to be vaccinated for smallpox, inform the doctor before he vaccinates you. There should be a wait between smallpox and yellow-fever vaccinations.

Cholera

No vaccination is required for your reentry into the United States, but it is required for entry into many other countries. It is relatively short-lived, and a booster every 6 months is recommended. Cholera vaccine gives only limited protection, so you should watch what you eat and drink in cholera areas. Do not swim off beaches that may be contaminated with human sewage.

Infectious hepatitis

Immune gamma globulin is given for protection against infectious hepatitis. It is short-lived, so get your vaccination as near to your date of departure as possible. If you have taken the Sabin (live virus) polio vaccine, wait at least 1 month before getting gamma globulin.

Malaria

If you are going to a malarious area, see your doctor soon enough for him to have you take antimalarial drugs at least 1 week before you leave home. Some doctors wish you to continue using the drugs for 1 month after you have left the malarious area. Have him explain any possible side effects from the drug he has prescribed.

Typhoid

No typhoid immunization is required for travelers. Immunization requires a short series of shots. If you might be in typhoid areas over a period of years, a booster every 3 years is recommended. Typhoid vaccine is not reliably effective, so watch what you eat and drink—don't drink your whisky in water or "on the rocks" in suspected areas.

General immunizations

Everyone traveling outside the United States should have all immunizations up to date before leaving the United States (see Appendix C). Your *tetanus-diphtheria* boosters should be up to date and a complete series of *poliomyelitis* vaccinations completed before your departure. If you are planning extended vacations or will be working or living abroad these immunizations along with one for *typhoid* may also be recommended. *Typhus* is not one of the four quarantinable diseases (smallpox, yellow fever, cholera, plague), but if you are going to work in an area where the local population is infected, such immunity would be wise. Two injections and a booster every 6 to 12 months is required for immunity.

Plague immunization is recommended only for Vietnam, Laos, and Cambodia. *Rabies* immunization may be suggested for American residents in South America, Africa, and Asia. It is not recommended for short-term visitors.

A phone call to your local public health department can answer many questions concerning the areas you are traveling in. If it does not have answers you are seeking, you may write or call the U.S. Government's Center for Disease Control, in Atlanta, Georgia (404-633-3311).

MEDICAL KIT

If you are planning to travel in remote areas where there are no up-to-date drugstores, ask your doctor to help you make up a medical kit. It should contain an antibiotic ointment for cuts and burns, a nasal decongestant, Dramamine or Marezine for motion sickness, Kaopectate or Lomotil for traveler's diarrhea, and some water-purifying tablets, such as Halazone or Globaline.

There is no known medical preventive of traveler's diarrhea (also called *turista*, Montezuma's revenge, the GIs, etc.), but Kaopectate or Lomotil may help relieve it. Purifying your drinking water and the water you brush your teeth in can help to prevent such diarrhea because the drinking of contaminated water is a major cause of infection.

Do not routinely use foreign over-the-counter drugs; many are worthless or dangerous. If you find yourself in need of a doctor, contact the nearest American embassy or consulate; they will help you find a competent physician.

Preventive-medicine schedule

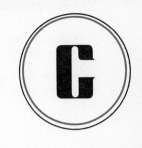

The modern trend in medicine is toward the prevention of diseases. The following tables are combined into a schedule which, if followed, would further this trend of preventive medicine.

Table C.1 *Typical immunization schedule*

age	preparation
2 months	DPT (diphtheria, whooping cough, tetanus)
	Trivalent OPV (oral vaccine containing types I, II, and III)
4 months	DPT
6 months	DPT
	Trivalent OPV
12 months	Live measles vaccine
12 months to puberty	German-measles vaccine
	Mumps vaccine
18 months	DPT
	Trivalent OPV
Before school entrance	DPT
	Trivalent OPV
15 years	TD (adult-type tetanus and diphtheria booster)
Over 15 years	TD boosters every 10 years for life

SOURCE: Public Health Service Advisory Committee on Immunization Practices, 1972 recommendations, National Communicable Disease Center Morbidity and Mortality report, Vol. 21, No. 25, June 24, 1972.

This schedule is recommended as a flexible guide: it may be modified, within limits, to meet the needs of the individual patient or physician. The U.S. Public Health Service withdrew its recommendation for routine smallpox vaccination in September, 1971. Smallpox immunizations are recommended only for persons traveling to countries where the disease still exists or where the International Certificate is required for entrance. Some individual physicians may still recommend routine smallpox vaccination.

Table C.2 *Typical examination and testing schedule*

age	recommendation
14 days or under	Exam, urinalysis (for infection or diabetes), PKU test
1 month	Exam
2 months	Exam
3 months	Exam, second PKU test
4 months	Exam
5 months	Exam
6 months	Exam
9 months	Exam
12 months	Exam, hemoglobin test, urinalysis, tuberculin test
18 months	Exam
2 years	Exam, urinalysis, tuberculin test
3 years	Regular dental care to begin Exam, hemoglobin test, urinalysis, tuberculin test
4 through 18 years	Yearly—exam, urinalysis, tuberculin test
19 through 40 years	Yearly—chest x-ray or tuberculin test Every 5 years—exam, blood count, urinalysis
40 years and up	Yearly—exam, blood count, urinalysis, check for rectal cancer, check eyes for glaucoma, chest x-ray Every 5 years—electrocardiogram
20 through 50 years	Females—yearly pelvic exam and pap smear for cancer of the cervix (plus monthly breast self-examination)
50 years and up	Females—pelvic exam and pap smear every six months

This schedule is recommended as a flexible guide: it may be modified within limits to meet the needs of the individual patient or physician.

Table C.3 *Immunization record*

		father	mother
Names			
Birth dates			
Polio	First		
	Second		
	Third		
	Fourth		
Diphtheria + Tetanus + Whooping Cough (DPT)	First		
	Second		
	Third		
	Boosters		
Smallpox	First		
	Second		
	Boosters		
Measles			
Mumps			
German measles			
Influenza	First		
	Boosters		
Other immunizations			

Table C.3 (*continued*)

children		

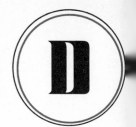

APPENDIX
Bibliography D

Emotional health   Chapter 2

Bischof, Ledford J., *Adult Psychology*. New York: Harper & Row, 1969.

Fullerton, Donald L., "Psychotherapy: Basic principles," *American Family Physician* (February 1964), 28–33.

Glasscote, R. M., et al., *The Community Mental Health Center*. Washington, D.C.: American Psychiatric Association and National Association for Mental Health, 1969.

Guttmacher, Jonathan A., and Lee Birk, "Group therapy: What specific therapeutic advantages?", *Mental Health Dig.* 4 (No. 6, June, 1972), 11–15.

Harris, Thomas, *I'm OK—You're OK: A Practical Guide to Transactional Analysis*. New York: Harper & Row, 1971.

Janov, Arthur, *The Primal Scream*. New York: Dell Publishing, 1970.

Jones, Kenneth L., Louis W. Shainberg, and Curtis O. Byer, *Emotional and Neurological Health*. San Francisco: Canfield Press, 1970.

Lazarus, Richard S., *Psychological Stress and the Coping Process*. New York: McGraw-Hill, 1966.

Levitt, Eugene E., *The Psychology of Anxiety*. Indianapolis: Bobbs-Merrill, 1967.

Maslow, Abraham H., *Motivation and Personality*, 2nd ed. New York: Harper & Row, 1970.

Maslow, Abraham H., *New Knowledge in Human Values*. New York: Harper & Row, 1959.

Maslow, Abraham H., *Toward a Psychology of Being*. New York: Van Nostrand, 1962.

Menninger, Karl A., Martin Mayman, and Paul Pruyser, *The Vital Balance: The Life Process in Mental Health and Illness.* New York: Viking, 1963.

Rogers, Carl, *Carl Rogers on Encounter Groups.* New York: Harper & Row, 1970.

Solomon, Philip, and Vernon Patch, *Handbook of Psychiatry,* 2nd ed. Los Altos, Calif.: Lange Medical, 1971.

Wiggins, Jerry, et al., *The Psychology of Personality.* Reading, Mass.: Addison-Wesley, 1971.

Structure and disorders of the nervous system   Chapter 3

Barr, Murray L., *The Human Nervous System: An Anatomical Viewpoint.* New York: Harper & Row, 1972.

Everett, N. B., *Functional Neuroanatomy,* 6th ed. Philadelphia: Lea & Febiger, 1971.

Gardner, Ernest, *Fundamentals of Neurology,* 5th ed. Philadelphia: Saunders, 1968.

Grollman, Sigmund, *The Human Body: Its Structure and Physiology,* 2nd ed. New York: Macmillan, 1969.

Guthrie, Robert, and Stewart Whitney, *Phenylketonuria, Detection in the Newborn Infant as a Routine Hospital Procedure.* Washington, D.C.: Department of Health, Education, and Welfare, Children's Bureau Publication No. 419–1964, Welfare Administration, 1964.

Guyton, Arthur C., *Textbook of Medical Physiology,* 4th ed. Philadelphia: Saunders, 1971.

Walton, John N., *Essentials of Neurology,* 3rd ed. Philadelphia: Lippincott, 1971.

Use and abuse of drugs   Chapter 4

Abood, L. G. "Recent development in the chemistry and biochemistry of narcotics," *Illinois Medical Journal,* 130 (October 1966), 450–452.

Bergersen, Betty S., and Elsie E. Krug, *Pharmacology in Nursing,* 11th ed. St. Louis: Mosby, 1971.

Birwood, George, *Willing Victim: A Parent's Guide to Drug Abuse.* New York: International Publishers, 1970.

Brenner, Joseph H., et al., *Drugs and Youth.* New York: Liveright, 1970.

Evans, Wayne O., "Mind-altering drugs and the future," *The Futurist,* 5 (No. 3, June 1971), 101–104.

"Exploring the nature of heroin addiction," *Medical World News,* 12 (No. 33, 10 Sept. 1971), 57–63, 66.

Gay, George R., "The next drug you'll see," *Emergency Medicine,* 4 (No. 2, Feb. 1972), 242, 243, 246, 248, 249.

Goode, Erich, *The Marijuana Smokers.* New York: Basic Books, 1970.

Hollister, Leo E., "Current research on marijuana," *J. Social Issues,* 27 (No. 3, 1971).

Lingeman, Richard, *Drugs from A to Z: A Dictionary.* New York: McGraw-Hill, 1969.

Lucas, B. G., *ABC of Drug Addiction.* Baltimore: Williams & Wilkins, 1970.

Maxwell, Kenneth E., "Mind modifiers," *Chemicals and Life.* Belmont, Calif.: Dickenson, 1970, pp. 104–107.

Merck Index. Rahway, N.J.: Merck, 1968.

Mirin, S. C., et al., "Casual vs. heavy use of marihuana, a redefinition of the marihuana problem," unpublished paper presented to the American Psychiatric Association in Washington, D.C., May 1970.

Williams, E. G., et al., "Studies on marijuana and pyrahexyl compound," *Public Health Reports,* 61 (No. 29, 16 July 1946), 1059–1083.

Use and abuse of alcohol   Chapter 5

Bergersen, Betty S., and Elsie E. Krug, *Pharmacology in Nursing,* 11th ed. St. Louis: Mosby, 1971.

Jellinek, E. M., *The Disease Concept of Alcoholism.* Highland Park, N.J.: Hill-House, 1960.

Jellinek, E. M., "Phases of alcohol addiction," *Quart. J. Studies on Alcohol,* Vol. 13, 1952, 673–678.

Phillipson, R., *Modern Trends in Drug Dependence and Alcoholism.* New York: Appleton, 1970.

Psychosocial aspects of drug abuse   Chapter 6

Baker, Stewart L., Jr., "U.S. Army heroin abuse identification program in Vietnam: Implications for a methadone program." *Am. J. Public Health,* 62 (No. 6, June 1972), 857–860.

Brecher, Edward M., *Licit and Illicit Drugs.* Mt. Vernon, N.Y.: Consumers Union, 1972.

Chayet, Neil, "Old laws for new junkies," *Emergency Medicine,* 3 (No. 4, April 1971), 217, 221.

Conn, Howard, ed., *Current Therapy, 1969.* Philadelphia: Saunders, 1969.

Haislip, Gene R., "*Law Enforcement and the Traffic in Illicit Drugs,*" *J. Drug Issues,* 1 (No. 1, Jan. 1971), 813.

Hentoff, Nat, *Doctor Among the Addicts.* Chicago: Rand McNally, 1968.

Huey, Florence L., "In a therapeutic community," *Am. J. Nursing,* 71 (No. 5, May 1971), 926–933.

Jaffee, Jerome H., and Edward C. Senay, "Methadone and methadly acetate: Use in management of narcotics addicts," *Mental Health Dig.,* 3 (No. 8, Aug. 1971), 38.

Nowlis, Helen, *Drugs on the College Campus.* New York: McGraw-Hill, 1969.

Nowlis, Helen, "Perspectives on drug use," *J. Social Issues,* 27 (No. 3, 1971), 7–21.

Rosenthal, Michael R., "Legal controls on mind- and mood-altering drugs," *J. Social Issues,* 27 (No. 3, 1971), 53–72.

Shafer, Raymond P., Chairman, *Marihuana: A signal of misunderstanding.* Washington, D.C.: 1972.

Foods and the digestive system   Chapter 7

Food for Us All, The Yearbook of Agriculture, 1969. Washington, D.C.: U.S. Department of Agriculture, 1969.

Food, The Yearbook of Agriculture, 1959. Washington, D.C.: U.S. Department of Agriculture, 1959.

Mazur, Abraham, and Benjamin Harrow, *Textbook of Biochemistry,* 10th ed. Philadelphia: Saunders, 1971.

Merck Manual of Diagnosis and Therapy, 12th ed. Rahway, N.J.: Merck, 1972.

Miller, J. J., *Nutritive Value of Foods,* rev., Washington, D.C.: U.S. Department of Agriculture, Home and Garden Bull. No. 72, Government Printing Office, 1964.

Tuttle, W. W., and B. A. Schottelius, *Textbook of Physiology,* 16th ed. St. Louis: Mosby, 1969.

Wohl, Michael G., and Robert S. Goodhart, *Modern Nutrition in Health and Disease,* 4th ed. Philadelphia: Lea & Febiger, 1968.

Diet and weight control   Chapter 8

"American Medical Association weighing guidelines for treating obesity," *Medical World News,* 9 (No. 3, 19 Jan. 1968), 24–26.

Benarde, Melvin A., and Norge W. Jerome, "Food quality and the consumer: A decalog," *Am. J. Public Health,* 62 (No. 9, Sept. 1972), 1199–1201.

"Fad diets: Major 'health pollutant'," *Medical World News,* 11 (No. 45, 6 Nov. 1970), 32DD.

Food for Us All, The Yearbook of Agriculture, 1969. Washington, D.C.: U.S. Department of Agriculture, 1969.

Food, The Yearbook of Agriculture, 1959. Washington, D.C.: U.S. Department of Agriculture, 1959.

Grollman, S., *The Human Body,* 2nd ed. New York: Macmillan, 1969.

How to Buy Food. Washington, D.C.: U.S. Department of Agriculture, 1969.

Mayer, Jean, *Overweight Causes, Cost, and Control.* Englewood Cliffs, N.J.: Prentice-Hall, 1968.

Nutritive Value of Foods. Washington, D.C.: U.S. Department of Agriculture, 1964.

Obesity and Health. Washington, D.C.: U.S. Department of Health, Education, and Welfare, Public Health Service, Publication No. 1485, 1966.

Protecting Our Food, The Yearbook of Agriculture, 1966. Washington, D.C.: U.S. Department of Agriculture, 1966.

Recommended Dietary Allowances, 7th ed. Washington, D.C.: Nat. Research Council, 1968.

Stare, Frederick J., *Eating for Good Health.* New York: Doubleday, 1964.

"The great American paradox," *Medical World News,* 10 (No. 48, 28 Nov. 1969), 24–33.

Wright, Carlton E., *Food Buying, Marketing Information for Consumers.* New York: Macmillan, 1962.

Population   Chapter 9

Appleman, Philip, *The Silent Explosion.* Boston: Beacon, 1966.

Berelson, Bernard, and Ronald Freeman, "A study in fertility control," *Scient. Am.,* 210 (No. 5, May 1964), 29–37.

Bogue, Donald J., *Principles of Demography.* New York: Wiley, 1969.

Bourgeois-Pichat, Jean, "Population growth and development," *Internat. Conciliation,* No. 556 (Jan. 1966), 1–81.

Chamberlain, Neil W., *Beyond Malthus.* New York: Basic Books, 1970.

Clark, C., "World power and population," *Nat. Rev.,* 21 (20 May 1969), 481–484.

Durand, John, *World Population Estimates, 1750–2000,* United Nations Doc., WPC/WP/289, 1965.

Ehrlich, Paul R., and Anne H. Ehrlich, *Population/Resources/Environment.* San Francisco: Freeman, 1970.

Ehrlich, Paul R., *The Population Bomb.* New York: Ballantine, 1968.

El-Badry, M. A., "Population projections for the world: 1965–2000," *Ann. Am. Acad. Sci.,* 369 (Jan. 1967), 9–15.

Fraser, Dean, *The People Problem: What You Should Know About Growing Population and Vanishing Resources.* Bloomington, Ind.: Indiana Univ. Press, 1971.

Harden, Garrett, *Population, Evolution, and Birth Control,* 2nd ed. San Francisco: Freeman, 1969.

Hauser, Philip M., "Demography and ecology," *Ann. Am. Acad. Polit. Social Sci.*, No. 362 (November 1965), 129–138.

"How U.S. is changing—People on the move," *U.S. News World Rep.*, 59 (No. 20, 15 Nov. 1965), 74–78.

Jaffe, Frederick S., and Steven Polgar, "Family planning and poverty," *Current*, 89 (Sep. 1968), 43–49.

Leisner, Robert S., and Edward J. Kormondy, *Population and Food*. Dubuque: Brown, 1971.

Miles, Rufus E., "Whose baby is the population problem?" *Population Bull.*, 16 (No. 1, Feb. 1970).

Mudd, Stuart, ed., *The Population Crisis and the Use of World Resources*. Bloomington, Ind.: Indiana Univ. Press, 1964.

Nortman, Dorothy L., *The Population Problem*. New York: National Educational Television, 1965.

Population Bulletin, Washington, D.C.: Population Reference Bureau, published six times yearly.

"World's number one worry, too many people," *U.S. News World Rep.*, 66 (17 Mar. 1969), 48.

Man and his environment   Chapter 10

Air Pollution Primer. New York: National Tuberculosis and Respiratory Disease Association, 1969.

Anderson, Walt, ed., *Politics and Environment*. Pacific Palisades, Calif.: Goodyear, 1970.

A Place to Live, The Yearbook of Agriculture. Washington, D.C.: U.S. Department of Agriculture, 1963.

Bresler, Jack B., *Environments of Man*. Reading, Mass.: Addison-Wesley, 1968.

Butrico, Frank A., "Environmental pollution in America," *Current Hist.*, 55 (Oct. 1968), 224–229.

Committee on Resources and Man, National Academy of Sciences, *Resources and Man*. San Francisco: Freeman, 1969.

Cox, George W., *Readings in Conservation Ecology*. New York: Appleton, 1969.

Darling, F. F., "Pollution: the number one problem," *UNESCO Courier*, 22 (Jan. 1969), 34–37.

Dasmann, Raymond F., *Environmental Conservation*, 3rd ed. New York: Wiley, 1972.

Dasmann, Raymond, *The U.S. Environment: A Time to Decide*. Washington, D.C.: Population Reference Bureau, 1968.

Davy, J., "Polluting the planet: Time to stop the blunder," *Current*, 103 (Jan. 1969), 59–62.

Ehrlich, Paul R., and Anne H. Ehrlich, *Population/Resources/Environment*. San Francisco: Freeman, 1970.

"Energy and power—The crisis in America." *Los Angeles Times*, 30 July 1972, pp. I-4,5.

Faltermayer, Edmund, "The energy 'joyride' is over," *Fortune*, Vol. 86 (No. 3, Sep. 1972), 99.

Friedman, Leo, "Safety of food additives," *FDA Papers*, 4 (No. 2, Mar. 1970), 4–8.

Glass, D. C., and J. E. Singer, *Urban Stress: Experiments in Noise and Social Stressors*. New York: Academic Press, 1972.

Goldman, Marshall, ed., *Controlling Pollution: The Economics of a Cleaner America*. Englewood Cliffs, N.J.: Prentice-Hall, 1969.

Henshaw, Paul S., *This Side of Yesterday: Extinction or Utopia.* New York: Wiley, 1971.

"How today's noise hurts body and mind," *Medical World News,* 10 (No. 24, 13 June 1969), 42–47.

Jackson, Wes, *Man and the Environment.* Dubuque: Brown, 1971.

Jennings, Burgess H., *Interactions of Man and His Environment.* New York: Plenum Press, 1966.

Johnson, Cecil E., *Human Biology: Contemporary Readings.* New York: Van Nostrand, 1970.

Kormondy, Edward, *Concepts of Ecology.* Englewood Cliffs, N.J.: Prentice-Hall, 1969.

Leinwand, Gerald, ed., *Air and Water Pollution.* New York: Washington Square Press, 1969.

Murdock, William W., *Environment: Resources, Pollution, and Society.* Stamford, Conn.: Sinauer Associates, 1971.

"Nuclear-arms race spreads despite superpower pacts," *U.S. News World Rep.,* 73 (No. 5, 31 July 1972), 56–58.

Odum, Eugene P., *Fundamentals of Ecology,* 3rd ed. Philadelphia: Saunders, 1971.

Scoby, Donald R., *Environmental Ethics: Studies of Man's Self-Destruction.* Minneapolis: Burgess, 1971.

Shillings, C. W., ed., *Atomic Energy Encyclopedia in the Sciences.* Philadelphia: Saunders, 1964.

"The toxicity of pesticides and their residues in food," *Nutr. Rev.* (Aug. 1965), 225–230.

Turk, Amos, Jonathan Turk, and Janet Wittes, *Ecology, Pollution, Environment.* Philadelphia: Saunders, 1972.

Wagner, Richard H., *Environment and Man.* New York: Norton, 1971.

Wallace, B., and T. H. Dobzhansky, *Radiation, Genes, and Man.* New York: Holt, Rinehart & Winston, 1965.

Warren, Charles E., *Biology and Water Pollution Control.* Philadelphia: Saunders, 1971.

Human reproduction   Chapter 11

Barish, Natalie, *The Gene Concept.* New York: Reinhold, 1965.

Bates, Jerome E., and Edward S. Zawadzki, *Criminal Abortion.* Springfield, Ill.: C. C Thomas, 1964.

Eastman, Nicholas J., *Expectant Motherhood,* 5th ed. Boston: Little, Brown, 1970.

Gardner, Eldon J., *Principles of Genetics,* 4th ed. New York: Wiley, 1972.

Grollman, Sigmund, *The Human Body,* 2nd ed. New York: Macmillan, 1969.

Guttmacher, Alan F., *Pregnancy, Birth, and Family Planning: A Guide for Expectant Parents in the 1970's.* New York: Viking, 1973.

Guyton, Arthur C., *Function of the Human Body,* 3rd ed. Philadelphia: Saunders, 1969.

Guyton, Arthur C., *Textbook of Medical Physiology,* 4th ed. Philadelphia: Saunders, 1971.

Havemann, Ernest, and Editors of Time-Life Books, *Birth Control.* New York: Time, 1967.

Hellman, L. M., and Jack A. Pritchard, *Williams Obstetrics,* 14th ed. New York: Appleton, 1971.

Herskowitz, Irwin J., *Genetics,* 2nd ed. Boston: Little, Brown, 1965.

Neubardt, Selig, *A Concept of Contraception.* New York: Trident Press, 1967.

Oster, Gerald, "Conception and contraception," *Nat. Hist.*, 81 (No. 7, Aug.–Sep. 1972), 47–77.

Stern, Curt, *Principles of Human Genetics*, 2nd ed. San Francisco: Freeman, 1960.

Tuttle, W. W., and B. A. Schottelius, *Textbook of Physiology*, 16th ed. St. Louis: Mosby, 1969.

Windle, William F., *Textbook of Histology*, 4th ed. New York: McGraw-Hill, 1969.

Ziegel, Emma, and Carolyn Van Blarcom, *Obstetric Nursing*, 6th ed. New York: Macmillan, 1972.

Success in marriage   Chapter 12

Aaron, Ruth, "Male contributions to female frigidity," *Medical Aspects Human Sexuality*, 5 (No. 5, May 1971), 42–57.

Auerback, Alfred, "Nymphomania," *Medical Aspects Human Sexuality*, 6 (No. 6, June 1972), 9.

Crawshaw, Ralph, "The psychology of the unwed mother," *Medical Aspects Human Sexuality*, 5 (No. 6, June 1971), 176–188.

Davids, Leo, "North American marriage: 1990," *Futurist* (Oct. 1971).

Davis, Keith, "Sex on campus: Is there a revolution?," *Medical Aspects Human Sexuality*, 5 (No. 1, Jan. 1971), 128–143.

Farber, Seymour M., and Roger H. L. Wilson, *Teen-age Marriage and Divorce*. Berkeley, Calif.: Diablo, 1967.

Gebhard, Paul, John Gagnon, Wardell B. Pomeroy, and Charles Christenson, *Sex Offenders*. New York: Harper & Row, 1965.

Grant, Igor, "Anxiety about orgasm," *Medical Aspects Human Sexuality*, 6 (No. 3, Mar. 1972), 14–16.

Jones, Kenneth L., Louis W. Shainberg, and Curtis O. Byer, *Sex*, 2nd ed. New York: Harper & Row, 1973.

Masters, William H., and Virginia E. Johnson, *Human Sexual Inadequacy*. Boston: Little, Brown, 1970.

Masters, William H., and Virginia E. Johnson, *Human Sexual Response*. Boston: Little, Brown, 1966.

Otto, Herbert A., *The Family in Search of a Future*. New York: Appleton, 1971.

Racy, John, "Ten misuses of sex." *Medical Aspects Human Sexuality*, 5 (No. 2, Feb. 1971), 136–145.

Salzman, Leon, "Female infidelity," *Medical Aspects Human Sexuality*, 6 (No. 2, Feb. 1972), 118–136.

Salzman, Leon. "Premature ejaculation," *Medical Aspects Human Sexuality*, 6 (No. 6, June 1972), 118–127.

Soloman, Philip, and Vernon Patch. *Handbook of Psychiatry*, 2nd ed. Los Altos, Calif.: Lange Medical, 1971.

Choosing and financing medical services   Chapter 13

A Brief Explanation of Medicare, U.S. Department of Health, Education, and Welfare, Social Security Administration, May 1969, Publication No. SSI–43.

A Buyer's Guide to Voluntary Health Insurance, Council on Medical Service, American Medical Association.

Blue Cross and Blue Shield Fact Book, 1972. Chicago: Blue Cross Association and National Association of Blue Shield Plans, 1972.

Crichton, Michael, "The high cost of cure," *Atlantic*, 225 (No. 3, Mar. 1970).

Health Resource Statistics, Health Manpower and Health Facilities, 1971, U.S. Department of Health, Education, and Welfare, Public Health Service, Publication (HSM) 72–1509.

Los Angeles County Health Department, Los Angeles, Division of Public Health Education, printed materials.

Occupational Outlook Handbook, 1972–1973 ed. Washington, D.C.: U.S. Department of Labor, 1972.

Pennell, Maryland Y., and David B. Hoover, *Health Manpower Source Book 21, Allied Health Manpower Supply and Requirements: 1950–80,* U.S. Department of Health, Education, and Welfare, Public Health Service Publication No. 263, Section 21.

"Sixty billion dollar crisis over medical care," *Business Week* (17 Jan. 1970).

Source Book of Health Insurance Data, 1972–73, 14th ed. New York: Health Insurance Institute, 1972.

State Licensing of Health Occupations, Washington, D.C.: U.S. Department of Health, Education, and Welfare, Public Health Service Publication No. 1758.

Quackery   Chapter 14

FDA Papers, The Official Magazine of the Food and Drug Administration, monthly. Washington, D.C.: U.S. Food and Drug Administration.

Food for Us All, The Yearbook of Agriculture, 1969. Washington, D.C.: U.S. Department of Agriculture, 1959.

Food, The Yearbook of Agriculture, 1959. Washington, D.C.: U.S. Department of Agriculture, 1959.

Magnuson, Warren G., *The Dark Side of the Marketplace.* Englewood Cliffs, N.J.: Prentice-Hall, 1968.

Michaelson, Mike, "Copper bracelets are a put-on," *Today's Health,* 48 (No. 6, June 1970), 27–29.

Miner, John, "A new dimension in murder," *Am. Cancer Soc. Volunteer,* 16 (No. 2, 1970), 4–5.

Protecting Our Food, The Yearbook of Agriculture, 1966, Washington, D.C.: U.S. Department of Agriculture, 1966.

The Medicine Show, Mount Vernon, N.Y.: Consumer Reports, 1963.

"The persistence of medical quackery in America," *Am. Scient.,* 60 (No. 3, May/June 1972), 318–326.

Young, Janes H., *The Medical Messiahs.* Princeton, N.J.: Princeton Univ. Press, 1967.

Your Money and Your Life. Washington, D.C.: Food and Drug Administration, Publication 19, 1964.

The meaning of physical fitness   Chapter 15

Bowerman, William J., and W. E. Harris, *Jogging* (paperback). New York: Grosset & Dunlap, 1967.

Cooper, Kenneth H., *New Aerobics.* New York: Bantam, 1970.

de Vries, Herbert A., "Exercise and fitness," *JOHPER,* The American Association for Health, Physical Education and Recreation, May, 1964.

Isola, Frank E., "Exercising for physical fitness," *CAHPER J.,* 32 (No. 3, Nov./Dec. 1969), 7, 28, 29.

Morgan, R. E., and G. T. Adamson, *Circuit Training,* 2nd ed. London: Bell, 1961.

Royal Canadian Air Force Exercise Plan For Physical Fitness. New York: Simon & Schuster, 1962.

The heart and circulation   Chapter 16

A Handbook of Heart Terms. Washington, D.C.: U.S. Department of Health, Education, and Welfare, Public Health Service Publication No. 1073.

American Heart Association, 44 E. 23rd St., New York, N.Y., 10010: pamphlets:
  Heart Attack
  Heart Disease Caused by Coronary Atherosclerosis
  The Framingham Heart Study
  Heart Disease in Children
  High Blood Pressure
  Heart Disease and Pregnancy

Arey, Leslie Brainerd, *Developmental Anatomy,* 7th ed. Philadelphia: Saunders, 1965.

Evans, William, *Diseases of the Heart and Arteries.* Baltimore: Williams & Wilkins, 1964.

Gefter, William I., Bernard H. Pastor, and Ralph M. Myerson, *Synopsis of Cardiology.* St. Louis: Mosby, 1965.

Grollman, Sigmund, *The Human Body,* 2nd ed. New York: Macmillan, 1969.

Guyton, Arthur C., *Textbook of Medical Physiology,* 4th ed. Philadelphia: Saunders, 1971.

Langley, L. L., E. Cheraskin, and Ruth Sleeper, *Dynamic Anatomy and Physiology,* 3rd ed. New York: McGraw-Hill, 1969.

MacBryde, Cyril Mitchell, *Signs and Symptoms,* 5th ed. Philadelphia: Lippincott, 1970.

Memmler, Ruth Lundeen, *The Human Body in Health and Disease,* 3rd ed. Philadelphia: Lippincott, 1970.

National Heart Institute. Washington, D.C.: U.S. Department of Health, Education, and Welfare, Public Health Service, National Institutes of Health.

"Sugar: Dangerous to the heart?," *Medical World News,* 12 (No. 6, 12 Feb. 1971), 38–47.

Winthrobe, Maxwell M., *Clinical Hematology,* 6th ed. Philadelphia: Lea & Febiger, 1967.

Wood, Paul, *Diseases of the Heart and Circulation,* 3rd ed. Philadelphia: Lippincott, 1968.

Cancer as a health problem   Chapter 17

Brecher, E., and R. Brecher, "Smoking and lung cancer," *Consumer Rep.,* 28 (No. 6, June 1963), 265–280.

Cameron, Charles S., *A Cancer Source Book for Nurses.* New York: American Cancer Society, 1971.

Cancer Facts and Figures, 1972. New York: American Cancer Society, 1972.

Friedman, Robert M., "Interferons and virus infections," *Am. J. Nursing,* 68 (No. 3, Mar. 1968), 542–546.

Hammond, Cuyler E., "The effects of smoking," reprint, *Scient. Am.,* 207 (No. 1, July 1962).

Holvey, D. N., ed., *The Merck Manual,* 12th ed. Rahway, N.J.: Merck, 1972.

Lyght, C. E., ed., *The Merck Manual,* 11th ed. Rahway, N.J.: Merck, 1966.

Mathe, G., ed., *Scientific Basis of Cancer Chemotherapy.* New York: Springer, 1969.

Sartwell, P. E., *Preventive Medicine and Public Health,* 9th ed. Des Moines: Meredith, 1965.

Seidman, Herbert, *Cancer of the Breast.* New York: American Cancer Society, 1972.

Smoking and the effects of tobacco   Chapter 18

Allen, W. A., et al., "Do parents care if their children smoke?," *Internat. J. Health Education,* 11 (July–Sep. 1968), 126–132.

Diehl, H. S., *Tobacco and Your Health.* New York: McGraw-Hill, 1969.

Godber, Sir George E., "Smoking disease: A self-inflicted injury," *Am. J. Public Health,* 60 (No. 2, Feb. 1970), 235–242.

Leone, L. A., and H. R. Musiker, et al., "A study of the effectiveness of the smoking deterrence clinic," *Rhode Island Med. J.,* 51 (No. 4, April 1968), 247–260.

Lussier, Richard, and A. J. Torribio, "The regional medical programs and the smoking problem," *Calif. School Health,* 4 (No. 3, Fall 1968), 12–17.

Mausner, J. S., and Bernard Mausner, "The physician and the control of smoking," *Ann. Internal Medicine,* 68 (June 1968), 1359–1362.

McGrady, Pat, *Cigarettes and Health,* Public Affairs Pamphlet No. 220A. New York: Public Affairs Committee, 1968.

Nolan, J. D., "Self-control procedures in the modification of smoking behavior," *J. Consulting Clinical Psychol.,* 32 (No. 1, 1968), 92–93.

Petterson, D. I., et al., "Results of a stop smoking program," *Arch. Environm. Health,* 16 (No. 2, Feb. 1968), 211–214.

Pollock, Marion B., "The drug abuse problem: Some implications for health education," *College Health,* 17 (No. 5, June 1969), 403–411.

"Proceedings of the National Forum on the Office Management of Smoking Problems," *Diseases Chest,* 54 (No. 3, Sep. 1968), complete issue.

Schwartz, J. L., and M. Dubitzky, "Clinical reduction of smoking: A California study," *Addictions,* 14 (No. 4, Winter 1967), 35–44.

Schwartz, J. L., and M. Dubitzky, "Maximizing success in smoking cessation methods," *Am. J. Public Health,* 59 (No. 8, Aug. 1969), 1392–1399.

Terry, L. L., Chairman, *11–12–13 World Conference on Smoking and Health.* New York: National Interagency Council on Smoking and Health, 1968.

The Health Consequences of Smoking, U.S. Public Health Service Publication No. 1696. Washington, D.C.: U.S. Government Printing Office, 1968.

Infectious disease   Chapter 19

Brock, Thomas D., *Biology of Microorganisms.* Englewood Cliffs, N.J.: Prentice-Hall, 1970.

Carpenter, Philip L., *Immunology and Serology,* 2nd ed. Philadelphia: Saunders, 1965.

Frobisher, Martin, *Fundamentals of Microbiology,* 8th ed. Philadelphia: Saunders, 1968.

Frobisher, Martin, Lucille Sommermeyer, and Robert Fuerst, *Microbiology in Health and Disease,* 12th ed. Philadelphia: Saunders, 1969.

Jones, Kenneth L., Louis W. Shainberg, and Curtis O. Byer, *Communicable and Noncommunicable Diseases.* San Francisco: Canfield Press, 1970.

Neter, Erwin, *Medical Microbiology,* 6th ed. Philadelphia: F. A. Davis, 1969.

Pelczar, Michael J., and Roger Reid, *Microbiology,* 3rd ed. New York: McGraw-Hill, 1972.

Rosebury, Theodor, *Life of Man.* New York: Viking Press, 1969.

Salle, A. J., *Fundamental Principles of Bacteriology,* 6th ed. New York: McGraw-Hill, 1967.

Top, Franklin H., *Communicable and Infectious Diseases,* 7th ed. St. Louis: Mosby, 1972.

Venereal disease   Chapter 20

Benenson, Anram S., ed., *Control of Communicable Diseases in Man*, 11th ed. New York: The American Health Association, 1970.

Brown, William J., *Typical Syphilis Lesions*. Washington, D.C.: U.S. Department of Health, Education, and Welfare, 1972.

"Chancroid," *Human Sexuality*, 5 (No. 11, Nov 1971), 141–143, 147.

"Congenital syphilis," *Human Sexuality*, 5 (No. 9, Sep. 1971), 70–72, 77, 78.

"Differential features of syphilis," *Human Sexuality*, 5 (No. 8, Aug. 1971), 90, 91, 94–96, 101.

"Gonorrhea epidemic and its control," *Human Sexuality*, 5 (No. 1, Jan. 1971), 96–115.

"Gonorrhea: Tougher than ever," *Medical World News*, 10 (No. 30, 8 Aug. 1969), 24.

"Granuloma Inguinale," *Human Sexuality*, 5 (No. 12, Dec., 1971), pp. 64–66, 70, 71, 73.

"Lymphogranuloma venereum," *Human Sexuality*, 6 (No. 1, Jan. 1972), 132–136, 138.

Morton, R. S., *Venereal Diseases*. Baltimore: Penguin, 1969.

"Other people's disease," *Emergency Medicine*, 3 (No. 3, Mar. 1971), 126–131.

Podair, S., *Venereal Disease: Man Against a Plague*. Palo Alto, Calif.: Dearon Press, 1969.

Sartwell, P. E., *Preventive Medicine and Public Health*, 9th ed. New York: Appleton, 1965.

"She may look clean, but—," *Emergency Medicine*, 3 (No. 3, Mar. 1971), 98–125.

Smartt, Walter H., "Prophylaxis of gonorrhea and syphilis," *Calif. Pharmacist*, Dec. 1969.

Smartt, Walter H., "Syphilis and gonorrhea—Epidemiological treatment," *County of Los Angeles Morbidity and Mortality Reports*, Feb. 14, 1970.

"Venereal disease," *Consumer Rep.* 35 (No. 2, Feb. 1970), 118–123.

Other diseases of man   Chapter 21

Benenson, Anram S., ed., *Control of Communicable Diseases of Man*, 11th ed. New York: The American Health Association, 1970.

Burdon, Kenneth L., and Robert P. Williams, *Microbiology*, 6th ed. New York: Macmillan, 1968.

Carpenter, Philip L., *Immunology and Serology*, 2nd ed. Philadelphia: Saunders, 1965.

Chandler, Asa C., *Introduction to Parasitology*, 10th ed. New York: Wiley, 1961.

Frobisher, Martin, Lucille Sommermeyer, and Robert Fuerst, *Microbiology in Health and Disease*, 12th ed. Philadelphia: Saunders, 1969.

Gordon, John E., ed., *Control of Communicable Diseases in Man*, 10th ed. New York: The American Public Health Association, 1965.

Neter, Erwin, *Medical Microbiology*, 6th ed. Philadelphia: F. A. Davis, 1969.

Sartwell, Philip E., ed., *Preventive Medicine and Public Health*, 9th ed. New York: Appleton, 1965.

Top, Franklin H., *Communicable and Infectious Diseases*, 7th ed. St. Louis: Mosby, 1972.

"WHO swings to environmental medicine," *Medical World News*, 10 (No. 27, 4 July 1969), 20B–20F.

Wilson, Marion E., and Helen Mizer, *Microbiology in Nursing Practice*. New York: Macmillan, 1969.

Accident prevention   Chapter 22

Accident Control in Environmental Health Programs. New York: American Public Health Association, 1966.

Accident Facts, National Safety Council, 425 N. Michigan Ave., Chicago, Ill., 60611, published annually, $2.65.

Creese, Angela, *Safety for Your Family.* New York: International Publications Service, 1968.

Seaton, Don C., *Administration and Supervision of Safety Education.* New York: Macmillan, 1969.

Strasser, Marland K., *Fundamentals of Safety Education.* New York: Macmillan, 1964.

Thygerson, Alton L., *Safety: Principle, Instruction, and Readings.* Englewood Cliffs, N.J.: Prentice-Hall, 1972.

Index